I0054931

Current Research in Drug Delivery

Current Research in Drug Delivery

Editor: Laurence Denton

FOSTER
ACADEMICS

www.fosteracademics.com

www.fosteracademics.com

FOSTER ACADEMICS

Cataloging-in-Publication Data

Current research in drug delivery / edited by Laurence Denton.
p. cm.
Includes bibliographical references and index.
ISBN 978-1-63242-478-5
1. Drug delivery systems. 2. Drug delivery devices. 3. Pharmaceutical technology. 4. Drugs--Administration.
I. Denton, Laurence.
RS199.5 .C87 2017
615.6--dc23

© Foster Academics, 2017

Foster Academics,
118-35 Queens Blvd., Suite 400,
Forest Hills, NY 11375, USA

ISBN 978-1-63242-478-5 (Hardback)

This book contains information obtained from authentic and highly regarded sources. Copyright for all individual chapters remain with the respective authors as indicated. All chapters are published with permission under the Creative Commons Attribution License or equivalent. A wide variety of references are listed. Permission and sources are indicated; for detailed attributions, please refer to the permissions page and list of contributors. Reasonable efforts have been made to publish reliable data and information, but the authors, editors and publisher cannot assume any responsibility for the validity of all materials or the consequences of their use.

Trademark Notice: Registered trademark of products or corporate names are used only for explanation and identification without intent to infringe.

Printed and bound in the United States of America.

Contents

Preface

Drug delivery is defined as the development of technology that enables the safe transportation of drugs to various parts of the human body. The route of administration of a drug facilitates its absorption and distribution throughout the body. This book elucidates the concepts and innovative models around prospective developments with respect to drug delivery. It elucidates new techniques and applications in a multidisciplinary approach. This book will be helpful for researchers and students in the field of biochemistry, pharmaceuticals, and medicinal chemistry.

This book is the end result of constructive efforts and intensive research done by experts in this field. The aim of this book is to enlighten the readers with recent information in this area of research. The information provided in this profound book would serve as a valuable reference to students and researchers in this field.

At the end, I would like to thank all the authors for devoting their precious time and providing their valuable contributions to this book. I would also like to express my gratitude to my fellow colleagues who encouraged me throughout the process.

Editor

1

Pharmacokinetics of BPA in Gliomas with Ultrasound Induced Blood-Brain Barrier Disruption as Measured by Microdialysis

Feng-Yi Yang[1,2]*, Yi-Li Lin[1], Fong-In Chou[3,4], Yu-Chuan Lin[4], Yen-Wan Hsueh Liu[4], Lun-Wei Chang[1], Yu-Ling Hsieh[1]

1 Department of Biomedical Imaging and Radiological Sciences, National Yang-Ming University, Taipei, Taiwan, **2** Biophotonics and Molecular Imaging Research Center, National Yang-Ming University, Taipei, Taiwan, **3** Nuclear Science and Technology Development Center, National Tsing Hua University, Hsinchu City, Taiwan, **4** Institute of Nuclear Engineering and Science, National Tsing Hua University, Hsinchu City, Taiwan

Abstract

The blood-brain barrier (BBB) can be transiently disrupted by focused ultrasound (FUS) in the presence of microbubbles for targeted drug delivery. Previous studies have illustrated the pharmacokinetics of drug delivery across the BBB after sonication using indirect visualization techniques. In this study, we investigated the in vivo extracellular kinetics of boronophenylalanine-fructose (BPA-f) in glioma-bearing rats with FUS-induced BBB disruption by microdialysis. After simultaneous intravenous administration of BPA and FUS exposure, the boron concentration in the treated brains was quantified by inductively coupled plasma mass spectroscopy. With FUS, the mean peak concentration of BPA-f in the glioma dialysate was 3.6 times greater than without FUS, and the area under the concentration-time curve was 2.1 times greater. This study demonstrates that intracerebral microdialysis can be used to assess local BBB transport profiles of drugs in a sonicated site. Applying microdialysis to the study of metabolism and pharmacokinetics is useful for obtaining selective information within a specific brain site after FUS-induced BBB disruption.

Editor: Jonathan A. Coles, Glasgow University, United Kingdom

Funding: This study was supported by grants from the National Science Council of Taiwan (no. NSC 102-2221-E-010-005-MY3 and NSC 101-2320-B-010-036-MY3), Cheng Hsin General Hospital Foundation (no. 102F218C11 and 103F003C17), Biophotonics & Molecular Imaging Research Center, and the Ministry of Education, Aim for the Top University Plan. The funders had no role in study design, data collection and analysis, decision to publish, or preparation of the manuscript.

Competing Interests: The authors have declared that no competing interests exist.

* E-mail: fyyang@ym.edu.tw

Introduction

The blood-brain barrier (BBB) is a highly specialized endothelial structure occurring along the brain capillaries [1]. The transport of many drugs from the blood into the brain tissue is limited by the BBB. Several methods have been developed to circumvent this barrier in order to enhance drug delivery into the brain, such as the chemical modification of drugs, the osmotic opening of tight junctions, and the direct injection of the therapeutic agent or agents into the targeted brain area [2]. Recent studies have shown that focused ultrasound (FUS) can enhance the delivery of chemotherapeutic drugs into brain tumors and improve antitumor effects due to FUS-induced BBB disruption [3,4]. As such, image-guided FUS technology may provide a novel strategy for targeted drug delivery in brain tumor treatment [5]. However, free drug concentrations cannot be measured if there is interference from signals produced by metabolites.

Patients with malignant gliomas have poor prognoses after radiation therapy and chemotherapy. Recently, several clinical studies have reported encouraging results in the treatment of patients with malignant brain tumors by boron neutron capture therapy (BNCT) [6–8]. For successful BNCT, sufficient neutrons and a selective accumulation of boron-10 (^{10}B) must be delivered to the tumor site [9,10]. The major challenge of boron delivery has been achieving sufficiently accurate tumor targeting to deliver therapeutic levels of boron to the tumor with minimal risk of toxicity to normal tissues. Therefore, chemical synthetic techniques and hyperosmotic BBB opening methods have been used to deliver the boron concentration into the brain tumor tissue for enhanced treatment efficacy [11–13]. However, these techniques produce dose-limiting side effects because they result in the boron concentration being increased throughout the whole brain.

The influx and efflux transport processes across the BBB are considered a key factor influencing the brain extracellular fluid (ECF) concentration of certain drugs. Intracerebral microdialysis is a tool to monitor the concentrations of free drugs and endogenous compounds at specific sites within the brain [14,15]. Drug concentrations in brain dialysate reflect concentrations in brain ECF. Using intracerebral microdialysis, simultaneous measurements of the brain ECF concentration and the plasma concentration can produce useful information for evaluating the pharmacokinetics of drugs that have crossed the BBB. In a previous study, microdialysis was used to continuously assess the concentration of boronophenylalanine (BPA) in the ECF of the brain tumor tissue in patients undergoing BNCT for glioblastoma treatment [16]. The data showed that the uptake of BPA in the ECF of the tumor tissue was clearly higher than in the ECF of normal brains.

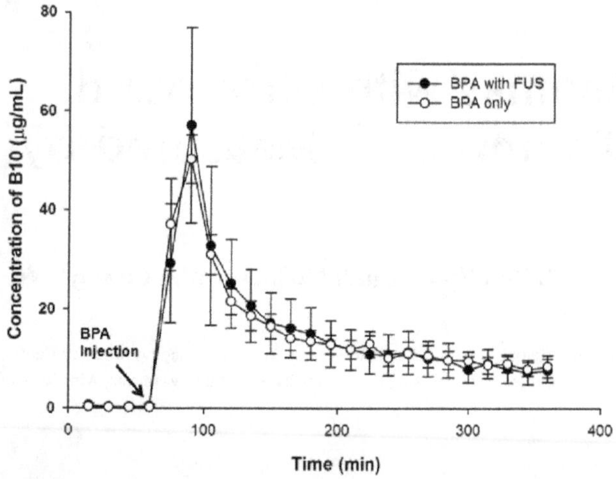

Figure 1. The boron concentration versus time profiles in the dialysate of the plasma after BPA administration at 500 mg/kg in glioma-bearing rats with or without FUS exposure. The concentration of boron measured in each 15-min sample of plasma represents the average concentration of that interval. Data are expressed as mean ± SEM, n = 6.

Previous studies have demonstrated that BPA-fructose (BPA-f) administration assisted by FUS can increase the accumulation of boron in brain tumors and elevate the tumor-to-normal-brain boron ratio [17,18]. The purpose of this study was to evaluate the concentration-time profile of boron in brain tumors with FUS exposure after intravenous administration of BPA-f. Furthermore, the pharmacokinetics of boron in sonicated brain tumors were compared with those in non-sonicated brain tumors.

Results

According to retrodialysis experiments, the in vivo relative recoveries were determined to be 48±7% (n = 3) for the plasma vascular probe and 30±5% (n = 4) for the brain tumor probe. The concentrations of BPA measured in the physiological samples were corrected for the relative recovery of the probe used.

The concentration versus time curves for boron in plasma before and after intravenous injection both with and without FUS exposure were almost identical (Fig. 1). The mean peak values were similar to those of the concentration profiles, in which the highest boron accumulation in the brain tumor ECF occurred at 30 min after drug injection and declined rapidly during the elimination phase.

The concentration versus time curves for boron in the brain tumor with and without FUS exposure after BPA (500 mg/kg) administration are shown in Fig. 2. The concentrations of boron in brain tumor dialysates were determined from the calibration curve. No significant difference in boron concentrations in the sonicated tumors and control tumors was found before intravenous bolus injection of BPA-f. Compared to the control tumors, a significant accumulation of boron can be seen in the sonicated tumors for a period of 5 h after BPA-f injection. The concentrations of boron in both types of tumors reached a peak at 30 min after drug administration and then declined rapidly. Furthermore, the mean peak value of boron in the ECF of the sonicated tumors was ~3.63-fold higher than in control tumor ECF.

Tables 1 and 2 show the pharmacokinetic parameters of boron with or without sonication in plasma and tumor ECF, respectively. Table 1 shows that no significant differences were found for the four parameters in plasma after FUS-induced BBB disruption as compared to the parameters for the BPA-alone group. Table 2 indicates that the maximum tumor ECF concentration (Ct_{max}), MRT, and area under the concentration versus time curve (AUC) values clearly increased after FUS exposure as compared with

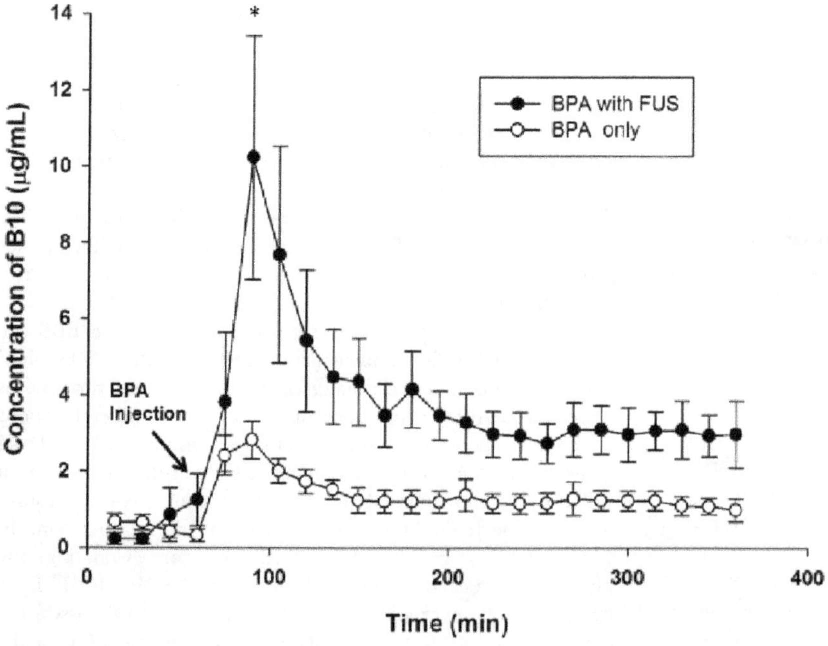

Figure 2. Representative data for boron concentration versus time profiles in tumor ECF after BPA administration at 500 mg/kg in glioma-bearing rats with or without FUS exposure. The concentration of boron measured in each 15-min sample of tumor ECF represents the average concentration of that interval. Data are expressed as mean ± SEM, n = 5. (*p<0.05).

Table 1. Pharmacokinetic Parameters of BPA in Plasma after Intravenous Injection.

Parameters	BPA 500 mg/kg only	BPA 500 mg/kg with FUS
Cp_{max} (μg/mL)	53.0±6.6	70.8±12.0
MRT (min)	208±29	209±46
AUC (min μg/mL)	6412±1030	7210±1430
AUC/dose	12.8±2.1	14.4±2.9

Cp_{max}: maximum plasma concentration ($n = 6$ for each group).
MRT: mean residence time.
AUC: area under the concentration.

those values for the BPA administration only group. The increases in MRT (from 313 to 503) and AUC/dose (from 1.8 to 3.8) show that the retention time of BPA in the tumor was extended with FUS exposure.

Discussion

BPA has been applied as a potential boron carrier in clinical trials with BNCT. BPA conjugated with fructose has been proven to enhance drug accumulation in the tumor due to increased solubility [19]. Non-invasive methods used for the in vivo determination of the local pharmacokinetics of a drug within the brain have been revolutionized by the development of positron emission tomography (PET) and nuclear magnetic resonance spectroscopy. In a previous study, PET was proposed to assess the biodistribution of ^{18}F-labeled BPA-f [20]. ^{18}F-FBPA-f showed specific tumor uptake in F98 glioma-bearing rats, indicating that PET can be used as a probe for BPA-f in BNCT [21]. Nevertheless, the key limitation of PET scanning is the instability of the isotope, and no free drug concentrations can be obtained. Furthermore, the spatial resolution of non-invasive PET imaging techniques is limited.

Since gliomas are highly infiltrative tumors, it actually would be highly desirable to have boron delivery to infiltrating tumor cells [22]. The barrier function of the BBB can become altered after FUS exposure. Thus, the further study as to whether FUS can enhance delivery to these infiltrating tumor cells in the F98 glioma model are needed to be investigated. Many studies have investigated the pharmacokinetics of BBB permeability in brains after FUS-induced BBB disruption using dynamic contrast-enhanced (DCE)-MRI [23–25]. In addition, ^{99m}Tc-DTPA micro-SPECT/CT shows that FUS not only increases the permeability of the BBB significantly at the sonicated site, but also elevates the lesion-to-normal brain ratio significantly in the focal region [26]. However, non-invasive imaging can provide neither chemical information nor information on the metabolites. Although intracerebral microdialysis has the disadvantage of being invasive, microdialysis sampling coupled to an appropriate analytical model can be used to study pharmacokinetics and metabolism in the target site. This technique has a temporal and spatial resolution suitable for evaluating neuropharmacokinetics in the brain ECF following drug administration with FUS exposure. Thus, such data may facilitate knowledge of the temporal features of pharmacological change after FUS-induced BBB disruption.

To our knowledge, this is the first *in vivo* study evaluating the local BBB transport profile in tumor ECF during FUS exposure. The BBB functionality is not significantly influenced by microdialysis probe implantation when experimental procedures are well-controlled. The results (Fig. 2) showed that FUS exposure increased the peak tumor ECF uptake value (10.23±3.19 μg/mL) while resulting in the same peak uptake time (at 30 min after BPA injection) compared with the control tumor (2.82±0.49 μg/mL). After FUS-induced BBB disruption, the boron concentration in tumor ECF followed the concentration in blood (Fig. 1), suggesting that neutron irradiation should be delivered as closely as possible to the time when the peak blood level is reached. In terms of the pharmacokinetic parameters (Table 2), the increases of Ct_{max} (from 3.8 to 6.8), MRT (from 313 to 503), and AUC/dose (from 1.8 to 3.8) imply that the absorption of BPA in the brain tumor was enhanced by FUS exposure. The major strength of intracerebral microdialysis lies in the fact that it not only measures the drug concentrations, but also monitors metabolite concentrations selectively within the targeted brain site. Thus, further investigations exploring the metabolism of BPA-f in the brain should be feasible.

This study demonstrated that the microdialysis technique is useful for the assessment of pharmacokinetics during FUS-induced BBB disruption while also not causing any severe side effects. The uptake of boron in the sonicated tumor ECF was clearly higher than that in the control tumor ECF, reaching a maximum of 3.63

Table 2. Pharmacokinetic Parameters of BPA in Tumor ECF after Intravenous Injection.

Parameters	BPA 500 mg/kg only	BPA 500 mg/kg with FUS
Ct_{max} (μg/mL)	3.8±0.5	6.8±1.9
MRT (min)	313±87	503±192
AUC (min μg/mL)	888±225	1887±600
AUC/dose	1.8±0.5	3.8±1.2

Ct_{max}: the maximum tumor ECF concentration ($n = 5$ for each group).
MRT: mean residence time.
AUC: area under the concentration.

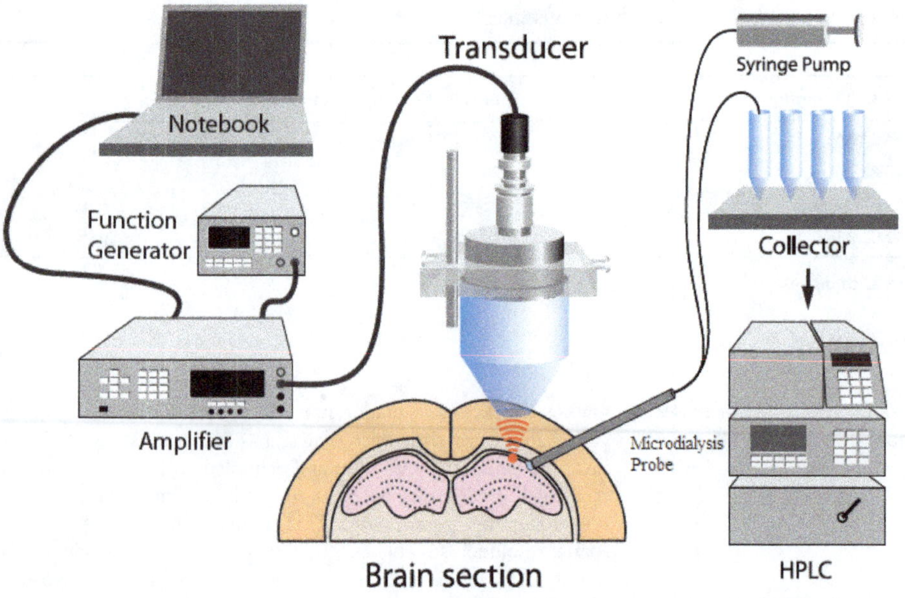

Figure 3. Schematic diagram illustrating the experimental setup for FUS and microdialysis.

times higher. The peak boron concentration in sonicated tumor ECF was reached at 30 min after BPA-f injection and at the same time as in blood. The boron concentration versus time profile in blood could thus be a good indicator of the optimal time for neutron irradiation when FUS exposure is applied in a brain tumor during BNCT.

Materials and Methods

Glioma Brain Tumors

Male Fischer 344 rats (11–13 wk, 250–280 g) were anesthetized with an intraperitoneal injection of pentobarbital at a dose of 40 mg/kg of body weight. Then, 1×10^5 F98 rat glioma cells (a generous gift from Dr. Rolf F. Barth, Ohio State University) in 10 μL Hanks' balanced salt solution without Mg^{2+} and Ca^{2+} were stereotactically injected into the right hemisphere (5.0 mm posterior and 3.0 mm lateral to the bregma) of each rat's brain at a depth of 5.0 mm from the brain surface. Finally, the hole in the skull was sealed with bone wax, and the wound was flushed with iodinated alcohol. The F98 rat glioma has been described in previous study [27]. All *in vivo* experiments were performed according to ARRIVE guidelines and were approved by the Animal Care and Use Committee of the National Yang-Ming University.

Focused Ultrasound Exposure

FUS was produced by a 1 MHz single-element focused transducer (A392S, Panametrics, Waltham, MA, USA) with a diameter of 38 mm and a radius of curvature of 63.5 mm. The half-maximum of the pressure amplitude of the focal zone had a diameter and length of 3 mm and 26 mm, respectively. The transducer was mounted on a removable cone filled with degassed water, and its tip was sealed with a polyurethane membrane. The FUS system setup was the same as described previously [28]. Animals were anesthetized intraperitoneally with urethane (1.2 g/kg) prior to the experiments. Ultrasound contrast agent (UCA, SonoVue, Bracco International, Amsterdam, the Netherlands) was injected into the femoral vein of the rats approximately 15 s before each sonication. The transducer was applied with a burst length of 50 ms at a 5% duty cycle and a repetition frequency of 1 Hz. The sonication time was 60 s at an acoustic power of 2.86 W and a UCA dose of 300 μL/kg. Ultrasound exposure was delivered to the tumor site on day 10 after tumor cell implantation.

Microdialysis

To evaluate the variability of BPA concentration within the brain tumor, a commercially available microdialysis probe (MAB 6, Stockholm, Sweden) was applied to sample the unbound BPA in the rat brain. Simultaneously, another microdialysis probe (MAB 7, Stockholm, Sweden) was implanted into the jugular vein toward the rat's right atrium. For brain ECF sampling, the rat was mounted on a stereotaxic frame. An incision was made in the scalp, and a small hole was drilled on the right side of the skull for implantation of the rigid microdialysis probe in the tumor. After implantation of the microdialysis probes, the probes were perfused with Ringer's solution (147 mM sodium chloride, 4 mM potassium chloride, 2.2 mM calcium chloride) by a microinjection pump (CMA 402, Stockholm, Sweden) at a flow rate of 2 μL/min. Dialysate samples were collected using a microfraction collector (MAB 85, Stockholm, Sweden). The entire experimental system is shown in Fig. 3.

Tumor progression was monitored by means of T2-weighted MR images (TRIO 3-T MRI, Siemens MAGNETOM, Germany) obtained on day 10 after tumor implantation (Fig. 4A). The maximum tumor size was about 0.125 cm^3. Moreover, the track of the probe within the tumor was verified by hematoxylin and eosin (H&E) staining (Thermo-Scientific, Waltham, MA, USA) (Fig. 4B) following microdialysis experiment. At the time of sacrifice, all rats were deeply anesthetized under isoflurane anesthesia (5%). After probe placement, 2 h were allowed to elapse so that probe and tumor ECF could equilibrate [29,30]. Subsequently, 24 sets of microdialysis samplings of tumor ECF and plasma were performed every 15 min for 6 h before and after intravenous bolus injection of BPA-fr (Taiwan Biotech Co., LTD., Taoyuan, Taiwan) at a dose of 500 mg/kg. These 24 sets of microdialysis samplings consisted of the four sets of samplings taken prior to BPA-fr

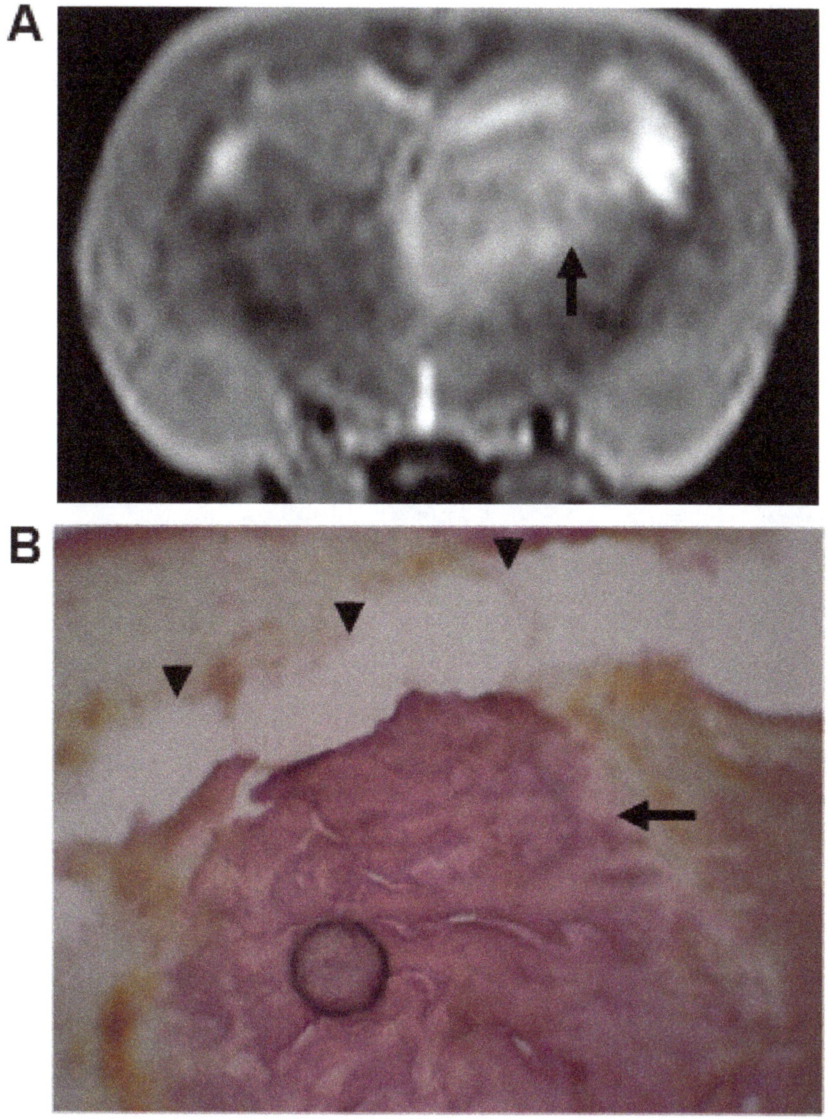

Figure 4. Tumor growth was monitored by MRI and histology. (A) Representative sample of tumor (arrow) by T2-weighted MR images on day 10 after implantation. (B) Hematoxylin-eosin-stained section shows the tunnel (arrow heads) punctured by the probe within the tumor tissue (arrow).

injection. Boron concentration in the tumor ECF and plasma were assayed by inductively coupled plasma mass spectroscopy (ICP-MS) and calibrated with the standard curve derived from the measurement of boric acid standard.

Recovery of the Microdialysate

To determine the unbound BPA concentration in the tumor ECF and plasma from the microdialysis data, the concentration of BPA in the microdialysis samples must be adjusted. A retrodialysis technique was used for the experiment of in vivo recovery [31]. One hour after probe implantation, Ringer's solution containing BPA (350 μg/mL) was perfused through the probes and separately into the rat's blood and brain at a constant rate of 2 μL/min. Furthermore, the dialysate (C_{dial}) and perfusate (C_{perf}) concentrations of BPA were measured by ICP-MS. The relative in vivo recovery of BPA across the dialysis membrane was calculated using the following equation: $R_{dial} = 1 - C_{dial}/C_{perf}$, where R_{dial} is the in vivo BPA recovery.

Pharmacokinetics

The pharmacokinetic parameters of boron in the plasma and tumor ECF were calculated for each set of sampled data using noncompartmental methods in the WinNonlin Version 5.2.1 software program (Pharsight, Montreal, Quebec, Canada). The area under the concentration versus the time curve extrapolated to infinity ($AUC_{0\text{-}\infty}$) was calculated using log-trapezoidal methods. Maximum observed concentration (C_{max}) and time to maximum concentration values were obtained directly from concentration versus time profiles. Mean residence time (MRT) extrapolated to infinity was calculated as $AUMC_{0\text{-}\infty}/AUC_{0\text{-}\infty}-(\text{infusion time})/2$, where $AUMC_{0\text{-}\infty}$ is the area under the first moment curve extrapolated to infinity.

Histological Observation

Two glioma-bearing rats were prepared for histological examination. The rats were perfused with saline and 10% neutral buffered formalin. The brains were removed, embedded in paraffin, and then serially sectioned into 30-μm-thick slices. The slices were stained with H&E to visualize their general cellular structure. Photomicrographs of 5 μm-thicknesses of the H&E stained tissues were obtained using a Mirax Scan digital microscope slide scanner (Carl Zeiss, Mirax 3D Histech) with a Plan-Apochromatic 20/0.8 objective lens.

Statistical Analysis

All data are shown as mean ± SEM. Data analysis was performed using an unpaired Student *t* test. Statistical significance was noted if $p \leq 0.05$.

Author Contributions

Conceived and designed the experiments: FYY YLL. Performed the experiments: FYY YLL YCL LWC YLH. Analyzed the data: FYY YLL LWC. Contributed reagents/materials/analysis tools: FYY FIC YWHL. Wrote the paper: FYY.

References

1. Rubin LL, Staddon JM (1999) The cell biology of the blood-brain barrier. Annu Rev Neurosci 22: 11–28.
2. Kroll RA, Neuwelt EA (1998) Outwitting the blood-brain barrier for therapeutic purposes: osmotic opening and other means. Neurosurgery 42: 1083–1099; discussion 1099–1100.
3. Yang FY, Teng MC, Lu M, Liang HF, Lee YR, et al. (2012) Treating glioblastoma multiforme with selective high-dose liposomal doxorubicin chemotherapy induced by repeated focused ultrasound. Int J Nanomedicine 7: 965–974.
4. Yang FY, Wong TT, Teng MC, Liu RS, Lu M, et al. (2012) Focused ultrasound and interleukin-4 receptor-targeted liposomal doxorubicin for enhanced targeted drug delivery and antitumor effect in glioblastoma multiforme. J Control Release 160: 652–658.
5. Hynynen K, McDannold N, Vykhodtseva N, Jolesz FA (2001) Noninvasive MR imaging-guided focal opening of the blood-brain barrier in rabbits. Radiology 220: 640–646.
6. Skold K, Gorlia T, Pellettieri L, Giusti V, B HS, et al. (2010) Boron neutron capture therapy for newly diagnosed glioblastoma multiforme: an assessment of clinical potential. Br J Radiol 83: 596–603.
7. Miyatake S, Kawabata S, Yokoyama K, Kuroiwa T, Michiue H, et al. (2009) Survival benefit of Boron neutron capture therapy for recurrent malignant gliomas. J Neurooncol 91: 199–206.
8. Kawabata S, Miyatake S, Kuroiwa T, Yokoyama K, Doi A, et al. (2009) Boron neutron capture therapy for newly diagnosed glioblastoma. J Radiat Res 50: 51–60.
9. Barth RF, Soloway AH, Brugger RM (1996) Boron neutron capture therapy of brain tumors: past history, current status, and future potential. Cancer Invest 14: 534–550.
10. Barth RF, Coderre JA, Vicente MG, Blue TE (2005) Boron neutron capture therapy of cancer: current status and future prospects. Clin Cancer Res 11: 3987–4002.
11. Barth R, Yang W, Rotaru J, Moeschberger M, Joel D, et al. (1997) Boron neutron capture therapy of brain tumors: enhanced survival following intracarotid injection of either sodium borocaptate or boronophenylalanine with or without blood-brain barrier disruption. Cancer Research 57: 1129.
12. Barth R, Yang W, Rotaru J, Moeschberger M, Boesel C, et al. (2000) Boron neutron capture therapy of brain tumors: enhanced survival and cure following blood-brain barrier disruption and intracarotid injection of sodium borocaptate and boronophenylalanine. International Journal of Radiation Oncology* Biology* Physics 47: 209–218.
13. Barth RF, Yang W, Bartus RT, Rotaru JH, Ferketich AK, et al. (2002) Neutron capture therapy of intracerebral melanoma: enhanced survival and cure after blood-brain barrier opening to improve delivery of boronophenylalanine. Int J Radiat Oncol Biol Phys 52: 858–868.
14. Westerink BH, Damsma G, Rollema H, De Vries JB, Horn AS (1987) Scope and limitations of in vivo brain dialysis: a comparison of its application to various neurotransmitter systems. Life Sci 41: 1763–1776.
15. Benveniste H, Huttemeier PC (1990) Microdialysis–theory and application. Prog Neurobiol 35: 195–215.
16. Bergenheim AT, Capala J, Roslin M, Henriksson R (2005) Distribution of BPA and metabolic assessment in glioblastoma patients during BNCT treatment: a microdialysis study. J Neurooncol 71: 287–293.
17. Yang FY, Chen YW, Chou FI, Yen SH, Lin YL, et al. (2012) Boron neutron capture therapy for glioblastoma multiforme: enhanced drug delivery and antitumor effect following blood-brain barrier disruption induced by focused ultrasound. Future Oncol 8: 1361–1369.
18. Alkins RD, Brodersen PM, Sodhi RN, Hynynen K (2013) Enhancing drug delivery for boron neutron capture therapy of brain tumors with focused ultrasound. Neuro Oncol 15: 1225–1235.
19. Yoshino K, Suzuki A, Mori Y, Kakihana H, Honda C, et al. (1989) Improvement of solubility of p-boronophenylalanine by complex formation with monosaccharides. Strahlenther Onkol 165: 127–129.
20. Kabalka GW, Nichols TL, Smith GT, Miller LF, Khan MK, et al. (2003) The use of positron emission tomography to develop boron neutron capture therapy treatment plans for metastatic malignant melanoma. J Neurooncol 62: 187–195.
21. Wang H, Liao A, Deng W, Chang P, Chen J, et al. (2004) Evaluation of 4-borono-2-18F-fluoro-L-phenylalanine-fructose as a probe for boron neutron capture therapy in a glioma-bearing rat model. Journal of Nuclear Medicine 45: 302.
22. Smith DR, Chandra S, Barth RF, Yang W, Joel DD, et al. (2001) Quantitative imaging and microlocalization of boron-10 in brain tumors and infiltrating tumor cells by SIMS ion microscopy: relevance to neutron capture therapy. Cancer Res 61: 8179–8187.
23. Vlachos F, Tung YS, Konofagou EE (2010) Permeability assessment of the focused ultrasound-induced blood-brain barrier opening using dynamic contrast-enhanced MRI. Phys Med Biol 55: 5451–5466.
24. Vlachos F, Tung YS, Konofagou E (2011) Permeability dependence study of the focused ultrasound-induced blood-brain barrier opening at distinct pressures and microbubble diameters using DCE-MRI. Magn Reson Med 66: 821–830.
25. Park J, Zhang Y, Vykhodtseva N, Jolesz FA, McDannold NJ (2012) The kinetics of blood brain barrier permeability and targeted doxorubicin delivery into brain induced by focused ultrasound. J Control Release 162: 134–142.
26. Yang FY, Wang HE, Lin GL, Teng MC, Lin HH, et al. (2011) Micro-SPECT/CT-based pharmacokinetic analysis of 99mTc-diethylenetriaminepentaacetic acid in rats with blood-brain barrier disruption induced by focused ultrasound. J Nucl Med 52: 478–484.
27. Barth RF (1998) Rat brain tumor models in experimental neuro-oncology: the 9L, C6, T9, F98, RG2 (D74), RT-2 and CNS-1 gliomas. J Neurooncol 36: 91–102.
28. Yang FY, Lin YS, Kang KH, Chao TK (2011) Reversible blood-brain barrier disruption by repeated transcranial focused ultrasound allows enhanced extravasation. J Control Release 150: 111–116.
29. Johansen MJ, Newman RA, Madden T (1997) The use of microdialysis in pharmacokinetics and pharmacodynamics. Pharmacotherapy 17: 464–481.
30. Kehr J (1993) A survey on quantitative microdialysis: theoretical models and practical implications. J Neurosci Methods 48: 251–261.
31. Evrard PA, Deridder G, Verbeeck RK (1996) Intravenous microdialysis in the mouse and the rat: development and pharmacokinetic application of a new probe. Pharm Res 13: 12–17.

2

A New Brain Drug Delivery Strategy: Focused Ultrasound-Enhanced Intranasal Drug Delivery

Hong Chen[1], Cherry C. Chen[1], Camilo Acosta[1], Shih-Ying Wu[1], Tao Sun[1], Elisa E. Konofagou[1,2]*

1 Department of Biomedical Engineering, Columbia University, New York, New York, United States of America, 2 Department of Radiology, Columbia University, New York, New York, United States of America

Abstract

Central nervous system (CNS) diseases are difficult to treat because of the blood-brain barrier (BBB), which prevents most drugs from entering into the brain. Intranasal (IN) administration is a promising approach for drug delivery to the brain, bypassing the BBB; however, its application has been restricted to particularly potent substances and it does not offer localized delivery to specific brain sites. Focused ultrasound (FUS) in combination with microbubbles can deliver drugs to the brain at targeted locations. The present study proposed to combine these two different platform techniques (FUS+IN) for enhancing the delivery efficiency of intranasally administered drugs at a targeted location. After IN administration of 40 kDa fluorescently-labeled dextran as the model drug, FUS targeted at one region within the caudate putamen of mouse brains was applied in the presence of systemically administered microbubbles. To compare with the conventional FUS technique, in which intravenous (IV) drug injection is employed, FUS was also applied after IV injection of the same amount of dextran in another group of mice. Dextran delivery outcomes were evaluated using fluorescence imaging of brain slices. The results showed that FUS+IN enhanced drug delivery within the targeted region compared with that achieved by IN only. Despite the fact that the IN route has limited drug absorption across the nasal mucosa, the delivery efficiency of FUS+IN was not significantly different from that of FUS+IV. As a new drug delivery platform, the FUS+IN technique is potentially useful for treating CNS diseases.

Editor: Mária A. Deli, Hungarian Academy of Sciences, Hungary

Funding: This study was supported by National Institutes of Health grants RO1 EB009041 and RO1 AG038961 and the Kinetics Foundation. The founders had no role in study design, data collection and analysis, decision to publish, or preparation of the manuscript.

Competing Interests: The authors have declared that no competing interests exist.

* Email: ek2191@columbia.edu

Introduction

Central nervous system (CNS) diseases are difficult to treat as most systemically administered therapeutic agents cannot penetrate the blood-brain barrier (BBB). The BBB prevents the access of ~100% of large-molecule drugs and ~98% of small-molecule drugs (usually defined as smaller than around 500–600 Da in molecular weight [1]) to the brain from the systemic circulation [2]. Various strategies have been developed for circumventing the BBB, such as invasive direct injection or infusion, modification of therapeutic agents, and carrier-mediated transport [3]. Among these strategies, intranasal (IN) delivery is a non-invasive approach for direct drug delivery to the brain via the nose, bypassing the BBB [4].

IN administration has emerged as a promising approach for drug delivery to the brain. Traditionally, it has been successfully used as a convenient method for drug delivery to the systemic circulation, because IN administered drugs can be absorbed through a rich vascular network in the nasal cavity into the systemic circulation [5]. Although most drugs absorbed into the blood circulation cannot enter the brain parenchyma because of the BBB, it has been demonstrated feasible in animal and clinical studies that drugs can be directly delivered from the nostrils to the brain, bypassing the BBB. A wide-range of therapeutics, such as peptides, proteins, gene vectors and stem cells, have been successfully delivered through IN administration to small animal brains and have shown efficacy in treating CNS diseases, such as Alzheimer's disease, Parkinson's disease, Huntington's disease, depression, anxiety, autism spectrum disorders, seizures, drug addiction, eating disorders, and stroke [6–8]. Moreover, a number of clinical trials have demonstrated CNS effects in humans following IN delivery of biologics, among which IN administration of insulin has been found to be a promising approach to slow down the progression of Alzheimer's disease [9].

Despite the fact that the mechanisms involved in IN drug delivery to the brain are still being elucidated, some of the pathways involved are known. The neural connections between the nasal mucosa and the brain through the olfactory and trigeminal nerves (involved in sensing odors and chemicals) have been found to provide unique pathways for the noninvasive delivery of therapeutic agents to the CNS [4,6]. IN administered drugs are most likely transported extracellularly along the olfactory and trigeminal nerves to the brain. The distribution of drugs from these brain entry points to other distant CNS sites may be envisioned to occur either by intracellular or extracelluar transport. The extracellular transport can occur via convective transport within the cerebral perivascular spaces, local diffusion at the entry points, and local diffusion from perivascular spaces into the parenchyma [4,6]. Although promising in brain drug delivery, the IN route has some disadvantages. One major drawback of this route is that the fraction of drug reaching the CNS from the nasal cavity is small, which has restricted its application to very potent substances [6,10]. The other disadvantage is that drugs are delivered to the whole brain through this route, while neurological diseases do not generally affect the brain in a global manner. Therefore, new strategies are needed for enhancing drug delivery efficiency at the sites requiring treatment while minimizing the exposure to other brain sites. Transcranial focused ultrasound (FUS) in combination with microbubbles may offer such a strategy.

FUS in combination with microbubbles can increase the BBB permeability for targeted brain drug delivery with no or minimal tissue damage [11,12]. The experimental design typically uses intravenous (IV) injection of therapeutic agents with microbubbles, and then applies FUS to induce BBB opening for drug delivery. The FUS focuses externally generated ultrasound pulses through the skull onto a small focal region (on the order of millimeters) deep into the subcortical structures, which allows highly precise and noninvasive targeting of brain regions where treatment is desired. Microbubbles are micron-scale gas bubbles stabilized by a lipid, protein, albumin or polymer shell. They have been used as ultrasound imaging contrast agents in the clinic for more than two decades and have shown great potential as drug delivery agents for therapeutic applications. The FUS technique has been successfully used in the delivery of various therapeutic agents, such as chemotherapeutic drugs [13], neurotrophins [14], antibodies [15], gene vectors [16], and cells [17]. Our group and others have shown that the BBB opening induced by FUS is reversible, and its closing time ranges from several hours to several days, depending on the acoustic parameters [18]. The volume of BBB opening can be controlled by adjusting the acoustic parameters or microbubble sizes [19]. Previous short-term (up to 5-hr survival) and long-term (up to 4-wk survival) safety assessment of the FUS technique demonstrated that, when appropriate ultrasound parameters are used, there is no or only minimal histological damage [20,21]. Nevertheless, although IV injection of therapeutic agents has high bioavailability, it is associated with systemic exposure and thus not suitable for the delivery of drugs with short half-lives in blood and/or high systemic side effects, such as neurotrophic factors, neuropeptides, and hormones [8,22]. In contrast, IN administration is a painless, simple, and noninvasive approach that allows direct drug delivery to the brain, eliminating the need for systemic delivery and thereby reducing associated side effects [7,8].

The physical mechanisms for FUS-enhanced drug delivery have been under extensive investigation [23,24]. Different from other contrast agents used in medical imaging, microbubbles are confined within the blood vessels after IV injection due to their relatively large sizes. When microbubbles pass through the FUS focal region, they cavitate, which is a broad term for ultrasound-induced activities of bubbles, including their oscillation and collapse. Cavitation is usually divided into two classes: stable cavitation (bubbles stably oscillate) and inertial cavitation (bubbles rapidly collapse). The cavitation emissions from microbubbles during FUS sonication can be detected, allowing real-time monitoring of the FUS treatment [25]. Microbubble cavitation generates mechanical effects on the nearby blood vessels, such as high shear stress, microstreaming, and microjetting, enabling transvascular delivery of drugs in the blood circulation [26]. Meanwhile, the oscillating microbubbles can push and pull on the blood vessels along with surrounding tissues, inducing expansion and contraction of the perivascular spaces [27]. The displacements of the perivascular spaces may induce convective bulk fluid flow, leading to enhanced drug penetration. Moreover, the radiation force generated by the FUS beam itself without microbubbles can generate shear stress on the tissue and increase hydraulic conductivity of the interstitial space, which can increase drug diffusion [26]. The mechanical effects exerted by the FUS beam in combination with microbubbles contribute to the enhanced brain delivery of IV-injected therapeutic agents. These same mechanical effects may also enhance the delivery of drugs administered through the IN route.

Therefore, we hypothesized that FUS can enhance IN drug delivery efficiency at the targeted brain sites. There were two objectives of this study: (1) to explore the feasibility of this new brain drug delivery strategy–FUS in combination with IN (FUS+IN); (2) to compare the drug delivery outcomes of this new strategy with the conventional approach–FUS coupled with IV injection (FUS+IV). Wild-type mice were used as the animal model and a 40 kDa fluorescently-labeled dextran was used as the model drug [28]. Dextrans are glucose polymers and the 40 kDa dextran was selected as the model drug because its molecular weight is on the same order of magnitude as many neurotrophic factors that have considerable potential in the treatment of CNS diseases [22]. The drug delivery outcomes using different strategies were evaluated based on fluorescence images of brain slices.

Materials and Methods

Animal preparation

This study was carried out in strict accordance with the recommendations in the Guide for the Care and Use of Laboratory Animals of the National Institutes of Health. The protocol was approved by the Columbia University Institutional Animal Care and Use Committee. All surgery was performed under isoflurane anesthesia, and all efforts were made to minimize animal suffering. The animal body temperature was maintained using a heating pad.

A total of 26 male C57BL/6 mice (20–25 g in weight; Harlan Laboratories, Indianapolis, IN) were used in this study. Among these 26 mice, 20 were divided into the following four experimental groups with n = 5 for each group. (1) Control group: no dextran delivery and no FUS. (2) IN sham group: IN administration of the dextran without FUS. (3) IN treatment group: IN administration of the dextran with FUS applied on the left side of the caudate putamen while the contralateral right side was not sonicated. (4) IV treatment group: IV injection of the dextran with FUS applied on the left side of the caudate putamen while the contralateral right side was not sonicated. The remaining 6 mice were treated following the same protocol as groups 3 and 4 with n = 3 for each group for the purpose of assessing the safety of the FUS treatment.

Microbubble generation

Microbubbles comprised of a 90 mol% 1,2-distearoyl-sn-glycero-3- phosphocholine (DSPC) and 10 mol% 1,2-distearoyl-sn-glycero-3- phosphoethanolamine-N-[methoxy(polyethylene glycol)2000] (DSPE-PEG2000) (Avanti Polar Lipids, Alabaster, AL, USA) lipid-shell and a perfluorobutane (FluoroMed, Round Rock, TX, USA) gas-core were manufactured in-house. Size-selected microbubbles with a median diameter of 4–5 μm were isolated from a poly-dispersed microbubble distribution using a differential centrifugation method [29]. Their size distributions and concentrations were determined by a particle counter (Multisizer III, Beckman Coulter Inc., Opa Locka, FL, USA). Before each injection into the mouse, their concentrations were diluted using sterile saline to a final concentration of approximately 8×10^8 number of microbubbles per mL.

Administration of the dextran

In the control group (group 1), no dextran was administered.

In the IN sham group (group 2) and IN treatment group (group 3), ~2 mg of 40 kDa Texas Red-labeled dextran (Life Technologies Inc, Grand Island, NY, USA) was administered intranasally following procedures used before [4,30]. The dextran was dissolved in saline at a concentration of 40 mg/mL. The anaesthetized mice were placed supine with the head position stabilized horizontally. A micropipette was used to intranasally administer 3 μL drops of the dextran solution to alternating nostril every 2 minutes. Drops were placed at the opening of the nostril, allowing the animal to snort each drop into the nasal cavity. A total of 51 μL dextran solution (~2 mg dextran) was delivered over a course of 34 min.

For the IV treatment group (group 4), the same amount of dextran (51 μL in volume, 40 mg/mL in concentration, and ~2 mg in dose) was administered by IV bolus injection through the tail vein.

Focused ultrasound sonication

For the IN treatment group (group 3) and IV treatment group (group 4), the mice were sonicated at a targeted brain location using an experimental setup illustrated in Fig. 1(A) and following an experimental timeline shown in Fig. 1(B).

A single-element FUS transducer (center frequency: 1.5 MHz, focal depth: 60 mm, diameter: 60 mm; Imasonic, Besancon, France) was driven by a function generator (33220A, Agilent, Palo Alto, CA, USA) through a nominal 50 dB gain power amplifier (325LA, E&I, Rochester, NY, USA). The lateral and axial dimensions of the FUS focal region measured in water were 1.2 mm and 13.0 mm. A custom-built truncated cone was attached to the transducer and filled with degassed water to provide acoustic coupling. The cone was immersed in a degassed-water container. The bottom of the water container had a window sealed with an almost acoustically and optically transparent membrane. The container was placed on the mouse head and coupled with degassed ultrasound gel. Acoustic emissions arising from microbubble cavitation were acquired by a pulse-echo transducer (center frequency 10 MHz; focal length 60 mm; Olympus NDT, Waltham, MA, USA). It was positioned through a central hole of the FUS transducer and confocally aligned with the FUS transducer. The signals received by the pulse-echo transducer were amplified by 20 dB (Model 5800, Panametrics-NDT, Waltham, MA, USA) and then digitized (Razor Express CompuScope 1422, Gage Applied Technologies, Inc., Lachine, QC, Canada) at a sampling frequency of 50 MHz.

Before FUS sonication, each mouse was positioned prone with its head immobilized by a stereotaxic frame (David Kopf Instruments, Tujunga, CA, USA). The fur on the mouse head was removed with an electric clipper and a depilatory cream. A modified 27G × ½ butterfly catheter (Terumo Medical, Somerset, NJ, USA) was inserted into the tail vein for IV injection. The FUS transducer was moved 2 mm lateral of the sagittal suture and 6 mm anterior of the lambdoid suture using a previously described grid positioning method [31]. Freshly diluted microbubble suspension (30 μL) was administered through a bolus injection via the tail vein prior to each sonication. For the IV treatment group (group 4), the microbubbles were co-injected with the dextran (Fig. 1B). Immediately after injection (~5 s), pulsed FUS (center frequency: 1.5 MHz; peak-negative pressure: 0.45 MPa; pulse length: 6.7 ms; pulse repetition frequency: 5 Hz; duration: 1 min) was applied transcranially to the left caudate putamen. The non-sonicated right caudate putamen served as control for IN administration only (group 3) or IV injection only (group 4). Additionally, prior to microbubble injection, a 30-s sonication using the same acoustic parameters was applied in order to measure the background cavitation signals, needed in the acoustic emission analysis described later.

For all the mice used in the current study, a 1-h period was allowed after finishing IN and IV dextran administration to enable the dextran to diffuse into the brain parenchyma (Fig. 1B). At the end of the allotted time, all mice were sacrificed by transcardial perfusion. The mouse brains were processed and prepared for either frozen (60 μm thick) or paraffin (6 μm thick) sections. The frozen sections were imaged by a fluorescence microscope (BX61; Olympus, Melville, NY, USA) and used later for quantifying dextran delivery outcomes. The paraffin sections were used for whole brain histological examinations by hematoxylin and eosin (H&E) staining [21].

Acoustic emission analysis

The acoustic emission analysis method was the same as that described previously [32–34]. To quantify the stable and inertial

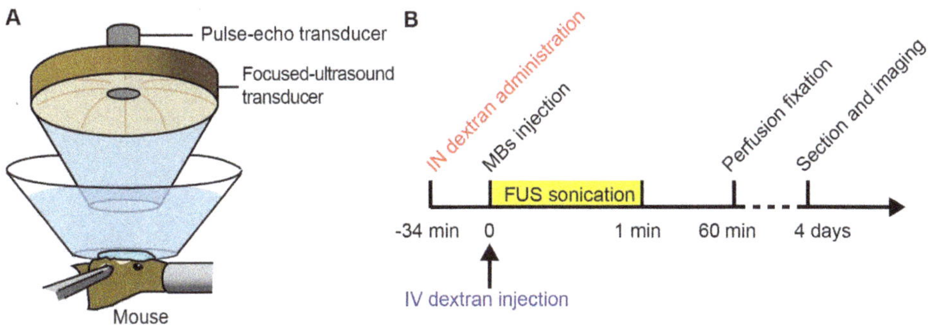

Figure 1. Illustration of experimental (A) setup and (B) timeline. For IN administration, the dextran was administered 3 μL at a time, alternating between the two nostrils, with a lapse of 2 min between each administration, over a total of 34 min.

cavitation behaviors of the microbubbles within the FUS targeted region, the stable cavitation dose and inertial cavitation dose were calculated, respectively.

For each ultrasound pulse, its frequency spectrum between 3 and 9 MHz was used for stable and inertial cavitation quantification to eliminate any contributions from the FUS beam (frequency = 1.5 MHz). The broadband emission from inertial cavitation was obtained using a comb filter, which had a cut-off band around each harmonic and ultraharmonic frequencies with bandwidths of 350 kHz and 100 kHz, respectively. The root mean square of the filtered spectra was calculated to represent the inertial cavitation level for each pulse. The stable cavitation level was obtained by first calculating the root mean square of the amplitudes of all harmonics and then subtracting the corresponding inertial cavitation level. The inertial cavitation activity was thus not included in the stable cavitation quantification. The stable and inertial cavitation doses were calculated by integrating the stable and inertial cavitation levels over the total ultrasound exposure time, respectively. The final doses were then calculated by subtracting baseline doses obtained based on signals acquired prior to microbubble injection.

Fluorescence analysis

The dextran delivery outcomes were determined by quantifying the fluorescence intensities within the targeted caudate putamen. Nine horizontal sections with four dorsal sections, four ventral sections, and a reference midline section were selected from each brain for the analysis. All the fluorescence images were first normalized by their corresponding exposure time. Then, a circular region-of-interest (ROI, diameter = 1.2 mm) was manually aligned with the sonicated and control caudate putamen on each section, and the spatial average fluorescence intensity within the ROI was calculated using ImageJ (National Institutes of Health; Bethesda, MD). The diameter of the ROI was selected to be the same as the FUS transducer lateral focal region dimension (1.2 mm). The reported fluorescence intensity for each side of the brain was the sum of the calculated fluorescence intensities within the ROI of all nine sections.

Statistical analysis

An unpaired two-tailed Student's t-test using GraphPad Prism (Version 5.01, La Jolla, CA, USA) was used to compare between groups. A P value of 0.05 was considered to represent a significant difference in all the analyses. All data were expressed as mean ± standard deviation.

Results

IN delivery to the brain

Figures 2A and 2B present representative fluorescence images of horizontal sections of the whole brain from the control group (group 1) and IN sham group (group 2). As shown in Fig. 2B, IN administration of the dextran without FUS resulted in an elevation of dextran concentration in the whole brain. A statistically significant increase in the fluorescence intensity was found in the IN sham group when compared with the control group (Fig. 2C), suggesting that the IN route enables direct access of drugs to the brain. Within each group, no difference was found between left and right caudate putamen regions, as expected. However, the delivered dextran did not accumulate in any particular brain region and the concentration achievable in different regions of the brain varied, which confirmed the non-targeted nature of IN administration.

FUS-enhanced IN delivery

Figures 3A and 3B show that FUS exposure in the presence of microbubbles significantly enhanced IN delivery at the targeted left caudate putamen (Fig. 3A) when compared with the contralateral right side with IN administration only (Fig. 3B). Quantification of the fluorescence intensities of mouse brains in the FUS+IN group found an 8-fold increase in the fluorescence intensity compared with the contralateral control side with IN only (Fig. 3E).

When IV injection was used for dextran delivery instead of IN, localized dextran accumulation was observed at the targeted caudate putamen. Figures 3C and 3D display representative fluorescence images from the FUS+IV treated (left) caudate putamen and contralateral non-treated (right) side with IV dextran injection only. The two mouse brains shown in Figs. 3A, B and 3C, D had fluorescence intensities of similar magnitude (27.2 and 19.4, respectively). When comparing across the entire FUS+IN and FUS+IV groups, the administration route did not appear to affect the delivery efficiency in the targeted caudate putamen as no significant difference in dextran accumulation was detected between FUS+IN and FUS+IV groups ($P = 0.48$; Fig. 3E). In addition, a significant increase in fluorescence intensity was found in the IN only group (Fig. 3B) compared with IV only group (Fig. 3D) ($P = 0.005$; Fig. 3E), further confirming that IN administration alone allows the dextran to gain direct access to the brain.

It should be noted that although the fluorescence intensities of FUS+IN and FUS+IV groups were at a similar level, distinct dextran distribution characteristics were observed, as representatively shown in Figs. 3A and 3C. Images shown in Fig. 3A–D were acquired at higher magnification than those presented in Fig. 2 to highlight the features of dextran distribution. A single sonication following IV dextran injection resulted in a more homogeneous dextran distribution within the FUS targeted region (Fig. 3C), while a less homogeneous dextran distribution with high intensity regions was observed in the FUS+IN group (Fig. 3A). Heterogeneous dextran distribution was also observed on the contralateral control side with IN administration only as shown in Fig. 3B as well as Fig. 2B. In addition, it was clearly observed in Fig. 3B that the vascular network was highlighted by the dextran, confirming that IN administered compounds can be transported within the perivascular spaces of cerebral blood vessels [7].

Preliminary safety assessment of FUS sonication was performed by histological analysis. Minor microhemorrhages were observed in both FUS+IN and FUS+IV groups. Figures 4C and 4D depict cases with the most severe damage from the FUS+IN and FUS+IV groups, respectively. Small clusters of erythrocyte extravasation were observed in both cases. Figure 5 shows the microbubble activities detected in these two groups, as quantified by stable and inertial cavitation doses. No significant difference in stable or inertial cavitation dose was found between the FUS+IN and FUS+IV groups.

Discussion

Our findings validated the hypothesis that FUS can enhance the delivery of IN-administered drugs at a targeted brain location. It is the first time that this novel combination of these two different platform techniques is proposed. Numerous studies have demonstrated that the IN route can provide a non-invasive approach for brain drug delivery, but none of them have shown that an enhanced delivery at a targeted location was possible. The FUS+IN technique offers a potentially useful drug delivery platform for treating CNS diseases.

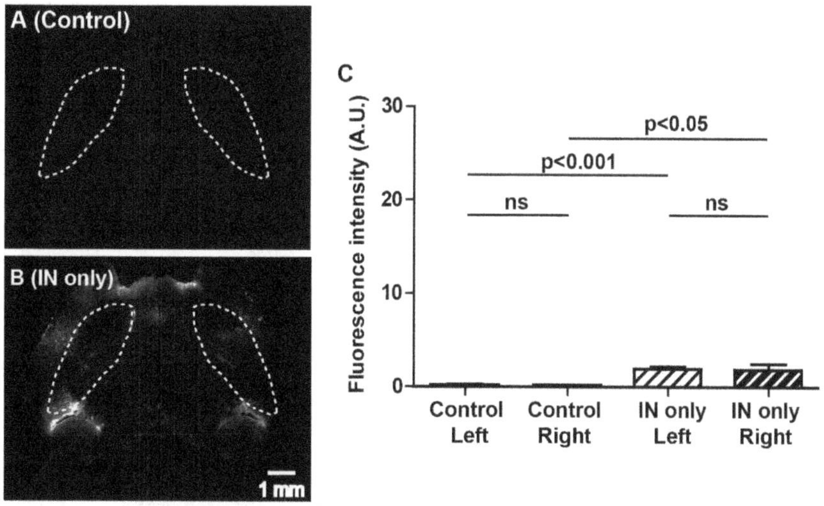

Figure 2. Fluorescently-labeled dextrans delivered to the whole brain through IN administration. (A) and (B) show the representative fluorescence images of horizontal sections of the whole brain from the control group (no FUS and no dextran administration) and the IN sham group (IN administration without FUS), respectively. The caudate putamen regions are highlighted by dash lines. (C) Quantitative analysis of the fluorescence intensities within the left and right caudate putamen regions for these two groups. IN administration resulted in a significant increase in the fluorescent intensity compared with the control. Scale bar represents 1 mm.

By combining FUS with IN drug delivery, we achieved a significant increase in drug accumulation in the targeted brain site, thus improving the bioavailability and biodistribution of the IN administered drug. We confirmed that IN-administered dextran could be delivered to the brain, bypassing the BBB, but it had low delivery efficiency and was non-targeted (Fig. 2). IN administration in combination with FUS achieved an 8-fold increase in drug delivery efficiency within the targeted region compared with IN administration only (Fig. 3E). In the past, the IN route could only be used for particularly potent substances because of limited absorption across the nasal epithelium [6]. FUS+IN may expand its application to a much broader range of drugs. Moreover, although IN administrated drugs are distributed to the whole brain, by decreasing the IN administration dose, FUS+IN has the potential to achieve therapeutic drug level only within the targeted site while keeping non-targeted sites at sub-therapeutic level. Therefore, the FUS technique would potentially overcome the major disadvantages of IN brain drug delivery: (1) overcome the restriction that the IN route can only be used for particularly potent substances and (2) achieve targeted brain drug delivery. FUS+IN can be applied in the future for the delivery of drugs that have been previously shelved from IN administration due to their

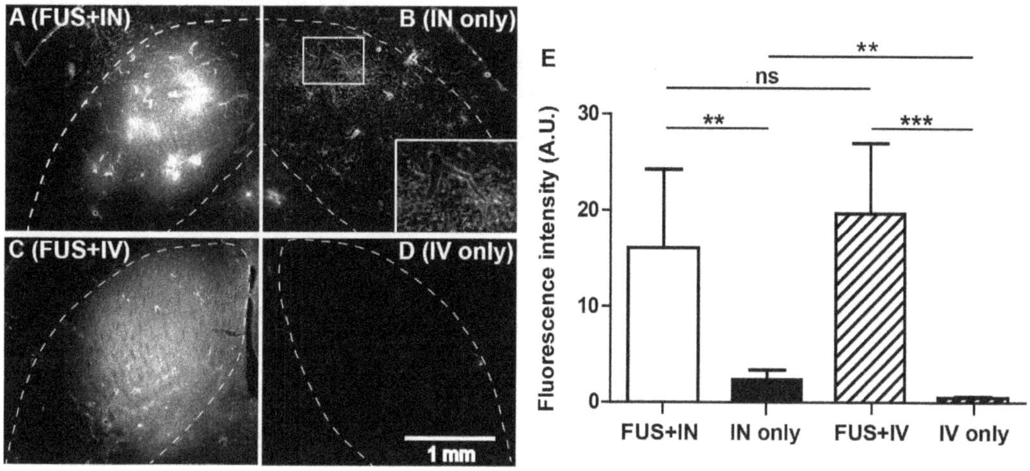

Figure 3. Focused ultrasound enhanced targeted delivery of the dextran administered through IN or IV route. (A) and (B) show fluorescence images of part of the left and right caudate putamen in one horizontal section from one mouse in the IN treatment group. (C) and (D) show part of the left and right caudate putamen in one horizontal section from one mouse in the IV treatment group. FUS was targeted at the left caudate putamen. The caudate putamen region in each image was highlighted by the dash line. The box insert in (B) is a blow up of the square area in (B), which shows that the vascular network was highlighted by the dextran, confirming that IN administered compounds can be transported within the perivascular spaces of cerebral blood vessels. (E) Quantitative fluorescence intensity analysis within the left and right caudate putamen regions for these two groups. FUS significantly enhanced IN delivery efficiency. No difference was found between FUS+IN and FUS+IV. Scale bar represents 1 mm.

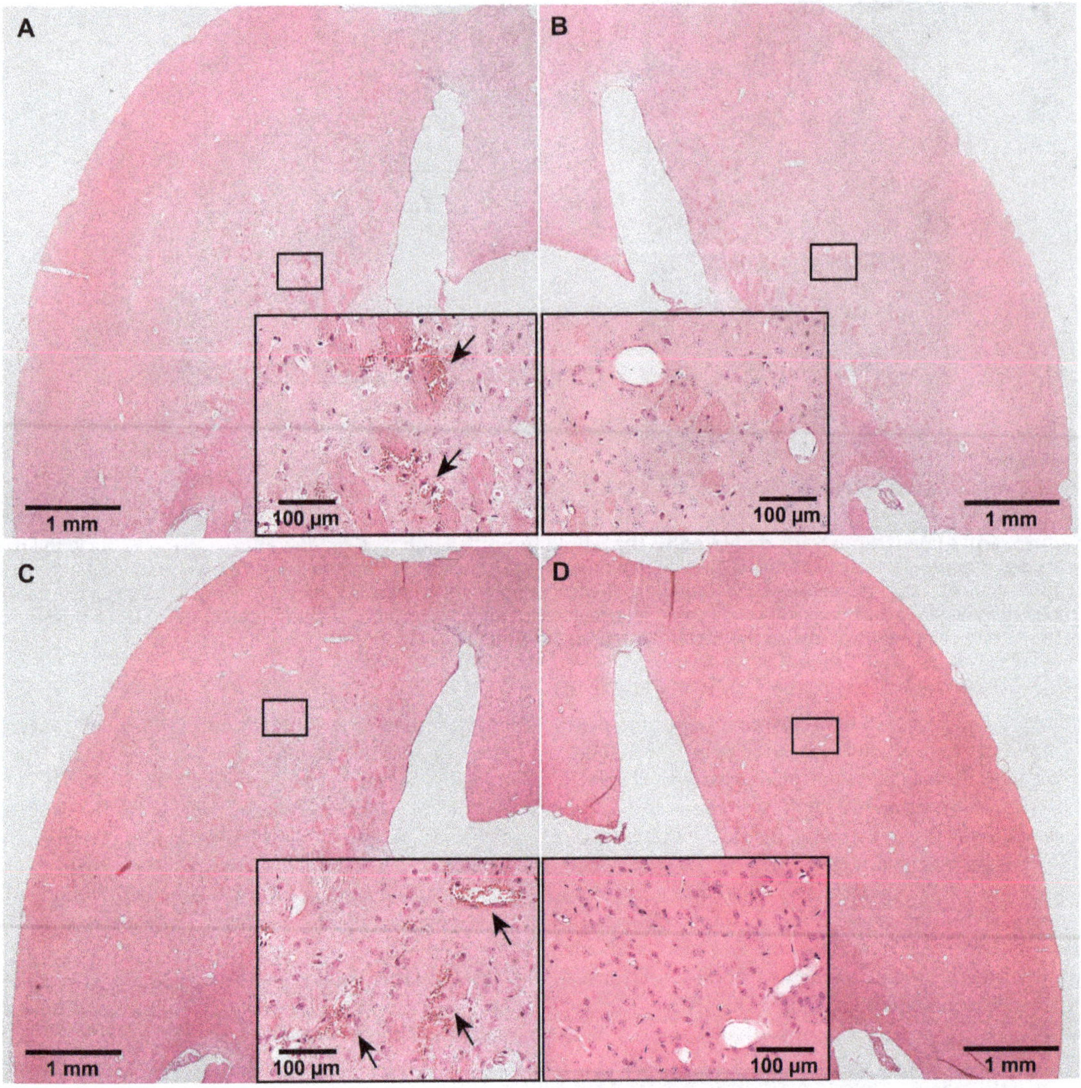

Figure 4. Whole brain histological examinations by hematoxylin and eosin (H&E) staining. Microscopic examination of (A, C) left (sonicated) and (B, D) the corresponding right (nonsonicated) caudate putamen in H&E stained horizontal sections. (A) and (B) were from the same section of a mouse brain with the most severe damage in the FUS+IN group. (C) and (D) were from the same section of a mouse brain with the most severe damage in the FUS+IV group. Minor microhemorrhages, as pointed out by arrows, were observed on the FUS targeted left caudate putamen in (A) and (C). No tissue damage was observed on the contralateral right caudate putamen without FUS sonication in (B) and (D).

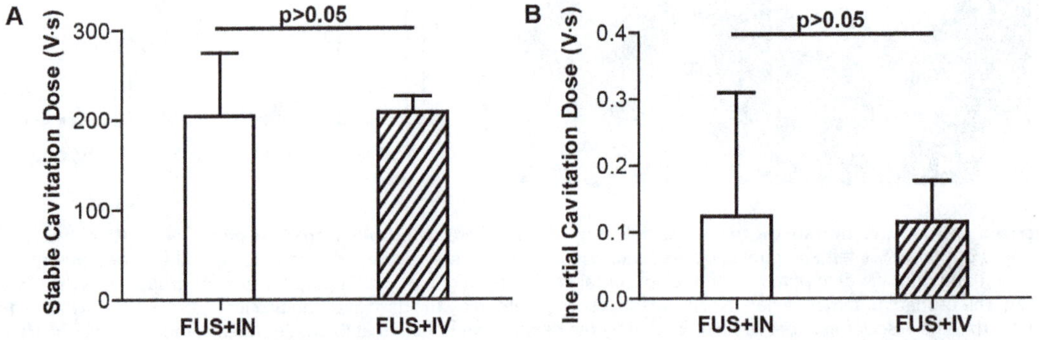

Figure 5. Quantification of microbubble cavitation activities in FUS+IN and FUS+IV groups. (A) Stable cavitation doses. (B) Inertial cavitation doses. No difference was found in both stable cavitation behavior and inertial cavitation behavior between these two groups.

poor pharmacokinetics. New CNS therapeutic strategies could emerge based on the FUS+IN technique.

Our findings should not be interpreted as if to establish that the IN administration when combined with FUS is superior for targeted brain drug delivery than FUS+IV. On the contrary, FUS+IV is better at targeted delivery than FUS+IN. IN administration is associated with drug delivery to the whole brain, whereas the dextran injected through IV can only be delivered at the FUS targeted region where the BBB was opened. Therefore, for drugs exhibiting high stability in circulation and low systemic side-effects, such as dextrans (the half-life of the 40 kDa dextran in blood is about 7.5 hours [35]) used in this study, FUS+IV remains an effective technique since it provides drug access only to the targeted location without affecting other CNS sites. However, IN administration offers a non-invasive alternative over the more conventional IV injection for brain drug delivery. It allows direct access to the CNS and has low systemic bioavailability [22]. Therefore, FUS+IN may become a viable alternative for FUS+IV in the delivery of therapeutics that have beneficial effects within the CNS, but short half-lives in the blood and/or high systemic side effects. IN delivery of such therapeutics, such as neurotrophic factors, neuropeptides, and hormones, have been shown promise in the treatment of CNS diseases and injuries, including Alzheimer's disease, stroke, Parkinson's disease, motor neuron diseases, demyelinating diseases and traumatic brain injury [6,8,22]. The combination of IN administration and FUS has great potential to improve treatment outcomes of these diseases compared with IN administration alone.

We clearly showed brain uptake of the IN administrated dextran in both the IN only group and FUS+IN group (Figs. 2B, 3A, and 3B). In addition, we found the FUS+IN group showed less homogeneous dextran distribution (Fig. 3A) than the FUS+IV group (Fig. 3C). Similar heterogeneous dextran distribution was also observed in the IN only group (Figs. 2B and 3B). For drug delivery by FUS+IV, the drug circulated throughout the body and significant CNS delivery can only be achieved in brain locations where BBB opening is induced by FUS with microbubbles through cellular mechanisms, including opening a part of the tight junctions, formation of channel and fenestration in endothelial cell cytoplasm, and enhancing transcytosis [36]. On the other hand, IN administered drugs are most likely transported along the olfactory and trigeminal nerves to the brain entry sites and then distribute to other distant CNS sites via convective and diffusive transport from the cerebral perivascular spaces into the parenchyma [4,6]. Figure 3B confirmed that IN-administered drugs can be transported within the perivascular spaces of cerebral blood vessels. The distribution of IN-administered drugs in the brain will be affected by the structural characteristics of the different brain compartments and the functional barriers between them [22], which may contribute to the observed heterogeneous dextran distribution. Future investigation is needed to better understand the pharmacokinetics of drug delivery by FUS+IN.

Further investigation is warranted on the mechanisms for FUS-enhanced IN drug delivery. It has been demonstrated that FUS and microbubbles can generate shear stress on the tissue and increase hydraulic conductivity of the interstitial space, leading to increased drug diffusion [26]. Thus, the diffusion of drugs in the perineural and perivascular spaces may be enhanced by the FUS technique. Meanwhile, it has been proposed that the most likely convective mechanism for the widespread distribution of IN administered drugs is the convective flow induced by the expansion and contraction of the perivascular spaces with the cardiac cycle, named "perivascular pump" [4,37]. Microbubble cavitation can cause expansion and contraction of the perivascular spaces, similar to the expansion and contraction induced by the cardiac cycle but at a much higher frequency [27]. The displacements of the perivascular spaces may induce bulk flow, leading to enhanced convective transport within cerebral perivascular spaces at the FUS targeted region. Furthermore, drugs that enter the systemic circulation through the IN route can cross the BBB at the FUS targeted regions. Therefore, the combination effects of FUS-enhanced local drug diffusion, convective transport, and BBB permeability may contribute to FUS-enhanced IN drug delivery. Ongoing efforts include unveiling the mechanisms by which FUS technique enhances the drug delivery after IN administration.

Whole brain histological examination showed minor microhemorrhages within the FUS targeted region. The damage induced by the FUS technique for FUS+IN and FUS+IV groups were similar (Fig. 4). Figure 5 confirmed that no difference was found in microbubble activities between these two groups. We note that the standard deviations of stable and inertial cavitation doses for FUS+IN group were higher than those for the FUS+IV group. The mice in the FUS+IV group were treated within one day using the same batch of microbubbles; while the mice in the FUS+IN group were treated on separate days using different batches of microbubbles, which could explain the higher standard deviations in microbubble activities observed in the FUS+IN group compared with the FUS+IV group. Nevertheless, these findings suggest that the likelihood of tissue damage by FUS was only correlated with the applied acoustic exposure, not the dextran administration route. The minor damaging effect is consistent with that observed in previous studies [20,21]. Previous short-term (up to 5-hr survival) and long-term (up to 4-wk survival) safety assessment of the FUS technique demonstrated that the damaging effect, characterized by the presence of a small number of extravasated blood cells within the sonicated region, were found to be transient as no evidence for continuous damage was seen [20,21]. Behavioral tests performed in non-human primates after repeated FUS sonication in combination with microbubbles showed that FUS did not cause any functional damage even in the presence of tiny clusters of extravasated blood cells [38]. Furthermore, the minimal microhemorrhage could be eliminated by decreasing the FUS exposure [39]. Future studies will optimize the FUS+IN treatment parameters for efficient drug delivery without any tissue damage and explore its potential as a new drug delivery platform in treating CNS diseases.

Conclusions

IN administration is a promising approach for brain drug delivery. The present study demonstrated for the first time that FUS can enhance IN drug delivery efficiency at the targeted brain location. Despite the fact that the IN route has limited drug absorption across the nasal mucosa, the FUS+IN technique achieved similar drug delivery efficiency within the targeted region compared with the conventional FUS+IV approach. Future studies will explore its potential as a drug delivery platform in treating CNS diseases.

Author Contributions

Conceived and designed the experiments: EEK HC CCC. Performed the experiments: CCC CA. Analyzed the data: HC CCC CA SYW TS. Wrote the paper: HC CCC EEK.

References

1. Workman P (2001) New drug targets for genomic cancer therapy successes, limitations, opportunities and future challenges. Curr Cancer Drug Targets 1: 33–47.
2. Pardridge WM (2005) The blood-brain barrier: bottleneck in brain drug development. NeuroRx 2: 3–14.
3. Gabathuler R (2010) Approaches to transport therapeutic drugs across the blood-brain barrier to treat brain diseases. Neurobiol Dis 37: 48–57.
4. Dhuria SV, Hanson LR, Frey WH II (2010) Intranasal delivery to the central nervous system: mechanisms and experimental considerations. J Pharm Sci 99: 1654–1673.
5. Pires A, Fortuna A, Alves G, Falcão A (2009) Intranasal drug delivery: how, why and what for? J Pharm Pharm Sci 12: 288–311.
6. Lochhead JJ, Thorne RG (2012) Intranasal delivery of biologics to the central nervous system. Adv Drug Deliv Rev 64: 614–628.
7. Hanson LR, Frey WH II (2008) Intranasal delivery bypasses the blood-brain barrier to target therapeutic agents to the central nervous system and treat neurodegenerative disease. BMC Neurosci 9 Suppl 3: S5.
8. Chapman CD, Frey WH II, Craft S, Danielyan L, Hallschmid M, et al. (2013) Intranasal treatment of central nervous system dysfunction in humans. Pharm Res 30: 2475–2484.
9. Freiherr J, Hallschmid M, Frey WH II, Brünner YF, Chapman CD, et al. (2013) Intranasal insulin as a treatment for Alzheimer's disease: a review of basic research and clinical evidence. CNS Drugs 27: 505–514.
10. Illum L (2004) Is nose-to-brain transport of drugs in man a reality. J Pharm Pharmacol 56: 3–17.
11. Konofagou EE, Tung Y-S, Choi J, Deffieuxa T, Baseria B, et al. (2012) Ultrasound-induced blood-brain barrier opening. Curr Pharm Biotechnol 13: 1332–1345.
12. Burgess A, Hynynen K (2013) Noninvasive and targeted drug delivery to the brain using focused ultrasound. ACS Chem Neurosci 8588: 1–7.
13. Treat LH, McDannold N, Zhang Y, Vykhodtseva N, Hynynen K (2012) Improved anti-tumor effect of liposomal doxorubicin after targeted blood-brain barrier disruption by MRI-guided focused ultrasound in rat glioma. Ultrasound Med Biol 38: 1716–1725.
14. Baseri B, Choi JJ, Deffieux T, Samiotaki G, Tung Y-S, et al. (2012) Activation of signaling pathways following localized delivery of systemically administered neurotrophic factors across the blood-brain barrier using focused ultrasound and microbubbles. Phys Med Biol 57: N65–81.
15. Jordão JF, Thévenot E, Markham-Coultes K, Scarcelli T, Weng Y-Q, et al. (2013) Amyloid-ß plaque reduction, endogenous antibody delivery and glial activation by brain-targeted, transcranial focused ultrasound. Exp Neurol 248: 16–29.
16. Huang Q, Deng J, Wang F, Chen S, Liu Y, et al. (2012) Targeted gene delivery to the mouse brain by MRI-guided focused ultrasound-induced blood-brain barrier disruption. Exp Neurol 233: 350–356.
17. Burgess A, Ayala-Grosso CA, Ganguly M, Jordão JF, Aubert I, et al. (2011) Targeted delivery of neural stem cells to the brain using MRI-guided focused ultrasound to disrupt the blood-brain barrier. PLoS One 6: e27877.
18. Samiotaki G, Konofagou EE (2013) Dependence of the reversibility of focused-ultrasound-induced blood–brain barrier opening on pressure and pulse length in vivo. IEEE Trans Ultrason Ferroelectr Freq Control 60: 2257–2265.
19. Tung Y-S, Vlachos F, Feshitan JA, Borden MA, Konofagou EE (2011) The mechanism of interaction between focused ultrasound and microbubbles in blood-brain barrier opening in mice. J Acoust Soc Am 130: 3059–3067.
20. McDannold N, Vykhodtseva N, Raymond S, Jolesz FA, Hynynen K (2005) MRI-guided targeted blood-brain barrier disruption with focused ultrasound: histological findings in rabbits. Ultrasound Med Biol 31: 1527–1537.
21. Baseri B, Choi JJ, Tung Y-S, Konofagou EE (2010) Multi-modality safety assessment of blood-brain barrier opening using focused ultrasound and definity microbubbles: a short-term study. Ultrasound Med Biol 36: 1445–1459.
22. Thorne RG, Frey WH II (2001) Delivery of neurotrophic factors to pharmacokinetic considerations. 40: 907–946.
23. Ferrara K, Pollard R, Borden M (2007) Ultrasound microbubble contrast agents: fundamentals and application to gene and drug delivery. Annu Rev Biomed Eng 9: 415–447.
24. Mitragotri S (2005) Healing sound: the use of ultrasound in drug delivery and other therapeutic applications. Nat Rev Drug Discov 4: 255–260.
25. Marquet F, Teichert T, Wu S-Y, Tung Y-S, Downs M, et al. (2014) Real-time, transcranial monitoring of safe blood-brain barrier opening in non-human primates. PLoS One 9: e84310.
26. Lai C-Y, Fite BZ, Ferrara KW (2013) Ultrasonic enhancement of drug penetration in solid tumors. Front Oncol 3: 204.
27. Chen H, Kreider W, Brayman AA, Bailey MR, Matula TJ (2011) Blood vessel deformations on microsecond time scales by ultrasonic cavitation. Phys Rev Lett 106: 034301.
28. Costantino HR, Illum L, Brandt G, Johnson PH, Quay SC (2007) Intranasal delivery: physicochemical and therapeutic aspects. Int J Pharm 337: 1–24.
29. Choi JJ, Feshitan JA, Baseri B, Wang S, Tung Y-S, et al. (2010) Microbubble-size dependence of focused ultrasound-induced blood-brain barrier opening in mice in vivo. IEEE Trans Biomed Eng 57: 145–154.
30. De Rosa R, Garcia AA, Braschi C, Capsoni S, Maffei L, et al. (2005) Intranasal administration of nerve growth factor (NGF) rescues recognition memory deficits in AD11 anti-NGF transgenic mice. Proc Natl Acad Sci U S A 102: 3811–3816.
31. Choi JJ, Pernot M, Brown TR, Small SA, Konofagou EE (2007) Spatio-temporal analysis of molecular delivery through the blood-brain barrier using focused ultrasound. Phys Med Biol 52: 5509–5530.
32. Chen CC, Sheeran PS, Wu S-Y, Olumolade OO, Dayton PA, et al. (2013) Targeted drug delivery with focused ultrasound-induced blood-brain barrier opening using acoustically-activated nanodroplets. J Control release 172: 795–804.
33. Wu S-Y, Tung Y-S, Marquet F, Downs ME, Sanchez CS, et al. (2014) Transcranial cavitation detection in primates during blood-brain barrier opening-a performance assessment study. IEEE Trans Ultrason Ferroelectr Freq Control 61: 966–978.
34. Chen H, Konofagou EE (2014) The size of blood-brain barrier opening induced by focused ultrasound is dictated by the acoustic pressure. J Cereb Blood Flow Metab 34: 1197–1204.
35. Quon CY (1988) Clinical pharmacokinetics and pharmacodynamics of colloidal plasma volume expanders. J Cardiothorac Anesth 2: 13–23.
36. Sheikov N, McDannold N, Vykhodtseva N, Jolesz F, Hynynen K (2004) Cellular mechanisms of the blood-brain barrier opening induced by ultrasound in presence of microbubbles. Ultrasound Med Biol 30: 979–989.
37. Hadaczek P, Yamashita Y, Mirek H, Tamas L, Bohn MC, et al. (2006) The "perivascular pump" driven by arterial pulsation is a powerful mechanism for the distribution of therapeutic molecules within the brain. Mol Ther 14: 69–78.
38. McDannold N, Arvanitis CD, Vykhodtseva N, Livingstone MS (2012) Temporary disruption of the blood-brain barrier by use of ultrasound and microbubbles: safety and efficacy evaluation in rhesus macaques. Cancer Res 72: 3652–3663.
39. Tung Y-S, Vlachos F, Choi JJ, Deffieux T, Selert K, et al. (2010) In vivo transcranial cavitation detection during ultrasound-induced blood-brain barrier opening. Phys Med Biol 55: 6141–6155.

3

Characterizations of Plasticized Polymeric Film Coatings for Preparing Multiple-Unit Floating Drug Delivery Systems (muFDDSs) with Controlled-Release Characteristics

Sheng-Feng Hung[1,¶], Chien-Ming Hsieh[1,3,¶], Ying-Chen Chen[1], Yu-Chun Wang[1], Hsiu-O Ho[1*], Ming-Thau Sheu[1,2*]

1 School of Pharmacy, College of Pharmacy, Taipei Medical University, Taipei, Taiwan, 2 Clinical Research Center and Traditional Herbal Medicine Research Center, Taipei Medical University Hospital, Taipei, Taiwan, 3 Department of Cosmetic Science, Providence University, Taiwan Boulevard, Shalu, Taichung, Taiwan, ROC

Abstract

Effervescent multiple-unit floating drug delivery systems (muFDDSs) consisting of drug (lorsartan)- and effervescent (sodium bicarbonate)-containing pellets were characterized in this study. The mechanical properties (stress and strain at rupture, Young's modulus, and toughness) of these plasticized polymeric films of acrylic (Eudragit RS, RL, and NE) and cellulosic materials (ethyl cellulose (EC), and Surelease) were examined by a dynamic mechanical analyzer. Results demonstrated that polymeric films prepared from Surelease and EC were brittle with less elongation compared to acrylic films. Eudragit NE films were very flexible in both the dry and wet states. Because plasticizer leached from polymeric films during exposure to the aqueous medium, plasticization of wet Eudragit RS and RL films with 15% triethyl citrate (TEC) or diethyl phthalate (DEP) resulted in less elongation. DEP might be the plasticizer of choice among the plasticizers examined in this study for Eudragit RL to provide muFDDSs with a short time for all pellets to float (TPF) and a longer period of floating. Eudragit RL and RS at a 1:1 ratio plasticized with 15% DEP were optimally selected as the coating membrane for the floating system. Although the release of losartan from the pellets was still too fast as a result of losartan being freely soluble in water, muFDDSs coated with Eudragit RL and RS at a 1:1 ratio might have potential use for the sustained release of water-insoluble or the un-ionized form of drugs from gastroretentive drug delivery systems.

Editor: Yuan-Soon Ho, Taipei Medical University, Taiwan

Funding: The authors have no funding or support to report.

Competing Interests: The authors have declared that no competing interests exist.

* Email: mingsheu@tmu.edu.tw (MTS); hsiuoho@tmu.edu.tw (HOH)

¶ These authors contributed equally to this work.

Introduction

Based on recently published literature and patents applied for, gastroretentive drug delivery systems (DDSs, GRDDSs) that are retained in the stomach for a prolonged and predictable period of time are one of the advanced approaches for novel drug-delivery systems [1,2]. GRDDSs are particularly appropriate for drugs with a narrow absorption window [3–5], drugs that act locally in a part of the gastrointestinal (GI) tract (GIT) such as antibiotic administration for *Helicobacter pylori* eradication to treat peptic ulcers [6–8], drugs which are unstable in intestinal fluids [3,9,10], and drugs that exhibit poor solubility in the intestinal tract [11,12]. The development of various approaches for GRDDSs, including low-density systems/floating systems, high-density systems/non-floating systems, mucoadhesive or bioadhesive systems, expansion systems, magnetic systems, supraporous hydrogels, and raft-forming systems, was reviewed [13,14]. Low-density systems or floating DDSs (FDDSs) are further divided into non-effervescent and effervescent systems based on the mechanism of buoyancy. If their bulk density is lower than that of gastric fluid, and they thus remain buoyant in the stomach for a prolonged period. From formulation and technological points of view, FDDSs are considerably easy and a logical approach for developing GRDDSs.

Upon contact of an effervescent FDDS with gastric fluid, the fluid penetrates its outer layer (or membrane) and reacts with the effervescent components (e.g., sodium bicarbonate alone or combined with citric acid or tartaric acid). Carbon dioxide (CO_2) is liberated causing the FDDS to float in the stomach due to its buoyancy effect and lower bulk density. Previously reported FDDSs were prepared as single-unit systems, such as tablets and capsules [15]. Nevertheless, the disadvantage of single-unit systems is the inter?/intra-subject variability of the GI transit time due to its all-or-nothing emptying processes [6,16–19], which raises the possibility of dose dumping [20]. Hence, the concept of multiple-unit dosage forms, such as granules, pellets, and mini-tablets, was developed. Various effervescent multiple-unit FDDSs (muFDDSs) were reported to prolong gastric residence times and increase the overall bioavailability of the dosage form. Those systems demonstrated that using Eudragit RL alone or a combination of Eudragit RL and RS as the polymeric layer could cause floating for desirable periods (in the stomach for about 5 h *in vivo*) and possessed controlled-release properties [21]. The development of effervescent muFDDSs is a promising area of pharmaceutical research for controlled release in the stomach. As flexible dose adjustment and reducing subject variatons are expected to achieve via the dosage form.

An ideal membrane for effervescent muFDDSs should allow water to permeate at a fast enough rate in order to immediately activate the effervescent reaction, thus preventing the individual unit from transiting to the small intestine [22]. But hydrated films should also be impermeable to the generated CO_2 to maintain floatation and remain sufficiently flexible to withstand the pressure of CO_2 to avoid rupture [23]. Therefore, with an optimal permeability for water, ideal coating polymeric films for effervescent muFDDSs should be strong and tough. In addition, they are expected to exhibit sufficient strain and resistance to rupture under high forces. Eudragit RL was the only single polymer that fulfilled all those requirements. However, a disadvantage of using Eudragit RL as the coating film to achieving pellet floating was the too-rapid release of the drug from this floating pellet system which should have a sustained-release pattern. Recently, it was reported that utilization of a combination of polymers with different physicochemical characteristics was able to overcome such limitations [21]. The optimized system of a mixture of Kollicoat SR with 5% each of triethyl citrate and polyethylene glycol (PEG) 600 at a 20% coating level began to completely float within 15 min and maintained its buoyancy over a period of 12 h with a sustained-release effect. However, none of those studies revealed the importance of mechanical properties of plasticized coating membrane on floating characteristics.

In this study, plasticized polymeric membranes for preparing effervescent muFDDSs with controlled-release characteristics were characterized based on mechanical properties (stress, strain, modulus, and toughness). Water-insoluble polymeric films (Eudragit NE, RL, and RS, Surelease, and ethyl cellulose (EC)) combined with various plasticizers at different percentages were evaluated in both dry and wet states. Spherical core pellets containing the model drug losartan [24] and an effervescent agent (sodium bicarbonate) were prepared by an extrusion-spheronization process followed by coating with a plasticized polymeric film. Schematic presentation of the structure of the effervescent muFDDSs was shown in **Fig. 1**. The floating ability (floating lag time and duration) and drug-release profiles of the resulting muFDDSs were characterized.

Materials and Methods

Materials

Losartan potassium (IPCA, Bangalore, India) was chosen as the model drug. Sodium bicarbonate ($NaHCO_3$, Merck, Darmstadt, Germany) was used as an effervescent agent to generate CO_2 gas, and microcrystalline cellulose (MCCPH102, Wei Ming Pharmaceutical, Taipei, Taiwan) was a pelletization aid. All aqueous colloidal polymethacrylate dispersions (Eudragit NE, RS 30D, and RL 30D) were obtained from Evonik Industries AG (Essen, Germany). EC powder (10 cP) was supplied by Aqualon (Wilmington, DE, USA). Surelease (25% ethycellulose aqueous dispersion, E-7-19040) was purchased from Colorcon (Dartford Kent, UK). Diethyl phthalate (DEP, water solubility 0.928 g/L), dibutyl phthalate (DBP, water solubility 0.011 g/L) and triethyl citrate (TEC, water solubility 65 g/L) were provided by Merck. Hydroxypropyl methylcellulose 60SH-50 (HPMC 60SH-50, with a methoxy content of 28%?30%, a hydroxypropyl content of 7%?12%, and a viscosity of 2% solution in water of 50 cps), HPMC 60SH-4000 (HPMC 60SH-50, with a methoxy content of 28%?30%, a hydroxypropyl content of 7%?12%, and a viscosity of 2% solution in water of 4000 cps), and low-substituted hydroxypropylcellulose (LH-22) were obtained from Shin-Etsu (Tokyo, Japan). HPMC 90SH-K100M (with a methoxy content of 19%?24%, a hydroxypropyl content of 7%?12%, and a viscosity of 2% solution in water of 80,000?120,000 cps) and HPMC60SH-E10M (with a methoxy content of 28%?30%, a hydroxypropyl content of 7%?12%, and a viscosity of 2% solution in water of 7500?14,000 cps) were supplied by Colorcon. Microtalc (IT extra) was provided by Mondo Minerals (Amsterdam, the Netherlands). Tween 80 (polysorbate 80, Riedel-de Haën, Germany) was used as a dispersing agent. All other reagents were of analytical grade.

Preparation and Characterization of Polymeric Films

Water-soluble plasticizers (TEC and DEP) and a water-insoluble plasticizer (DBP) were first thoroughly mixed in an aqueous solution and methanol, respectively. Then water-insoluble polymers (Eudragit RS and RL, and Surelease) were added as an aqueous dispersion at a final polymer level of 10% (w/w) and blended for 24 h for plasticization. In order to increase the water absorption, the powder form of EC dissolved in an 95% w/w of ethanol containing 20% of either of three plasticizers was further added with different grades of HPMC (60SH-50, 60SH-4000, E10M, and K100M) at 30% w/w with respect to the corresponding EC amount with or without extra water to completely dissolve the HPMC. Dried polymeric films were prepared by pouring the resultant mixture onto the parafilm-sealed bottom of a polyacrylic column, drying at 40°C for 8 h, and further curing at 50°C for 12 h. Wet films were prepared by soaking the dried polymeric films in 500 mL of simulated gastric fluid (SGF, 0.1 N HCl solution) at 37°C for 24 h. Polymeric films cut in a circle with a diameter of 30 mm were placed on a glass filter of a modified Enslin apparatus [25] at a temperature of 37°C. The water uptake profile was monitored by following the volume change reading from a graduated pipette with time ($n = 4$). The mechanical strengths of all polymeric films (10×3 mm with a thickness of 0.25?0.30 mm) were measured using a Dynamic Mechanical Analyzer (DMA7e, Perkin-Elmer, Waltham, MA, USA) by monitoring the time-modulus curve conducted at ambient temperature. The initial applied force was 5 mN, with an extension rate of 100 mN/min. The stress-strain curves for polymeric films were obtained, and the strain (%) and stress (MPa) at the rupture point were both recorded. The slope at the origin of the stress-strain curve gives Young's modulus (MPa/%) and the

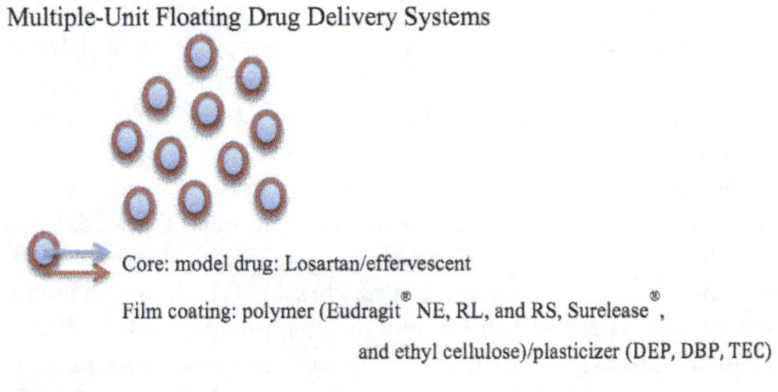

Figure 1. Schematic illustration of the structure of the effervescent multiple-unit floating drug delivery systems (muFDDSs).

total area under the stress-strain curve up to rupture is termed the modulus of toughness (MJ/m^3) ($n = \geq 4$) [26].

Preparation and Floating Ability Test of Pellets

The pellet cores according to Table 1 were produced by extrusion (radial-basket type) through a screen size of 1 mm and spheronization at 700 rpm for 5 min (Shang Yuh Machine, New Taipei City, Taiwan), and the so-obtained pellets were dried at 40°C for 12 h. Since L-HPC was reported to be more advantageous in terms of water absorbability and swelling tendency than MCC, it was included in B formulations to examine its influence [27]. The coating solution was prepared by the same method as for polymeric films with a slight modification of adding 10% talc (w/w based on polymer solids) as an anti-adhesive to prevent coalescence during pellet coating. Pellets were coated using a rotor-type fluidized-bed system (GPCG-1, Glatt, Binzen, Germany) at respective optimal conditions (an inlet temperature of 44~48°C, an outlet temperature of 34~37°C, spray pressure of 15 psi, rotor speed of 180 rpm, and a flow rate of 4.5~5.0 g/min) to a designated weight gain (% w/w). All coating efficiencies were found to exceed 90%. After coating, pellets were further cured at 50°C for 12 h, and pellets in the size range of 0.71?1.25 mm were collected for further experiments. A detailed formulation design of pellets and coating films and their respective code names are given in Table 2.

For the floating study, 100 pellets were placed in the medium (SGF, 0.1 N HCl), and the time for all pellets to float (TPF) and floating duration (the duration when a certain percentage had pellets floated (%)) were determined by visual counting. The TPF was defined as the time that 100 pellets completely floated to the top surface of 900 ml of SGF at 37°C and a stirring rate of 50 rpm. The percentage of floating pellets was defined as the floating pellets (%) based on the following equation (1):

$$\text{Floating Pellet (\%)} = \frac{\text{number of floating pellets at the measured time}}{\text{initial number of the pellets}} \times 100 \quad (1)$$

Drug-Release Studies

Drug dissolution from the coated pellets was conducted in 900 mL of SGF at 37±0.5°C and 50 rpm based on the apparatus II method (USP XXIX) (VK7020, Agilent Technologies Inc, Santa Clara, CA, USA). The medium (5 mL) was sampled at predetermined times and replaced with fresh medium of the same volume. The drug concentration was measured with an ultraviolet/visible spectrophotometer (V-550, Jasco, Tokyo, Japan) at a wavelength of 254 nm that had been validated to have acceptable precision and accuracy. Each *in vitro* release study was performed in at least triplicate.

Table 1. Pharmaceutical composition of the core pellets.

	A	B	A20	C20
Losartan (mg)	50	50	50	50
MCC (mg)	200	100	150	75
L-HPC (mg)		100		75
$NaHCO_3$ (mg)			50	50
Total (mg)	250	250	250	250

Theoretical Consideration of the Minimal Strain of Polymeric Films to Make Pellets Floats

At equilibrium of floating pellets, the magnitude and direction of the force, F_{net}, corresponded to the vectorial sum of the buoyancy (F_{buoy}) and gravitational (F_{grav}) forces acting on the pellet [28]. By definition, the more positive F_{net} is (forces directed upward), the faster and longer a pellet floats. As described by the following equation, where F_{net} is the net vertical force, g the acceleration of gravity, d_F the fluid density, d_P the pellet density, M the pellet mass, V_P and V_{SP} the pellet volume before and after swelling, respectively, and ε_v and ε_d the strain of pellet volume and pellet diameter, respectively:

$$\begin{aligned} F_{net} &= F_{buoy} - F_{grav} = d_F \cdot g \cdot V_{SP} - d_P \cdot g \cdot V_P = d_F \cdot g \cdot \varepsilon_v \cdot V_P - (M/V_P) \cdot g \cdot V_P \\ &= (d_F \cdot \varepsilon_v \cdot V_P - M) \cdot g \\ &= (d_F \cdot \varepsilon_v \cdot (M/d_P) - M) \cdot g \\ &= (d_F \cdot \varepsilon_v / d_P - 1) \cdot M \cdot g. \end{aligned} \quad (2)$$

To be able to float, F_{net} must be greater than zero. Assuming $d_F = 1.0$ for the water medium, the minimal value for the strain of pellet volume (ε_v) and the strain of pellet diameter (ε_d) can be predicted as related to the pellet density (d_P:

$$\begin{aligned} &d_F \cdot \varepsilon_v / d_P \geq 1.0 \\ &\varepsilon_v \geq d_P \text{ and } \varepsilon_d \geq (d_P)^{1/3}. \end{aligned} \quad (3)$$

Based on Eq. 3, a theoretical plot of d_p in the range of 1.0?5.0 versus the corresponding minimal ε_d ($\varepsilon_d = (d_P)^{1/3}$) is illustrated in **Fig. 2**. It demonstrates that for a pellet with the density of 1.5 or 2.0, its minimal elongation of polymeric thin film to make pellet floating is about 14% or 26%, respectively.

Statistical Analysis

The analysis was done with a linear regression (PASW Statistics 18.0, Chicago, IL, USA) to assess the relationship between independent variables (water permeability or strain in the wet state) with all dependent variables (TPF, floating duration, and drug-release rate) of different formulations by multi-variant analysis with a stepwise regression. A p value of <0.05 was considered statistically significant.

Results and Discussion

Preparation and Characterization of Polymeric Films

An ideal coating film on pellets for floating DDSs requires that (1) the water permeability of the coating film should be fast enough to generate enough CO_2 gas for a buoyancy effect to make the pellet float, with sooner being better; (2) the flexibility of the coating film should be sufficient to withstand disruptive forces exerted by the CO_2 gas generated inside the pellet core; and (3) the permeability of the CO_2 gas generated across the coated film should be limited to maintaining a longer duration of floating. Since plasticizers play an important role in determining not only the water permeability and flexibility of polymeric film but also the permeability of CO_2. The influences of the three most commonly used plasticizers (TEC, DEP, and DBP) added at various levels on the mechanical properties of water insoluble polymers (Eudragit RS, RL, NE, Surelease, and EC) were examined. The stress-strain curve for polymeric films was obtained by applying a tensile force at a uniform rate and constant temperature. The mechanical properties measured included Young's modulus (slope at the origin, E), stress at break (σ), elongation (strain) at break (ε), and

Table 2. Pharmaceutical composition of floating pellets with a film coating.

Formulation	Coating layer[a]			Core pellets
	Polymer	Plasticizer[b]	Coating level (%)	
A-RS TEC 15 10%	Eudragit RS	TEC 15%	10	A
A-RS TEC 15 20%		TEC 15%	20	A
B-RS TEC 15 3%		TEC 15%	3	B
B-RS TEC 15 6%		TEC 15%	6	B
B-RS TEC 15 9%		TEC 15%	9	B
B-RS TEC 15 12%		TEC 15%	12	B
A20-RS TEC 15 10%		TEC 15%	10	A20
A20-RS TEC 15 15%		TEC 15%	15	A20
A20-RS TEC 15 20%		TEC 15%	20	A20
A20-RL TEC 15 10%	Eudragit RL	TEC 15%	10	A20
A20-RL TEC 15 20%			20	A20
A20-RL TEC 15 30%			30	A20
A20-RL TEC 15 40%			40	A20
A20-RL DEP15 20%		DEP 15%	20	A20
A20-RL DEP15 30%			30	A20
A20-RL DEP15 40%			40	A20
A20-RL DBP15 20%		DBP 15%	20	A20
A20-RL DBP15 30%			30	A20
A20-RL DBP15 40%			40	A20
A20-1S1LDEP15 10%	Eudragit RL: RS = 1:1	DEP 15%	10	A20
A20-1S1LDEP15 15%			15	A20
A20-1S1LDEP15 20%			20	A20

[a]Diluted with water (the final suspension had a concentration of 10% of solid polymer and plasticizer) and the addition of 10% talc (w/w based on polymer solids).
[b]w/w based on polymer solids.

the modulus of toughness of the polymeric films (the total area up to break, *T*) for polymeric coating films are listed in Tables 3–5 for Eudragit RS, RL, and Surelease (EC aqueous dispersion, EC_{sure}), respectively, and is illustrated in Fig. 3 for EC (dissolved in 95% w/w of ethanol, EC_{sol}).

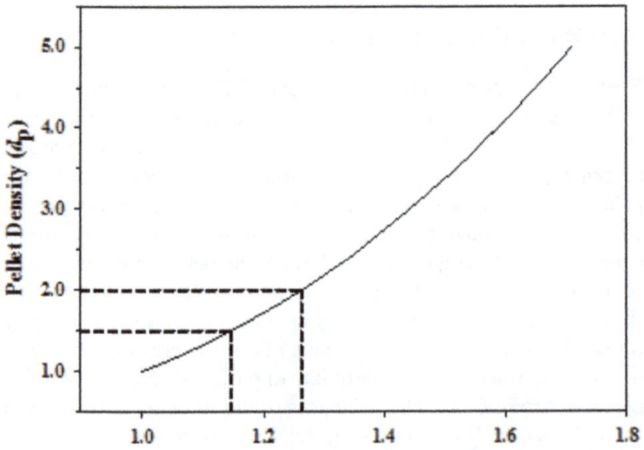

Figure 2. Theoretical plot of the pellet density versus the minimal elongation ratio of the pellet diameter based on ($\varepsilon_d = (d_P)^{1/3}$).

As shown in Tables 3 and 4, respectively, both Eudragit RS and RL films measured in the dry state demonstrated that ε increased with an increasing addition level of all three plasticizers (except DEP as a plasticizer), whereas *E*, *σ*, and *T* decreased with an increasing addition level. Among the three plasticizers used, TEC expressed the highest plasticizing effect to cause a greater extent of elongation. However, when mechanical properties of both Eudragit RL and RS films were measured in the wet state, the plasticizing effect of water obviously decreased their mechanical strengths. Further, adding TEC as plasticizer caused a greater decreasing extent of ε in the wet state, and also resulted in a less elongation tendency compared to the dry state. This phenomenon is comparable to that reported by Bodmeier and Paeratakul [27]. It was due to differences in the water solubilities among the three plasticizers. Since TEC has a water solubility of 65 g/L, a greater amount of TEC could be released in comparison to the two other plasticizers when soaking polymeric films in the GIF medium leading to a disappearance of the plasticizing effect of TEC. Further, the decreasing extent of a plasticizing effect of TEC was expected to be more obvious when the level added increased from 15% to 30%. Regarding DEP, less influence on the plasticizing effect was seen at an addition level of 15%, whereas a profound decrease in ε from 690.75% and 601.88% to 299.64% and 66.46% for Eudragit RS and RL, respectively, was observed at the 30% addition level. This seems to indicate that such a release amount of DEP was still able to have a greater influence on mechanical properties when the added amount of DEP was

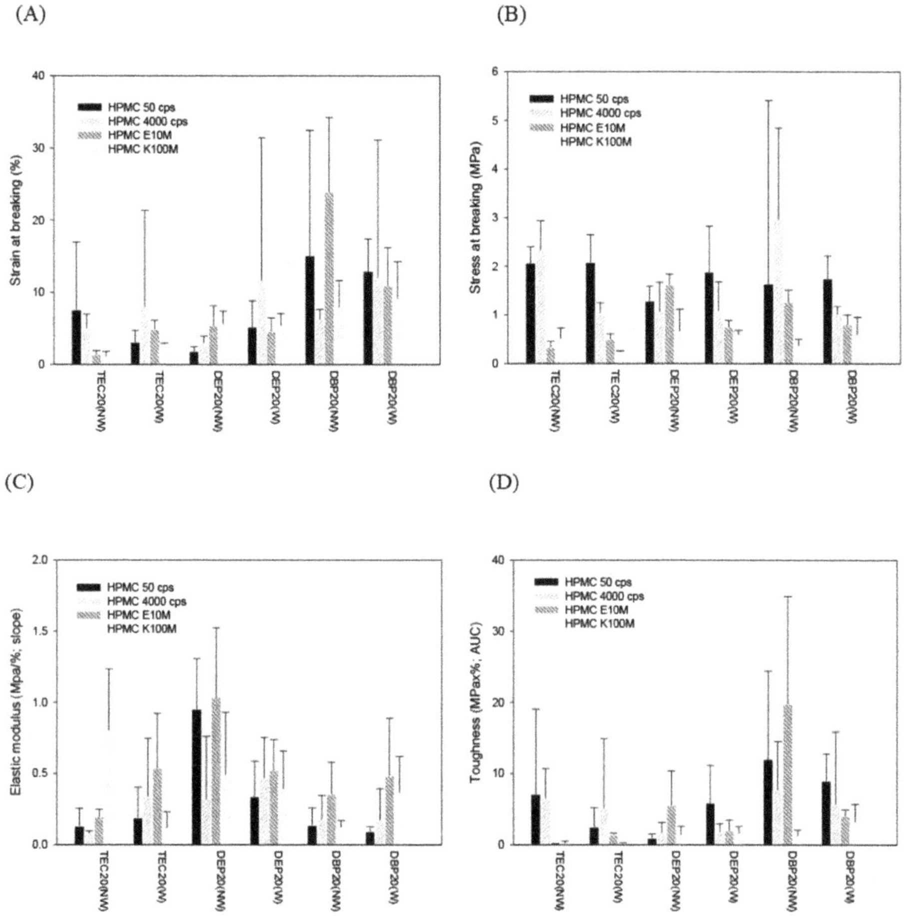

Figure 3. Mechanical properties of wet-state films composed of ethyl cellulose and different grades of HPMC. (A) Strain at breaking (%), (B) stress at breaking (MPa), (C) elastic modulus (MPa/%; slope), (D) toughness (MPa×%; AUC) ($n=4$).

higher. Further, at both 15% and 30% addition levels of DBP in Eudragit RS and RL films, an insignificant change in mechanical properties was seen when measured in the wet state. Obviously, this can be explained by there being the least amount of DBP released from the polymeric film during soaking since DBP is only slightly soluble in water. It was concluded that the volume of plasticized RS- and RL-coated pellets might be expanded without rupture under the tensile stress (which should be equal to or greater than the tensile stress that could be exerted by a 5-mN force applied by DMA) exerted by the CO_2 gas pressure which generated sufficient buoyancy to make the pellets float.

Compared to the Eudragit RS film, the RL film was more highly permeable to water because it was composed of a higher fraction of hydrophilic quaternary ammonium groups in the structure. This higher water permeability not only made RL film able to absorb more water to enhance the plasticizing effect, but also made water-soluble plasticizers leak at a greater amount and a faster rate from RL film than water-insoluble plasticizers. Hence, a greater extent of changes presented in mechanical properties between measurements in the dry and wet states for water-soluble plasticizers. In addition, a higher permeability of RL membranes to water should enable RL-coated pellets to generate CO_2 gas faster, leading to a shortened TPF.

Surelease is a commercially available product containing an EC aqueous dispersion at a 25% w/w solids content and already optimally plasticized with medium-chain triglycerides (MCTs). The same as shown by Table 5, EC films prepared from Surelease (EC_{Sure}) showed a similar tendency for the influence of the three plasticizers at two different levels on their mechanical properties as that of Eudragit RS and RL in both the dry and wet states. However, the strain (%) of EC_{Sure} films so prepared regardless of which plasticizer was used at two levels were observed to be obviously lower than those of corresponding formulations of both Eudragit RL and RS. The intermolecular hydrogen bonds and sugar-based three-dimensional hindrances might have resulted in the poor extendibility of EC. This was also confirmed by Sungthongjeen et al. [15], who determined that the EC_{Sure} membrane is a mechanically weak and brittle polymer and not flexible and hence can easily rupture once CO_2 pressure is generated. This means that the volume expansion of EC_{Sure}-coated pellets under stress exerted by the CO_2 gas generated might not be able to reach a significant extent with a sufficient buoyant force to make the pellets float.

When the polymeric film of Eudragit NE without adding any plasticizer was measured in both the dry and wet states, it was found that polymeric film of Eugragit NE was already too ductile to break (over the instrument limit of static strain, 1064.82%) (data not shown). This is because Eudragit NE is a neutral ester polymer (ethyl acrylate and methyl methacrylate in a 2:1 ratio) with no hydrogen bonds or other intermolecular forces, and the glass transition temperature (T_g) value is approximately 5°C; therefore, it has high flexibility (static strain >600%) at room temperature.

Table 3. Mechanical properties of dry and wet Eudragit RS films to which different plasticizers were added (mean±SD; $n=4$).

	Strain at breaking (%)	Stress at breaking (MPa)	Elastic modulus (MPa/%; slope)	Toughness (MPa×%; AUC[a])
Dry state				
TEC15	446.47±229.41	3.0039±0.4342	0.1239±0.0169	989.68±594.70
TEC30	786.30±181.64	0.4139±0.1560	0.0030±0.0006	211.88±157.09
DEP15	690.75±113.42	2.2363±0.3941	0.0743±0.0341	1129.6±379.37
DEP30	299.64±27.43	0.5430±0.0484	0.0076±0.0025	73.306±15.436
DBP15	434.27±279.76	4.1246±0.6028	0.1512±0.0543	1247.1±915.99
DBP30	558.33±289.40	0.6571±0.0975	0.0053±0.0029	222.10±152.37
Wet state				
TEC15	314.86±81.359	1.5674±0.0759	0.0520±0.0190	246.24±100.07
TEC30	157.77±56.59	0.8202±0.1402	0.0265±0.0102	63.989±24.066
DEP15	203.31±21.52	0.9995±0.0406	0.0573±0.0625	114.74±16.126
DEP30	363.94±133.48	0.5906±0.0872	0.0142±0.0075	109.59±57.422
DBP15	683.17±415.88	1.0441±0.2547	0.0198±0.0099	429.30±288.65
DBP30	485.74±205.13	0.3493±0.1106	0.0061±0.0024	106.97±72.246

[a]AUC: area under curve.

Our results were consistent with those reported by Sungthongjeen et al. [15], for which an Eudragit NE film was observed to have the highest elongation values in both the dry and wet states. This polymer dispersion has a low minimum film formation temperature and does not require plasticizers, resulting in flexible films [23]. In the wet state, the strain of Eudragit NE films decreased to a lesser extent than that in the dry state. This can be explained by the hydrophobic character of Eudragit NE [29]. It was concluded that the lower permeability of Eudragit NE for water due to its hydrophobic character might be a hindrance to generating CO_2 gas faster for shortening the TPF although the volume expansion of NE-coated pellets might be large enough to generate sufficient buoyancy to promote pellet floating.

Table 6 illustrates the mechanical properties of EC films (EC_{sol}) cast from the 95% w/w of ethanol supplemented with either one of three plasticizers (TEC, DEP, and DBP) at the 20% level and 30% (w/w, with respect to the EC amount) of various grades of HPMC as a water-permeation enhancer with or without a sufficient quantity of water (W/NW) to dissolve the added HPMC. Results demonstrated that except for the static strain of the EC_{sol} film (NW-DBP20) plasticized with DBP and incorporating HPMC E10M without adding water which was around 30%, those for the other EC_{sol} films remained <10%. This indicates that the addition of various grades of HPMC was unable to enhance the flexibility of EC_{sol} membranes to accommodate pellet expansion.

Water-Uptake Rate and Amount

Permeation of a liquid through the polymeric film into the core and the subsequent generation of CO_2 may play major roles in the floating and drug-release characteristics. The gastric emptying

Table 4. Mechanical properties of dry and wet Eudragit RL films to which different plasticizers were added (mean±SD; $n=4$).

	Strain at breaking (%)	Stress at breaking (MPa)	Elastic modulus (MPa/%; slope)	Toughness (MPa×%; AUC)
Dry state				
TEC15	580.14±122.55	2.1692±1.1637	0.0412±0.0284	862.52±570.94
TEC30	797.47±124.37	0.3895±0.0550	0.0041±0.0018	183.31±38.917
DEP15	601.88±66.87	3.1674±1.4374	0.0659±0.0164	470.12±301.73
DEP30	66.46±21.46	0.4918±0.1306	0.0092±0.0018	63.841±78.045
DBP15	109.81±36.13	3.6164±0.3243	0.0766±0.0253	259.74±136.77
DBP30	282.84±38.11	0.5294±0.4627	0.0068±0.0058	76.560±69.535
Wet state				
TEC15	226.50±167.23	2.5874±0.9953	0.1612±0.1111	480.60±545.52
TEC30	221.79±146.83	1.5295±0.2939	0.0867±0.0408	257.40±267.62
DEP15	411.46±275.43	1.5275±0.5158	0.0947±0.1314	525.01±505.54
DEP30	115.02±79.574	0.4414±0.4031	0.0147±0.0161	44.717±70.662
DBP15	431.97±211.87	0.3773±0.1334	0.0011±0.0012	93.873±78.816
DBP30	642.82±324.24	0.0845±0.0181	0.00015± 0.0003	15.443±7.7931

Table 5. Mechanical properties of dry and wet Surelease films to which different plasticizers were added (mean±SD; $n=4$).

	Strain at breaking (%)	Stress at breaking (MPa)	Elastic modulus (MPa/%; slope)	Toughness (MPa×%; AUC)
Dry state				
TEC15	6.7361±2.8417	0.8079±0.2859	0.1788±0.0326	2.7533±2.3976
TEC30	16.523±8.0149	0.6695±0.2050	0.0678±0.0287	6.6291±4.0169
TEC40	29.101±13.149	0.4456±0.0765	0.0192±0.0083	6.4249±4.9425
DEP15	24.903±2.2796	0.8544±0.0708	0.0755±0.0216	10.784±3.3239
DEP30	47.954±28.124	0.1863±0.0467	0.0084±0.0023	4.6311±2.9695
DEP40	48.567±30.050	0.1056±0.0678	0.0033±0.0036	1.8308±1.5193
DBP15	48.190±13.677	0.9065±0.0523	0.0583±0.0280	24.029±12.256
DBP30	59.332±26.369	0.1763±0.0432	0.0051±0.0041	5.9398±4.6835
DBP40	105.18±81.586	0.1297±0.0336	0.0027±0.0007	6.5892±5.9964
Wet state				
TEC15	13.645±5.7402	1.1292±0.2477	0.1294±0.0619	6.5684±5.4072
TEC30	27.250±11.057	1.1020±0.4379	0.0706±0.0387	15.468±16.032
DEP15	23.583±6.0892	1.5542±0.3462	0.3647±0.3092	20.372±10.613
DEP30	79.160±19.205	1.9423±0.7567	0.0984±0.0760	91.969±60.517
DBP15	52.389±14.903	0.3327±0.0456	0.0114±0.0067	7.6282±4.5475
DBP30	118.53±56.976	0.0999±0.0473	0.0014±0.0013	4.7794±5.3844

time ranges from 15 min to 3 h, so FDDSs should float within 15 min. The water uptake rate was evaluated for EC_{sol} films with various grades of HPMC added at 30% w/w with respect to the EC weight, and results are illustrated in **Fig. 4**. It demonstrates that the addition of any grade of HPMC led to faster uptake of greater amounts of water. An insignificant effect of adding water to make HPMC completely dissolve was seen on the water-uptake rate and amount taken up.

Preparation and Floating Characterization of Coated Pellets

The muFDDS systems consisted of a drug (lorsartan)-containing core pellet with an effervescent ($NaHCO_3$) and pelletization aid (MCC), and a gas-entrapping polymeric membrane. Developing a successful effervescent muFDDS requires rapid formation of a low-density system within minutes after contact with gastric fluid and maintenance of the buoyancy in the stomach with controlled release. The integrity of coated films on the pellet surface with uneven texture would be a prerequisite for achieving these goals. SEM photographs shown in **Fig. 5** demonstrate that the integrity of coated films improved with an increasing coated level. It clearly illustrates that at least a 9% coated level is required to fully cover with an uneven surface of pellets produced by the extrusion-spheronization process (B-RS TEC15). Therefore, a coating level of >10% was selected for all coated polymeric films in the following experiment.

Floating Ability

As shown in **Table 6**, when using Eudragit RS 30D as the coating polymer with 15% TEC as the plasticizer, core A pellets (MCC as pelletization aid) coated at the 10% and 20% levels, core B pellets (MCC+L-HPC as pelletization aid) coated at 3%~12%, and core A20 pellets ($NaHCO_3$ for gas generation) coated at 10%~20% were found to be unable to float during the 24-h observation period. However, when using Eudragit RL 30D as the coating polymer on A20 core pellets, TEC and also DEP and DBP could make the pellets float within 20 min in 0.1 N HCl medium even at a coating level of as high as 40%. This result conforms to that reported by Sungthongjeen et al. [15]. It was attributed to the difference in the permeability of the acidic medium and the extent of elongation as a result of expansion of the CO_2 gas generated when $NaHCO_3$ was neutralized by the inward-permeating acidic medium. As predicted by **Fig. 2**, coated pellets must expand to some extent in order to increase the volume, which in turn decreases the density of the pellets to make them floatable as a result of a more-positive upward F (the vectorial sum of the F_{buoy} and F_{grav} forces). Expansion of the pellets was observed for those floating on the surface of 0.1 N HCl medium as shown by **Fig. 6A and 6B** respectively for pellets (A20-RL DEP15 20%) coated with Eudragit RL and those (A20-1S1L DEP15 20%) coated with Eudragit RL:RS at 1:1. Those photographs clearly illustrate that there is a white core suspended inside the pellet and a translucent space between the coated membrane and center core, which was apparently created by the expansion of the CO_2 gas generated. This phenomena was not observed when Eudragit RS was used as the coating polymer (data not shown), and we found that no pellets coated with Eudragit RS were able to float. It was concluded that Eudragit RL coating films, but not Eudragit RS, were able to allow a faster permeation of the acidic medium into the pellets. This resulted in elongation of the Eudragit coating films under outward expansion of the CO_2 gas generated from neutralization of the inward-permeating acidic medium with $NaHCO_3$. Consequently, sufficient CO_2 then make the pellets less dense and thus to float.

Results of the TPF measurements and the percentage of floating pellets for both Eudragit RL and Eudragit RS:RL at 1:1 coating films with different plasticizers at various levels on A20 core pellets are shown in **Fig. 7**. As shown in **Fig. 7A and 7E**, TPFs for both coating films increased with an increasing coating level for all plasticizers examined. Also **Fig. 7A** further indicates that the lower solubility of the plasticizer in water was (TEC>DEP>DBP), the longer the TPF results were (DBP>DEP>TEC). Theoreti-

Table 6. Diameter and volume changes of pellets after immersion in gastric fluid.

Formulation	Pre-immersion (0 min)		After 1 h	
	Diameter (mm)	Volume (ml)	Diameter (mm)	Volume (ml, $\times 10^4$)
A-RS TEC 15 10%	1.05±0.07	6.06×10^{-4}	NF	
A-RS TEC 15 20%	1.09±0.10	6.78×10^{-4}	NF	
B-RS TEC 15 3%	1.00±0.05	5.24×10^{-4}	NF	
B-RS TEC 15 6%	1.03±0.04	5.72×10^{-4}	NF	
B-RS TEC 15 9%	1.02±0.04	5.56×10^{-4}	NF	
B-RS TEC 15 12%	1.05±0.06	6.06×10^{-4}	NF	
A20-RS TEC 15 10%	1.07±0.06	6.41×10^{-4}	NF	
A20-RS TEC 15 15%	1.09±0.06	6.78×10^{-4}	NF	
A20-RS TEC 15 20%	1.12±0.09	6.34×10^{-4}	NF	
A20-RL TEC15 20%	1.03±0.11	5.72×10^{-4}	1.62±0.20	22.26
A20-RL TEC15 30%	1.01±0.08	5.39×10^{-4}	1.34±0.09	12.60
A20-RL TEC15 40%	1.05±0.07	6.06×10^{-4}	1.55±0.16	19.50
A20-RL DEP15 20%	1.01±0.09	5.39×10^{-4}	2.22±0.19	57.29
A20-RL DEP15 30%	1.06±0.12	6.24×10^{-4}	2.80±0.20	114.94
A20-RL DEP15 40%	1.10±0.05	6.97×10^{-4}	2.69±0.28	101.92
A20-RL DBP1520%	1.11±0.04	7.16×10^{-4}	2.39±0.23	71.48
A20-RL DBP15 30%	1.14±0.06	7.76×10^{-4}	2.50±0.24	81.81
A20-RL DBP15 40%	1.13±0.05	7.55×10^{-4}	2.67±0.31	99.67
A20-1S1L DEP15 10%	1.06±0.12	6.24×10^{-4}	1.94±0.10	38.23
A20-1S1L DEP15 15%	1.06±0.05	6.24×10^{-4}	2.07±0.17	46.44
A20-1S1L DEP15 20%	1.08±0.05	6.60×10^{-4}	1.97±0.15	40.03

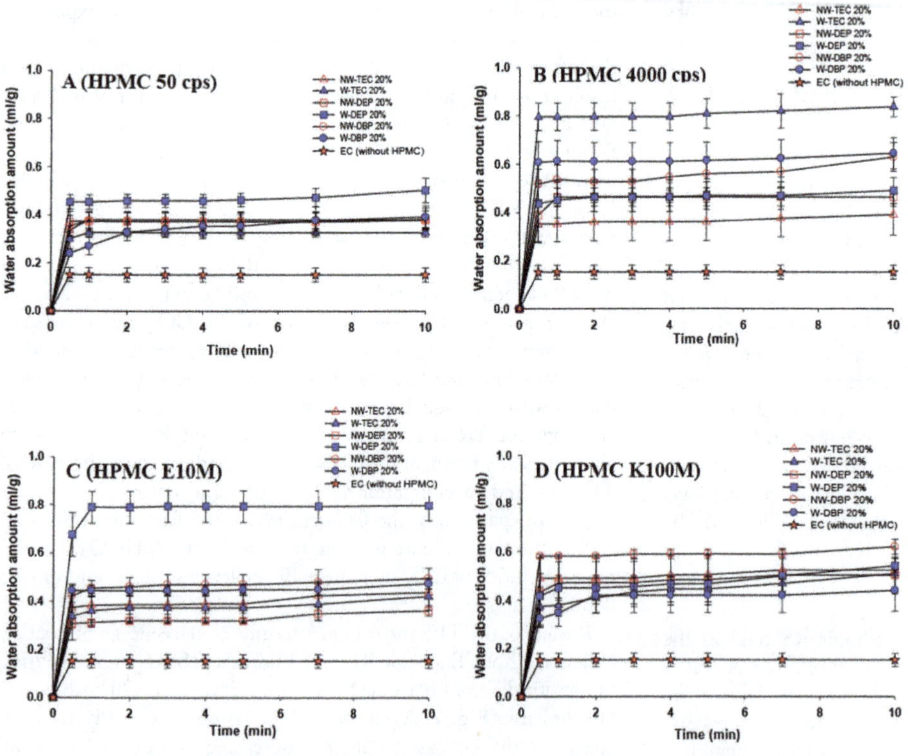

Figure 4. Water uptake plots of ethyl cellulose film samples plasticized with various plasticizers at 20% w/w and after adding 30% w/w of (A) HPMC 50 cps, (B) HPMC 4000 cps, (C) HPMC E10M, (D) HPMC K100M (n=4).

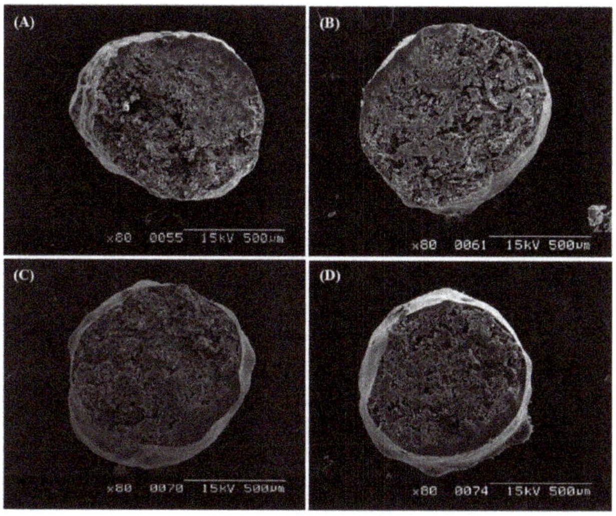

Figure 5. SEM photos of pellets (B-RS TEC15) at various coating levels (w/w) of (A) 3%, (B) 6%, (C) 9%, and (D) 12%.

cally, the water permeation rate per unit area ($dQ/(A*dt) = D*\Delta C/h$) is proportionally inverse to the thickness of the coating film (h) and is proportional to the diffusion coefficient (D), which could be influenced by the hydrophilicity of the coated membrane. Since increasing the thickness of coating films with an increasing coating level theoretically leads to a decrease in the water-permeation rate, this results in the slower generation of CO_2 gas to expand the pellet such that it has a density low enough to float and in turn a longer TPF. The addition of hydrophobic plasticizers within the coated films creating a more-hydrophobic environment for water permeation probably decreases the diffusion coefficient of water in those plasticized coated films. As a result, the lower permeation rate of the acidic medium through the coated films due to a decreasing diffusion coefficient with increasing hydrophobicity of the added plasticizer more likely causes slower generation of CO_2 gas to expand the pellet until it has a density low enough to float and in turn a longer TPF.

Furthermore, **Fig. 7B–7D** demonstrate the time course of percent pellets floating for Eudragit RL coating films plasticized with 15% TEC, DEP, and DBP, respectively, at three coating levels (20%, 30%, and 40%), and **Fig. 7F** illustrates Eudragit RS:RL at 1:1 coating films plasticized with 15% DEP at three coating levels (10%, 15%, and 20%). When comparing among the percent pellet floating time plots for Eudragit RL coating films plasticized with three different plasticizers (**Fig. 7B**, TEC; **Fig. 7C**, DEP, and **Fig. 7D**, DBP), almost all pellets coated with Eudragit RL plasticized with DEP and DBP could maintain floating for as long as 24 h, whereas the percent pellet floating for pellets coated with Eudragit RL films plasticized with TEC decreased with increasing time. As observed by **Fig. 7B**, it was found that the percent pellets floating for pellets coated with Eudragit RL plasticized with 15% TEC at three different coating levels all decreased with increasing time. The extent of percent pellets floating at the same time point decreased with a decreasing coating level (20%>30%>40%), and the corresponding extents of percent pellets floating at the end of 24 h were 47%, 49%, and 54%, respectively for coating levels of 20%, 30%, and 40%. However, **Fig. 7C and 7D** show that using Eudragit RL plasticized with DEP and DBP as the coating films could maintain pellets floating for as long as 24 h, and even when increasing the coating level from 20% to 30%, and even further to 40%, the pellets still maintained their floatability. All of these phenomena might be attributed to differences in water solubility. TEC with the highest solubility in water could make the permeation rate of acidic medium faster in the initial period to shorten the TPF as described above. But the higher water solubility could also cause a greater amount of TEC to be released with increasing time resulting in the decay of its plasticized effect on the coated film and in turn a gradual loss of its floatability over time. However, both DEP and DBP have lower water solubilities and are released at such a lower level that they could not deteriorate the plasticized effect on the coated film and in turn effectively maintained the floatability of pellets over time. Overall, it was concluded that a plasticizer like DEP with its water solubility is optimal for use in combination with Eudragit RL as the coated film on pellets to produce an appropriate TPF of as short as 15 min and a floating period as long as 24 h.

Table 6 further compares the expansion extents of the pellet diameter and volume after immersion in 0.1 N HCl medium for 1 h (the time to reach equilibrium of expansion) with that of pellets before immersion for various coated films with different plasticizers added at the same 15% level. It reveals that all three core pellets (A, B, and A20 cores) coated with Eudragit RS with 15% of TEC as the plasticizer were unable to expand after immersion leading to no pellets floating. On the contrary, Eudragit RL with the same 15% TEC as the plasticizer coated on A20 core pellets was able to allow acidic medium to permeate into the pellet to generate CO_2 gas for expansion and then floating. When two other plasticizers, DEP and DBP, were added at the same 15% level, an expansion of the pellet volume was observed but to different extents. In comparison to the extent of volume expansion

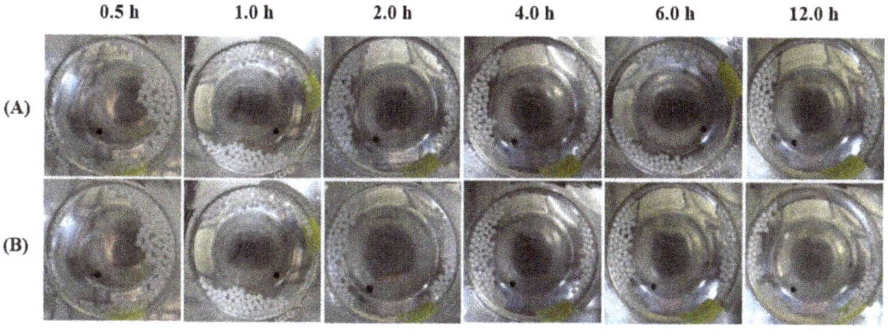

Figure 6. Photographs of pellets (A20-RL DEP15 20%) (A) and (A20-1S1L DEP15 20%) (B) after immersion in pH 1.2 buffer for specific times.

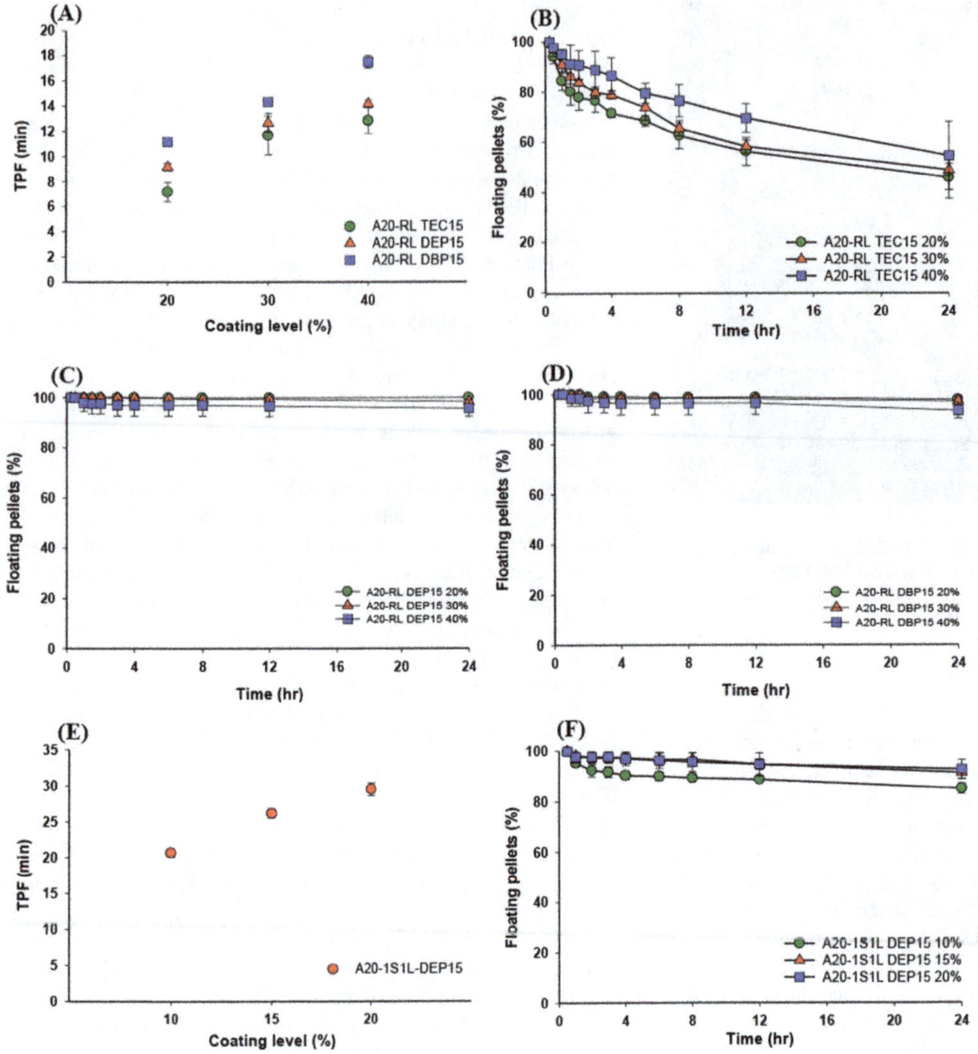

Figure 7. Effect of the coating level of Eudragit RL 30D (A) or Eudragit RL 30D RS 30D at 1:1 (E) and different plasticizers on the time to float of pellets in pH 1.2 buffer at 37°C. Floating patterns of the pellets coated with Eudragit RL 30D (B, C, and D) or Eudragit RL 30D: Eudragit RS 30D at 1:1 (F) after immersion in pH 1.2 buffer at 37°C.

after 1 h of immersion, 4-, 11-, and 10-fold expansions of the pellet volume were observed when using TEC, DEP, and DBP as the plasticizer, respectively, at the same 20% coating level of Eudragit RL. This clearly shows that the expansion of coated Eudragit RL films was the least when using TEC as the plasticizer, and greater extents of increases in volume expansion occurred when using DEP and DBP as plasticizers. These data further confirm that the plasticized effects of both DEP and DBP in a wet state are greater than that of TEC leading to a greater extent of elongation as discussed above. These data also support longer floating periods when using DEP and DBP as plasticizers than when using TEC.

In order to search for alternative coated films suitable for muFDDSs, a combination of Eudragit RS:RL at 1:1 was examined using DEP as the plasticizer in consideration of its effect on the TPF and floating period. As illustrated in **Fig. 7E**, all pellets coated with Eudragit RS:RL at 1:1 with 15% DEP as the plasticizer at the 10% coating level were observed to float within 20 min (TPF). However, when increasing the coating level to 15% and 20%, TPFs were prolonged to 25 and 30 min, respectively. A 6?7-fold increase in pellet volume after 1 h of immersion in 0.1 N HCl was observed for those pellets with the same coating film at a coating level of 10%?20% as shown in **Table 6**. However, maintaining a longer floating period was observed for those pellets with the same coating film at a coating level of 10%?20% as shown in **Fig. 7F**. Prolongation of the TPF and a lower extent of volume expansion were expected for pellets coated with Eudragit RS:RL at 1:1 since a lower permeability of water and a lower elongation for Eudragit RS than that for Eudragit RL occurred with the same plasticizer and added amount. Nevertheless pellets coated with Eudragit RS:RL at 1:1 (15% DEP) at the 10% level still achieved 86% pellets floating for 24 h. Therefore, this film composition could be an alternative to Eudragit RL as a coating film for muFDDSs.

Drug-Release Studies

The drug-release profiles for those muFDDS formulations were characterized in simulated gastric fluid of pH 1.2 HCl dissolution medium using losartan as a model drug, and results are shown by **Figs. 8** and **9**. Results in **Fig. 8** show that when Eudragit RS was

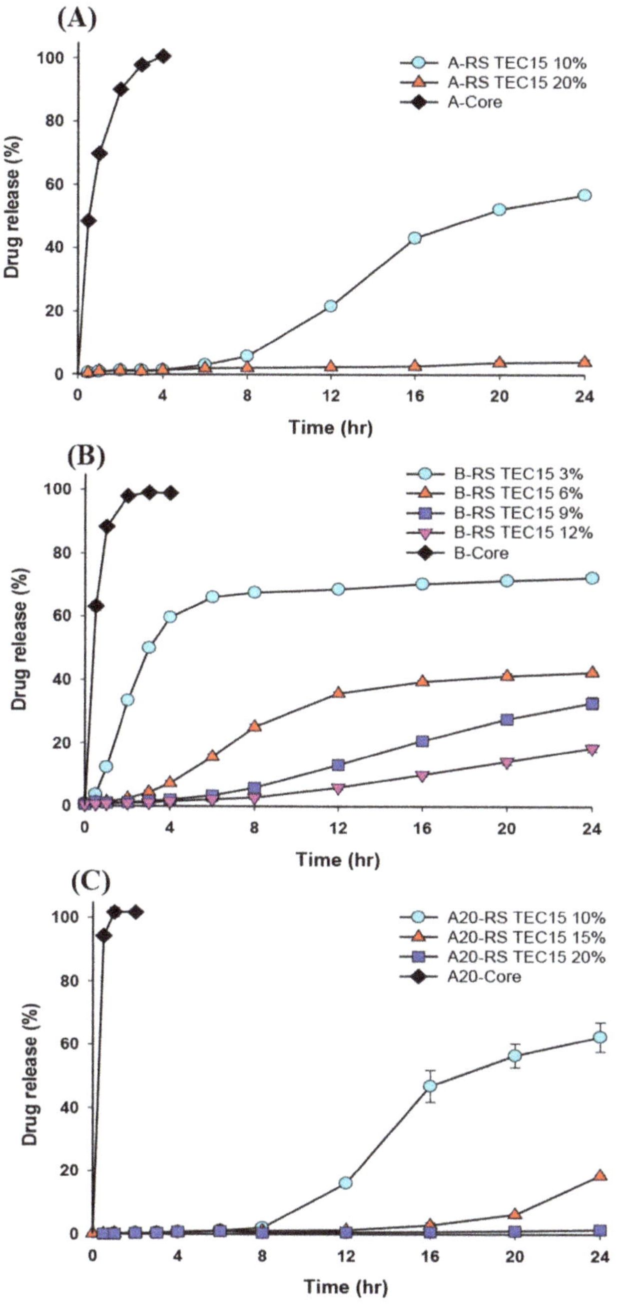

Figure 8. Losartan release profiles of formulations (A) A-RS TEC15 and A-Core, (B) B-RS TEC15 and B-Core, and (C) A20-RS TEC15 and A20-Core in pH 1.2 buffer.

used as the coating film with the same plasticizer of TEC at 15%, a long sustained release profile of losartan with a coating level-dependent lag time was observed regardless of which core pellets (core A: **Fig. 8A**; core B; **Fig. 8B**; A20: **Fig. 8C**) were sprayed on. The lag time was obviously extended with an increasing coating level. This phenomenon was attributed to the lag time for membrane diffusion being proportional to the square of the thickness of the coating film ($t_L = h^2/6D$). Because of that, a complete release of 100% drug amount was not achievable within a 24-h period for any drug-containing pellets coated with Eudragit RS. On the contrary, faster release of losartan (complete release within 2?3 h) from A20 core pellets coated with Eudragit RL plasticized with TEC, DEP, and DBP at 15% was observed for all coating levels up to 40% (**Fig. 9A–C**). Apparently, a higher permeability of acidic medium across the Eudragit RL coating film than that of the Eudragit RS coating film accompanied by the freely soluble characteristic of losartan HCl in acidic medium was responsible for the difference in the release rates. Sungthongjeen et al. [15] reported that sustained release was able to completely release all drug within 11 h from pellets coated with Eudragit RL observed for theophylline, which has a lower solubility (sparely soluble) than losartan (freely soluble). Therefore, this muFDDS system is still potentially promising to deliver a sustained-release pattern for model drugs with lower solubilities or in a un-ionized form (acidic or basic form).

In consideration of the higher permeability of the Eudragit RL coating film (15% DEP as the plasticizer) having a shorter TPF and a longer period of floating and the lower permeability of Eudragit RS coating film having a greater extent of sustained release manner, a 1:1 combination of Eudragit RS and RL was used as the coating film. **Figure 7E and 7F** demonstrate that an optimal TPF and a longer period of floating were achieved at a 10% coating level of Eudragit RS:RL at 1:1 coating film. The drug release profile shown in **Fig. 9D** for a 10% coating level of Eudragit RS:RL at 1:1 coating film was completed within 4 h, and the release rate also decreased with an increased coating level. At the same coating level of 20% as shown in **Fig. 9E**, the drug release from pellets coated with Eudragit RL: RS at 1:1 was observed to be slower than that from pellets coated with Eudragit RL. This confirms that the combination of Eudragit RL and Eudragit RS had lower water permeability and was correspondingly expected to decrease the drug-release rate.

Conclusions

Plasticized polymeric coating films for achieving rapid floating and a longer period of floating in a sustained-release manner were characterized for the effervescent muFDDSs developed in the present study. The water solubility of the plasticizer and its plasticized effect on the elongation of the polymeric coating film were the greatest influencing factors on the TPF and period of floating. The water solubility of the plasticizer in terms of water permeability is responsible for how soon the acidic medium can penetrate into the pellet core to generate CO_2 gas by neutralizing the incorporated $NaHCO_3$. The effect of the plasticizer on the polymeric coating film determines how easy it is for the resulting polymeric film to expand by the CO_2 gas generated to a volume having a pellet density low enough for floating. The overall effects will determine the TPF. The water solubility also determines how long a pellet can float, since a plasticizer with optimal water solubility can be preserved in the coating film long enough to maintain its plasticized effect for the same expanded volume that has a density low enough for floating. It was concluded that DEP might be the plasticizer of choice among the plasticizers examined in this study for Eudragit RL to provide muFDDSs with a short TPF and a longer period of floating. However, the drug-release rate from muFDDSs using Eudragit RL plasticized with DEP was not sustainable by adjusting the coating level of the polymeric film. Alternatively, using a combination of Eudragit RL:RS of 1:1 as the coating film prolonged drug release for a longer period. Drugs with a lower solubility or in an un-ionized form (acidic or basic form) would be another choice to prolong or sustain drug release rates from muFDDSs designed in this study.

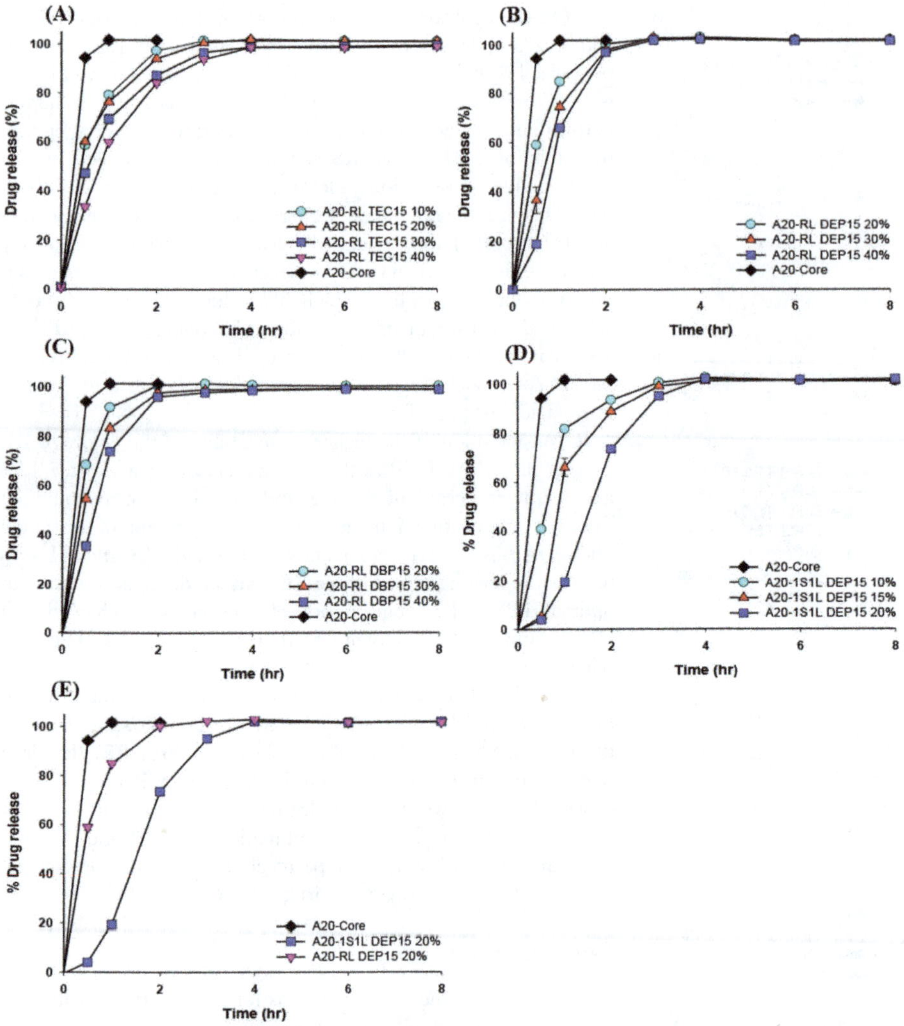

Figure 9. Losartan release profiles of A20-Core and formulations (A) A20-RL TEC15, (B) A20-RL DEP15, (C) A20-RL DBP15, and (D) A20–1S1L DEP15 in pH 1.2 buffer. (E) Effect of the coating membrane (Eudragit RL 30D: RS 30D at 1:1 versus Eudragit RS 30D) on release profiles.

Author Contributions

Conceived and designed the experiments: MTS HOH. Performed the experiments: SFH CMH. Analyzed the data: SFH CMH YCC YCW. Contributed reagents/materials/analysis tools: MTS HOH. Contributed to the writing of the manuscript: CMH HOH MTS. Interpretation of data for the work: CMH YCC YCW.

References

1. Pawar VK, Kansal S, Garg G, Awasthi R, Singodia D, et al. (2011) Gastroretentive dosage forms: a review with special emphasis on floating drug delivery systems. Drug delivery 18: 97–110.
2. Waterman KC (2007) A critical review of gastric retentive controlled drug delivery. Pharmaceutical development and technology 12: 1–10.
3. Singh BN, Kim KH (2000) Floating drug delivery systems: An approach to oral controlled drug delivery via gastric retention. J Controlled Release 63: 235–259.
4. Rouge N, Buri P, Doelker E (1996) Drug absorption sites in the gastrointestinal tract and dosage forms for site-specific delivery. Int J Pharm 136: 117–139.
5. Sato Y, Kawashima Y, Takeuchi H, Yamamoto H (2004) *In vitro* and *in vivo* evaluation of riboflavin-containing microballoons for a floating controlled drug delivery system in healthy humans. Int J Pharm 275: 97–107.
6. Umamaheshwari RB, Jain S, Bhadra D, Jain NK (2003) Floating microspheres bearing acetohydroxamic acid for the treatment of *Helicobacter pylori*. J Pharm Pharmacol 55: 1607–1613.
7. Bardonnet PL, Faivre V, Pugh WJ, Piffaretti JC, Falson F (2006) Gastroretentive dosage forms: Overview and special case of Helicobacter pylori. J Controlled Release 111: 1–18.
8. Yang L, Eshraghi J, Fassihi R (1999) A new intragastric delivery system for the treatment of *Helicobacter pylori* associated gastric ulcer: *In vitro* evaluation. J Controlled Release 57: 215–222.
9. Seta Y, Higuchi F, Kawahara Y, Nishimura K, Okada R (1988) Design and preparation of captopril sustained-release dosage forms and their biopharmaceutical properties. Int J Pharm 41: 245–254.
10. Jain SK, Awasthi AM, Jain NK, Agrawal GP (2005) Calcium silicate based microspheres of repaglinide for gastroretentive floating drug delivery: Preparation and *in vitro* characterization. J Controlled Release 107: 300–309.
11. Wurster DE, Alkhamis KA, Matheson LE (2003) Prediction of the adsorption of diazepam by activated carbon in aqueous media. J Pharm Sci 92: 2008–2016.
12. Munday DL (2003) Film coated pellets containing verapamil hydrochloride: Enhanced dissolution into neutral medium. Drug Dev Ind Pharm 29: 575–583.
13. Prajapati VD, Jani GK, Khutliwala TA, Zala BS (2013) Raft forming system-an upcoming approach of gastroretentive drug delivery system. Journal of controlled release : official journal of the Controlled Release Society 168: 151–165.
14. Dixit N (2011) Floating Drug Delivery System. Journal of Current Pharmaceutical Research 7: 6–20.
15. Sungthongjeen S, Sriamornsak P, Puttipipatkhachorn S (2008) Design and evaluation of floating multi-layer coated tablets based on gas formation. Eur J Pharm Biopharm 69: 255–263.

16. Ichikawa M, Watanabe S, Miyake Y (1991) A new multiple-unit oral floating dosage system. I: Preparation and *in vitro* evaluation of floating and sustained-release characteristics. J Pharm Sci 80: 1062–1066.
17. Kawashima Y, Niwa T, Takeuchi H, Hino T, Ito Y (1991) Preparation of multiple unit hollow microspheres (microballoons) with acrylic resin containing tranilast and their drug release characteristics (*in vitro*) and floating behavior (*in vivo*). J Controlled Release 16: 279–289.
18. Streubel A, Siepmann J, Bodmeier R (2003) Multiple unit gastroretentive drug delivery systems: A new preparation method for low density microparticles. J Microencapsul 20: 329–347.
19. Talukder R, Fassihi R (2004) Gastroretentive delivery systems: Hollow beads. Drug Dev Ind Pharm 30: 405–412.
20. Bechgaard H, Ladefoged K (1978) Distribution of pellets in the gastrointestinal tract. The influence on transit time exerted by the density or diameter of pellets. J Pharm Pharmacol 30: 690–692.
21. Chen YC, Lee LW, Ho HO, Sha C, Sheu MT (2012) Evaluation of water uptake and mechanical properties of blended polymer films for preparing gas-generated multiple-unit floating drug delivery systems. Journal of pharmaceutical sciences 101: 3811–3822.
22. Iannuccelli V, Coppi G, Bernabei MT, Cameroni R (1998) Air compartment multiple-unit system for prolonged gastric residence. Part I. Formulation study. Int J Pharm 174: 47–54.
23. Krögel I, Bodmeier R (1999) Floating or pulsatile drug delivery systems based on coated effervescent cores. Int J Pharm 187: 175–184.
24. Sica DA, Gehr TWB, Ghosh S (2005) Clinical pharmacokinetics of losartan. Clin Pharmacokinet 44: 797–814.
25. Wu JS, Ho HO, Sheu MT (2001) A statistical design to evaluate the influence of manufacturing factors on the material properties and functionalities of microcrystalline cellulose. Eur J Pharm Sci 12: 417–425.
26. Kawano Y, Wang Y, Palmer RA, Aubuchon SR (2002) Stress-Strain Curves of Nafion Membranes in Acid and Salt Forms. Polímeros: Ciência e Tecnologia 12: 96–101.
27. Bi Y, Sunada H, Yonezawa Y, Danjo K, Otsuka A, et al. (1996) Preparation and evaluation of a compressed tablet rapidly disintegrating in the oral cavity. Chemical & pharmaceutical bulletin 44: 2121–2127.
28. Hamdani J, Moes AJ, Amighi K (2006) Development and in vitro evaluation of a novel floating multiple unit dosage form obtained by melt pelletization. International journal of pharmaceutics 322: 96–103.
29. Bodmeier R, Paeratakul O (1994) Mechanical properties of dry and wet cellulosic and acrylic films prepared from aqueous colloidal polymer dispersions used in the coating of solid dosage forms. Pharm Res 11: 882–888.

4

RGDechi-hCit: $\alpha v\beta 3$ Selective Pro-Apoptotic Peptide as Potential Carrier for Drug Delivery into Melanoma Metastatic Cells

Domenica Capasso[1]❾, Ivan de Paola[2]❾, Annamaria Liguoro[3]❾, Annarita Del Gatto[2], Sonia Di Gaetano[2], Daniela Guarnieri[4], Michele Saviano[5], Laura Zaccaro[2]*

1 Department of Pharmacy, University of Naples "Federico II", Naples, Italy, 2 Institute of Biostructures and Bioimaging -CNR, Naples, Italy, 3 Diagnostic and Molecular Pharmaceutics -Scarl, Naples, Italy, 4 Center for Advanced Biomaterials for Health Care @ CRIB- Italian Institute of Technology, Naples, Italy, 5 Institute of Crystallography -CNR, Bari, Italy

Abstract

$\alpha v\beta 3$ integrin is an important tumor marker widely expressed on the surface of cancer cells. Recently, we reported some biological features of RGDechi-hCit, an $\alpha v\beta 3$ selective peptide antagonist. In the present work, we mainly investigated the pro-apoptotic activity of the molecule and its ability to penetrate the membrane of WM266 cells, human malignant melanoma cells expressing high levels of $\alpha v\beta 3$ integrin. For the first time we demonstrated the pro-apoptotic effect and the ability of RGDechi-hCit to enter into cell overexpressing $\alpha v\beta 3$ integrin mainly by clathrin- and caveolin-mediated endocytosis. Furthermore, we deepened and confirmed the selectivity, anti-adhesion, and anti-proliferative features of the peptide. Altogether these experiments give insight into the biological behavior of RGDechi-hCit and have important implications for the employment of the peptide as a new selective carrier to deliver drugs into the cell and as a therapeutic and diagnostic tool for metastatic melanoma. Moreover, since the peptide shows a pro-apoptotic effect, a great perspective could be the development of a new class of selective systems containing RGDechi-hCit and pro-apoptotic molecules or other therapeutic agents to attain a synergic action.

Editor: A Ganesan, University of East Anglia, United Kingdom

Funding: This study was supported by FIRB MIUR "RENAME" 2010-RBAP114AMK and Programma Operativo Nazionale Ricerca e Competitività 2007-2013 PON 01_02388. The funders had no role in study design, data collection and analysis, decision to publish, or preparation of the manuscript.

Competing Interests: The authors have declared that no competing interests exist.

* Email: lzaccaro@unina.it

❾ These authors equally contributed to this work.

Introduction

The $\alpha v\beta 3$ receptor is a member of the integrin family, heterodimeric membrane glycoproteins, with a prominent role in angiogenesis and metastatic dissemination [1,2]. Interaction between $\alpha v\beta 3$ integrin and the extracellular matrix (ECM) proteins has been identified as the most important survival system for nascent vessels, by controlling different cellular functions, including survival, proliferation, migration and apoptosis [3,4]. Since this integrin is expressed at high levels on the surface of many cancer cells [5,6,7] as well as tumor-associated endothelial cells [8], it has become an important target in the development of new anticancer strategies.

Integrin $\alpha v\beta 3$ performs its function by interacting with several ECM proteins containing the RGD motif, recognized by membrane-bound adhesion molecules, playing a key role as cell adhesion mediator [4]. Peptides containing this motif show potent anti-adhesion effects, since they compete for the integrin-matrix interaction and show anti-proliferative, antichemotactic and pro-apoptotic effects [9,10].

In the last twenty years, a large number of $\alpha v\beta 3$ antagonists, including antibodies, small molecules, peptidomimetics, and cyclic RGD peptides, have been developed with the aim of selectively inhibiting $\alpha v\beta 3$-mediated processes [11,12,13]. Most importantly, Kessler and colleagues in 1996 reported the development of cRGDf[N(Me)]V, an $\alpha v\beta 3$/$\alpha v\beta 5$ antagonist known as Cilengitide [14] that was in phase III clinical study as anti-angiogenic drug for glioblastoma therapy [15,16,17,18]. Unfortunately, very recently (News/Press release from Merck, February 25, 2013) it was announced that the Phase III trial of the investigational integrin inhibitor Cilengitide did not meet its primary endpoint of significantly increasing overall survival when added to the current standard chemoradiotherapy regimen (temozolomide and radiotherapy). Furthermore, neither Cilengitide nor all known antagonists are able to discriminate between $\alpha v\beta 3$ and other type of integrins.

Over the last few years, we reported the development of a new and selective peptide named RGDechi-hCit [19]. It proved able to selectively bind to $\alpha v\beta 3$ integrin and did not cross-react with $\alpha v\beta 5$ and $\alpha IIb\beta 3$ in adhesion and competitive binding assays on stably transfected K562 cells expressing $\alpha v\beta 3$. This selectivity is a fundamental feature for the design of new systems with reduced side effects and dosage. In agreement with in vitro findings, imaging studies on human glioblastoma U87MG also indicated that RGDechi-hCit allows selective visualization of αvβ3 expression [20]. Furthermore, very recently we showed the ability of RGDechi-hCit to significantly inhibit some intracellular pathways acting as an αvβ3 integrin inhibitor, and its role as an antiangiogenic agent *in vitro* and in *vivo* [21].

In melanomas, a number of studies have shown malignant transformation to be associated with a general up-regulation of cell adhesion molecules [22,23]. In particular, it is well-known that over-expression of αvβ3 heterodimer is often associated in melanoma with the transition to a metastatic phenotype [24,25]. Indeed, while in normal epithelial cells the αvβ3 heterodimer is expressed at very low levels or is even absent, it is highly over-expressed in MM (metastatic melanoma) cells, and this increased expression is correlated with the degree of tumor progression.

Importantly, MM is highly resistant to conventional radio and chemotherapies and remains a disease of poor prognosis, with a survival times of a few months. Different chemotherapeutic agents, alone or in combination, have been employed over the last few years resulting, unfortunately, in limited activity with relatively low response rates [26,27], and providing so far only a small impact on overall survival. As chemoresistance remains a serious concern for melanoma therapy, a great challenge is the development of molecules, to use alone or in combination with other drugs, having the ability to interfere with systems involved in angiogenesis and metastatic dissemination processes and so be remarkably effective in shrinking melanoma tumors.

Very recently [28], we evaluated the *in vitro* antitumor efficacy of RGDechi-hCit peptide on melanoma cell lines differently expressing αvβ3 integrin. The data obtained showed that RGDechi-hCit induces a significant inhibition of proliferation only on the WM266 cell line, in accordance with its very high surface expression of αvβ3.

On the basis of these promising data and taking into account the key role played by integrin αvβ3 in melanoma progression, the aim of this paper was to thoroughly investigate the biological behavior of RGDechi-hCit on the WM266 metastatic cell line to reinforce its potential as an anticancer drug and as carrier for drug delivery. In particular, adhesion, binding, uptake, proliferation and apoptosis studies by flow cytometry and confocal microscopy were performed.

Materials and Methods

Peptide Synthesis, Cyclization and Labelling

Polypropylene reaction vessels and sintered polyethylene frits were supplied by Alltech Italy. MeIm, MSNT, TFA and scavengers were purchased from Fluka; NovaSyn TGA resins, coupling reagents and all amino acids were from Novabiochem. DIPEA was purchased from Romil; piperidine, $PhSiH_3$ and $Pd(PPh_3)_4$, NBD-Cl and FITC from Sigma-Aldrich.

RGDechi-hCit (c(KRDGe)MDDPGRNPHHocitGPAT-OH) and the scrambled sequence (Ac-KPGRGHNDPDPGHocitDeM-HAT-OH) were synthesized in solid phase by Fmoc chemistry basically as previously reported [19], but introducing some synthetic improvements and a different Lys functionalisation procedure [29]. Briefly, assembly of fully protected peptides was carried out manually in a polypropylene reaction vessel fitted with a sintered polyethylene frit using NovasynTGA resin (0.21 mmol/g) and all standard amino acids, except for D-Glu. The first amino acid was bound to the support by treatment with Fmoc-Thr(tbu)-OH (5 equiv)/MSNT (5 equiv)/MeIm (3.75 equiv) in DCM for 3 h. The Fmoc protecting group was removed by treatment with 30% piperidine in DMF (3×10 min). Coupling reactions of the following amino acids were performed by using 10 equiv of Fmoc protected derivative activated in situ with HBTU (9.8 equiv)/HOBt (9.8 equiv)/DIPEA (20 equiv) or COMU or HATU (9.8 equiv)/DIPEA (20 equiv) in DMF for 30 min. The coupling efficiency was assessed by the Kaiser test. Each step was followed by resin washings (3×5 min). For RGDechi-hCit, before the final Fmoc deprotection, selective α-carboxyl deprotection of the D-Glu residue from the allyl group was carried out by treatment of the peptidyl resin with $PhSiH_3$ (24 equiv)/$Pd(PPh_3)_4$ (0.25 equiv) in DCM (2×30 min). The cyclisation between αNH of D-Glu and αCO of Lys was performed with PyBop (1.5 equiv)/HOBt (1.5 equiv)/DIPEA (2 equiv) in DMF for 5 h at millimolar pseudo-dilution. For both peptides Fmoc-Lys(ivDde)-OH was employed as the last amino acid with the orthogonal ivDde protecting group in order to selectively remove it onto the resin and carry on the following functionalisation with the NBD-Cl (4-Chloro-7-nitro-1,2,3-benzoxadiazole) or FITC (fluorescein isothiocyanate) ivDde group which was removed from Lys by using a solution of 2% hydrazine in DMF (10×2 min); coupling reactions were performed with 3 equiv of NBD-Cl or FITC and 6 equiv DIPEA in DMF overnight. Finally the peptides were cleaved off the resin and deprotected using a mixture of TFA/H_2O/EDT/TIS (94:2.5:2.5:1 *v/v/v/v*) for 3 h. The resins were then filtered, and the white solid peptides were obtained by precipitation from cold anhydrous diethyl ether. The crude products were purified by preparative RP-HPLC on the Shimadzu LC-8A system, equipped with an UV-Vis detector SPD-10A using a Phenomenex Jupiter Proteo column (21.2×250 mm; 4 μm; 90 Å) and a linear gradient of H_2O (0.1% TFA)/CH_3CN (0.1% TFA) from 5 to 70% of CH_3CN (0.1% TFA) in 30 min at a flow rate of 20 mL/min. The purified peptides were analysed and characterised by an ESI-LC-MS instrument (ThermoFinnigan) equipped with a diode array detector combined with an electrospray ion source and a quadrupole mass analyzer, using a Phenomenex Jupiter Proteo column (4.60×150 mm; 4 μm; 90 Å) at a flow rate of 0.8 mL/min and the same gradient used for the purification step.

Cell lines and culture conditions

Human adenocarcinoma cells line (HeLa) (ATCC U.S.) were grown in DMEM supplemented with 10% fetal bovine serum (FBS), 2 mM glutamine, 100 U/mL penicillin and 100 μg/mL streptomycin (Euroclone, Italy). Human metastatic melanoma cells line (WM266), kindly provided by Dr. Gentilcore (IRCCS-Fondazione Pascale, Naples Italy), were grown in RPMI, supplemented with heat-inactivated 10% fetal bovin serum (FBS), 1% glutamine, 100 U/mL penicillin and 100 μg/mL streptomycin. The cells were maintained in humidified air containing 5% CO_2 at 37°C.

FACS analysis for αvβ3 integrin

Adherent cells at about 70% confluence were detached using 0.1 mM EDTA in PBS (Sigma Aldrich), centrifuged and suspended in PBS containing 0.2% BSA. Cell aliquots (2.5×10^5 cells) were treated with primary monoclonal antibody, clone LM609 (Millipore MA, USA) or isotype control (Santa Cruz Biotechnology, Germany), at the same concentrations for 30 min at 4°C. After washing, the cells were incubated with secondary antibody FITC-conjugated (Santa Cruz Biotechnology, Germany), washed and analysed by using a flow cytometer equipped with a 488 nm argon laser (FACScan, Becton Dickinson, USA). A total of 20000 events per sample were collected. Values of fluorescence intensity were obtained from the histogram statistic of CellQuest software.

Cell adhesion and detachment assays

NUNC MaxiSorp 96 well plates (Dasit Sciences, Italy) were coated overnight at 4°C with vitronectin, fibronectin or collagen type I (Millipore, USA), at 10 μg/mL concentration diluted in PBS, pH 7.4; then a blocking step for nonspecific binding was performed with 1.5% BSA in PBS for 1 h at room temperature. WM266 cells were suspended and mixed in Hank's balanced salt solution (HBSS: 50 mM HEPES, 1 mg/ml BSA, 1 mM $CaCl_2$, 1 mM $MgCl_2$, 1 mM $MnCl_2$, pH 7.4, Sigma Aldrich, Italy) with peptides (50 μM) or anti-αvβ3 antibody (10 μg/mL) for 30 min at 4°C and then plated on pre-coated plates (1.5×10^4cells/well). Non adherent cells were gently removed by repeated washings. After 1 h of incubation, the adherent cell number was evaluated by crystal violet (Sigma Aldrich, Italy) assay, which correlates optical density with cell number [30]. Briefly, cells were washed with PBS and fixed by adding 10% formalin solution. After 15 min cells were washed with deionized water and stained with 100 μl of 0.1% crystal violet solution in water for 30 min. Excess dye was removed by washing with deionised water and plates were air-dried prior to bound dye solubilisation in 200 μL of 10% acetic acid. The optical density of dye extracts was measured directly in plates at 595 nm (BioRad microplate reader model 680). The mean value ± SE of adherent cells for each treatment was expressed as relative percentage of cell number *vs* cells not treated (control). Statistical differences were determined by Student's t test, unpaired, two-sided. All experiments were performed in triplicate and repeated at least 3 times; a p value less than 0.05 was considered to be significant.

Cell proliferation assay and apoptosis

WM266 cells were seeded at 4×10^3 cells/mL in 96 well plates in RPMI 10% FCS. After 24 h the cells were starved (4% FCS in RPMI) for 4 h and incubated with increasing concentrations (10, 25 and 50 μM) of peptides. The proliferation was evaluated after 24 h using crystal violet assay.

The apoptosis assay was analysed on WM266 cells seeded at 2×10^5 cells/well in a 6 well plate and starved as described above. Next, the cells were incubated at 37°C with different peptides at 50 μM concentration, and apoptosis was analysed after 16 h by staining with annexin V/FITC and Propidium iodine (PI) (eBioscience, USA). Briefly, after incubation, the untreated and treated cells were detached with Accutase solution (eBioscience), harvested and washed with cold PBS. Subsequently, the cells were treated following the manufacturer' instructions. The percentage of cell undergoing apoptosis or necrosis was quantified using a flow cytometer (Becton Dickinson, USA) equipped with Cell Quest software.

Cell binding and uptake of peptides by FACS

WM266 cells were detached with 0.1 mM EDTA in PBS, washed and incubated with peptides. In detail, 2.5×10^5 cells were treated with 10 μM NBD-labeled RGDechi-hCit or 10 μM scrambled peptide, in 100 μL of 20 mM $CaCl_2$/HBSS at room temperature in slow agitation for 30 min. Then, the cells were washed in 20 mM $CaCl_2$/HBSS and resuspended in the same buffer to perform FACS analysis. The NBD-labeled peptides were excited at 465 nm and fluorescence was measured at 530 nm. After the analysis, 5 μL of dithionite (Sigma Aldrich, Italy) stock solution (1 M freshly prepared in 1 M Tris-HCl pH 10) was added to cells at 4°C for 5 min and the fluorescence of internalised peptides was detected by FACS.

Cellular uptake of peptides by confocal microscopy

WM266 and HeLa cells were seeded on a 35 mm diameter Fluorodish Cell Culture Dish (World Precision Instruments, Inc., Florida) at the concentration of about 5×10^4 cells/mL. 24 h after seeding, cells were incubated with FITC-RGDechi-hCit and FITC-RGD scrambled at the final concentration of 50 μM in HBSS buffer for 30 min at 37°C. Cells were rinsed twice with PBS to remove peptide excess and fixed with 4% paraformaldehyde at room temperature. Samples were then observed with a confocal microscope (Leica SP5) with a 63× oil immersion objective with a 488 nm wavelength laser line and transmitted light.

Indirect immunofluorescence

For co- localization experiments, after peptide incubation, cells were first rinsed twice with PBS to remove non-internalised peptide and fixed with paraformaldehyde 4% for 20 min. The cells were washed for 10 min in 10 mM PBS/20 mM glycine, permeabilised with 10 mM PBS/20 mM glycine containing 0.005% saponin for 7 min, and blocked with PBS/20 mM glycine 1% albumin. αvβ3 integrin was performed by using mouse anti-human integrin αvβ3 primary antibodies (Chemicon) and Alexa-fluor 568 goat anti-mouse secondary antibodies (Molecular Probes, Invitrogen). Endocytic vesicles were localised by incubating samples first with mouse anti-clathrin monoclonal (ABR) and rabbit anti-caveolin 1 (Abcam) primary antibodies and then with Alexa-fluor 568 goat anti-mouse and anti-rabbit secondary antibodies (Molecular Probes, Invitrogen), respectively. Lysosomes were localised with rabbit anti-LAMP 2 polyclonal (Abcam) primary antibodies and with 568 goat anti-rabbit secondary antibodies (Molecular Probes, Invitrogen).

All samples were then observed with a confocal microscope with a 63× oil immersion objective. Co-compartimentalisation between the peptide and the endocytic markers was analysed with ImageJ analysis software plugin.

Inhibition of clathrin- and caveolin-mediated endocytosis

Hypertonic challenge was carried out by incubating the WM266 cells with 0.45 M sucrose for 20 minutes at 37°C [31] in order to inhibit the clathrin-mediated endocytosis. Treatment aimed at inhibiting caveolae-mediated endocytosis was evaluated by incubating cells with filipin at 5 μg/mL for 30 minutes at 37°C. After both treatments, cells were incubated with 50 μM RGDechi-hCit solution in HBSS buffer for 30 minutes at 37°C. Then, cells were washed twice with PBS. Some samples were fixed with paraformaldehyde for the confocal microscopy observations and other ones were lysed with 1% Triton ×100 in PBS for the quantitative analysis. To this aim, the intensity fluorescence of cell lysates was measured at an excitation wavelength of 488 nm by a spectrofluorimeter (Perkinelmer). Results reported as percentage of cellular uptake were normalized with respect to non-treated control cells (expressed as 100%).

Results

Synthesis of functionalized RGDechi-hCit and scrambled peptides

Peptides were synthesized by the solid-phase method using Fmoc chemistry. All amino acids were coupled according to the HBTU/HOBt/DIPEA/DMF procedure [32]. To improve the overall yield of RGDechi-hCit over that previously reported (24%) [19], in the case of more difficult reactions a double coupling procedure was performed or more efficient coupling reagents were employed, e.g. COMU or HATU/DIPEA DMF. Before the Fmoc deprotection of Lys^1, α-carboxyl-selective deprotection of the

D-Glu[5] residue from the allyl group was carried out by the treatment of the peptidyl resin with a solution of $PhSiH_3$/$Pd(PPh_3)_4$ in DCM [33]. The cyclisation between the αNH group of Lys[1] and the αCO group of D-Glu[5] was performed with PyBop/HOBt/DIPEA [34] in DMF.

For both peptides, Fmoc-Lys(ivDde)-OH was employed as the last amino acid with the orthogonal ivDde protecting group in order to selective remove it onto the resin and carry out the subsequent functionalisation with NBD-Cl or FITC. The ivDde group was removed from Lys by using a solution of 2% hydrazine in DMF. The coupling reactions were performed using NBD-Cl or FITC and DIPEA in DMF overnight. Final deprotection and cleavage from the resin were achieved with TFA and scavengers.

The peptides were purified by preparative RP-HPLC; the purity and identity of the peptides were confirmed by analytical RP-HPLC and ESI-LC-MS mass spectrometry. The used synthetic conditions permitted the increase of the overall yield of the peptide up to 30%. This is a good result considering the chimeric nature of a molecule having both a cycle and linear motif and a lysine residue for its functionalization in view of its specific applications.

Expression of αvβ3 integrin on human melanoma cells (WM266) and human adenocarcinoma cells (HeLa)

Evaluation of the expression levels of αvβ3 integrin on the membrane surface of WM266 and HeLa cell lines was performed by flow cytometric analysis using the monoclonal antibody LM609. To maintain surface marker integrity, cells were detached using 0.1 mM EDTA in PBS. Data showed that WM266 cells expressed αvβ3 at high level, while HeLa cells displayed low levels of αvβ3. Specifically, the relative percentage of fluorescence is about 5% on HeLa cells and 85% on WM266 (Figure 1). Therefore we used WM266 and HeLa cell lines as positive and negative controls for αvβ3 integrin expression, respectively.

Effect of RGDechi-hCit on WM266 adhesion

The influence of RGDechi-hCit on the adhesion of WM266 cells seeded onto vitronectin (a matrix able to recognise both αvβ3 and αvβ5 integrins), fibronectin (recognising αvβ3) or collagen type I (not recognising either αvβ3 or αvβ5 integrins) [35,36,37] was investigated in a specific cells adhesion buffer [38] containing fundamental bivalent ions for integrin activity, such as Mg^{2+} or Ca^{2+}, to perform the assay under optimal conditions.

In order to prevent receptor internalisation, cells were preincubated at 4°C in adhesion buffer with peptides or monoclonal antibody anti αvβ3 integrin and then seeded into plates previously coated with different matrices. As shown in Figure 2A, RGDechi-hCit decreased the adhesion of WM266 plated onto vitronectin (~70%) and fibronectin (~40%), but did not have significant effect on adhesion to collagen type I. Similar data were obtained with cilengitide used as positive control and with the monoclonal antibody LM609 used to demonstrate the specificity of αvβ3 -dependent adhesion.

Incubation of cells with scrambled peptide, used as negative control, did not decrease WM266 adhesion onto matrix proteins. Furthermore, it is worth noting that the inhibition of adhesion by RGDechi-hCit occurred in a concentration-dependent manner giving an IC50 of 25.5 μM and 53 μM for vitronectin and fibronectin, respectively (Figure 2B).

In addition, the effect of RGDechi-hCit on cell detachment from vitronectin was tested 1 h after attachment of cells to vitronectin, the peptide was added and a significant cell detachment was observed (50%); an analogous effect was obtained using Cilengitide (60%) and antibody LM609 (50%), while using a scrambled peptide, no significant effect was observed (Figure 3), further confirming the RGDechi-hCit specific activity on αvβ3-dependent adhesion.

RGDechi-hCit inhibits proliferation and induces apoptosis in WM266 cells

To evaluate cell proliferation, starved WM266 were incubated with Cilengitide (50 μM) or with RGDechi-hCit peptide at different concentrations (10-50 μM) for 24 h. The inhibition of cell proliferation results in a dose-dependent manner. At the higher concentration used, RGDechi-hCit peptide induced a significative inhibition of proliferation (~45%) in respect to the untreated cells (Figure 4) and comparable to the Cilengitide (~60%)

In the same conditions of starvation, after 16 h of treatment with RGDechi-hCit or Cilengitide (both 50 μM), apoptosis was evaluated with annexin V-FITC/PI double staining by flow cytometry analysis. Starved WM266 cells, treated with RGDechi-hCit, exhibited 8.5% early apoptotic cells, 3.9% late apoptotic and

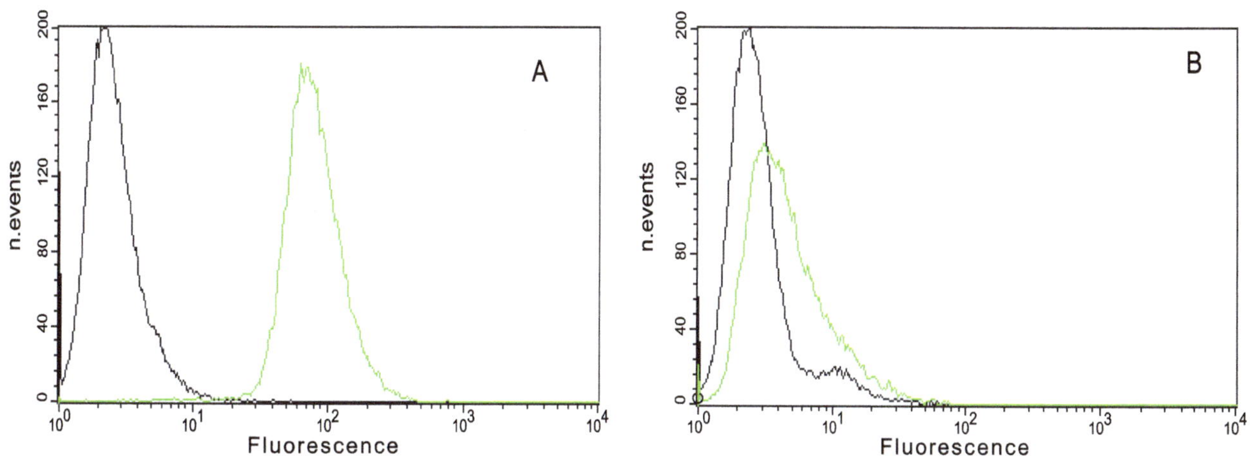

Figure 1. Analysis of expression of αvβ3 integrin in WM266 and HeLa cells by flow cytometry. Pre-confluence cells (WM266 cells (A), HeLa cells(B)) were detached by 0.1 mM EDTA in PBS and incubated with anti αvβ3 antibody (green curve) or isotype (black curve) and then with secondary antibody FITC conjugate.

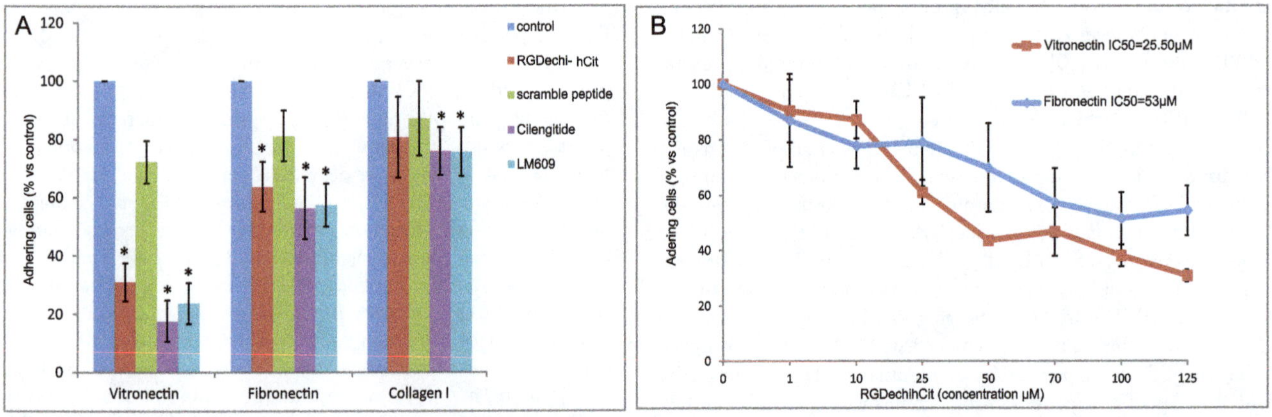

Figure 2. Inhibition of adhesion of WM266 on different extracellular matrix coated plates (A). Cells were pre-incubated with peptides (50 μM) or anti-αvβ3 antibody (10 μg/mL) for 30 min at 4°C and then seeded on extracellular matrix pre-coated plates. Cell adhesion was evaluated after 1 h of incubation using crystal violet reagent. The results are presented as the percentage of adherent cells respect to the control (untreated cells) and are expressed as means ± SE of three independent experiments performed in triplicate. Statistical significance was analyzed using Student's t test, unpaired, two-sided (*$p<0.05$). RGDechi-hCit dose-effect on WM266 cell adhesion (B). Cells were pre-incubated with increasing concentrations of RGDechi-hCit for 30 min at 4°C and then seeded on vitronectin or fibronectin (10 μg/mL) pre-coated plates at 37°C. The cell adhesion was evaluated after 1 h of incubation using crystal violet reagent. The results are presented as the percentage of adherent cells respect to the control (untreated cells) and are expressed as mean ± DS from three independent experiments performed in triplicate.

3.7% of necrotic cells; whereas using Cilengitide, 16.0% early apoptotic cells, 5.0% late apoptotic and 2.0% of necrotic cells were obtained (Figure 5). The same experiment conducted on starved cells in the absence of peptides displayed 0.7% early apoptotic cells, 1.4% late apoptotic and 5.6% necrotic cells.

RGDechi-hCit cellular uptake by flow cytometry analysis and confocal microscopy

The uptake of NBD-RGDechi-hCit into WM266 cells was determined by flow cytometry. The trans-bilayer distribution of NBD-peptides was determined by comparing the fluorescence intensity before and after addition of sodium dithionite, an essentially membrane-impermeant molecule, which irreversibly suppresses the fluorescence of the accessible NBD-moiety localised on the external cell surface [39]. The NBD-RGDechi-hCit (10 μM) was incubated with WM266 cells for 30 min at 37°C and then its quenching by dithionite treatment, was measured. To avoid dithionite diffusion in the biological membranes, this reaction was performed at 4°C. The addition of dithionite determined a strong increase of fluorescence compared to the intrinsic fluorescence of the cells. This result showed that a remarkable percentage of peptide (~90%) was internalised. In the same experimental conditions, NBD-scrambled peptide was used to exclude the non-specific fluorescence signal (data not show).

To confirm the peptide cell penetration and to collect information about the mechanism of internalisation in WM266 cells, confocal studies were also performed.

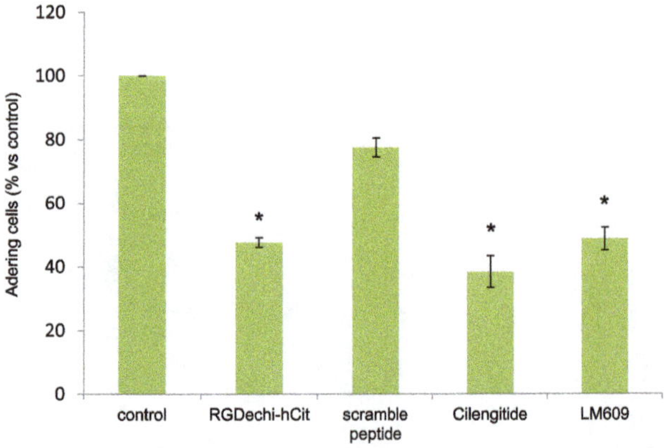

Figure 3. Detachment of WM266 cells from vitronectin coated plates. Cells were plated onto vitronectin (10 μg/mL) pre-coated wells and were allowed to adhere for 1 h. Peptides (50 μM) or anti-αvβ3 antibody (10 μg/mL) were added and the incubation was continued for 2 h. Cell adhesion was determined by crystal violet assay. Results are presented as percentage of adherent cells respect to the control (untreated cells) and are expressed as means ± SE of three independent experiments performed in triplicate. Statistical significance was analyzed using Student's t test, unpaired, two-sided (* $p<0.05$).

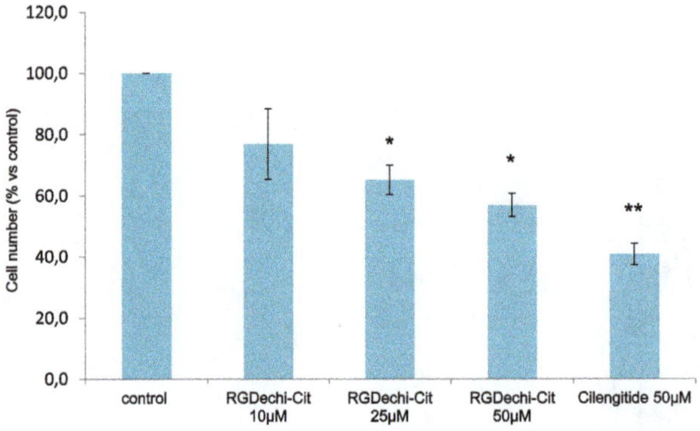

Figure 4. Cytotoxicity assay. WM266 were treated with starvation conditions (4% FCS) for 4 h and then peptides at different concentrations were added and incubated for 24 h. The proliferation was evaluated using crystal violet assay. The results are presented as the percentage of proliferating cells respect to the control (untreated cells) and are expressed as means ± SE of three independent experiments performed in triplicate. Statistical significance was analyzed using Student's t test, unpaired, two-sided (* $p<0.05$, **$p<0.01$).

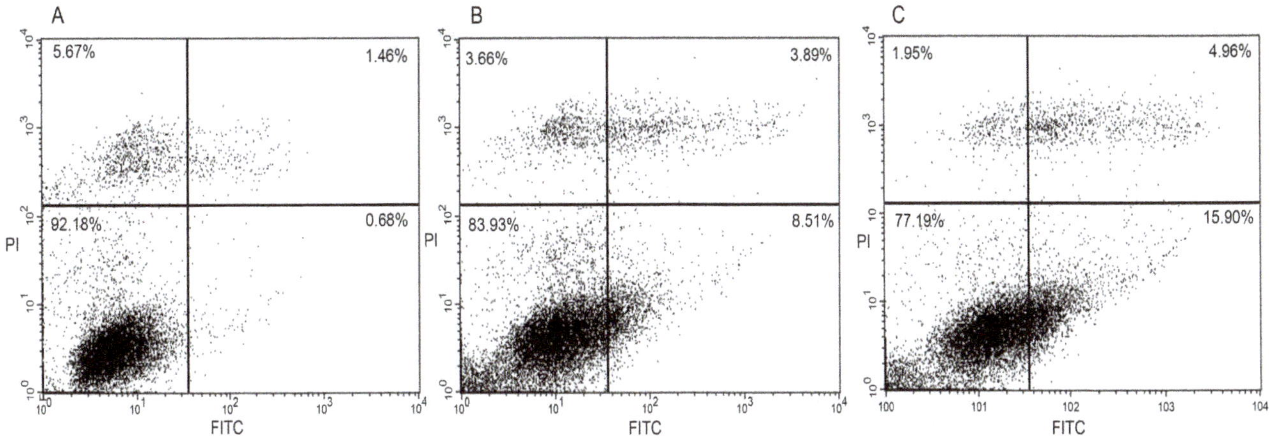

Figure 5. Apoptosis analyses with annexin V-FITC/PI double staining on WM266 cells. Untreated cells (A); cilengitide treated cells (B); RGDechi-hCit treated cells (C). Upper left quadrant: necrotic cells; upper right: advanced apoptotic cells; lower left: viable cells; lower right: early apoptotic cells. These pictures are representative of three independent experiments.

FITC-RGDechi-hCit was efficiently internalised after 30 min of incubation at 37°C (Figure 6A). Indeed, confocal images show that the peptide was localised within cell cytoplasm and mainly distributed into discrete spots suggesting its confinement in vesicular structures. Conversely, no cellular uptake was observed for FITC-scrambled peptide in WM266 cells (Figure 6B) and also for FITC-RGDechi-hCit in HeLa cells (Figure 6C) not expressing αvβ3 integrin receptor.

In order to investigate the mechanism of RGDechi-hCit peptide uptake, co-localisation experiments by using anti-αvβ3 integrin antibody were carried out. Figure 7A shows a partial co-localisation of FITC-RGDechi-hCit with αvβ3 integrin along cell boundaries (white arrows), suggesting a possible interaction between the peptide and the receptor at the cell membrane level.

Endocytosis of αvβ3 integrin was described to occur through clathrin-dependent [40] or caveolae endocytosis [41]. Therefore, to determine whether RGDechi-hCit peptide uptake followed the same endocytic pathways, we performed indirect immunofluorescence analyses using anti-clathrin and anti-caveolin 1 antibodies. Results showed a partial co-compartimentalisation of RGDechi-hCit both with caveolin 1 (Figure 7B) and clathrin (Figure 7C) proteins. A clear co-compartimentalisation of RGDechi-hCit with LAMP2 (Lysosome-Associated Membrane Proteins, whose function is mainly related to the protection, maintenance, and adhesion of the lysosome) was found, indicating an accumulation of this peptide in lysosomes (Figure 7D), as a possible consequence of receptor-mediated endocytic pathway.

To further elucidate the mechanism of RGDechi-hCit peptide uptake, WM266 cells were treated with sucrose and filipin which inhibit clathrin- and caveolin-mediated endocytosis, respectively. Confocal images showed a decrease of intracellular peptide fluorescence after both treatments compared to non-treated cells (Figure 8 A–F). A quantitative analysis indicated a reduction of about 40% and 20% RGDechi-hCit cellular uptake upon sucrose and filipin treatments, respectively (Figure 8 G). These results confirmed that the uptake of RGDechi-hCit peptide partially involves clathrin- and caveolin-mediated endocytic mechanisms.

Discussion and Conclusion

Several ECM proteins, enclosing the RGD motif, play a crucial role in integrin-mediated cell adhesion and consequently, in cell proliferation, survival and migration [4,42,43]. So far a huge variety of RGD peptides and mimetics are reported in the literature as potential candidates for tumor imaging, cell-targeting and therapy [44,45,46,47] thanks to their ability to recognise integrin receptors and eventually to internalise into different cell types, including endothelial and melanoma cells [42,48,49,50,51]. Many studies have identified marked differences in the surface expression and distribution of integrins in malignant tumor cells [52]. In particular αvβ3 integrin is expressed strongly on the

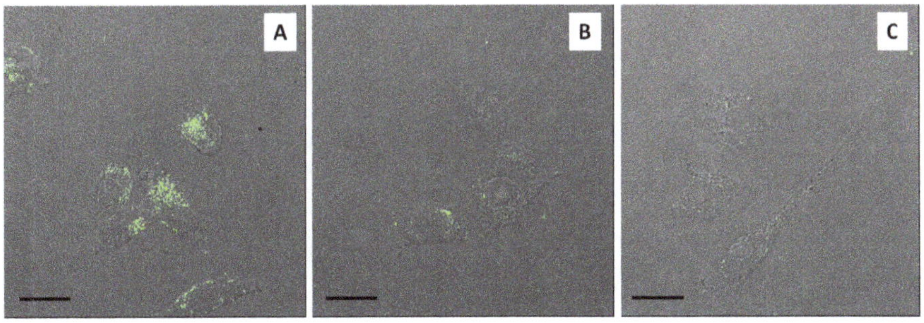

Figure 6. Merge of confocal and transmitted light images of peptide cellular uptake. WM266 cells after 30 min incubation with 50 μM RGDechi-hCit (A) and scrambled peptide(B). HeLa cells after 30 minute incubation with 50 μM RGDechi-hCit (C). Green fluorescence indicates peptides. Magnification bar: 20 μm.

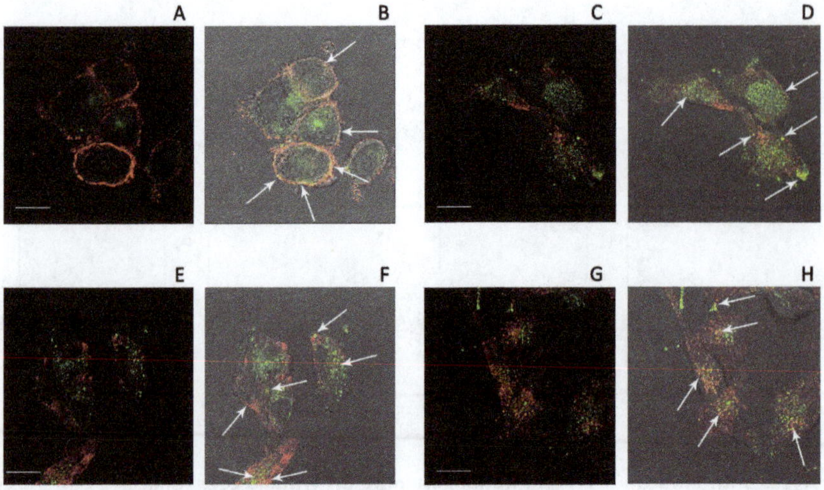

Figure 7. Co-localization areas (white arrows) of RGDechi-hCit peptide (green) with $\alpha v\beta 3$ integrin (red)(A), caveolin 1 (red)(B), clathrin (red)(C) and LAMP 2 (red)(D) in WM266 cells after 30 minute incubation. (A, C, E, G) fluorescence images; (B, D, F, H) transmitted and fluorescence image overlapping. Magnification bar: 20 μm.

surface of malignant melanoma cells and angiogenic blood vessels, but weakly on pre-neoplastic melanomas and quiescent blood vessels [30,38]. So a high expression of $\alpha v\beta 3$ integrin seems to be correlated to the increase of the metastatic potential of the melanoma cell line [19,28,39,40].

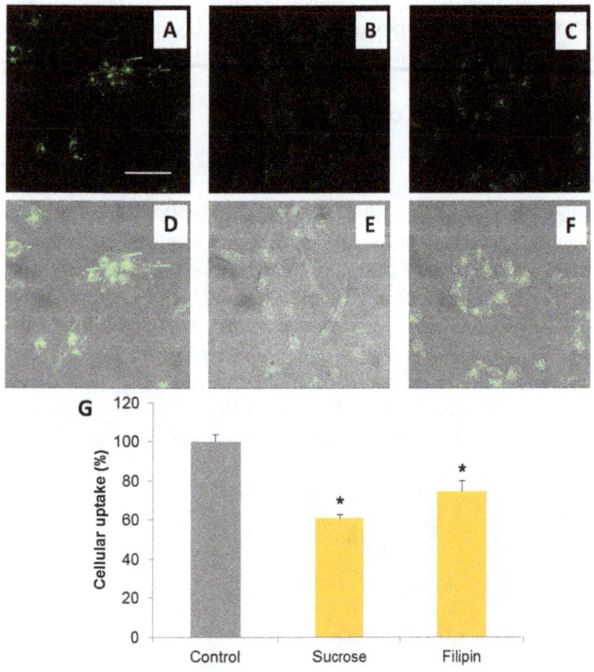

Figure 8. RGDechi cellular uptake inhibition experiments. A–F, Confocal microscope images of WM266 cells after 30 minutes of incubation with 50 μM RGDechi. A and D control non-treated cells; B and E cells treated with 0.45 M sucrose; C and F cells treated with 5 μg/ml filipin. A–C fluorescence images; D–F merge of fluorescence and transmitted light images. Magnification bar 50 μm. G, quantitative analysis of RGDechi cellular uptake by spectrofluorimeter measurements. Data are expressed as mean ± standard deviation (* $p<0.05$).

Over the last few years we focused our attention on the study of the biological features of a highly selective chimeric $\alpha v\beta 3$ antagonist named RGDechi-hCit. Very recently [28], we reported some data on *in vitro* antitumor efficacy of RGDechi-hCit on melanoma cell lines differently expressing $\alpha v\beta 3$ integrin. In particular, the data showed that the peptide induces a significant inhibition of proliferation only on the WM266 cell line, in accordance with its very high surface expression of $\alpha v\beta 3$.

Here we mainly investigated the pro-apoptotic activity of RGDechi-hCit peptide and its ability to penetrate the WM266 cell membrane. Simultaneously we deepened the selectivity, anti-adhesion, and anti-proliferative features of the peptide. Interestingly, for the first time we demonstrated the ability of RGDechi-hCit to enter cells overexpressing $\alpha v\beta 3$ integrin. This exciting result opens the way to consider this peptide as a new potential carrier to deliver drugs into the cell also confirming its selectivity.

In detail, to reinforce the evidence regarding the receptor selectivity of the molecule, we investigated the adhesion effect of RGDechi-hCit on WM266 cells, using vitronectin, fibronectin and collagen I as different matrix proteins. Remarkably, we observed that peptide activity depends on the matrix used; it evidently inhibits cell adhesion to vitronectin and somewhat to fibronectin in contrast to the effect on collagen I, which does not interact with αv integrin and protects cells from the RGDechi-hCit anti-adhesion activity. The higher effect observed on cells seeded on vitronectin with respect to fibronectin is very likely to be ascribed to the different level of receptor expression on the WM266 cell surface, where the presence of the $\alpha v\beta 3$ receptor dominates over that of $\alpha v\beta 5$ ($\alpha v\beta 3$:$\alpha v\beta 5$, 10:1 ratio, data not shown).

Since vitronectin interacts with $\alpha v\beta 3$ as well as $\alpha v\beta 5$ receptors while fibronectin interacts with $\alpha 5\beta 1$, $\alpha IIb\beta 3$ and $\alpha v\beta 3$, we have strong reasons to believe that the different behavior of RGDechi-hCit on the various matrices is due to the capability of the WM266 cells to bind fibronectin most efficiently, ascribable to the presence of other integrins not directly interacting with RGDechi-hCit. The inhibition of adhesion by RGDechi-hCit occurs in a concentration-dependent manner for vitronectin and fibronectin and the ability to detach adherent cells from vitronectin is very similar to that of the anti-$\alpha v\beta 3$ antibody, reinforcing our findings that the action of the peptide is integrin specific. Additional experiments confirmed our previous data [28] that RGDechi-hCit significantly inhibits the growth of melanoma cells. The anti-proliferative effect of the peptide on cancer cells is comparable to Cilengitide used as positive control and to other RGD–based systems reported in the literature [9,10].

Interestingly, studies by FACS indicated that RGDechi-hCit is also able to induce apoptosis in a similar way to Cilengitide on other cell lines [53] and in accordance with other reports indicating that cells detached by treatment with RGD molecules go on to apoptosis. This outcome enhances the value of the RGDechi-hCit peptide even if the principal criterion for its success was the evidence of its cell entry ability. For this reason, particular attention was paid to the investigation of the mechanism of internalisation both by flow cytometric and confocal microscopy studies. Generally, RGD-based peptides are able to cross the cell membrane both by passive diffusion [54,55] and receptor specific mechanism. Here we reported that our peptide is able to enter cells overexpressing αvβ3 integrin and shows a partial co-localisation with anti-αvβ3 integrin antibody, suggesting very likely an αvβ3 receptor-mediated uptake.

Actually, indirect immunofluorescence analysis highlighted a partial co-compartimentalisation of RGDechi-hCit both with caveolin 1 and clathrin proteins. This result was confirmed by using inhibitors of clathrin- and caveolin-mediated endocytosis which induce a clear reduction of peptide cellular uptake. What is more, an evident co-compartimentalisation of RGDechi-hCit with LAMP2 was observed by the accumulation of peptide in lysosome, clear consequence of a receptor-mediated endocytic pathway. Altogether these findings strongly suggest the uptake of RGDechi-hCit occurs mainly through the internalisation of αvβ3 receptor *via* an endocytic pathway. Further investigations will be necessary to confirm such data.

The observed uptake poses the question regarding the mechanism of apoptosis induced by RGDechi-hCit. Studies on RGD peptides have led to several models of antagonist-induced cell death including a type of caspase-dependent apoptosis known as anoikis [42,56] due to the cells loosing adherence and subsequent detachment caused by interaction with integrins. In our case, the apoptosis could be ascribed both to anoikis and/or to activation of an intracellular pathway consequent to the peptide entrance into the cell. Further studies will be needed to address likely intracellular targets mediating the apoptosis.

All results here reported give some convincing evidence that RGDechi-hCit is able to penetrate cells mainly by αvβ3 integrin-dependent endocytosis and could be considered a novel carrier to deliver selectively drugs into the cell. What is more, we discovered that the peptide displays an apoptotic effect *per se*. This consideration and the previous data on the ability to inhibit some intracellular pathways [21], suggest that RGDechi-hCit can be potentially considered a true αvβ3 integrin inhibitor.

In conclusion, a great challenge to evaluate the achievable application of RGDechi-hCit molecule in vivo is the development of new selective systems containing both our peptide and pro-apoptotic molecules or different therapeutic agents to induce a synergic action.

Author Contributions

Conceived and designed the experiments: DC ADG LZ. Performed the experiments: DC IdP AL DG. Analyzed the data: DC IdP AL ADG SDG DG MS LZ. Wrote the paper: DC SDG ADG MS LZ.

References

1. Hynes RO (2002) Integrins: bidirectional, allosteric signaling machines. Cell 110: 673–687.
2. Zaccaro L, Del Gatto A, Pedone C, Saviano M (2007) Integrin receptor family: promising target for therapeutic and diagnostic applications. Current Topics in Biochemical Research 9: 45–56.
3. Brooks PC, Clark RA, Cheresh DA (1994) Requirement of vascular integrin alpha v beta 3 for angiogenesis. Science 264: 569–571.
4. Giancotti FG, Ruoslahti E (1999) Integrin signaling. Science 285: 1028–1032.
5. Gladson CL, Cheresh DA (1991) Glioblastoma expression of vitronectin and the alpha v beta 3 integrin. Adhesion mechanism for transformed glial cells. The Journal of clinical investigation 88: 1924–1932.
6. Liapis H, Adler LM, Wick MR, Rader JS (1997) Expression of alpha(v)beta3 integrin is less frequent in ovarian epithelial tumors of low malignant potential in contrast to ovarian carcinomas. Human pathology 28: 443–449.
7. Albelda SM, Mette SA, Elder DE, Stewart R, Damjanovich L, et al. (1990) Integrin distribution in malignant melanoma: association of the beta 3 subunit with tumor progression. Cancer research 50: 6757–6764.
8. Zhaofei L (2008) Integrin avb3-Targeted Cancer Therapy. Drug Development Research 69: 329–339.
9. Aguzzi MS, D'Arcangelo D, Giampietri C, Capogrossi MC, Facchiano A (2011) RAM, an RGDS analog, exerts potent anti-melanoma effects in vitro and in vivo. PloS one 6: e25352.
10. Oliveira-Ferrer L, Hauschild J, Fiedler W, Bokemeyer C, Nippgen J, et al. (2008) Cilengitide induces cellular detachment and apoptosis in endothelial and glioma cells mediated by inhibition of FAK/src/AKT pathway. Journal of experimental & clinical cancer research: CR 27: 86.
11. Zaccaro L, Del Gatto A, Pedone C, Saviano M (2009) Peptides for tumour therapy and diagnosis: current status and future directions. Current medicinal chemistry 16: 780–795.
12. Chen K, Chen X (2011) Integrin targeted delivery of chemotherapeutics. Theranostics 1: 189–200.
13. Millard M, Odde S, Neamati N (2011) Integrin targeted therapeutics. Theranostics 1: 154–188.
14. Dechantsreiter MA, Planker E, Matha B, Lohof E, Holzemann G, et al. (1999) N-Methylated cyclic RGD peptides as highly active and selective alpha(V)beta(3) integrin antagonists. Journal of medicinal chemistry 42: 3033–3040.
15. Reardon DA, Neyns B, Weller M, Tonn JC, Nabors LB, et al. (2011) Cilengitide: an RGD pentapeptide alphanubeta3 and alphanubeta5 integrin inhibitor in development for glioblastoma and other malignancies. Future oncology 7: 339–354.
16. Tabatabai G, Weller M, Nabors B, Picard M, Reardon D, et al. (2010) Targeting integrins in malignant glioma. Targeted oncology 5: 175–181.
17. Yin AA, Cheng JX, Zhang X, Liu BL (2013) The treatment of glioblastomas: a systematic update on clinical Phase III trials. Critical reviews in oncology/hematology 87: 265–282.
18. Scaringi C, Minniti G, Caporello P, Enrici RM (2012) Integrin inhibitor cilengitide for the treatment of glioblastoma: a brief overview of current clinical results. Anticancer research 32: 4213–4223.
19. Del Gatto A, Zaccaro L, Grieco P, Novellino E, Zannetti A, et al. (2006) Novel and selective alpha(v)beta3 receptor peptide antagonist: design, synthesis, and biological behavior. Journal of medicinal chemistry 49: 3416–3420.
20. Zannetti A, Del Vecchio S, Iommelli F, Del Gatto A, De Luca S, et al. (2009) Imaging of alpha(v)beta(3) expression by a bifunctional chimeric RGD peptide not cross-reacting with alpha(v)beta(5). Clinical cancer research: an official journal of the American Association for Cancer Research 15: 5224–5233.
21. Santulli G, Basilicata MF, De Simone M, Del Giudice C, Anastasio A, et al. (2011) Evaluation of the anti-angiogenic properties of the new selective alphaVbeta3 integrin antagonist RGDechiHCit. Journal of translational medicine 9: 7.
22. Fogel M, Mechtersheimer S, Huszar M, Smirnov A, Abu-Dahi A, et al. (2003) L1 adhesion molecule (CD 171) in development and progression of human malignant melanoma. Cancer letters 189: 237–247.
23. Haass NK, Smalley KS, Li L, Herlyn M (2005) Adhesion, migration and communication in melanocytes and melanoma. Pigment cell research/ sponsored by the European Society for Pigment Cell Research and the International Pigment Cell Society 18: 150–159.
24. Marshall JF, Rutherford DC, Happerfield L, Hanby A, McCartney AC, et al. (1998) Comparative analysis of integrins in vitro and in vivo in uveal and cutaneous melanomas. British journal of cancer 77: 522–529.
25. McGary EC, Lev DC, Bar-Eli M (2002) Cellular adhesion pathways and metastatic potential of human melanoma. Cancer biology & therapy 1: 459–465.
26. Jilaveanu LB, Aziz SA, Kluger HM (2009) Chemotherapy and biologic therapies for melanoma: do they work? Clinics in dermatology 27: 614–625.
27. Garbe C, Peris K, Hauschild A, Saiag P, Middleton M, et al. (2010) Diagnosis and treatment of melanoma: European consensus-based interdisciplinary guideline. European journal of cancer 46: 270–283.
28. Pisano M, I dP, Nieddu V, Sassu I, Cossu S, et al. (2013) In vitro activity of the alphavbeta3 integrin antagonist RGDechi-hCit on malignant melanoma cells. Anticancer research 33: 871–879.

29. Monfregola L, De Luca S (2011) Synthetic strategy for side chain mono-N-alkylation of Fmoc-amino acids promoted by molecular sieves. Amino acids 41: 981–990.
30. Gillies RJ, Didier N, Denton M (1986) Determination of cell number in monolayer cultures. Analytical Biochemistry. 159: 109–113.
31. Hansen SH, Sandvig K, van Deurs B (1993) Clathrin and HA2 adaptors: effects of potassium depletion, hypertonic medium, and cytosol acidification. The Journal of cell biology 121: 61–72.
32. Fields CG, Lloyd DH, Macdonald RL, Otteson KM, Noble RL (1991) HBTU activation for automated Fmoc solid-phase peptide synthesis. Peptide research 4: 95–101.
33. Coste J, Le-Nguyen D, Castro B (1990) PyBOP: a new peptide coupling.
34. reagent devoid of toxic byproduct. Tetrahedron Lett 31: 205–208.
35. Davis GE (1992) Affinity of integrins for damaged extracellular matrix: $\alpha v \beta 3$ binds to denatured collagen type I through RGD sites. Biochem Biophys Res Comm 182: 1025–1031.
36. Kanda S, Kuzuya M, Ramos MA, Koike T, Yoshino K, et al. (2000) Matrix metalloproteinase and alphavbeta3 integrin-dependent vascular smooth muscle cell invasion through a type I collagen lattice. Arteriosclerosis, thrombosis, and vascular biology 20: 998–1005.
37. Barczyk M, Carracedo S, Gullberg D (2010) Integrins. Cell and tissue research 339: 269–280.
38. Seiffert D, Smith JW (1997) The cell adhesion domain in plasma vitronectin is cryptic. The Journal of biological chemistry 272: 13705–13710.
39. Angeletti C, Nichols JW (1998) Dithionite quenching rate measurement of the inside-outside membrane bilayer distribution of 7-nitrobenz-2-oxa-1,3-diazol-4-yl-labeled phospholipids. Biochemistry 37: 15114–15119.
40. De Deyne PG, O'Neill A, Resneck WG, Dmytrenko GM, Pumplin DW, et al. (1998) The vitronectin receptor associates with clathrin-coated membrane domains via the cytoplasmic domain of its beta5 subunit. Journal of cell science 111 (Pt 18): 2729–2740.
41. Alam MR, Dixit V, Kang H, Li ZB, Chen X, et al. (2008) Intracellular delivery of an anionic antisense oligonucleotide via receptor-mediated endocytosis. Nucleic acids research 36: 2764–2776.
42. Maubant S, Saint-Dizier D, Boutillon M, Perron-Sierra F, Casara PJ, et al. (2006) Blockade of alpha v beta3 and alpha v beta5 integrins by RGD mimetics induces anoikis and not integrin-mediated death in human endothelial cells. Blood 108: 3035–3044.
43. Plow EF, Cierniewski CS, Xiao Z, Haas TA, Byzova TV (2001) AlphaIIbbeta3 and its antagonism at the new millennium. Thrombosis and haemostasis 86: 34–40.
44. Rosenow F, Ossig R, Thormeyer D, Gasmann P, Schluter K, et al. (2008) Integrins as antimetastatic targets of RGD-independent snake venom components in liver metastasis [corrected]. Neoplasia 10: 168–176.
45. White DE, Muller WJ (2007) Multifaceted roles of integrins in breast cancer metastasis. Journal of mammary gland biology and neoplasia 12: 135–142.
46. Ellerby HM, Arap W, Ellerby LM, Kain R, Andrusiak R, et al. (1999) Anti-cancer activity of targeted pro-apoptotic peptides. Nature medicine 5: 1032–1038.
47. Andersen MH, Svane IM, Becker JC, Straten PT (2007) The universal character of the tumor-associated antigen survivin. Clinical cancer research: an official journal of the American Association for Cancer Research 13: 5991–5994.
48. Adderley SR, Fitzgerald DJ (2000) Glycoprotein IIb/IIIa antagonists induce apoptosis in rat cardiomyocytes by caspase-3 activation. The Journal of biological chemistry 275: 5760–5766.
49. Matsuki K, Sasho T, Nakagawa K, Tahara M, Sugioka K, et al. (2008) RGD peptide-induced cell death of chondrocytes and synovial cells. Journal of orthopaedic science: official journal of the Japanese Orthopaedic Association 13: 524–532.
50. Zaffaroni N, Pennati M, Daidone MG (2005) Survivin as a target for new anticancer interventions. Journal of cellular and molecular medicine 9: 360–372.
51. Grossman D, Altieri DC (2001) Drug resistance in melanoma: mechanisms, apoptosis, and new potential therapeutic targets. Cancer metastasis reviews 20: 3–11.
52. Mizejewski GJ (1999) Role of integrins in cancer: survey of expression patterns. Proceedings of the Society for Experimental Biology and Medicine Society for Experimental Biology and Medicine 222: 124–138.
53. Lautenschlaeger T, Perry J, Peereboom D, Li B, Ibrahim A, et al. (2013) In vitro study of combined cilengitide and radiation treatment in breast cancer cell lines. Radiation oncology 8: 246.
54. Castel S, Pagan R, Mitjans F, Piulats J, Goodman S, et al. (2001) RGD peptides and monoclonal antibodies, antagonists of alpha(v)-integrin, enter the cells by independent endocytic pathways. Laboratory investigation; a journal of technical methods and pathology 81: 1615–1626.
55. Aguzzi MS, Fortugno P, Giampietri C, Ragone G, Capogrossi MC, et al. (2010) Intracellular targets of RGDS peptide in melanoma cells. Molecular cancer 9: 84.
56. Frisch SM, Ruoslahti E (1997) Integrins and anoikis. Current opinion in cell biology 9: 701–706.

5

Formulation Optimization and *In Vivo* Proof-of-Concept Study of Thermosensitive Liposomes Balanced by Phospholipid, Elastin-Like Polypeptide, and Cholesterol

Sun Min Park[1], Jae Min Cha[1¤], Jungyong Nam[1], Min Sang Kim[1], Sang-Jun Park[1], Eun Sung Park[1], Hwankyu Lee[2], Hyun Ryoung Kim[1]*

1 Drug Delivery System Group, Bio Research Center, Samsung Advanced Institute of Technology (SAIT), Yongin, Gyeonggi-do, South Korea, **2** Department of Chemical Engineering, Dankook University, Yongin, Gyeonggi-do, South Korea

Abstract

One application of nanotechnology in medicine that is presently being developed involves a drug delivery system (DDS) employing nanoparticles to deliver drugs to diseased sites in the body avoiding damage of healthy tissue. Recently, the mild hyperthermia-triggered drug delivery combined with anticancer agent-loaded thermosensitive liposomes was widely investigated. In this study, thermosensitive liposomes (TSLs), composed of 1,2-dipalmitoyl-*sn*-glycero-3-phosphocholine (DPPC), 1,2-distearoyl-*sn*-glycero-3-phosphoethanolamine-*N*-[methoxy(polyethyleneglycol)-2000] (DSPE-PEG), cholesterol, and a fatty acid conjugated elastin-like polypeptide (ELP), were developed and optimized for triggered drug release, controlled by external heat stimuli. We introduced modified ELP, tunable for various biomedical purposes, to our thermosensitive liposome (e-TSL) to convey a high thermoresponsive property. We modulated thermosensitivity and stability by varying the ratios of e-TSL components, such as phospholipid, ELP, and cholesterol. Experimental data obtained in this study corresponded to results from a simulation study that demonstrated, through the calculation of the lateral diffusion coefficient, increased permeation of the lipid bilayer with higher ELP concentrations, and decreased permeation in the presence of cholesterol. Finally, we identified effective drug accumulation in tumor tissues and antitumor efficacy with our optimized e-TSL, while adjusting lag-times for systemic accumulation.

Editor: Efstathios Karathanasis, Case Western Reserve University, United States of America

Funding: The simulation part of this research was supported by the Basic Science Research Program through the National Research Foundation of Korea (NRF), funded by the Ministry of Education, Science, and Technology (2012R1A1A1001196), and by the National Institute of Supercomputing and Networking/Korea Institute of Science and Technology Information with supercomputing resources, including technical support (KSC-2013-C2-18). The funders had no role in study design, data collection and analysis, decision to publish, or preparation of the manuscript.

Competing Interests: Sun Min Park, Jae Min Cha, Min Sang Kim, Sang-Jun Park, Eun Sung Park, and Hyun Ryoung Kim have declared their affiliation to a commercial company (Samsung Advanced Institute of Technology).

* Email: hyunryoung.kim@samsung.com

¤ Current address: Samsung Biomedical Research Institute, Samsung Advanced Institute of Technology (SAIT), Samsung Electronics Co., Ltd., Seoul, South Korea

Introduction

A drug delivery system (DDS), developed for the highest efficacy of clinical drugs, provides damaged/diseased sites in a body with a therapeutic dosage of drugs, while reducing side effects caused by undesired delivery to normal tissues. The development of nanotechnologies has enabled specific tailoring of the properties of drug delivery carriers for currently existing medical issues and problems. Accordingly, the range of DDS applications in biomedical and clinical fields has expanded with the creation of unprecedented therapeutic approaches in the area of nanomedicine [1]. A platform technology of DDS has been adopted to potentiate a variety of diagnostic methodologies using biomarkers/bioimaging, tissue engineering/regenerative medicine, and gene therapy, as well as pharmaceutical industries [2–4].

Advances in nanotechnology have allowed for the fabrication of nano-sized particles that are capable of carrying a variety of drugs [5]. Selective drug targeting through the use of drug-loaded nanocarriers allows nanoparticles to effectively extravasate and accumulate in tumorous tissues exhibiting the enhanced permeability and retention (EPR) effect, constituted by leaky vasculature and poor lymphatic drainage [6]. Local mild hyperthermia, which conditions the treated site at about 42°C (39–42°C), has been applied clinically, in order to increase vascular permeability and interstitial microconvection of the drug within the sites of disease. This enhances the EPR effect, further elevating drug accumulation. Moreover, many researchers have developed thermosensitive nanovehicles to control drug release within the diseased region under locally-treated mild hyperthermia [6–13]. This could yield a synergistic effect with EPR, and provide abrupt exposure of highly concentrated drugs specifically to diseased tissues, further maximizing the therapeutic effects. Approved for clinical use, liposomes are currently one of the most versatile nano-sized drug carriers; thus, thermosensitive liposome (TSL) has been widely studied for transitioning laboratory findings to the clinic [1,7,9,14].

Herein, we report the development of novel temperature-sensitive liposomes, a short chain elastin-like polypeptide-incorporating TSL (e-TSL), which is composed of 1,2-dipalmitoyl-*sn*-

glycero-3-phosphocholine (DPPC), 1,2-distearoyl-*sn*-glycero-3-phosphoethanolamine-*N*-[methoxy(polyethyleneglycol)-2000] (DSPE-PEG), cholesterol, and a fatty acid conjugated elastin-like polypeptide (ELP). By incorporating ELP, consisting of a [VPGVG]n pentapeptide repeat, e-TSLs could possess high thermosensitivity and biocompatibility for use in various biomedical applications [15–18]. In this study, the component optimization of e-TSL was conducted as a thermosensitive drug carrier under mild hyperthermia. To select ELP-lipid conjugates for incorporation into the thermosensitive liposome bilayer, their transition temperature were obtained at different concentrations. To optimize the composition, the cargo-release from various liposomes, consisting of different molar ratios of main lipid (DPPC and DSPC), cholesterol, and selected ELP, was investigated. A simulation study supported the experimental data, which demonstrated the change of lateral diffusion coefficients with different ratios of ELP and cholesterol. Finally, the e-TSLs formulated with the optimized components were loaded with doxorubicin, and applied to tumor-bearing mice via intravenous injection, in order to obtain the largest amount of drug accumulation and better antitumor effect.

Materials and Methods

Ethics Statement

All animal protocols were reviewed and approved by the Institutional Animal Care and Use Committee at the Sahmyook University (Approval ID: SYUIACUC2013-010), and experiments were conducted according to institutional guideline.

Materials

We purchased 1,2-dimyristoly-*sn*-glycero-3-phosphocholine (DMPC), 1,2-dipalmitoyl-*sn*-glycero-3-phosphocholine (DPPC), 1,2-distearoyl-*sn*-glycero-3-phosphocholine (DSPC), 1,2-distearoyl-*sn*-glycero-3-phosphoethanolamine-*N*-[methoxy(polyethylene glycol)-2000] (DSPE-PEG), and cholesterol from Avanti Polar Lipid, Inc. (Alabaster, AL). Chemically-synthesized ELP, $[VPGVG]_n$, and ELP-lipid conjugates were provided by Peptron, Inc. (Daejeon, Korea). Doxorubicin (DOX) and calcein were purchased from Sigma-Aldrich (USA).

Phase transition temperature of ELP-lipid conjugates

The transition temperatures of ELP-lipid conjugates were identified by measuring transmittance at 280 nm in the temperature range of 20–55°C, using a scan rate of 1°C per minute, in triplicate. The ELP-lipid conjugates were expressed as SA-Vn. The lipid moiety, stearyl group, was introduced to N-terminus of ELP peptide by amide bond and abbreviated to SA. The ELP (VPGVG) unit and repeating number were considered as Vn. The C-terminus of ELP was amidated to control the physical property of ELP- lipid conjugates. The details of ELP-lipid conjugate were summarized in Table 1. The transmittance profiles were checked for different concentrations of ELP-lipid conjugates from 0.1mM to 1 mM in phosphate-buffered saline (PBS) buffer. The data were collected on a Cary 300 Bio UV-visible spectrophotometer equipped with a multi-cell thermoelectric temperature controller from Varian (Palo Alto, CA). The transition temperature (Tt) was considered to be the temperature corresponding to the maximum of the first derivative of transmittance versus temperature.

Preparation of DOX-loaded liposome

Liposomes were prepared using a previously reported method with minor modifications [19]. The general formulation of the liposome was phosphocholine lipid:DSPE-PEG:cholesterol:ELP-lipid conjugates = 55:2:X:Y (molar ratio). We encapsulated small molecules, calcein or doxorubicin (DOX), according to the experiment. In summary, lipids and modified ELPs were dissolved in chloroform, and the solvent was removed under reduced pressure. The thin film of lipids/ELP-lipid conjugates was dispersed in the calcein solution by vortexing and sonication. The liposome suspension was extruded through a polycarbonate membrane with 100-nm pores to facilitate formation of homogeneous liposomes and was followed by removal of uncapsulated calcein with PBS by size-exclusion chromatography (SEC) using a Sepadex (G-50) column. Calcein was encapsulated into the liposome during the hydration step, after lipid film formation. In the case of DOX encapsulation, DOX was loaded into liposomes using the ammonium sulfate (250 mM) gradient method. After film formation, 250 mM ammonium sulfate solution was added and the solution was vortexed and sonicated, followed by extrusion through polycarbonate membrane with 100 nm pores. Next, the exterior buffer of the liposome suspension was exchanged with 25 mM Tris·HCl (pH 9.0) by size exclusion chromatography (SEC) using a Sepadex (G-50) column. DOX was added to the liposome suspension at 1:0.2 (w/w, phospholipid:DOX), and the mixture of liposome suspension and DOX was incubated at 37°C for 1 hr. Finally, unloaded DOX was removed by SEC, using PBS, pH 7.4 as eluent. The encapsulation efficiency of DOX by liposome was estimated from the absorbance of the liposome dissolved in dimethyl sulfoxide (DMSO) at 490 nm (UV-VIS Spectrometer), before and after purification with the Sephadex (G-50) column. The loading efficiency (LE) was empirically found to be variable depending on the amount of drugs contained in the liposome solution. In case that 1 mL of liposome suspension contains more than 500 μg of DOX, 50~60% of LE was shown; whereas, 95% of LE was obtained when 300 μg of DOX was mixed with the same volume of liposome suspension.

Drug release from liposomes

Thermosensitive drug release was measured using the fluorescent quenching property of calcein or DOX. Each aliquot of liposome suspension was incubated in a preheated chamber for 5 min, followed by ice bath quenching. The fluorescent intensity was monitored at 520 nm (for calcein) or 615 nm (for DOX), with excitation at 490 nm, by a fluorescence spectrometer (PerkinElmer, Envision 2104-multilabel reader). The drug release percentage was calculated according to the following equation: $(F_t - F_i)/(F_f - F_i) \times 100\%$, where F_t and F_i denote the fluorescent intensities of the heated and initial (at room temperature) liposome suspension, respectively. Here, F_f is the fluorescent intensity of the liposome solution after addition of 1% TritonX-100 containing ethanol to disrupt the liposome completely.

Size and morphology of liposomes

The size of liposome was measured by dynamic light scattering (DLS) at 25°C using a Zetasizer Nano ZS (Malvern instrument, UK) with a He-Ne laser at a wavelength of 633 nm and a detection angle of 90 degrees.

Liposome morphology was observed using a cryo-transmission electron microscope (cryo-TEM). Samples for cryo-TEM were prepared on carbon film-supported grids with holes. Thin aqueous film, blotted with filter paper, was fabricated by Vitrobot (FEI) and immediately plunged into liquid ethane. The resulting grids were stored in liquid nitrogen and transferred to a cryotransfer holder (Gatan). Images were obtained using a CCD camera (2 k, Gatan) with a Tecnai F20 field emission gun electron microscope operated at 200 kV (FEI) in low dose mode.

Table 1. List of ELP-lipid conjugates.

ELP-lipid conjugate	Sequence
SA-V2	Stearoyl-$(VPGVG)_2$-NH_2
SA-V3	Stearoyl-$(VPGVG)_3$-NH_2
SA-V4	Stearoyl-$(VPGVG)_4$-NH_2
SA-V5	Stearoyl-$(VPGVG)_5$-NH_2
SA-V6	Stearoyl-$(VPGVG)_6$-NH_2

Molecular dynamics simulations of lipid bilayers

All coarse-grained (CG) molecular dynamics (MD) simulations and analyses were performed using the GROMACS4.5.5 simulation package [20–22] with the "MARTINI" CG force field (FF) [23–25], which lumps 3 or 4 heavy atoms into each CG bead. Models for DPPC, DSPE-PEG, cholesterol, and ELP were taken directly from the MARTINI FF. All simulated systems are listed in Table 2. For the system with ELP molecules, ELPs of three different lengths ($[VPGVG]_n$, where n = 1, 2, and 3) were simulated.

The lipid bilayer, which consists of DPPC, DSPE-PEG, cholesterol, and ELP molecules at different molar ratios, was solvated with ~35,000 CG water molecules (representing ~140,000 real water molecules) in a periodic box of size $20\times20\times16$ nm^3. Since a single DSPE-PEG has a net charge of −1, 48 counterions (Na^+) were added to neutralize the bilayer system. A cutoff of 12 Å was used for Lennard-Jones (LJ) and electrostatic interactions. The LJ and Coulomb potentials were shifted to 0 between 9 and 12 Å, and between 0 and 12 Å, respectively. Since the transition temperature for MARTINI DPPC is 295 K [26], which is ~20 K lower than the experiment value, a temperature of 295 K and a pressure of 1 bar were maintained by applying the Berendsen thermostat and barostat in the $NP_{xy}P_zT$ ensemble [27]. Simulations were performed for 2 μs with a time step of 8 fs, which is lower than the typical time step of 20–40 fs because of the inclusion of PEG dihedral potentials. The last 500 ns were used for analyses.

Animals and tumor implantation

Six-week-old male BALB/c nude mice were used in this study. To produce tumors, the murine mammary tumor cell line, EMT-6, was cultured in RPMI media (Sigma-Aldrich Co. St Louis, MO) supplemented with 10% fetal bovine serum and 1% antibiotics. For *in vivo* injections, EMT-6 cells were trypsinized and centrifuged at 1,200 rpm for 3 min at 4°C, washed twice with PBS, and reconstituted in Dulbecco's phosphate-buffered saline (D-PBS; Gibco, Carlsbad, CA). EMT-6 cells (1.0×10^6 cells/50 μL of D-PBS) were injected subcutaneously into both thigh areas.

Drug accumulation and antitumor efficacy study

Tumor-bearing mice (n = 4) were anesthetized by ventilation with isoflurane (Forane; Baxter, Deerfield, IL) and fixed on a custom-made holder. The temperature in the water bath was maintained at 42°C by a thermostat (NTT-2200, Eyela, Tokyo, Japan).

These experiments were carried out when the average tumor volume was approximately 500 mm^3 (300–350 mg in mass, ±10%). The tumor tissues of mice were initially preheated for 30 min using a water bath. After removal from the water bath, the drugs (5 mg/kg of free DOX or its equivalent) were administered through the tail vein of mice in the DOX and DOX-encapsulated liposome groups. The same volume of PBS was injected intravenously to mice in the control group. At different time points (1, 6, and 12 hr) after drug administration, mice were anesthetized and sacrificed for tumor tissue collection. Tumor tissues isolated from mice were dissociated in nuclear lysis buffer composed of 0.25 mol/L sucrose, 5 mmol/L Tris-HCl, 1 mmol/L $MgSO_4$, 1 mmol/L $CaCl_2$ (pH 7.6) by a homogenizer. After the addition of 10% (v/v) Triton X-100, the sample was then centrifuged for 10 min at 12,000×g and the supernatant was loaded onto a 96-well plate for determination of fluorescence at Ex 490 nm/Em 615 nm by a fluorescence spectrometer (PerkinElmer, Envision 2104-multilabel reader). DOX concentration was obtained by comparing fluorescence with a calibration curve generated from known amounts of DOX in tumor tissue homogenates, and the amount of DOX accumulated from free DOX and the liposome group was determined as μg doxorubicin/g tissue.

For detecting intratumoral distribution of DOX, 8 mg/kg of the drug was introduced to reinforce the visibility of DOX accumulated in tumor tissues. Tumor tissues were collected at 6 hr-post injection of drugs, embedded immediately in OCT compound,

Table 2. List of all simulations.

No. of molecules				Molar ratio
DPPC	DSPE-PEG	Cholesterol	ELP	
1296	48	360	0	55:2:15:0
1296	48	360	6	55:2:15:0.25
1296	48	0	10	55:2:0:0.41
1296	48	240	10	55:2:10:0.41
1296	48	360	10	55:2:15:0.41

and frozen in liquid nitrogen. Upon the histological analysis, samples were cryosectioned as 10 μm tissue sections and imaged by a confocal laser scanning microscope (LSM710, Carl Zeiss). Subsequent to imaging of DOX, tumor tissue sections were fixed in acetone for 10 minutes, stained with anti-CD31 (MAB1398Z, Millipore) and Hoechst (Sigma-Aldrich), and mounted in Vectashield mounting medium (Vector Laboratories).

The maximized drug accumulation was shown in 6 hrs after drug administration among the different time points (1, 6, and 12 hrs). We chose this time course for the anti-tumor efficacy study, and compared with free DOX and control groups in the presence/absence of mild hyperthermia. Briefly, the tumor tissues of mice were initially preheated for 30 min as described above and the DOX-loaded liposome or free DOX (5 mg of DOX/kg of mouse) was administered through the tail vein of mice. 6 hrs of lag-time was given to obtain the maximized accumulation of drug-encapsulated liposomes in the tumor tissues. Subsequently, the tumor tissues of mice were stimulated with another heating treatment for 30 min using a water bath in order for bursting-out of drugs from the thermosensitive liposomes accumulated in the tumor tissues. The tumor size was measured on day 0, 1, 2, 3, 5, 7, 9, 11, 13, and 15 by vernire calipers, and the volume was calculated by the following formula: Volume = $(\text{width of tumor})^2 \times (\text{length of tumor}) \times \pi/6$.

Statistical analysis

The data obtained in our anticancer efficacy study was analyzed statistically with two-tailed unpaired *t*-test using a one-way analysis of variance (ANOVA) test implemented by SigmaPlot 11 software.

Results

Concept design of ELP-incorporated thermosensitive liposome (e-TSL)

To develop the TSL under mild hyperthermia (39–42°C), we introduced a short chain elastin-like polypeptide modified with lipid moieties (ELP-lipid conjugate). An elastin-like polypeptide (ELP) consisting of a [VPGXG]n pentapeptide repeat, where X can be any amino acid except proline, possesses thermosensitivity and a transition temperature that is adjustable according to length, sequence, concentration, pH, and ionic strength [15–18]. The mechanism of this phenomenon is known: a hydrogen bonding interaction between ELP and a water molecule dominates in aqueous solution below the transition temperature (Tt), while an intramolecular ELP hydrophobic interaction is predominant in aqueous solution above the Tt, resulting in a conformational change from a random coil to a β-turn. In the present study, we utilized ELP as a heat-triggered moiety, and a single hydrocarbon tail (stearyl group) was conjugated at the N-terminus of ELP for incorporation into the bilayer of the liposome. The expected ELP-liposome hybrid vesicle is depicted in Figure 1.

ELP-lipid conjugates screening

ELPs are smart biopolymers, which exhibit reversible precipitation above a certain temperature, called inverse phase T_t. We analyzed the T_t of modified ELPs using UV spectrometry. ELPs, thermally sensitive polypeptides with a repeating unit (VPGVG), undergo an inverse temperature phase transition above a certain Tt. Depending on the concentration and the length of the repeating unit (length of peptide), the ELP shows unique features of intermolecular interaction. We prepared five ELP-lipid conjugates with different ELP lengths and identified their T_t, according to the concentration and the number of repeating units. Figure 2 shows the transmittance of ELP-lipid conjugates as a function of temperature and concentration. The phase transition of the ELP-lipid conjugate was observed in all groups undergoing a change of turbidity. Depending on the number of repeating units (the length of ELP) and the concentration, we observed different phase transition behaviors. In the case of a longer ELP-conjugated lipid, a sharp phase transition was observed, whereas a relatively short ELP-conjugated lipid showed a somewhat smooth phase transition. Tt decreased as concentration increased and the sequence became longer, as expected. This is most likely because the intermolecular hydrophobic interaction of ELPs is readily occurred even at the lower temperature. We also confirmed that the temperature-responsive behavior of ELP was maintained, even after modification of the N-terminal peptide.

Drug release study dependent on liposome formulation

We designed the e-TSL composed of four different components, phospholipid, cholesterol, DSPE-PEG, and ELP-lipid conjugates. The temperature-dependent release profile of liposome was investigated using calcein and DOX, which is fluorescent and easy to detect upon release from the liposome.

The effect of main lipid. We prepared five liposomes with different ratios of DPPC and DSPC, in order to investigate the effect of the main lipid on temperature-responsive release of liposomes. The liposomes were formulated with phospholipid (DPPC, DSPC, and DPPC/DSPC), DSPE-PEG, cholesterol, and SA-V6 (phospholipid:DSPE-PEG:cholesterol:SA-V6 = 55:2:10:0.55). Figure 3 shows that while T_t increased as the ratio of DPPC decreased, it remained lower than the original melting temperature of DSPC because of the other elements (DSPE-PEG, ELP, and cholesterol). Compared to other liposomes with different formulations, liposomes composed of DPPC and DPPC with 25% DSPC showed similar calcein leakage profiles.

Cholesterol effect. Next, we verified the effect of cholesterol on the release profile. It is well known that cholesterol is a major factor of membrane stability and fluidity. The release profile of 6 different liposomes with different ratios of cholesterol was identified. As expected, the release of encapsulated molecules was delayed by increasing the ratio of cholesterol. Additionally, the maximum released amount was lower in accordance with higher cholesterol content (Figure 4).

ELP effect. The length of ELP, based on the repeating unit (VPGVG), caused variations in the release profile. With a shorter ELP-lipid incorporated liposome, the T_t of release from the liposome was increased. It correlated well with the trends of reverse T_t of ELP, depending on the length of peptide and temperature. Presumably, because of the destabilization of the liposome membrane induced by the conformational change of ELP from random coil to β-turn, the encapsulated molecules are released from the liposome. With the longer ELP, the T_t of the liposome is lower than that of the liposome with the shorter ELP (data not shown).

The role of ELP was investigated as a heat trigger in this liposome system. The amount of DOX release from the liposome was determined by ELP above 37°C. According to the formulation, the DOX release was different from about 70 to 100% over mild hyperthermic temperature (Figure 5). There was an inverse relationship between T_t and the amount of ELP for drug release: the higher the amount of ELP, the lower the T_t. At the same time, the liposomes with higher percentage of ELP showed ~40% of drug leakage below 40°C (Figure 5).

Optimized liposome formulation for mild hyperthermia

Generally, the temperature range of clinically relevant mild hyperthermia is from 39–42°C. The first requisite of TSL for mild

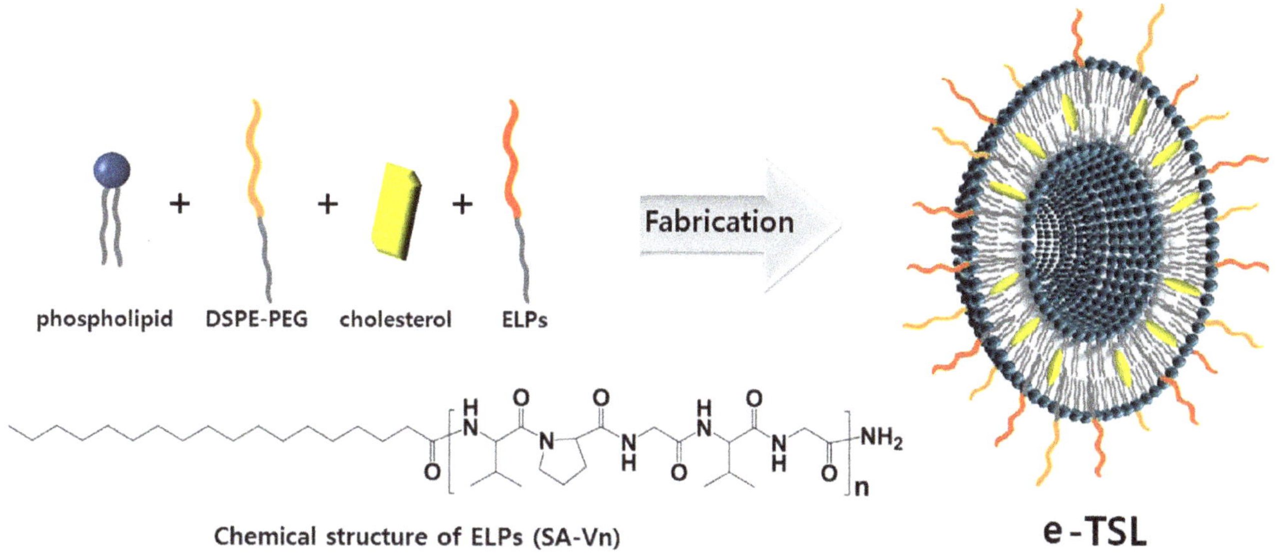

Figure 1. Schematic diagram of e-TSL and the chemical structure of ELP-lipid conjugates.

hyperthermia is a very sharp drug release within 3–4°C. Formulation screening for e-TSL identified the DPPC only or DPPC/DSPC (75/25) as a main lipid, cholesterol as a stabilizer, and SA-V3 as a trigger. With the 3 factors for thermosensitive peptide-incorporated liposome, further optimization studies were carried out to refine and improve the performance of liposome. As we already identified, the observed maximum drug release percentage at 42°C decreased by increasing the mol% content of cholesterol. In most of the tested liposome formulations, the influence of SA-V3 on temperature dependent drug release at 42°C was observed and it was more than 80% within 5 minutes. With higher amounts of SA-V3, the temperature sensitivity for

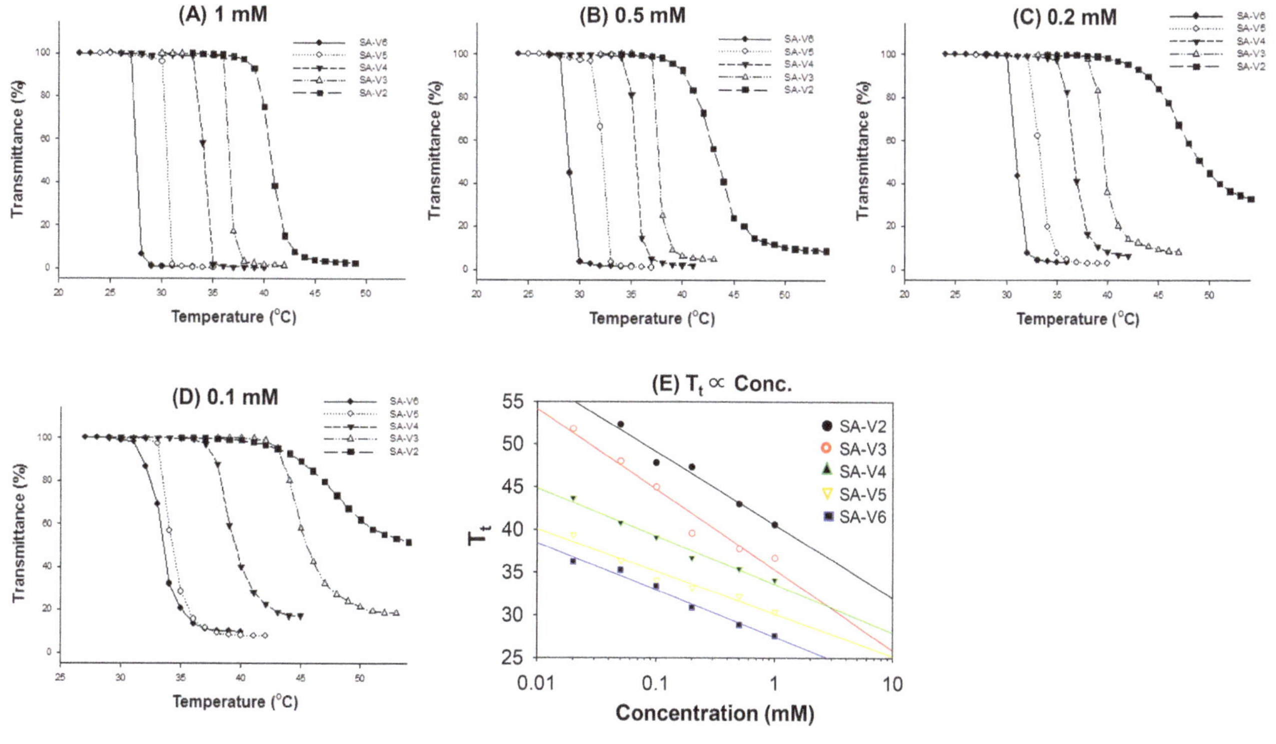

Figure 2. Transmittance profile of ELP-lipid conjugates of (A) 1 mM, (B) 0.5 mM, (C) 0.2 mM, and (D) 0.1 mM in PBS at pH 7.4., and transition temperature as function of the concentration (mM) of various ELP-lipid conjugates (E). The turbidity of ELP-lipid conjugates were characterized by monitoring transmittance at 280 nm as a function of temperature. Solution of ELP-lipids conjugates were heated at a constant rate of 1°C/min. The transition temperature (Tt) was defined as the temperature at which the solution of ELP-lipid conjugate reached 50% of transmittance. Data is shown as mean ± S.D. (n = 3).

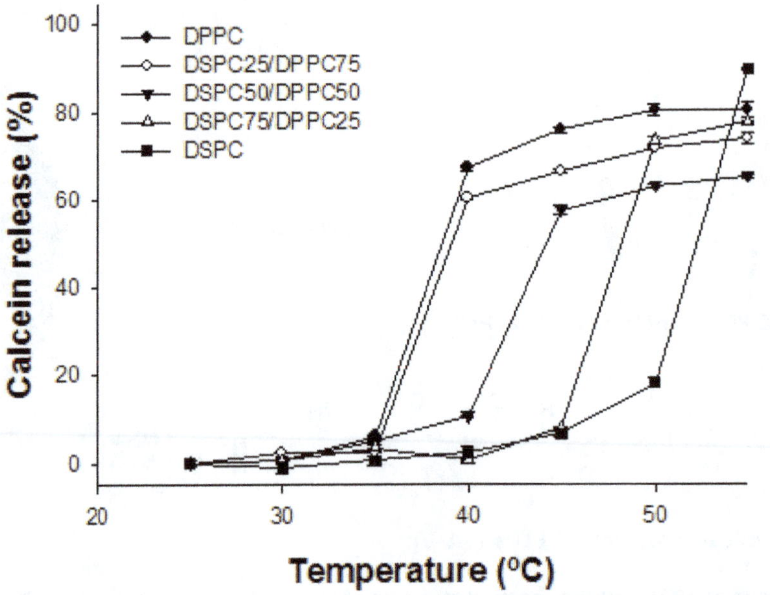

Figure 3. Calcein release profile of the liposome with the formulations of varied phospholipid compositions. Phospholipid (DPPC/DSPC = 100-X/X):DSPE-PEG:cholesterol:SA-V6 = 55:2:10:0.55 (X = 0, 25, 50, 75, and 100). Samples were measured after 5 min incubation at desired temperatures from 25 to 55°C by fluorometry at Ex. 493 nm/Em. 513 nm. Data is shown as mean ± S.D. (n = 3).

drug release increased. However, drug leakage in the temperature range of 37–39°C occurred as the mol% contents of SA-V3 increased, especially for the DPPC liposome. By considering the effect of cholesterol and SA-V3, the optimal formulation was finalized as the liposome composed of DPPC/DSPE-PEG/cholesterol/SA-V3 (= 55/2/15/0.41) for stable blood circulation and effective drug release under mild hyperthermia. Actually, the liposome composed of DPPC showed phase transition under hyperthermia, even without ELP. To confirm the effect of ELP as a trigger on a screened formulation, liposomes were prepared with or without SA-V3, and their drug release profiles were checked (Figure 6). As shown in Figure 6, the liposome in the absence of SA-V3 showed a drug release of less than 10% of encapsulated DOX under mild hyperthermia. However, the maximum amount of drug release and the temperature sensitivity of the ELP-free liposome were much lower than that of the ELP-incorporated liposome.

Size and morphology of e-TSL

With the optimized ELP-incorporated liposome, the size and morphology of the liposomes were identified. The diameter of the liposome was 161 ± 4 nm and polydispersity index (PdI) value was relatively good (less than 0.05). To visualize the DOX-encapsulated liposome, transmission electron microscopy (TEM) was utilized. TEM is a powerful tool for the structural analysis of nano-sized materials. It clearly showed round-shaped liposomes, and

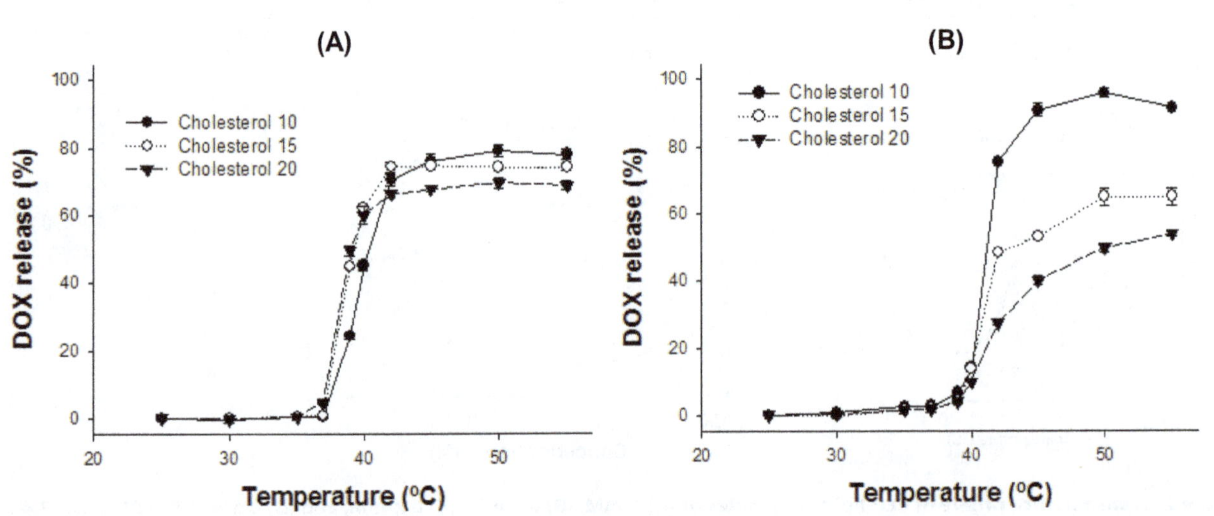

Figure 4. DOX release profile of the liposome with the formulations. (A) DPPC:DSPE-PEG:cholesterol:SA-V3 = 55:2:X:55 and (B) DPPC/DSPC (75/25):DSPE-PEG:cholesterol:SA-V3 = 55:2:X:55 (X = 10, 15, or 20). The amounts of DOX release were measured after 5 min incubation at desired temperature from 25 to 55°C by fluorometry at Ex. 490 nm/Em. 615 nm. Data is shown as mean ± S.D. (n = 3).

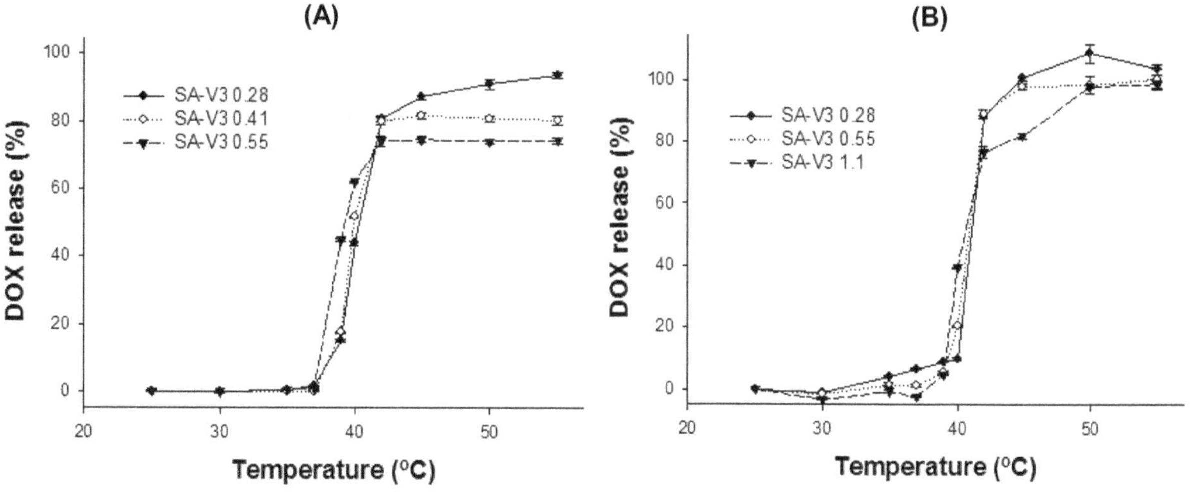

Figure 5. DOX release profile of the liposome with the formulations. (A) DPPC:DSPE-PEG:cholesterol:SA-V3 = 55:2:15:Y_1 (Y_1 = 0.28, 0.41, or 0.55) and (B) DPPC/DSPC (75/25):DSPE-PEG:cholesterol:SA-V3 = 55:2:10:Y_2 (Y_2 = 0.28, 0.55, or 1.1). The amounts of DOX release were measured after 5 min incubation at desired temperature from 25 to 55°C by fluorometry at Ex. 490 nm/Em. 615 nm. Data is shown as mean ± S.D. (n = 3).

visualized the presence of DOX as an electron-opaque band, which was loaded into the liposome by ammonium sulfate gradient procedures. The size of liposomes visualized by TEM corresponded to the DLS results. Liposomes with varying contents of DOX had different distributions in the TEM images (Figure 7). Encapsulated DOX was bundled with relatively low loading amounts of DOX. However, encapsulated DOX became looped in liposomes with a high content of DOX. The mean size of each liposome determined by DLS was 171±3 nm (bundle type type) and 177±2 nm (loop type). We also observed structural changes of DOX-encapsulated liposomes at 25, 37, and 42°C. The TEM images indicated drug encapsulation and release from the liposome. As we had already confirmed, over 80% of the encapsulated amount of DOX in the liposome was released at 42°C. The looped form of DOX disappeared in the image obtained for the liposome group incubated at 42°C (Figure 8).

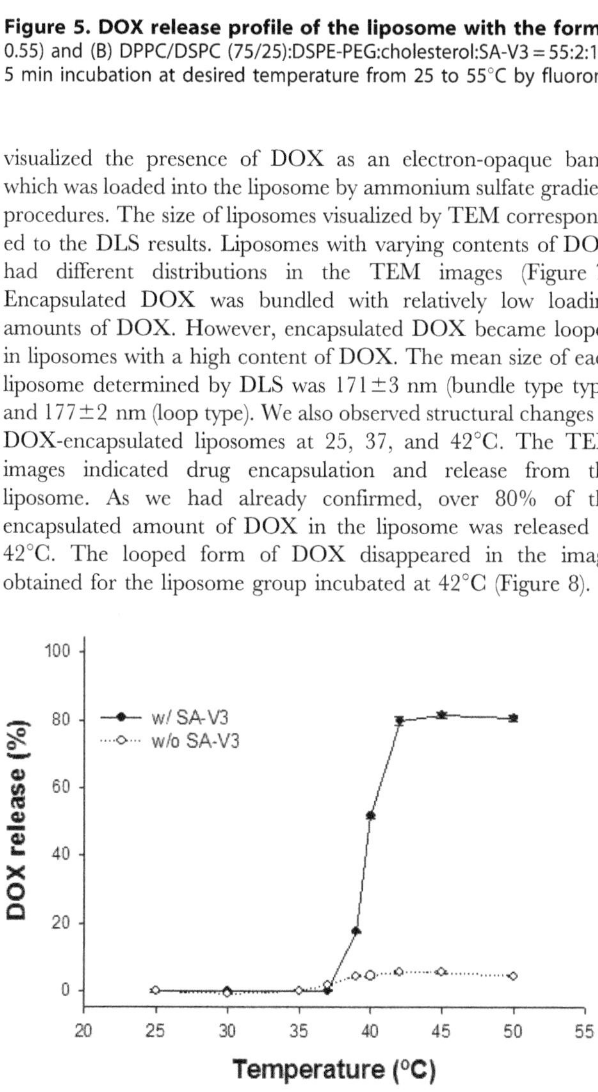

Figure 6. DOX release profile of the liposome with the formulations. DPPC:DSPE-PEG:cholesterol = 55:2:15 in the presence/absence of SA-V3 (molar ratio:0.41). The amounts of DOX release were measured after 5 min incubation at desired temperature from 25 to 55°C by fluorometry at Ex. 490 nm/Em. 615 nm. Data is shown as mean ± S.D. (n = 3).

Molecular dynamics simulations of lipid bilayers

Lipid bilayers, which consist of DPPC, DSPE-PEG, cholesterol, and ELP-lipid conjugates (SA-Vn, n = 1, 2, and 3), were simulated at 5 different molar concentrations of cholesterol and ELP for 2 μs. Figure 9 shows snapshots from the beginning and end of the simulation (at the molar ratio of liposome formulation, DPPC:DSPE-PEG:cholesterol:SA-Vn = 55:2:15:0.41). The peptide chains of ELP, which were initially positioned on the bilayer surface, insert into the bilayer because of the interaction between hydrophobic amino acids and lipid tails, as observed in our previous all-atom simulations [28]. The xy-plane areas (the bilayer surface) and energies for each system reach steady-state values within 1.5 μs, indicating that the simulations are equilibrated within the simulated time scales (Supplementary data, Figure S1). Note that our previous all-atom simulations showed that ELPs in water become more collapsed and folded as temperature increases, while those in lipid bilayers become linearly swollen with mostly random conformation at increased temperature, indicating the structural difference of ELPs in aqueous and membrane environments. This implies that the bilayer may be disrupted more effectively by extended random coils of ELPs than by the compact ELPs.

Experiments have shown that the lateral mobility of lipids significantly depends on the bilayer phase, indicating that the phase of lipid bilayers can be characterized by calculating lateral diffusion coefficients of lipids [30,31]. Since the MARTINI FF has successfully predicted the experimentally observed lateral diffusivities of DPPC lipids at different phases [26], we calculated lateral diffusion coefficients (D) of lipids from the slopes of the mean-square displacements (MSD) of lipids as a function of time. Figure 10 shows that D drastically increase at higher concentrations of SA-V3, indicating an effect of ELP on the lipid mobility, presumably because the inserted ELP disorders the bilayer, as observed in our previous all-atom simulation. SA-V1 and SA-V2, which consist of shorter ELPs, show that lateral diffusivities do not change much at different ELP concentrations, indicating that shorter ELPs do not significantly increase the lipid dynamics. This implies that lipids are more disordered by longer ELPs than by shorter ones, and thus the lipid bilayer with shorter ELPs should have the higher Tt, consistent with our experimental observation of higher Tt of the liposome with shorter ELP chains. For the

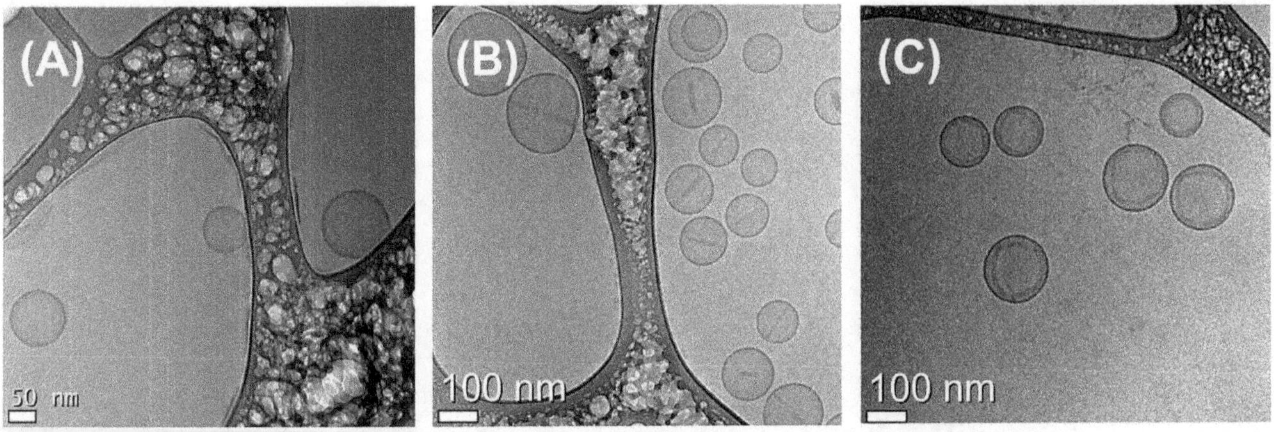

Figure 7. Cryo-TEM images with varying amounts of DOX in the liposome. DPPC:DSPE-PEG:cholesterol:SA-V3 = 55:2:15:0.41, with (A) liposome only, (B) 300 μg DOX/mL and (C) 500 μg DOX/mL.

effect of cholesterols, lateral diffusion coefficients were significantly reduced in the presence of cholesterol, indicating that cholesterol inhibits the dynamic motion and permeation of the bilayer. This effect of cholesterol on lipid dynamics is not influenced by the ELP length.

In vivo drug accumulation and antitumor efficacy study

To investigate DOX delivery *in vivo*, we carried out a drug accumulation study in the tumor. The available drug amount in a tumor site is closely related with antitumor efficacy. We confirmed that the blood circulation of the DPPC-based liposome decreased gradually with time, and that the half-life of the DOX-encapsulated liposome *in vivo* was about 2.5 hr, as shown in a previous study [19]. Because tumors have inherently leaky vessels, nano-sized particles are easy to accumulate by EPR. In this study, we induced enhanced EPR by locally heating (42°C) the tumor site for 30 min before i.v. injection; the detailed procedures are described in Figure 11. As shown in Figure 11, we identified drug accumulation in the tumor at 1, 6, and 12 hr time points after injection (Figure 12). Compared to the free DOX-treated group, liposomal DOX (e-TSL-DOX) showed better accumulation in tumors at every time point with or without preheating. In particular, the group of e-TSL-DOX with preheating showed significant drug accumulation at 6 hr after i.v. injection; the difference was 5 fold with e-TSL without preheating, 11 fold with free DOX without preheating, and 31 fold with free DOX with preheating. In case of free DOX, the group without preheating resulted in more drug accumulation than its preheated group contrary to e-TSL group. To support the drug accumulation data, the histological observation of intratumoral distribution of doxorubicin was carried out. The significant fluorescence of DOX was detected only in the group of e-TSL-DOX with preheating (6 hr lag time), which was in alignment with aforementioned drug accumulation results (Figure 13).

Finally, we evaluated the antitumor efficacy of e-TSL with optimized hyperthermia protocol based on the results of drug accumulation study (preheating and 6 hr lag time). In the presence/absence of the mild hyperthermia, the tumor regression effect of e-TSL is shown in Figure 14. The mice group treated with e-TSL showed better antitumor efficacy than other groups and delayed tumor growth, especially with mild hyperthermia. The trend of antitumor effect was similar with the result of drug accumulation study. The more doxorubicin was accumulated, the more effective antitumor efficacy was outcome.

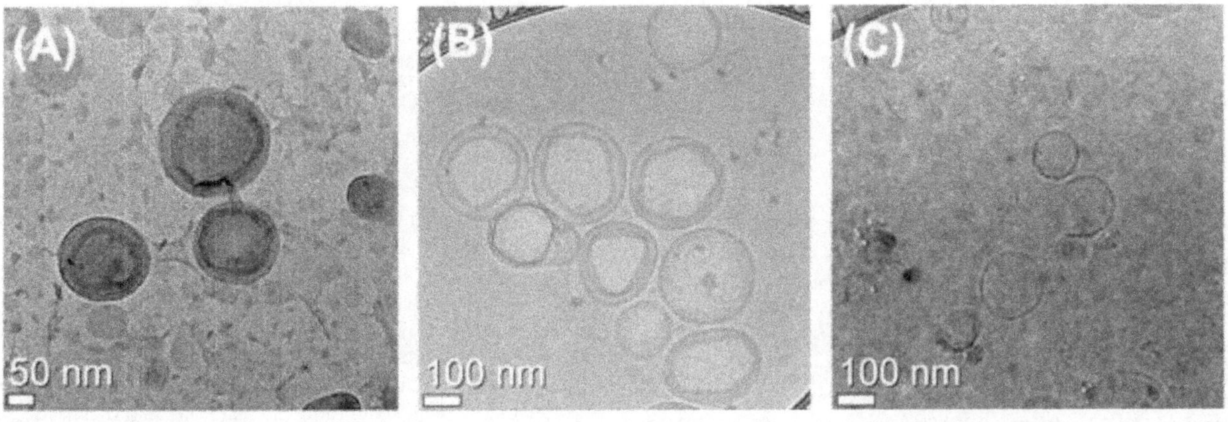

Figure 8. Cryo-TEM images of the liposome at (A) 25°C, (B) 37°C, and (C) 42°C. Liposomes were composed of the formulation DPPC:DSPE-PEG:cholesterol:SA-V3 = 55:2:15:0.41 and heat-treated for 5 min at indicated temperature in advance and followed by general cryo-TEM measurement.

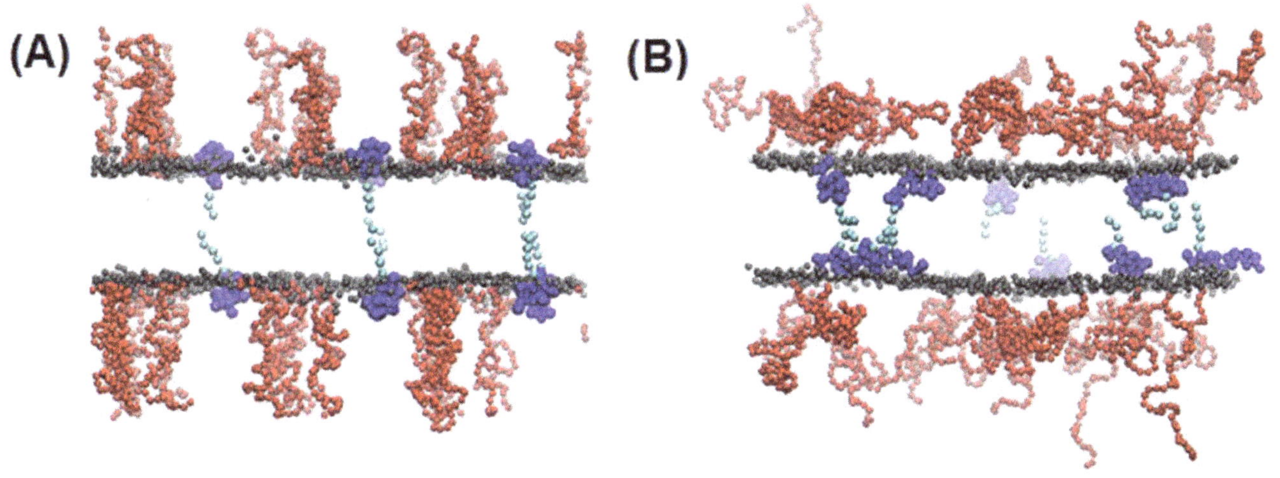

Figure 9. Snapshots at the (A) beginning (0 ns) and (B) end (2 μs) of the simulation of the bilayer system. The molar ratio of liposome formulation is DPPC:DSPE-PEG:cholesterol:SA-Vn 55:2:15:0.41. Gray, red, dark-, and light-blue colors respectively represent the lipid-head phosphate, PEG, ELP head (peptide), and tail (carbon chain) groups. For clarity, lipid tail, water, and ion beads are omitted. The images were created with Visual Molecular Dynamics [29].

Discussion

For an ideal antitumor treatment, enhanced drug delivery at the target site with minimized toxicity at off target sites, the TSLs have to be stable in circulating blood (at 37°C) and burst-released as soon as they are exposed to mildly hyperthermic temperatures. The most clinically-advanced TSL, lysolipid-containing temperature sensitive liposome (LTSL), was developed by Needham and Dewhirst and is now under clinical trials. LTSL is formulated with lyso-phospholipid, DSPE-PEG, and DPPC. Lysolipid has only one acyl chain, and tends to form a micelle structure. Due to these characteristics, lysolipid induces stabilization of grain boundaries, which are formed between the solid and liquid domain of a liposome upon heating. Rapid drug release from the LTSL occurred through lysolipid-stabilized pores when mild hyperthermia was applied. Despite the high responsiveness to heating, LTSL was reported to have the low stability of LTSL in *in vitro* serum-containing media (37°C) and *in vivo* blood circulation [32,33]. To realize TSL formulation that allows for both physiological stability and high responsiveness to heating, we introduced cholesterol as membrane stabilizer and ELP as heat-triggered moiety to liposome. By controlling the liposome composition of DPPC (or DSPC), cholesterol, DSPE-PEG, and ELP, the Tt and amount of drug release was tunable.

To rapidly test thermosensitivity of e-TSL, calcein fluorescent dye-loaded and various ELP-lipid conjugates incorporating e-TSLs were prepared and checked calcein release. Of these, SA-V6- loaded e-TSL exhibited the optimal release (data not shown). Even if Tt of SA-V6 itself was shown to be below 36°C (Figure 2), it was shifted above 36°C after calcein loading (Figure 3). Because calcein was added to the hydration buffer before extrusion in the liposome preparation procedure, it happened to be inserted into the lipid bilayer membrane and also encapsulated inside the inner core of liposome. The inserted calcein molecules probably interfere with the hydrophobic interaction of ELP, resulting in the shift of Tt. On the other hand, to load DOX into liposome, the

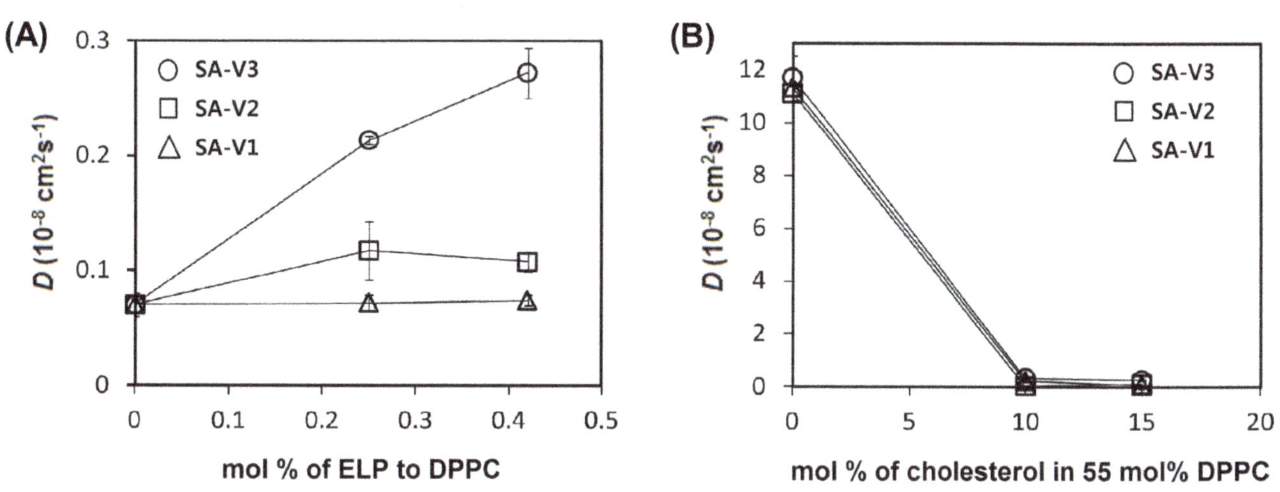

Figure 10. Average lateral diffusion coefficients (*D*) of DPPC lipids. *D* was calculated from the slopes of the mean-square displacements in the xy-plane (the direction perpendicular to the bilayer normal), for the simulation systems with different ELP lengths (SA-V1, -V2, and V3) as functions of the molar ratio of (A) ELP and (B) cholesterol.

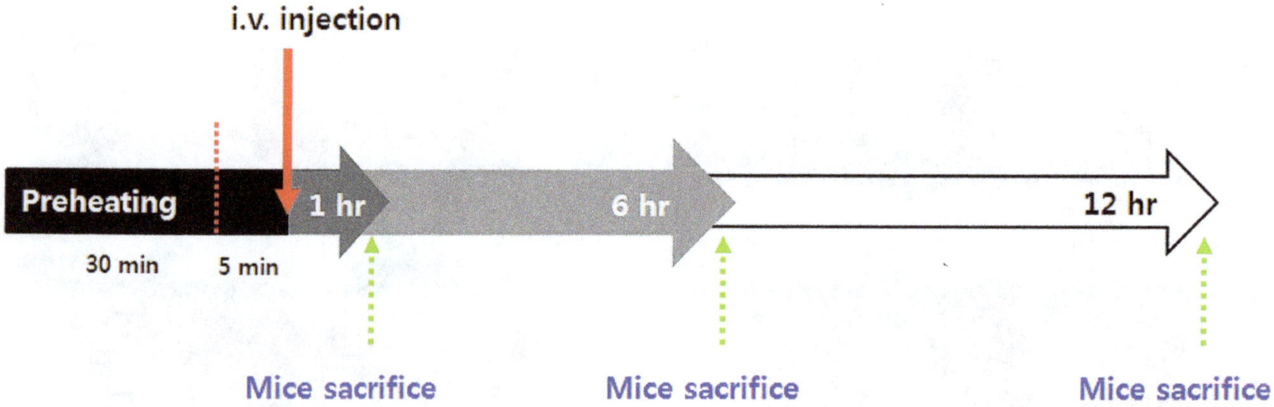

Figure 11. The protocol of the drug accumulation study with e-TSL-DOX and free DOX, administered under mild hyperthermia.

remote loading method using ammonium sulfate gradient was employed, inducing the encapsulation of DOX inside the inner core as crystallized, and the encapsulated DOX did not influence on the properties of ELP conjugated lipid bilayer membrane. As shown by Figure 2E, SA-V2, SA-V3, and SA-V4 were evaluated as the relevant candidates for thermally triggered moiety under the mild hyperthermia temperature (40~45°C). We assessed the DOX release profile of e-TSL comprising SA-V2, SA-V3, and SA-V4 (data not shown). Among these, SA-V3 was chosen for further *invitro* and *invivo* studies as highly potent profile was shown.

We found that the amount of drug release was related to cholesterol content, and the T_t could be finely tuned by the

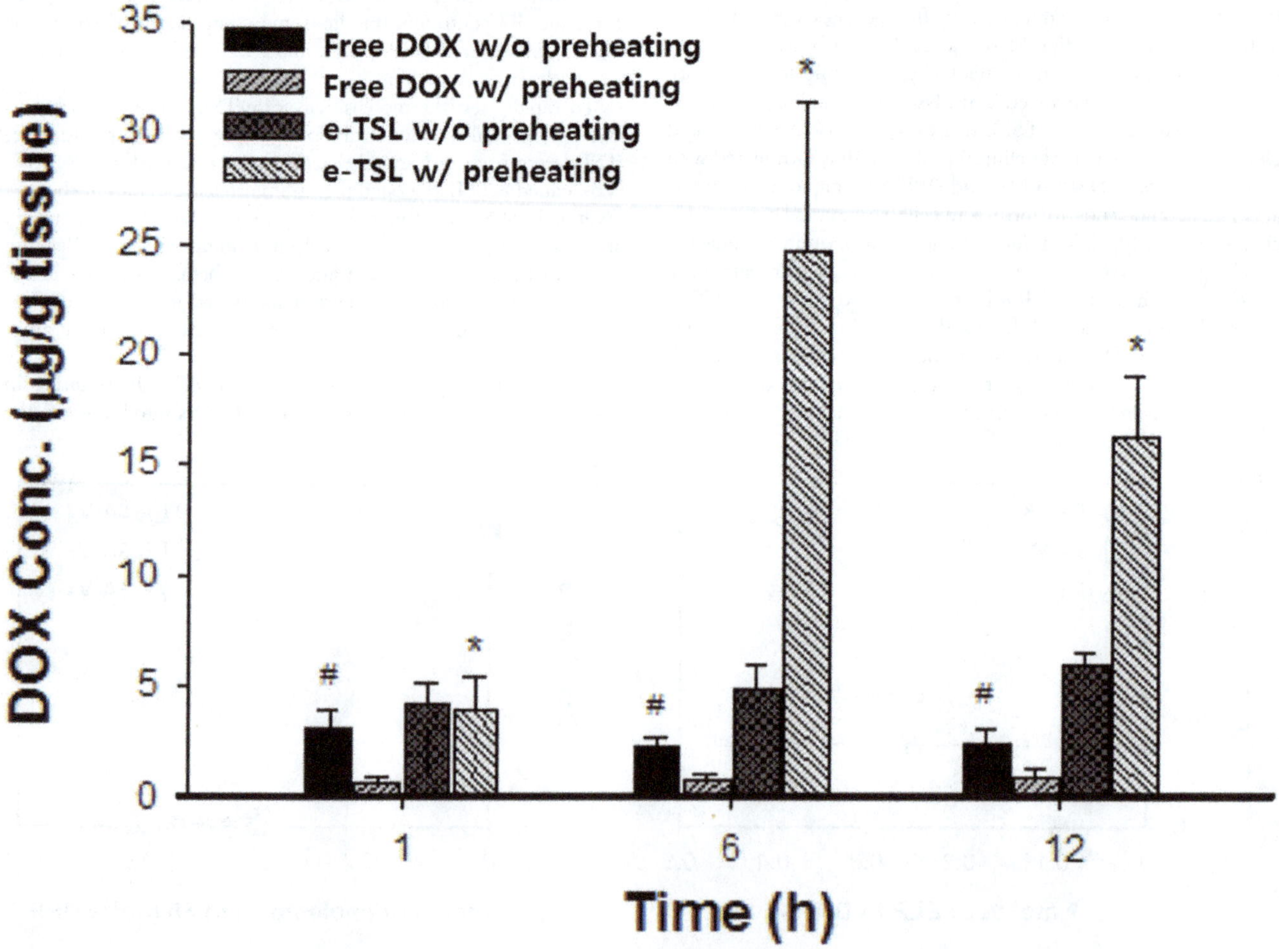

Figure 12. DOX accumulation in the tumor at 1, 6, and 12 hr after i.v. injection combined with preheating. *, $p<0.005$, #, $p<0.001$, significant difference compared to e-TSL without preheating and free DOX with preheating.

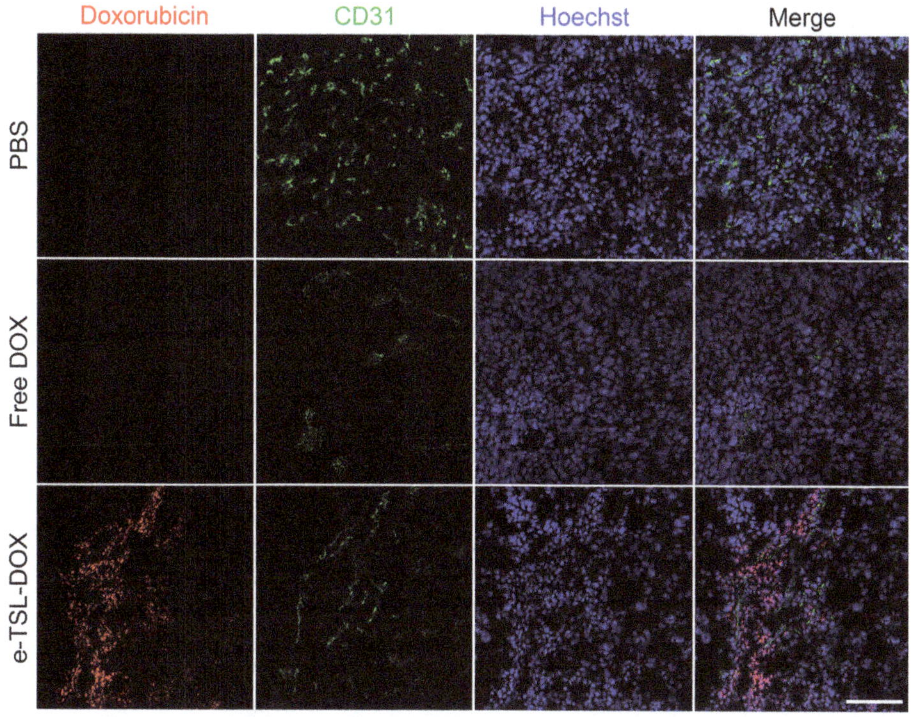

Figure 13. Intratumoral distribution of DOX. Red, DOX; green, CD31 (endothelial marker); blue, Hoechst (nuclear marker). Scale bar, 100 μm.

length/amount of ELP-lipid conjugate in the liposome. For thermosensitive liposome-based therapy under mild hyperthermia, we carefully analyzed and selected the formulation after screening. To avoid large leakages of the encapsulated drug during blood circulation, a higher concentration of cholesterol was necessary for a stable liposome. The T_t of drug release was increased with incorporation of a minor amount of ELP. Taken together, the balance between the two factors, cholesterol and ELP-lipid conjugate, was important for preparation of a certain-temperature sensitive liposome formulation. When the amount of cholesterol in a tested formulation was more than 10 mol%, drug release at 42°C was less than 70%. While the addition of more ELP-lipid conjugate in the formulation could compromise maximum drug release, drug leakage was observed at 37–39°C. Drug leakage is thought to be mainly dependent on the amount of cholesterol, but is partly affected by relatively a higher incorporation of ELP-lipid conjugate (>1.1 mol%). The effect of ELP-lipid conjugate on the drug release of liposomes is not only the control of T_t but also of drug leakage. The findings of our simulation study compared favorably with our experimental observations, which showed that the extent of DOX or calcein release increased at a higher concentration of ELP but decreased at a higher concentration of cholesterol.

The optimized liposome formulation showed somewhat long blood circulation (>2.5 hr) [15]. To maximize antitumor efficacy, with optimized formulation of e-TSL, we set up the treatment protocol combined with mild hyperthermia in mice. The advantage of tumor tissue for drug accumulation is an EPR effect, which we enhanced by heating the tumor prior to i.v. injection of the DOX-encapsulated liposome. The hyperthermia in tumors may have increased vascular permeability by widening the gaps of endothelial walls which were preserved for some time after heat treatment [34]. We utilized mild hyperthermia as the stimulus for drug release as well as a booster for the EPR effect. The optimized liposome formulation (DPPC/DSPE-PEG/Cholesterol/SA-V3 = 55/2/15/0.41) was stable enough to circulate in the blood for a relatively longer period. The improved EPR phenomenon was obtained with e-TSL but not with free DOX. With e-TSL-DOX, induction of increased drug accumulation by improved EPR was evident by 6 hr. These opposing trends in drug accumulation with EPR and preheating between free DOX and e-TSL-DOX is likely because the behavior of a small molecule and a nanoparticle is different in the tissue; tumor perfusion resulting from hyperthermia increases perfusion both in and out of the tissue, and a small molecule like DOX can easily diffuse out of the tumor. And the blood half-life of free DOX in mice (12 min) is significantly shorter than e-TSL (2.03±0.77 hr) [35]. Therefore e-TSL that possesses the long circulating property may have more chances to extravasate into tumor site. In the case of LTSL, the heat treatment was carried out immediately after i.v. injection, and drug accumulation and delayed tumor growth were improved compared to that with local heat exposure after 24 hr. e-TSL with high thermal sensitivity and stability exhibited superior drug accumulation in tumors with increased time (by 6 hr). Similar with the drug accumulation result, the effect of tumor growth delay of e-TSL was better than free DOX–treated groups. Therefore, determination of a treatment schedule is an important factor in yielding improved therapeutic effects with TSLs. High stability under physiological conditions would enable TSLs carrying desired biological factors to stably circulate through blood vessels in a body. Subsequently, external stimulation to the defective site to induce mild hyperthermia could trigger the release of cargo-content in a spatially- and temporally-controlled manner with therapeutically available amounts that assist the self-healing potential of the diseased tissue.

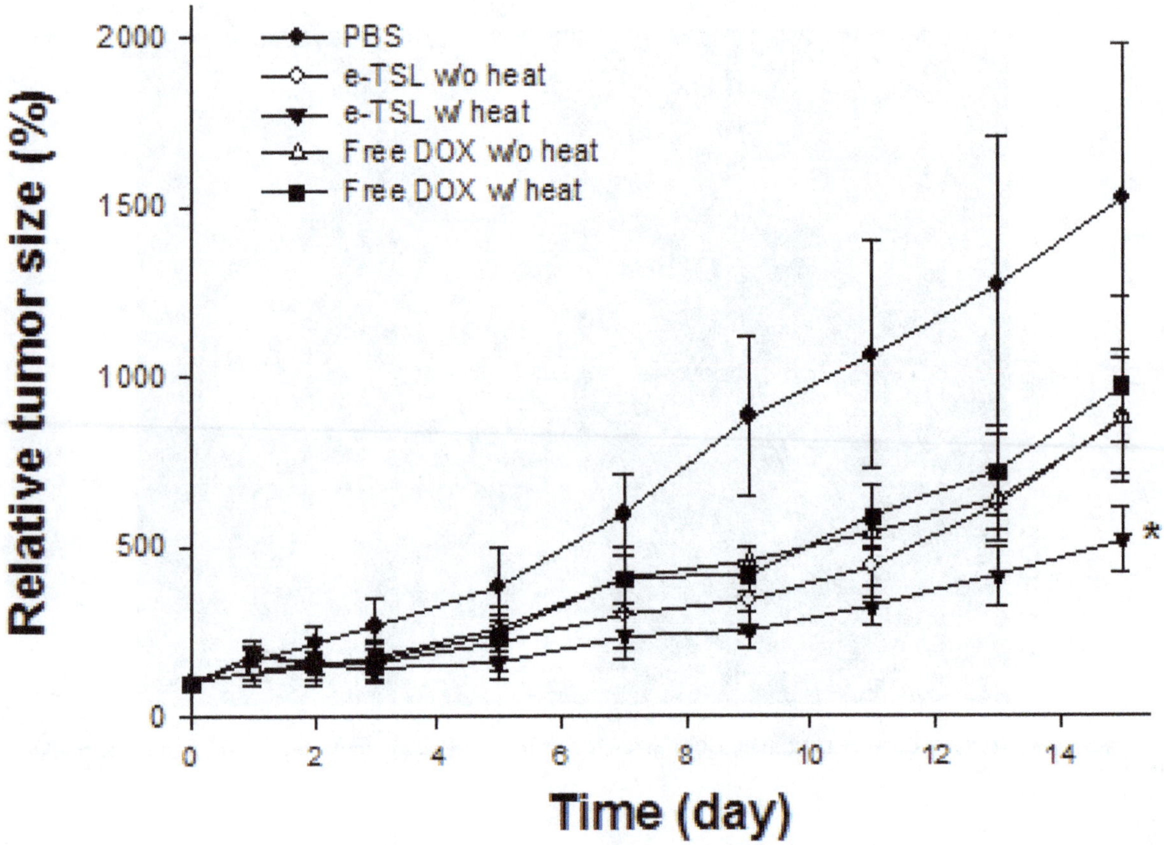

Figure 14. Antitumor efficacy of e-TSL and free DOX in the presence/absence of mild hyperthermia. e-TSL and free DOX were administered (5 mg DOX/kg) into tumor bearing BALB/c mice 5 min after preheating (30 min of water bath) and followed by mild hyperthermia (42°C, water bath) after 6 hrs. *, $p<0.05$, significant difference compared to free DOX and PBS (control).

Conclusion

We have designed and optimized the formulations of highly thermosensitive liposomes by control of DPPC, DSPC, DSPE-PEG, cholesterol, and ELP-lipid conjugates. During the optimization of formulation, we found that the concentration and balance of cholesterol and ELP-lipid conjugates were the main factors in the amount and temperature of drug release. The characteristics of selected formulations were investigated *in vitro* drug release, cryo-TEM analysis, simulation study, DOX accumulation study, and antitumor efficacy study. The results demonstrated that, in our system, e-TSL was very versatile for the modulation of amount and temperature of drug release, as we intended. Our liposome system was confirmed to be highly stable in physiological environments. It is expected that mild hyperthermia before i.v. injection and lag time after i.v. injection would play important role for maximize the drug accumulation. We found that treatment protocol optimization, in addition to the formulation of the liposome, is important for reflecting the advantage of TSL formulation.

Supporting Information

Figure S1 The bilayer size in xy dimension (top), which equals the bilayer surface areas, and energies (bottom) of simulation systems as functions of time.

Author Contributions

Conceived and designed the experiments: HRK SMP ESP. Performed the experiments: SMP JMC MSK SJP JN. Analyzed the data: SMP JMC HL HRK . Contributed reagents/materials/analysis tools: SJP MSK JMC JN. Wrote the paper: SMP HRK.

References

1. Salata O (2004) Applications of nanoparticles in biology and medicine. J Nanobiotechnology 2: 1–6.
2. Manzoor AA, Linder LH, Landon CD, Park JY, Simnick AJ, et al. (2012) Overcoming limitations in nanoparticle drug delivery: Triggered, intravascular release to improve drug penetration into tumors. Cancer Res 72: 5566–5575.
3. Haidar ZS (2010) Bio-inspired/-functional colloidal core-shell polymeric-based nanosystems: Technology promise in tissue engineering, bioimaging and nanomedicine. Polymers 2: 323–352.
4. Tabata Y (2009) Biomaterial technology for tissue engineering applications. J R Soc Interface 6: S311–S324.
5. Koo OM, Rubinstein I, Onyuksel H (2005) Role of nanotechnology in targeted drug delivery and imaging: a concise review. Nanomedicine: Nanotechnology, Biology, and Medicine 1: 193–212.
6. Li L, Hagen TLM, Bolkestein M, Gasselhuber A, Yatvin J, et al. (2013) Improved intratumoral nanoparticle extravasation and penetration by mild hyperthermia. J Control Release 167: 130–137.
7. Li L, Hagen TLM, Hossann M, Süss R, van Rhoon GC, et al. (2013) Mild hyperthermia triggered doxorubicin release from optimized stealth thermosensitive liposomes improves intratumoral drug delivery and efficacy. J Control Release 168: 142–150.

8. Kong G, Anyarambhatla G, Petros WP, Braun RD, Colvin OM, et al. (2000) Efficacy of liposomes and hyperthermia in a human tumor xenograft model: Importance of triggered drug release. Cancer Res 60: 6950–6957.
9. Tagami T, Ernsting MJ, Li SD (2011) Efficient tumor regression by a single and low dose treatment with a novel and enhanced formulation of thermosensitive liposomal doxorubicin. J Control Release 152: 303–309.
10. Jeong B, Bae YH, Lee DS, Kim SW (1997) Biodegradable block copolymers as injectable drug delivery systems. Nature 388: 860–862.
11. Bae YH, Okano T, Hsu R, Kim SW (1987) Thermo-sensitive polymers as on-off switches for drug release. Makromol Chem Rapid Commun 8: 481–485.
12. Unezaki S, Maruyama K, Takahashi N, Koyama M, Yuda T, et al. (1994) Enhanced delivery and antitumor activity of doxorubicin using long-circulating thermosensitive liposomes containing amphiphatic polyethylene glycol in combination with local hyperthermia. Pharm Res 11: 1180–1185.
13. Maruyama K, Unezaki S, Takahashi N, Iwatsuru M (1993) Enhanced delivery of doxorubicin to tumor by long-circulating thermosensitive liposomes and local hyperthermia. Biochim Biophys Acta 1149: 209–216.
14. Allen TM, Cullis PR (2013) Liposomal drug delivery systems: From concept to clinical applications. Adv Drug Deliv Rev 65: 36–48.
15. Betre H, Ong SR, Guilak F, Chilkoti A, Fermor B, et al. (2006) Chondrocytic differentiation of human adipose tissue-derived adult stem cells in elastin-like polypeptide. Biomaterials 27: 91–99.
16. Nettles DL, Chilkoti A, Setton LA (2010) Applications of elastin-like polypeptides in tissue engineering. Adv Drug Deliv Rev 62: 1479–1485.
17. Dreher MR, Raucher D, Balu N, Colvin OM, Ludeman SM, et al. (2003) Evaluation of an elastin-like polypeptide–doxorubicin conjugate for cancer therapy. J Control Release 91: 31–43.
18. Liu W, Dreher MR, Furgeson DY, Peixoto KV, Yuan H, et al. (2006) Tumor accumulation, degradation and pharmacokinetics of elastin-like polypeptides in nude mice. J Control Release 116: 170–178.
19. Park SM, Kim MS, Park S-J. Park ES, Choi K-S, et al. (2013) Novel temperature-triggered liposome with high stability: Formulation, in vitro evaluation, and in vivo study combined with high-intensity focused ultrasound (HIFU), J Control Release 170: 373–379.
20. Hess B, Kutzner C, van der Spoel D, Lindahl E (2008) Gromacs 4: Algorithms for highly efficient, load-balanced, and scalable molecular simulation. J Chemical Theory and Computation 4: 435–447.
21. Lindahl E, Hess B, van der Spoel D (2001) Gromacs 3.0: A package for molecular simulation and trajectory analysis. J Mol Modelin 7: 306–317.
22. Van Der Spoel D, Lindahl E, Hess B, Groenhof G, Mark AE, et al. (2005) Gromacs: Fast, flexible, and free. J Comp Chem 26: 1701–1718.
23. Marrink SJ, de Vries AH, Mark AE (2004) Coarse grained model for semiquantitative lipid simulations. J Phys Chem B 108: 750–760.
24. Marrink SJ, Risselada HJ, Yefimov S, Tieleman DP, de Vries AH (2007) The Martini force field: coarse grained model for biomolecular simulations. J Phys Chem B 111: 7812–7824.
25. Monticelli L, Kandasamy SK, Periole X, Larson RG, Tieleman DP, et al. (2008) The Martini coarse-grained force field: extension to proteins. J Chem Theory and Comp 4: 819–834.
26. Marrink SJ, Risselada J, Mark AE (2005) Simulation of gel phase formation and melting in lipid bilayers using a coarse grained model. Chem Phys Lipids. 135: 223–244.
27. Berendsen HJC, Postma JPM, van Gunsteren WF, DiNola A, Haak JR (1984) Molecular-dynamics with coupling to an external bath. J Chem Phys. 81: 3684–3690.
28. Lee H, Kim HR, Larson RG, Park JC (2012) Effects of the size, shape, and structural transition of thermosensitive polypeptides on the stability of lipid bilayers and liposomes. Macromolecule 45: 7304–7312.
29. Humphrey W, Dalke A, Schulten K (1996) Vmd: Visual molecular dynamics. J Mol Graph 14: 33–38.
30. Nagle JF, Tristram-Nagle S (2000) Structure of lipid bilayers. Biochimica Et Biophysica Acta-Reviews on Biomembranes 1469: 159–195.
31. Koynova R, Caffrey M (1998) Phases and phase transitions of the phosphatidylcholines. Biochimica Et Biophysica Acta 1376: 91–145.
32. Sandström NC, Ickenstein LM, Mayer LD, Edwards K (2005) Effect of lipid segregation and lysolipid dissociation on drug release from thermosensitive liposomes. J Control Release 107: 131–142.
33. Banno B, Ickenstein LM, Chiu GN, Bally MB, Thewalt J, et al. (2010) The functional roles of poly(ethylene glycol)-lipid and lysolipid in the drug retention and release from lysolipid-containing thermosensitive liposomes invitro and invivo. J Pharm Sci 99(5): 2295–2308.
34. Huang SK, Stauffer PR, Hong K, Guo JWH, Philips TL, et al. (1994) Liposomes and hyperthermia in mice: Increased tumor uptake and therapeutic efficacy of doxorubicin in sterically stabilized liposomes. Cancer Res 54: 2186–2191.
35. Gabizon AA (1992) Selective tumor localization and improved therapeutic index of anthracyclines encapsulated in long-circulating liposomes. Cancer Res 52: 891–896.

6

Codelivery of Chemotherapeutics via Crosslinked Multilamellar Liposomal Vesicles to Overcome Multidrug Resistance in Tumor

Yarong Liu[1]❡, Jinxu Fang[1]❡, Kye-Il Joo[1], Michael K. Wong[2], Pin Wang[1,3,4]*

1 Mork Family Department of Chemical Engineering and Materials Science, University of Southern California, Los Angeles, California, United States of America, 2 Division of Medical Oncology, Norris Comprehensive Cancer Center, Keck School of Medicine, University of Southern California, Los Angeles, California, United States of America, 3 Department of Biomedical Engineering, University of Southern California, Los Angeles, California, United States of America, 4 Department of Pharmacology and Pharmaceutical Sciences, University of Southern California, Los Angeles, California, United States of America

Abstract

Multidrug resistance (MDR) is a significant challenge to effective cancer chemotherapy treatment. However, the development of a drug delivery system that allows for the sustained release of combined drugs with improved vesicle stability could overcome MDR in cancer cells. To achieve this, we have demonstrated codelivery of doxorubicin (Dox) and paclitaxel (PTX) *via* a crosslinked multilamellar vesicle (cMLV). This combinatorial delivery system achieves enhanced drug accumulation and retention, in turn resulting in improved cytotoxicity against tumor cells, including drug-resistant cells. Moreover, this delivery approach significantly overcomes MDR by reducing the expression of P-glycoprotein (P-gp) in cancer cells, thus improving antitumor activity *in vivo*. Thus, by enhancing drug delivery to tumors and lowering the apoptotic threshold of individual drugs, this combinatorial delivery system represents a potentially promising multimodal therapeutic strategy to overcome MDR in cancer therapy.

Editor: Bing Xu, Brandeis University, United States of America

Funding: This work was supported by National Institutes of Health grants (R01AI068978, R01CA170820 and P01CA132681), a translational acceleration grant from the Joint Center for Translational Medicine, the National Cancer Institute (P30CA014089), and a grant from the Ming Hsieh Institute for Research on Engineering Medicine for Cancer. The funders had no role in study design, data collection and analysis, decision to publish, or preparation of the manuscript.

Competing Interests: The authors have declared that no competing interests exist.

* Email: pinwang@usc.edu

❡ These authors contributed equally to this work.

Introduction

The development of multidrug resistance (MDR) against a variety of conventional and novel chemotherapeutic agents has been a major impediment to the success of cancer therapy [1,2]. One of the most important mechanisms involved in MDR is the overexpression of P-glycoprotein (P-gp) in the plasma membrane of various cancer cells. P-gp, an active drug efflux transporter, is capable of effluxing a broad range of anticancer agents, such as taxanes and anthracyclines [3]. For example, the efficacy of doxorubicin (Dox) and paclitaxel (PTX), two of the most widely used agents for the treatment of various cancers, is often compromised by P-gp-mediated MDR [4,5]. Therefore, a strategy to inhibit P-gp expression has been developed to overcome MDR. For instance, a large number of P-gp inhibitors and siRNAs targeting the gene encoding P-gp have been delivered in combination with anticancer agents to downregulate P-gp expression, thereby enabling drugs to reach sufficient concentrations to induce cytotoxicity [6,7]. However, P-gp inhibitors, either functional inhibitors or siRNA, have yielded disappointing clinical trials resulting from their high systemic toxicities and enhanced side effects of chemotherapy in normal cells [8,9].

Combination therapy with multiple chemotherapeutics provides an alternative strategy to suppress MDR. Different drugs may attack cancer cells at varying stages of their growth cycles, thus decreasing the concentration threshold for individual drugs that is otherwise required for cytotoxicity [10]. It has been reported that various drug combinations have successfully induced synergistic antitumor activities and prevented disease recurrence [11,12]. For example, a Dox and PTX cocktail is now considered a standard anthracycline-taxane combination treatment for various tumors by their ability to overcome drug resistance [13,14,15]. However, a major challenge of combination therapy is coordinating the pharmacokinetics and cellular uptake of combined therapeutics. This obstacle has limited the clinical success of combination therapy [16,17].

To overcome this challenge, novel strategies that allow loading of multiple therapeutics into a single drug-delivery vehicle for concurrent delivery at the site of action have been extensively explored [18,19]. Several drug delivery systems have been able to intercalate multiple drugs for site-specific delivery to tumors and, hence, improve antitumor activities, potentially overcoming drug resistance, while, at the same time, reducing the dosage of individual drugs [20,21,22]. Indeed, nanoparticle delivery systems are known to deliver therapeutics efficiently to the tumor sites through the enhanced permeability and retention (EPR) effect, thereby enhancing the concentration of therapeutics in tumors [23,24]. Moreover, these nanoparticles can enter cancer cells through endocytosis in a manner independent of the P-gp pathway, thereby enhancing cellular accumulation of therapeutics [25,26,27]. Thus, a nanoparticle delivery system capable of mediating high efficiency of cellular entry and subsequent triggering of intracellular release of multiple anticancer drugs to overcome MDR is highly desirable.

Liposomes are one of the most popular nanoparticle delivery systems for combinatorial delivery of multiple drugs based on their ability to efficiently load both hydrophilic and hydrophobic drugs [24,28]. We previously developed a robust crosslinked multilamellar liposomal vesicle (cMLV), with enhanced vesicle stability, to efficiently codeliver hydrophilic (Dox) and hydrophobic (PTX) drugs and induce ratio-dependent synergistic antitumor activity, both *in vitro* and *in vivo* [29,30,31]. Moreover, it was shown that cMLV particles are mainly internalized by cells through caveolin-dependent endocytosis and are then trafficked through the endosome-lysosome network for release of drugs [30]. In this study, we have examined the potential of cMLV as a combinatorial delivery system aimed at overcoming P-gp-mediated drug resistance, both *in vitro* and *in vivo*. Indeed, we have demonstrated that the combination of Dox and PTX, when administered at 1:1 weight ratio in cMLV formulations, shows significant enhancement of cytotoxicity and antitumor activities. Combining these drugs through the use of cMLV formulations contributes to these antitumor activities by enhancing systemic delivery efficiency and lowering tumor apoptotic threshold.

Materials and Methods

Mice

Female BALB/c mice (6–10 weeks old) were purchased from Charles River Breeding Laboratories (Wilmington, MA). All mice were held under specific pathogen-reduced conditions in the Animal Facility of the University of Southern California (USA). All experiments were performed in accordance with the guidelines set by the National Institutes of Health and the University of Southern California on the Care and Use of Animals. This study was approved by the Committee on the Ethics of Animal Experiments of the University of Southern California.

Cell culture

B16 tumor cells (B16–F10, ATCC number: CRL-6475) and 4T1 tumor cells (ATCC number: CRL-2539) were maintained in a 5% CO_2 environment with Dulbecco's modified Eagle's medium (Mediatech, Inc., Manassas, VA) supplemented with 10% FBS (Sigma-Aldrich, St. Louis, MO) and 2 mM of L-glutamine (Hyclone Laboratories, Inc., Omaha, NE). B16-R and 4T1-R cells were produced by continuously treating B16 and 4T1 cells with 5 μg/ml PTX for 4 days. The cells were then recovered by replacing medium with fresh medium without drugs for 7 days. The remaining cells formed drug resistance for PTX. JC cells (ATCC number: CRL-2116) were used as a model drug-resistant tumor cell line because it has been shown that JC cells overexpress P-gp and exhibit a drug-resistant phenotype, both *in vitro* and *in vivo* [32].

Synthesis of cMLVs

Liposomes were prepared based on the conventional dehydration-rehydration method. All lipids were obtained from the NOF Corporation (Japan). 1.5 μmol of lipids 1,2-dioleoyl-sn-glycero-3-phosphocholine (DOPC), 1,2-dioleoyl-sn-glycero-3-phospho-(1′-rac-glycerol) (DOPG), and maleimide-headgrouplipid1,2-dioleoyl-sn-glycero-3-phosphoeth-anolamine-N-[4-(p-maleimidophenyl) butyramide (MPB-PE) were combined in chloroform at a molar lipid ratio of DOPC:DOPG:MPB = 4:1:5, and the organic solvent in the lipid mixture was evaporated under argon gas. The lipid mixture was further dried under vacuum overnight to form dried thin lipid films. To prepare cMLV(PTX) and cMLV(Dox+PTX) at a molar ratio of 0.2:1 (drugs:lipids), paclitaxel in organic solvent was mixed with the lipid mixture to form dried thin lipid films. The resultant dried film was hydrated in 10 mM Bis-Tris propane at pH 7.0 with (cMLV(Dox) or cMLV(Dox+PTX)) or without doxorubicin (cMLV(PTX)) at a molar ratio of 0.2:1 (drugs:lipids) with vigorous vortexing every 10 min for 1 h, followed by applying 4 cycles of 15-s sonication (Misonix Microson XL2000, Farmingdale, NY) on ice in 1-min intervals of each cycle. To induce divalent-triggered vesicle fusion, $MgCl_2$ was added at a final concentration of 10 mM. The resulting multilamellar vesicles were further crosslinked by addition of Dithiothreitol (DTT, Sigma-Aldrich) at a final concentration of 1.5 mM for 1 h at 37°C. The resulting vesicles were collected by centrifugation at 14,000 g for 4 min and then washed twice with PBS. For pegylation of cMLVs, the particles were incubated with 1 μmol of 2 kDa PEG-SH (Laysan Bio Inc., Arab, AL) for 1 h at 37°C. The particles were then centrifuged and washed twice with PBS. The final products were stored in PBS at 4°C. The mean diameter of all cMLVs is around 220 nm determined by dynamic light scattering (DLS), and around 160 nm estimated by cryo-electron microscopy. The loading efficiency, and stability of cMLVs were similar to that demonstrated previously [30,31].

In vitro cytotoxicity and data analysis

B16–F10, 4T1, B16–R, 4T1-R, and JC cells were plated at a density of 5×10^3 cells per well in D10 media in 96-well plates and grown for 6 h. The cells were then exposed to a series of concentrations of cMLV (single drug) or cMLV (drug combinations) for 48 h. The cell viability was assessed using the Cell Proliferation Kit II (XTT assay) from Roche Applied Science according to the manufacturer's instructions. Slope m and IC_{50} were obtained from median effect model, and IIP_{Cmax} was calculated via the following equation: $IIP_{Cmax} = \log(1+(Cmax/IC_{50})^m)$. Cmax is the maximum plasma drug concentrations for the commonly recommended dose for each drug.

Cellular uptake of doxorubicin and paclitaxel in cells

4T1 cells were seeded in 24-well plates at a density of 2×10^5 cells per well and grown overnight. The cells were then exposed to empty cMLVs (control), cMLV(Dox), cMLV(PTX), cMLV(Dox+PTX), and Dox+PTX. The final concentrations of Dox and PTX were 1 μg/ml for each group. JC cells were seeded at a density of 10^5 cells per well in D10 media in 96-well plates. The cells were exposed to empty cMLVs, cMLV(Dox), cMLV(PTX), cMLV(Dox+PTX), and Dox+PTX. The final concentrations of Dox and PTX were 5 μg/ml for each group. At 48 h after treatment, the cells were washed twice with PBS and lysed with PBS containing 1% Triton X-100. Doxorubicin and paclitaxel in cell lysates were extracted by 1:1 (v/v) Chloroform/isopropyl alcohol or ethyl acetate, respectively. Paclitaxel concentrations in cell lysates were measured by HPLC C18 column and detected at 227 nm (flow rate 1 ml/min), and doxorubicin was detected by fluorescence with 480/550 nm excitation/emission. The concentrations of Dox and PTX were normalized for protein content as measured with BCA assay (Pierce).

In vivo antitumor activity study

BALB/c female mice (6–10 weeks old) were inoculated subcutaneously with 0.2×10^6 4T1 breast tumor cells. The tumors were allowed to grow for 8 days to a volume of ~50 mm^3 before treatment. After 8 days, the mice were injected intravenously through the tail vein with cMLV(2 mg/kg Dox), cMLV(2 mg/kg PTX), cMLV(2 mg/kg Dox)+cMLV(2 mg/kg PTX), or cMLV(2 mg/kg Dox + 2 mg/kg PTX) every three days (six mice per group). Tumor growth and body weight were monitored for 40 days or to the end of the experiment. The length and width of the tumor masses were measured with a fine caliper every three days after injection. Tumor volume was expressed as 1/2 × (length × $width^2$). Survival end point was set when the tumor volume reached 1000 mm^3. The survival rates are presented as Kaplan-Meier curves. The survival curves of individual groups were compared by a log-rank test.

Immunohistochemistry of tumors and confocal imaging

BALB/c female mice (6–10 weeks old) were inoculated subcutaneously with 0.2 × 10^6 4T1 or JC tumor cells. The tumors were allowed to grow for 20 days to a volume of ~500 mm^3 before treatment. On day 20, the mice were injected intravenously through the tail vein with cMLV (5 mg/kg Dox), cMLV(5 mg/kg PTX), 5 mg/kg Dox + 5 mg/kg PTX, or cMLV(5 mg/kg Dox + 5 mg/kg PTX). Three days after injection, tumors were excised, fixed, frozen, cryo-sectioned, and mounted onto glass slides. Frozen sections were fixed and rinsed with cold PBS. After blocking and permeabilization, the slides were washed by PBS and then incubated with TUNEL reaction mixture (Roche, Indianapolis, Indiana) for 1 h. For P-gp expression, the slides were stained after permeabilization with mouse monoclonal anti-P-gp antibody (Abcam, Cambridge, MA) for 1 h, followed by staining with Alexa488-conjugated goat anti-mouse immunoglobulin G (IgG) antibody (Invitrogen, Carlsbad, CA) and counter-staining with DAPI (Invitrogen, Carlsbad, CA). Fluorescence images were acquired by a Yokogawa spinning-disk confocal scanner system (Solamere Technology Group, Salt Lake City, UT), using a Nikon Eclipse Ti-E microscope. Illumination powers at 405, 491, 561, and 640 nm solid-state laser lines were provided by an AOTF (acousto-optical tunable filter)-controlled laser-merge system with 50 mW for each laser. All images were analyzed using Nikon NIS-Elements software. To quantify TUNEL and P-gp-positive cells, 4 regions of interest (ROI) were randomly chosen per image at ×2 magnification. Within one region, area of TUNEL, or P-gp-positive nuclei, and area of nuclear staining were counted by Nikon NIS-Element software. The data are expressed as % total nuclear area stained by TUNEL or P-gp in the region.

Hematoxylin and Eosin staining of heart sections

Mice bearing 4T1 tumors were i.v. injected with 5 mg/kg Dox + 5 mg/kg PTX or cMLV(5 mg/kg Dox+5 mg/kg PTX). Three days after injection, heart tissues were harvested and fixed in 4% formaldehyde. The tissues were frozen, cut into sections, and mounted onto glass slides. The frozen sections were stained with hematoxylin and eosin. Histopathologic specimens were examined by light microscopy.

Statistics

Differences between two groups were determined with Student's *t* test. The differences among three or more groups were determined with a one-way ANOVA.

Results

In vitro efficacy study by XTT assay

To achieve combination delivery of doxorubicin (Dox) and paclitaxel (PTX), a previously developed crosslinked multilamellar liposomal vesicle (cMLV) was used to incorporate PTX in the lipid membrane and encapsulate Dox in the aqueous core at a 1:1 ratio to form cMLV(Dox+PTX) [30]. We chose this combination ratio because our previous study showed that it could induce synergy combination effect both *in vitro* and *in vivo* [31]. It has been reported that drug combinations can overcome drug resistance that would otherwise limit the potential application of various monotherapeutics [10]. To determine whether codelivery of Dox and PTX could overcome drug resistance, an *in vitro* cytotoxicity assay was performed at a wide range of concentrations of single drug-loaded or dual drug-loaded cMLVs. As shown in Figure 1A and 1B (left panel), both B16 cells and 4T1 cells developed drug resistance to single drug-loaded cMLVs, but this resistance was inhibited by applying the combined formulation, cMLV(Dox+PTX). The maximal cytotoxicity of single drug-loaded cMLV observed in these two tumor cells was between 60%–80%, while cells treated with dual drug-loaded cMLV(Dox+PTX) showed significantly more growth inhibition (~95%).

To further confirm the efficiency of dual drug-loaded cMLVs in overcoming drug resistance, drug-resistant cell lines B16-R and 4T1-R were generated by continuously treating parental B16 or 4T1 with a high concentration of paclitaxel (5 μg/ml). Various concentrations of single drug-loaded cMLV and dual drug-loaded cMLV(Dox+PTX) were incubated with these two drug-resistant cell lines for 48 h, and the cytotoxicity was measured by a standard XTT assay. As shown in Figure 1D and 1E, both B16-R and 4T1-R cells showed a high tolerance when treated with cMLV(PTX) or cMLV(Dox), indicating that multidrug resistance had been developed in these cells. In contrast, cMLV(Dox+PTX) triggered significantly more cell death (90–100%) compared to that of single drug-loaded cMLVs, confirming that a codelivery system could overcome drug resistance induced by a high concentration of single drug. Furthermore, *in vitro* cytotoxicity studies demonstrated therapeutic efficacy of cMLV(Dox+PTX) in JC cells, a model drug-resistant tumor cell line, corroborating the weaker potency of single drug-loaded cMLVs compared to the dual drug-loaded cMLVs. As shown in Figure 1C (left panel), the maximal cytotoxicity of cMLV(Dox) and cMLV(PTX) was in the range of 60–70%, while peak cMLV(Dox+PTX) cytotoxicity was about 90% in JC cells.

IC_{50}, which indicates drug concentration that causes 50% inhibitory effect on cell proliferation, can provide information on the efficacy of drugs. The IC_{50} values of the individual drugs and combined drugs through cMLVs in B16, 4T1 and JC cells are provided in Figure S1. However, it has also been reported that slope m, a parameter mathematically analogous to the Hill coefficient, may also have a significant effect on cytotoxicity [33,34]. Therefore, a new model has been developed to evaluate drug activity by incorporating three parameters (IC_{50}, drug concentration, and m) from the median effect model into a single-value IIP (potential inhibition) with an intuitive meaning, i.e., the log reduction in inhibitory effect [34]. Accordingly, to increase the trustworthiness of our experiment, IIP was used to evaluate the efficiency of dual drug-loaded cMLVs on cell viability. As shown in Figure 1A to 1C (middle and right panels), Dox and PTX in the dual drug-loaded cMLVs displayed a significantly larger IIP_{Cmax} value in the cell lines studied compared to that of the single drug-loaded cMLVs, indicating that

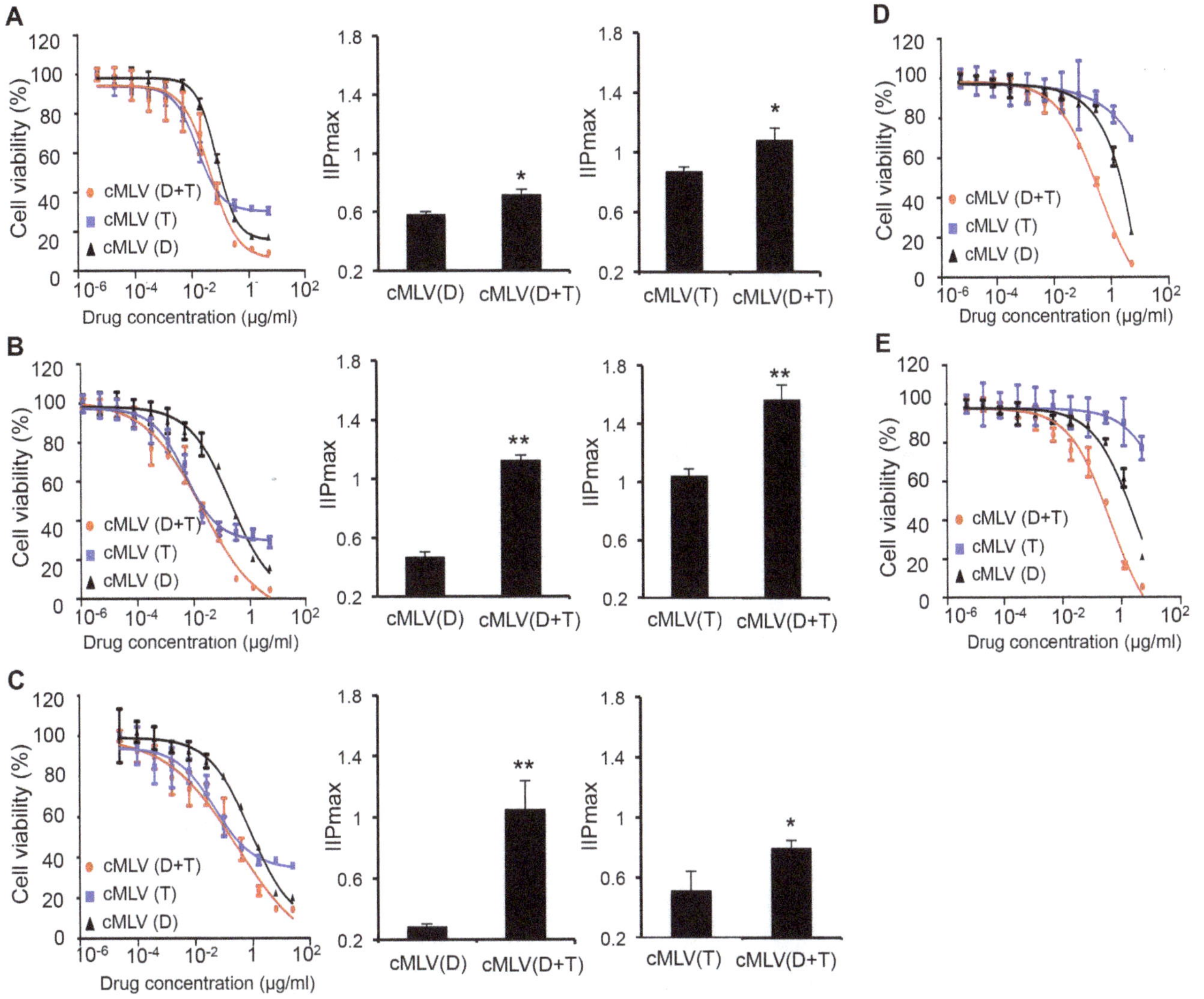

Figure 1. Overcoming drug resistance by codelivery of Dox and PTX via cMLVs (D: Dox; T: PTX). (A, B) *In vitro* cytotoxicity of cMLV(single drug) and cMLV(drug combinations) in B16 melanoma tumor cells (A) and 4T1 breast tumor cells (B). (C, D, E) *In vitro* cytotoxicity of cMLV(single drug) and cMLV(drug combinations) in drug-resistant JC cells (C), B16-R cells (D) and 4T1-R cells (E). IIP_{Cmax} was determined by incorporating three parameters (IC_{50}, *D* and m) in the median effect model into the following equation: $IIP_{Cmax} = \log(1+(Cmax/IC_{50})^m)$. Data are represented as mean ± SD (n = 3). Asterisks indicate statistical significance between two groups (*$P < 0.05$, **$P < 0.01$).

combinatorial cMLVs were more potent in cancer treatment than single drug-loaded cMLVs.

Cellular uptake study of doxorubicin and paclitaxel

To investigate the mechanism of enhanced cytotoxicity observed with cMLV combination therapy, we evaluated the effect of dual drug-loaded cMLVs on rates of drug influx/efflux in cells. The intracellular accumulation of Dox and PTX was examined by HPLC in 4T1 cells following exposure to Dox (1 μg/ml) and PTX (1 μg/ml) in cMLVs, both individually and in combination, and in JC cells with higher dose of Dox and PTX (5 μg/ml). After 3 h incubation, the extracellular medium was discarded, and intracellular drug (Dox or PTX) accumulation was quantitatively determined by drug concentration in the cell lysates, normalized by total cellular protein content of the cells. As seen in Figure 2A and 2B, cMLV(Dox+PTX) significantly increased both Dox and PTX accumulation in 4T1 cells compared to that of single drug-loaded cMLVs ($p < 0.05$), suggesting that combination treatments may overcome drug resistance. In addition, compared to the administration of drug in solution, cMLV combination treatment resulted in higher cellular accumulation of Dox and PTX, an outcome most likely resulting from the internalization of cMLVs by cells through endocytosis [30] and, consequently, effectively bypassing the P-gp efflux pumps. The enhanced cellular accumulation of drugs in dual drug-loaded cMLVs was also observed in drug-resistant JC cells (Figure 2C and 2D) compared to single drug-loaded cMLVs and drug combination in solution. These data suggest that cMLV(Dox+PTX) significantly enhanced the intracellular accumulation of anticancer drugs through mechanisms involving both combination treatment and nanoparticle delivery.

Effect of codelivered nanoparticles on P-gp expression

Having shown that dual drug-loaded cMLVs enhance cellular accumulation of drugs, we next sought to verify that this did, indeed, result from the modulation of membrane pumps, which

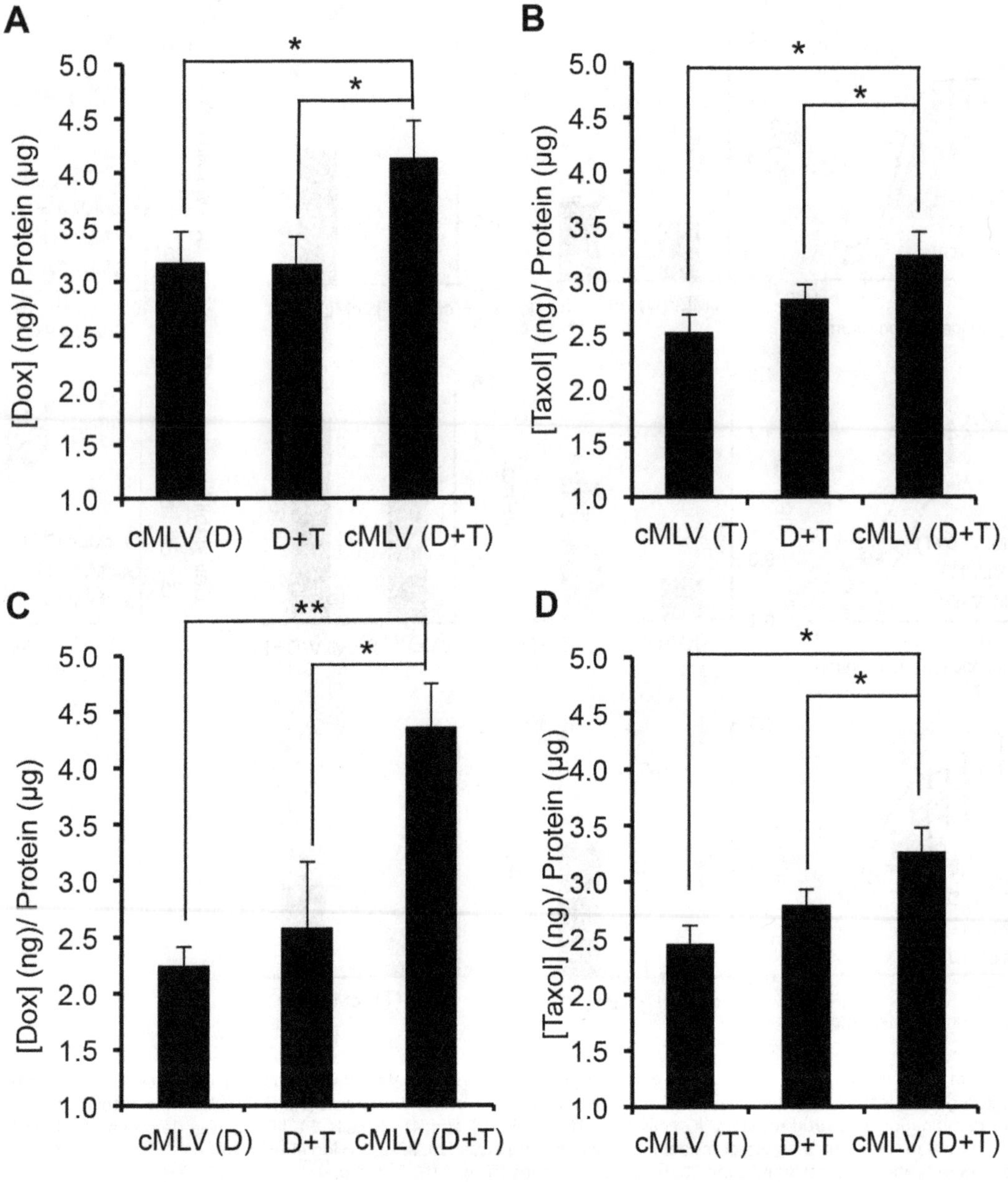

Figure 2. Cellular uptake of Dox and PTX (D: Dox; T: PTX). (A, B) Total cellular uptake of Dox (A) and PTX (B) into 4T1 cells. 4T1 cells were exposed to cMLV(D), cMLV(T), cMLV(D+T), and D+P in solution. The final concentrations of Dox and PTX were 1 μg/ml for each group. (C, D) Total cellular uptake of Dox (C) and PTX (D) in JC cells. JC cells were exposed to cMLV(D), cMLV(T), cMLV(D+T), and D+T. The final concentrations of Dox and PTX were 5 μg/ml for each group. The uptake of Dox and PTX was normalized to protein content measured with the BCA assay. All data are shown as the means of triplicate experiments from three different nanoparticle preparations. Asterisks indicate statistical significance between two groups (*$P < 0.05$, **$P < 0.01$).

are responsible for multidrug resistance. We first measured the expression of P-gp by flow cytometry in 4T1 cells treated with various nanoparticle formulations for 48 h to test if these cMLV formulations were responsible for altering P-gp involvement in multidrug resistance, along with decreased drug accumulation, in cells [3,35]. As shown in Figure 3A, with the single drug-loaded cMLV treatment, the expression of P-gp (in terms of integrated mean fluorescence intensity) increased significantly in 4T1 cells ($p < 0.01$), possibly leading, in turn, to the development of drug resistance in 4T1 cells. However, dual drug-loaded cMLVs significantly inhibited expression of P-gp when compared to that of the single drug-loaded cMLVs and drug combination in solution ($p < 0.01$), suggesting that the combinatorial delivery of Dox and PTX *via* cMLVs could efficiently suppress P-gp expression, thereby overcoming MDR. We next investigated whether cMLV(Dox+PTX) could inhibit multidrug resistance in JC cells, which exhibit drug-resistant phenotype by overexpression of P-gp [32]. As shown in Figure 3B, the expression of P-gp decreased after 48 h of incubation with JC cells ($p < 0.05$) when treated with single drug-loaded cMLV, indicating that the nanoparticle drug delivery system could, at least partially, suppress MDR. However, the codelivery formulation of cMLV(Dox+PTX) significantly inhibited P-gp expression compared to that of single drug-loaded cMLVs and drug combination in solution ($p < 0.01$).

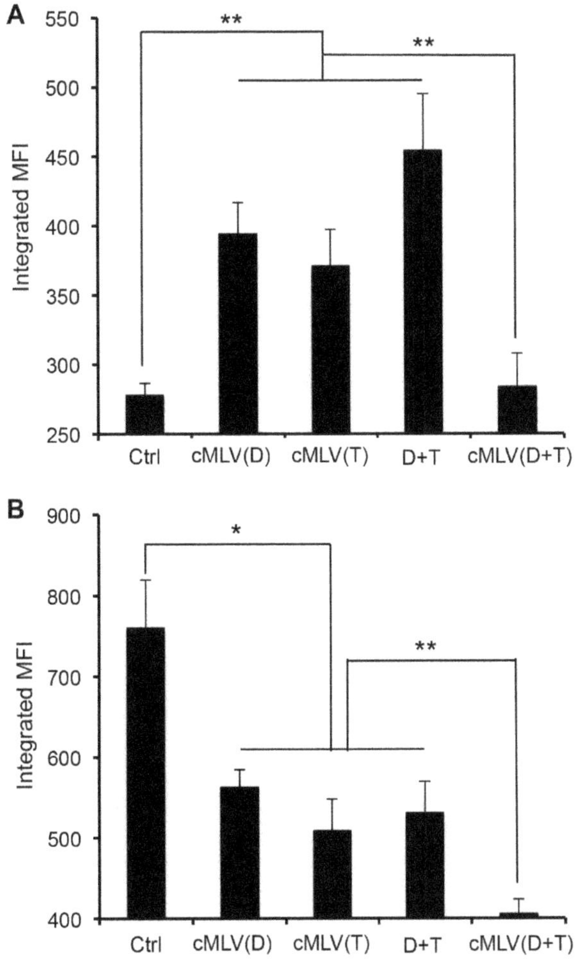

Figure 3. Effect of codelivered nanoparticles on P-gp expression (D: Dox; T: PTX). (A) 4T1 cells were exposed to empty cMLVs (Ctrl), cMLV(D), cMLV(T), cMLV(D+T), and D+T with the same concentration of Dox and PTX (1 μg/ml). (B) JC cells were exposed to empty cMLVs (Ctrl), cMLV(D), cMLV(T), cMLV(D+T), and D+T with the same concentration of Dox and PTX (5 μg/ml). P-gp expression was detected by P-gp-specific antibody *via* flow cytometry. Data are represented as mean ± SD (n = 3). Asterisks indicate statistical significance between two groups (*$P < 0.05$, **$P < 0.01$).

Taken together, these results indicated that the codelivery of Dox and PTX via cMLVs could inhibit the expression of P-gp and increase cellular accumulation of drugs, leading to enhanced drug action in cells, including drug-resistant cells.

Efficacy of dual drug-loaded cMLVs against a murine breast cancer model

It has been demonstrated that codelivery of Dox and PTX via cMLVs is able to overcome drug resistance *in vitro*. However, since the *in vivo* environment is considerably more complicated, it remains unknown if this effect could be translated to an animal cancer model. Therefore, in this experiment, a mouse breast tumor model was used to evaluate the therapeutic efficacy of dual drug-loaded cMLVs compared with that of single-drug liposomal formulations. At day 0, BALB/c mice were inoculated subcutaneously with 4T1 breast tumor cells. On day 8, mice bearing tumors were randomly sorted into six groups, and each group was treated with one of the following: PBS (control), cMLV(2 mg/kg Dox), cMLV(2 mg/kg PTX), cMLV(2 mg/kg Dox)+ cMLV(2 mg/kg PTX), or cMLV(2 mg/kg Dox + 2 mg/kg PTX) every three days. Tumor growth and body weights were monitored until the end of the experiment (Figure 4A).

As shown in Figure 4B, mice in groups receiving cMLV(Dox), cMLV (PTX) or cMLV(Dox)+cMLV(PTX) exhibited tumor inhibition compared to those in the control group ($p < 0.01$). Even more significantly, cMLV(Dox+PTX) treatment induced a greater inhibition than that of cMLV encapsulating a single drug and that of cMLV(Dox)+cMLV(PTX), indicating that codelivery of Dox and PTX through single nanoparticle is essential for overcoming drug resistance ($p < 0.01$). As one indication of systemic toxicity, no weight loss was seen for the cMLV formulation over the duration of the experiment (Figure 4C). The *in vivo* efficacy of dual drug-loaded cMLVs against the 4T1 tumor model was further confirmed by a survival test. As shown in Figure 4D, the groups treated with cMLV(Dox), cMLV(PTX), or cMLV(Dox)+cMLV(PTX) had a prolonged lifespan compared to the control group, while the mice in the group treated with cMLV(Dox+PTX) had a significantly increased lifespan compared to the groups treated with single drug-loaded cMLVs and the group treated with cMLV(Dox) + cMLV(PTX) ($p < 0.01$).

Histology study

To study the antitumor mechanism *in vivo*, a TUNEL assay was carried out to detect tumor cell apoptosis in tumors treated with Dox (5 mg/kg) and/or PTX (5 mg/kg) in various formulations for 3 days. As shown in Figure 5A and Figure 5C, 4T1 tumors treated with cMLV(Dox), cMLV(PTX), and Dox+PTX in solution showed significantly more apoptotic cells compared with controls ($p < 0.01$). The apoptosis index was also significantly higher in the cMLV(Dox+PTX)-treated group as compared with other groups ($p < 0.05$). Thus, the efficacy of cMLV(Dox+PTX) as an antitumor treatment could be explained by data suggesting increased tumor cell apoptosis. To further confirm the induction of cell apoptosis in treated groups, the TUNEL assay was performed in drug-resistant JC tumors treated with various formulations for 3 days. As shown in Figure 5B and 5D, cMLV(Dox), cMLV(PTX), and Dox+PTX induced more apoptotic cells compared to control JC tumors ($p < 0.01$). Dual drug-loaded cMLV-treated JC tumors showed a remarkably higher apoptosis index compared with other groups ($p < 0.01$), again confirming the enhanced antitumor activity of cMLV(Dox+PTX).

To further investigate the innate characteristics of treated tumors, both 4T1 and JC tumor sections from each treatment group were analyzed for the expression of P-gp protein. As shown in Figure 6A, P-gp expression level was moderate in the control group. There appeared to be a significant enhancement of P-gp expression in the cMLV(Dox) and cMLV(PTX) groups, with an even more significant enhancement in Dox+PTX group compared to controls. However, a marked decrease was observed in the cMLV(Dox+PTX)-treated group when compared to the cMLV(Dox), cMLV(PTX), and Dox+PTX groups, as further confirmed by the quantification data in Figure 6C ($p < 0.01$). Interestingly, P-gp was very high in the JC tumor control group, as shown in Figure 6B. However, a significant decrease appeared in the cMLV(Dox), cMLV(PTX), and Dox+ PTX groups, as further confirmed by the quantification data in Figure 6D ($p < 0.05$). An even more significant decrease of P-gp expression was seen in the cMLV(Dox+PTX) group ($p < 0.01$), indicating that dual drug-loaded cMLVs might be able to alter the innate characteristics of the multidrug-resistant tumor cells such as JC cells. Taken together, these data show that drug-loaded nanoparticles can partially bypass the P-gp efflux

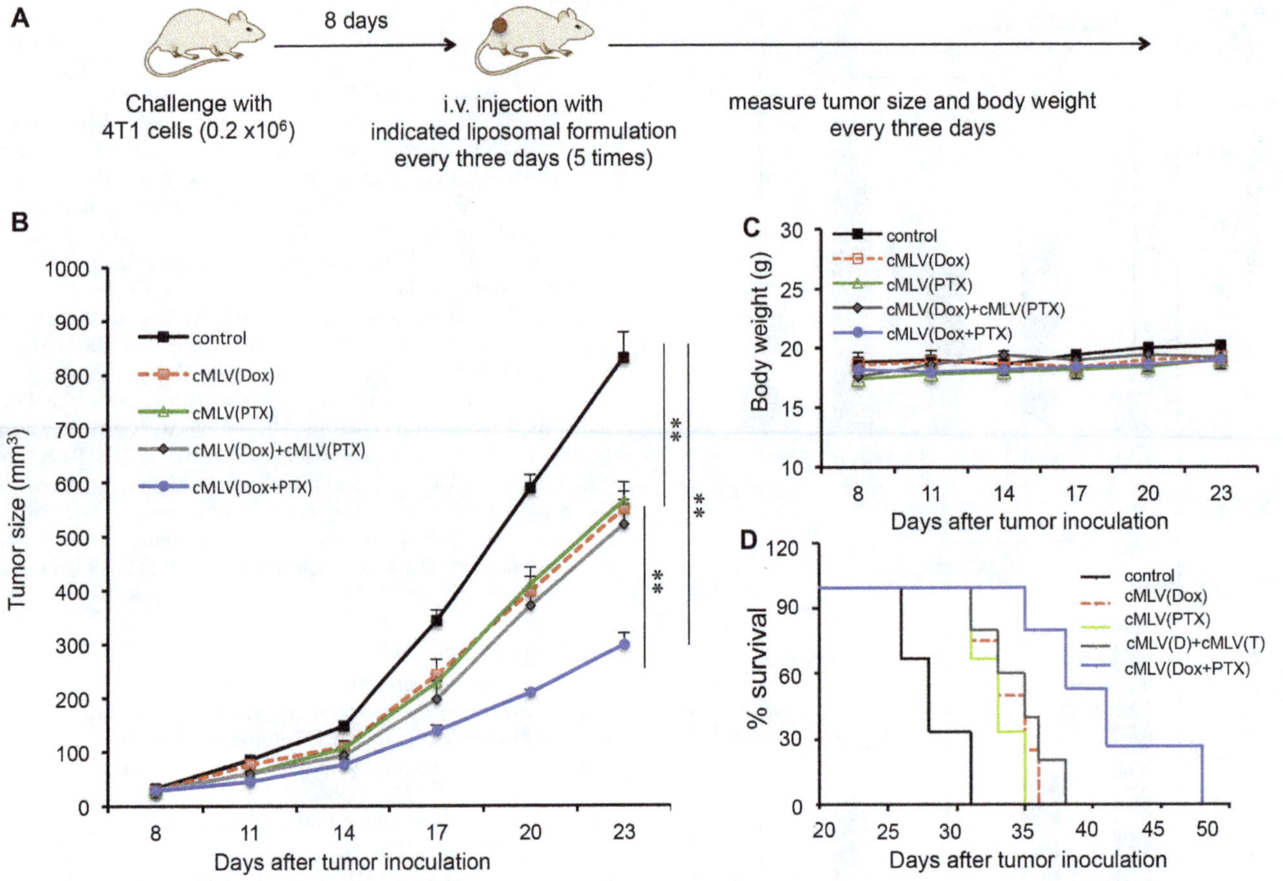

Figure 4. *In vivo* efficacy of drug combinations *via* cMLVs in a 4T1 tumor model. (A) Schematic diagram of the experimental protocol for *in vivo* 4T1 tumor study in BALB/c mice. (B) Tumor growth was measured after treatment with PBS (control, black solid line), cMLV (2 mg/kg Dox) (red dashed line), cMLV (2 mg/kg PTX) (green solid line), cMLV(2 mg/kg Dox)+cMLV(2 mg/kg PTX) (grey solid line), or cMLV (2 mg/kg Dox+2 mg/kg PTX) (blue solid line). Error bars represent standard error of the mean, n = 6 for each treatment group (**$p < 0.01$). (C) Average mouse weight loss over the duration of the experiment. (D) Survival curves for 4T1-bearing mice treated with PBS (black solid line), cMLV 2 mg/kg Dox) (red dashed line), cMLV (2 mg/kg PTX) (green solid line), cMLV(2 mg/kg Dox)+cMLV(2 mg/kg PTX) (grey solid line), or cMLV (2 mg/kg Dox+2 mg/kg PTX) (blue solid line). Survival end point was set when the tumor volume reached 1000 mm^3. The survival rates were presented as Kaplan-Meier curves. The survival curves of individual groups were compared by a log-rank test.

pumps to increase cellular uptake of Dox and PTX, sufficiently inducing cytotoxicity in cancer cells.

It has been reported that Dox treatment results in severe irreversible cardiotoxicity, leading to myocyte apoptosis [36]. In addition, cardiac toxicity, an unexpected clinical outcome of combinatorial Dox and PTX treatment, has been reported [37]. Therefore, systemic toxicity of free Dox+PTX and cMLV(Dox+PTX) was evaluated to determine whether codelived cMLVs could decrease this side effect of combination drug treatment. To accomplish this, a single intravenous dose of either Dox+PTX in solution or cMLV(Dox+PTX) was administered to mice bearing 4T1 tumors. Next, hematoxylin and eosin-stained cardiac tissue sections from each treatment group were examined (Figure S2). Treatment with free Dox (5 mg/kg) and PTX (5 mg/kg) in solution did cause cardiac toxicity, as indicated by myofibril loss, disarray, and cytoplasmic vacuolization. However, when cMLV(5 mg/kg Dox+5 mg/kg PTX) was administered under the same experimental conditions *via* cMLVs, no visible loss of myocardial tissue was observed.

Discussion

Chemotherapeutics are crucial to combating a variety of cancers; however, clinical outcomes are always poor, as cancer cells develop a multidrug resistance (MDR) phenotype after several rounds of exposure to the chemotherapeutics. Many efforts have been made to develop a therapeutic strategy to overcome tumor MDR through the use of combined therapeutics to enhance the efficiency of systemic drug delivered to the tumor site and lower the apoptotic threshold. In this study, we have examined augmentation of therapeutic efficacy upon co-administration of Dox and PTX using a crosslinked multilamellar liposomal vesicle (cMLV) in breast cancer cells and drug-resistant JC cells. We demonstrated that combination therapy of Dox and PTX, especially when codelivered in cMLV formulations, was effective in enhancing the cytotoxicity in both wild-type and drug-resistant cells by elevating the cellular accumulation and retention of the drugs. We also showed that the dual therapeutic strategy efficiently suppressed tumor growth by enhancing apoptotic response.

P-glycoprotein (P-gp), a membrane-bound active drug efflux pump, is considered one of the most important mechanisms involved in MDR [3,35]. As a result, growing interest has been

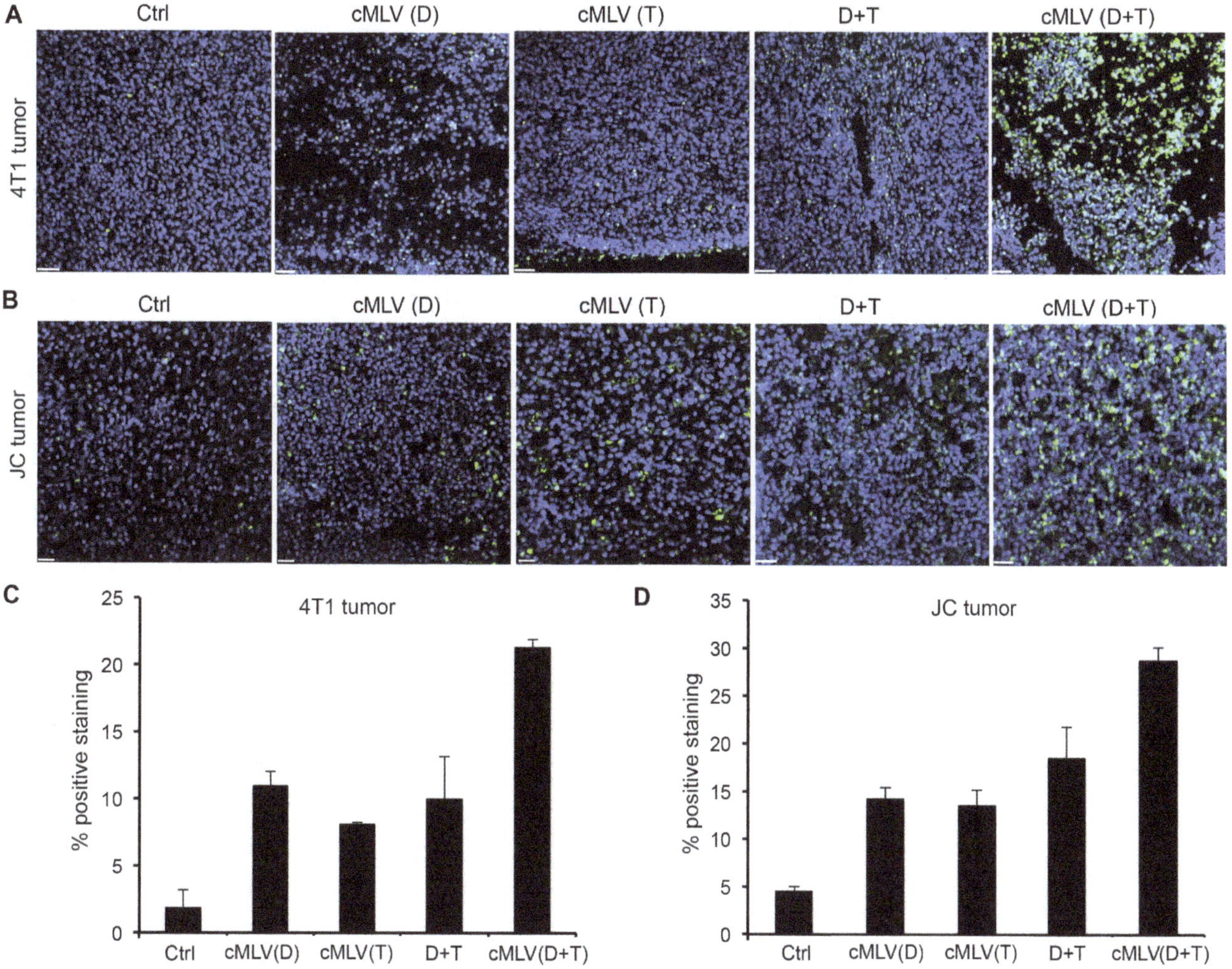

Figure 5. Effect of codelivered cMLVs on tumor apoptosis (D: Dox; T: PTX). (A, B) Mice bearing either 4T1 tumor (A) or multidrug-resistant JC tumor (B) were injected intravenously through the tail vein with cMLV (5 mg/kg Dox), cMLV (5 mg/kg PTX), 5 mg/kg Dox + 5 mg/kg PTX, or cMLV (5 mg/kg Dox+5 mg/kg PTX). Three days after injection, tumors were excised. Apoptotic cells were detected by a TUNEL assay (green), followed by nuclear costaining with DAPI (blue). Scale bar represents 50 μm. (C, D) Quantification of apoptotic cells in 4T1 (C) and JC (D) tumors. To quantify TUNEL-positive cells, 4 regions of interest (ROI) were randomly chosen per image at ×2 magnification. Within one region, area of TUNEL-positive nuclei and area of nuclear staining were counted. The data are expressed as % total nuclear area stained by TUNEL in the region. Data are represented as mean ± SD (n = 3).

shown in the development of nanoparticle drug delivery systems to overcome MDR. With their unique properties, nanoparticles are able to passively target the tumor mass through the enhanced permeability and retention (EPR) effect, enhancing the accumulation of chemotherapeutics at target sites [23,24]. In addition, nanoparticles can enter cells through the endocytosis pathway, which is thought to be independent of the P-gp pathway, thus increasing the cellular uptake and retention of therapeutics in resistant cancer cells [26,27]. Previously, we demonstrated the advantage of cMLVs in cancer therapy over conventional liposomal formulations based on their sustained drug release, enhanced vesicle stability and improved drug release, resulting in improved therapeutic activity with reduced systemic toxicity [30]. Further investigation of this novel liposomal formulation showed that it enable to translate the synergistic combination effect from in vitro to in vivo antitumor efficiency [31]. Moreover, cMLVs are internalized by tumor cells through caveolin-mediated endocytosis [30], suggesting that cMLVs could be an efficient drug carrier to overcome MDR. In this study, our *in vitro* and *in vivo* results demonstrated that the co-administration of Dox and PTX at the synergistic ratio (1:1) *via* cMLVs efficiently suppressed P-gp expression in both wild-type and drug-resistant cancer cells.

In addition to nanodelivery, another potential strategy to overcome MDR has resulted from combining multiple drugs. For example, the combination of Dox and PTX in a cocktail is a standard anthracycline-taxane treatment regimen and was found to be efficacious in treating a variety of tumors by reducing the individual drug concentration that would otherwise be required to achieve cytotoxicity, thus overcoming drug resistance [13,14,15]. However, its clinical outcome was limited by the un-coordinated biodistribution of combined drugs [16,17] and increase in cardiac cytotoxicity [37]. In this study, the pharmacokinetics of Dox and PTX was unified through the encapsulation of both drugs into a single cMLV particle, resulting in dual drug-loaded cMLVs which successfully reduced P-gp expression, increased the cellular accumulation of drugs, and enhanced cytotoxicity in cancer cells, including drug-resistant cells, as compared to single drug-loaded cMLVs. Moreover, combination therapy of Dox and PTX

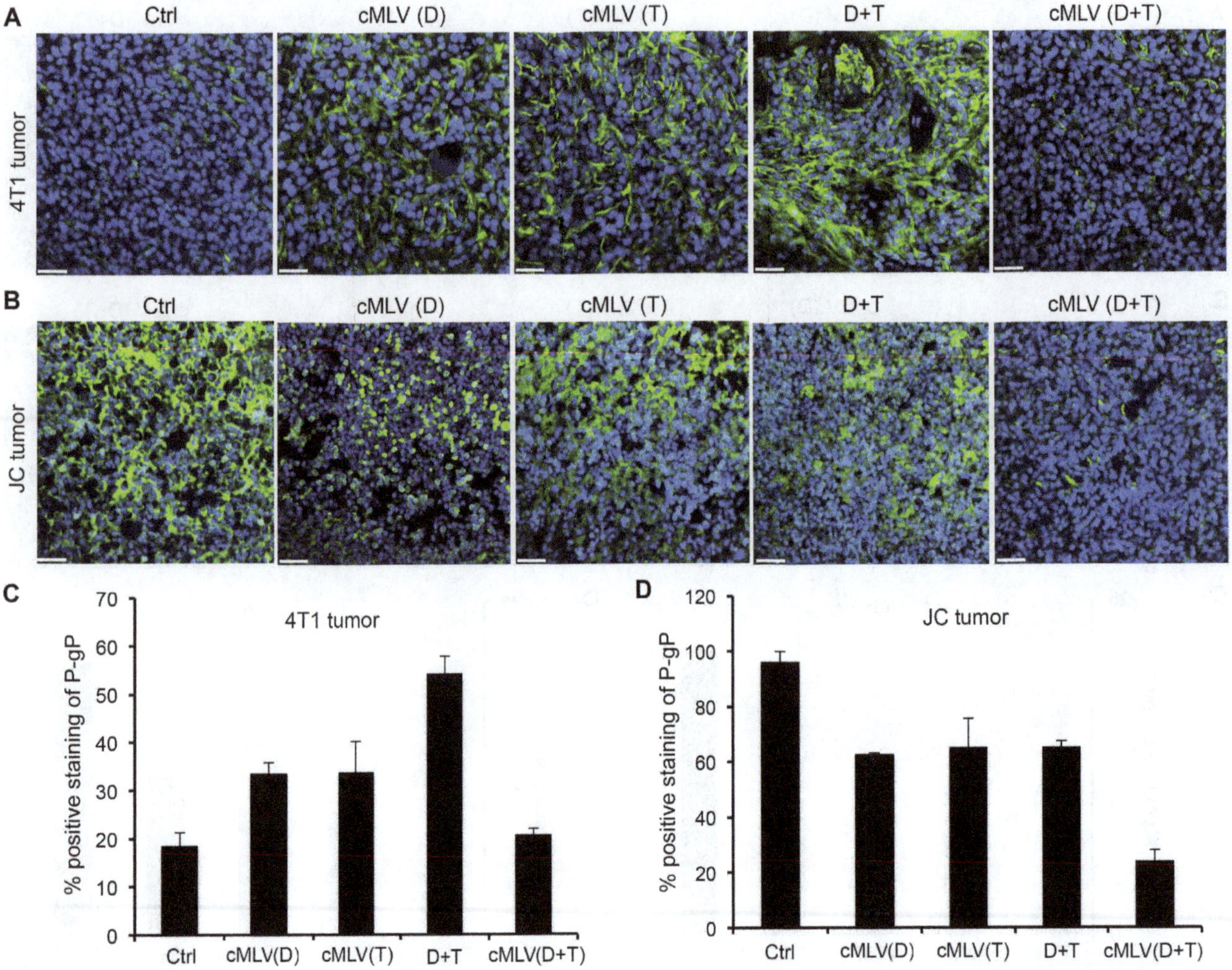

Figure 6. Effect of codelivered cMLVs on P-gp expression in tumors. (A, B) Mice bearing 4T1 tumor (A) and multidrug-resistant tumor JC (B) were injected intravenously through the tail vein with cMLV (5 mg/kg Dox), cMLV (5 mg/kg PTX), 5 mg/kg Dox + 5 mg/kg PTX, or cMLV (5 mg/kg Dox+5 mg/kg PTX). Three days after injection, tumors were excised, and stained by P-gp-specific antibody (green), followed by nuclear costaining with DAPI (blue). Scale bar represents 50 μm. (C, D) Quantification of P-gp-positive cells in 4T1 (C) and JC (D) tumors. To quantify P-gp-positive cells, 4 regions of interest (ROI) were randomly chosen per image at ×2 magnification. Within one region, area of P-gp-positive nuclei and area of nuclear staining were counted. The data are expressed as % total nuclear area that is P-gp-positive in the region. Data are represented as mean ± SD (n = 3).

administered in cMLV formulations showed increased efficacy over cMLV monotherapy in the suppression of tumor growth by promoting apoptotic response *in vivo*.

Conclusion

In summary, we have developed a multimodal therapeutic strategy to overcome tumor MDR by codelivery of Dox and PTX *via* a crosslinked multilamellar liposomal vesicle. We demonstrated that such combinatorial delivery system increased therapeutic efficacy by enhancing delivery efficiency to tumors and lowering the apoptotic threshold of individual drugs, thus overcoming drug resistance. The properties of cMLVs, such as improved stability and sustained release of drugs, enable the nanoparticles to sufficiently accumulate at tumor sites, subsequently entering tumor cells *via* endocytosis to release therapeutics, thus potentially bypassing the P-gp pathway to enhance cellular retention of therapeutics. Moreover, cMLVs enable multidrug delivery to the same action site, thereby lowering the tumor apoptotic threshold of individual therapeutics and potentially inhibiting the MDR. Taken together, this dual drug-loaded cMLV approach shows promise for reducing MDR in cancer therapeutics.

Supporting Information

Figure S1 IC50 values of cMLV(Dox), cMLV(PTX) and cMLV(Dox+PTX) in B16 melanoma, 4T1 breast tumor cells, or drug-resistant JC cancer cells.

Figure S2 Histologic appearance (hematoxylin and eosin staining) of heart tissues by light microscopy isolated on day 3 after a single intravenous injection of PBS (left), 5 mg/kg Dox+5 mg/kg PTX in solution (middle) and cMLV(5 mg/kg Dox+5 mg/kg PTX) (right).

Acknowledgments

We thank the USC NanoBiophysics Core Facility. We also thank Jennifer Rohrs for critical reading of the manuscript.

Author Contributions

Conceived and designed the experiments: YL PW. Performed the experiments: YL JF KJ. Analyzed the data: YL JF KJ. Contributed reagents/materials/analysis tools: MW PW. Contributed to the writing of the manuscript: YL PW.

References

1. Szakács G, Paterson JK, Ludwig JA, Booth-Genthe C, Gottesman MM (2006) Targeting multidrug resistance in cancer. Nat Rev Drug Discov 5: 219–234.
2. Teicher BA (2009) Acute and chronic in vivo therapeutic resistance. Biochem Pharmacol: 1665–1673.
3. Fletcher JI, Haber M, Henderson MJ, Norris MD (2010) ABC transporters in cancer: more than just drug efflux pumps. Nat Rev Cancer 10: 147–156.
4. Schöndorf T, Kurbacher C, Göhring U, Benz C, Becker M, et al. (2002) Induction of MDR1-gene expression by antineoplastic agents in ovarian cancer cell lines. Anticancer Res 22: 2199–2203.
5. Lespine A, Ménez C, Bourguinat C, Prichard RK (2012) P-glycoproteins and other multidrug resistance transporters in the pharmacology of anthelmintics: Prospects for reversing transport-dependent anthelmintic resistance. Int J Parasitol Drugs Drug Resist 2: 230–270.
6. Chen Y, Bathula SR, Li J, Huang L (2010) Multifunctional nanoparticles delivering small interfering RNA and doxorubicin overcome drug resistance in cancer. J Biol Chem 285: 22639–22650.
7. Xu D, McCarty D, Fernandes A, Fisher M, Samulski RJ, et al. (2005) Delivery of MDR1 small interfering RNA by self-complementary recombinant adeno-associated virus vector. Mol Ther 11: 523–530.
8. Hubensack M, Müller C, Höcherl P, Fellner S, Spruss T, et al. (2008) Effect of the ABCB1 modulators elacridar and tariquidar on the distribution of paclitaxel in nude mice. J Cancer Res Clin Oncol 134: 597–607.
9. Liu Y, Rohrs J, Wang P (2014) Development and challenges of nanovectors in gene therapy. Nano LIFE 4: 1441007.
10. Lehar J, Krueger AS, Avery W, Heilbut AM, Johansen LM, et al. (2009) Synergistic drug combinations tend to improve therapeutically relevant selectivity. Nat biotechnol 27: 659–666.
11. Calabrò F, Lorusso V, Rosati G, Manzione L, Frassinet iL, et al. (2009) Gemcitabine and paclitaxel every 2 weeks in patients with previously untreated urothelial carcinoma. Cancer 115: 2652–2659.
12. Mamounas EP, Sledge GW Jr (2001) Combined anthracycline-taxane regimens in the adjuvant setting. Semin Oncol 28: 24–31.
13. Dean-Colomb W, Esteva F (2008) Emerging agents in the treatment of anthracycline- and taxane-refractory metastatic breast cancer. Semin Oncol 35(2 Suppl 2): S31–38.
14. De Laurentiis M, Cancello G, D'Agostino D, Giuliano M, Giordano A, et al. (2008) Taxane-based combinations as adjuvant chemotherapy of early breast cancer: a meta-analysis of randomized trials. J Clin Oncol 26: 44–53.
15. Kataja V, Castiglione M (2008) ESMO Guidelines Working Group Locally recurrent or metastatic breast cancer: ESMO clinical recommendations for diagnosis, treatment and follow-up. Ann Oncol 19(2 suppl): ii11–ii13.
16. Grasselli G, Viganò L, Capri G, Locatelli A, Tarenzi E, et al. (2001) Clinical and pharmacologic study of the epirubicin and paclitaxel combination in women with meta-static breast cancer. J Clin Oncol 19: 2222–2231.
17. Gustafson DL, Andrea L Merz, Long ME (2005) Pharmacokinetics of combined doxorubicin and paclitaxel in mice. Cancer Letters 220: 161–169.
18. Ahmed F, Pakunlu RI, Brannan A, Bates F, Minko T, et al. (2006) Biodegradable polymersomes loaded with both paclitaxel and doxorubicin permeate and shrink tumors, inducing apoptosis in proportion to accumulated drug. J Control Release 116: 150–158.
19. Sengupta S, Eavarone D, Capila I, Zhao G, Watson N, et al. (2005) Temporal targeting of tumour cells and neovasculature with a nanoscale delivery system. Nature 436: 568–572.
20. Wang H, Zhao Y, Wu Y, Hu Y-l, Nan K, et al. (2011) Enhanced anti-tumor efficacy by co-delivery of doxorubicin and paclitaxel with amphiphilic methoxy PEG-PLGA copolymer nanoparticles. Biomaterials 32: 8281–8290.
21. Gao H, Zhang Z, Yu Z, He Q (2014) Cell-penetrating peptide based intelligent liposomal systems for enhanced drug delivery. Curr Pharm Biotechnol 15: 210–219.
22. Yu Z, Schmaltz RM, Bozeman TC, Paul R, Rishel MJ, et al. (2013) Selective tumor cell targeting by the disaccharide moiety of bleomycin. J Am Chem Soc 135: 2883–2886.
23. Cho K, Wang X, Nie S, Chen ZG, Shin DM (2008) Therapeutic nanoparticles for drug delivery in cancer. Clin Cancer Res 14: 1310–1316.
24. Ferrari M (2005) Cancer nanotechnology: opportunities and challenges. Nat Rev Cancer 5: 161–171.
25. Dobson PD, Kell DB (2008) Carrier-mediated cellular uptake of pharmaceutical drugs: an exception or the rule? Nat Rev Drug Discov 7: 205–210.
26. Hillaireau H, Couvreur P (2009) Nanocarriers' entry into the cell: relevance to drug delivery. Cell Mo Life Sci 66: 2873–2896.
27. Sahay G, Alakhova DY, Kabanov AV (2010) Endocytosis of nanomedicines. J Control Release 145: 182–195.
28. Torchilin VP (2005) Recent Advances with Liposomes as Pharmaceutical Carriers. Nat Rev Drug Discov 4: 145–160.
29. Liu Y, Ji M, Wong MK, Joo K-I, Wang P (2013) Enhanced therapeutic efficacy of iRGD-conjugated crosslinked multilayer liposomes for drug delivery. BioMed Research International 2013: 378380.
30. Joo K, Xiao L, Liu S, Liu Y, Lee C, et al. (2013) Crosslinked multilamellar liposomes for controlled delivery of anticancer drugs. Biomaterials 34: 3098–3109.
31. Liu Y, Fang J, Kim Y-J, Wong MK, Wang P (2014) Codelivery of doxorubicin and paclitaxel by cross-linked multilamellar liposome enables synergistic antitumor activity. Mol Pharmaceutics 11: 1651–1661.
32. Lee B, French K, Zhuang Y, Smith C (2003) Development of a syngeneic in vivo tumor model and its use in evaluating a novel P-glycoprotein modulator, PGP-4008. Oncol Res 14: 49–60.
33. Goutelle S, Maurin M, Rougier l, Barbaut X, Bourguignon L, et al. (2008) The Hill equation: a review of its capabilities in pharmacological modelling. Fundam Clin Pharmacol 22: 633–648.
34. Shen L, Peterson S, Sedaghat AR, McMahon MA, Callender M, et al. (2008) Dose-response curve slope sets class-specific limits on inhibitory potential of anti-HIV drugs. Nat Med 14: 762–766.
35. Robey RW, To KK, Polgar O, Dohse M, Fetsch P, et al. (2009) ABCG2: a perspective. Adv Drug Deliv Rev 61: 3–13.
36. Rahman AM, Yusuf SW, Ewer MS (2007) Anthracycline-induced cardiotoxicity and the cardiac-sparing effect of liposomal formulation. Int J Nanomedicine 2: 567–583.
37. Bird B, Swain S (2008) Cardiac toxicity in breast cancer survivors: review of potential cardiac problems. Clin Cancer Res 14: 14–24.

7

Brain-Targeted Delivery of Trans-Activating Transcriptor-Conjugated Magnetic PLGA/Lipid Nanoparticles

Xiangru Wen[1,5], Kai Wang[2], Ziming Zhao[3], Yifang Zhang[2], Tingting Sun[2], Fang Zhang[4], Jian Wu[4], Yanyan Fu[4], Yang Du[4], Lei Zhang[6], Ying Sun[6], YongHai Liu[6], Kai Ma[5,7], Hongzhi Liu[4]*, Yuanjian Song[1,4]*

1 Jiangsu Key Laboratory of Brain Disease Bioinformation, Xuzhou Medical College, Xuzhou, Jiangsu Province, China, **2** College of Animal Science and Technology, Yunnan Agricultural University, Yunnan, Kunming Province, China, **3** School of Pharmacy, Xuzhou Medical College, Xuzhou, Jiangsu Province, China, **4** Research Center for Neurobiology and Department of Neurobiology, Xuzhou Medical College, Xuzhou, Jiangsu Province, China, **5** School of Basic Education Sciences, Xuzhou Medical College, Xuzhou, Jiangsu Province, China, **6** Department of Neurology, Affiliated Hospital of Xuzhou Medical College, Xuzhou, Jiangsu Province, China, **7** Department of Medical Information, Xuzhou Medical College, Xuzhou, Jiangsu Province, China

Abstract

Magnetic poly (D,L-lactide-co-glycolide) (PLGA)/lipid nanoparticles (MPLs) were fabricated from PLGA, L-α-phosphatidylethanolamine (DOPE), 1,2-distearoyl-sn-glycero-3-phosphoethanolamine-N-amino (polyethylene glycol) (DSPE-PEG-NH_2), and magnetic nanoparticles (NPs), and then conjugated to trans-activating transcriptor (TAT) peptide. The TAT-MPLs were designed to target the brain by magnetic guidance and TAT conjugation. The drugs hesperidin (HES), naringin (NAR), and glutathione (GSH) were encapsulated in MPLs with drug loading capacity (>10%) and drug encapsulation efficiency (>90%). The therapeutic efficacy of the drug-loaded TAT-MPLs in bEnd.3 cells was compared with that of drug-loaded MPLs. The cells accumulated higher levels of TAT-MPLs than MPLs. In addition, the accumulation of QD-loaded fluorescein isothiocyanate (FITC)-labeled TAT-MPLs in bEnd.3 cells was dose and time dependent. Our results show that TAT-conjugated MPLs may function as an effective drug delivery system that crosses the blood brain barrier to the brain.

Editor: Bing Xu, Brandeis University, United States of America

Funding: This work was supported by Jiangsu Key Laboratory of Brain Disease Bioinformation (Jsbl1102), the Priority Academic Program Development of Jiangsu Higher Education Institutions, the Education Departmental Natural Science Research Funds of Jiangsu Provincial Higher School of China (13KJB310021), the National Natural Science Foundation of China (31100762, 81371300), the Foundation of President of Xuzhou Medical College (2012KJZ06), and the Qing Lan Project of Jiangsu Province. The funders had no role in study design, data collection and analysis, decision to publish, or preparation of the manuscript.

Competing Interests: The authors have declared that no competing interests exist.

* Email: xzmclhz@126.com (HL); biosongyuanjian@126.com (YJS)

These authors contributed equally to this work.

Introduction

Developing an effective drug delivery system with the ability of crossing the blood brain barrier (BBB) is the crucial point in treating diseases of the human central nervous system (CNS) effectively. Many potential drugs have been abandoned during their development for their poor ability to cross the BBB in sufficient quantities to produce a therapeutic effect [1]. The BBB is not only an anatomical barrier to the free movement of solutes between the blood and brain, but also a transport and metabolic barrier [2]. Consequently, developing tools and methods that allow the therapeutic agents to delivery to the brain safely and effectively *in vivo* is important.

Nanocarrier systems, such as micelles, liposomes [3,4], and polymeric nanoparticles [5,6], have been investigated for delivering therapeutic agents to the brain [7]. Magnetically driven Nanocarrier drug delivery systems are powerful tools for delivering drugs, genes and cells to a target organ, and may be suitable for delivering drugs to the brain. These systems have many unique characteristics, including the delivery of a range of biomolecules *in vivo*, such as DNA and siRNA [8]; non-invasive magnetic targeting with therapeutic biomolecules by using external magnetic fields over the target organ or injury site, and trackability *in vivo* with various imaging systems [9–11]. Furthermore, carrying capacity could be improved by magnetic guidance to target the drug to the brain parenchyma. In order to increase the uptake efficiency, magnetic nanoparticles can be modified with specific ligands such as cationic albumin [12], thiamine [13], or transferrin [14], surfactant coatings [15], proteins and peptides [16–18]. The HIV-1 trans-activating transcriptor (TAT) peptide [19], which is a cell penetrating peptide, has been widely used to increase the transport efficiency of drug-loaded NPs across the BBB to the CNS [20]. TAT has been used to form the Chitosan-PEG-TAT nanoparticles for complexing siRNA to be delivered in neuronal cells [21]. TAT-GS nanoparticle-mediated calcitonin gene-related peptide (CGRP) gene delivery has been proposed to be an innovative strategy for cerebral vasospasm [22]. Therefore, normal brain drugs combining with peptides, nanotechnology and magnetic targeting may greatly improve the treatment of brain disorders [23].

Magnetic poly (D,L-lactide-co-glycolide) (PLGA)/lipid NPs (MPLs) combine the advantages of PLGA and magnetic liposomes, such as a well-defined biocompatible coating and

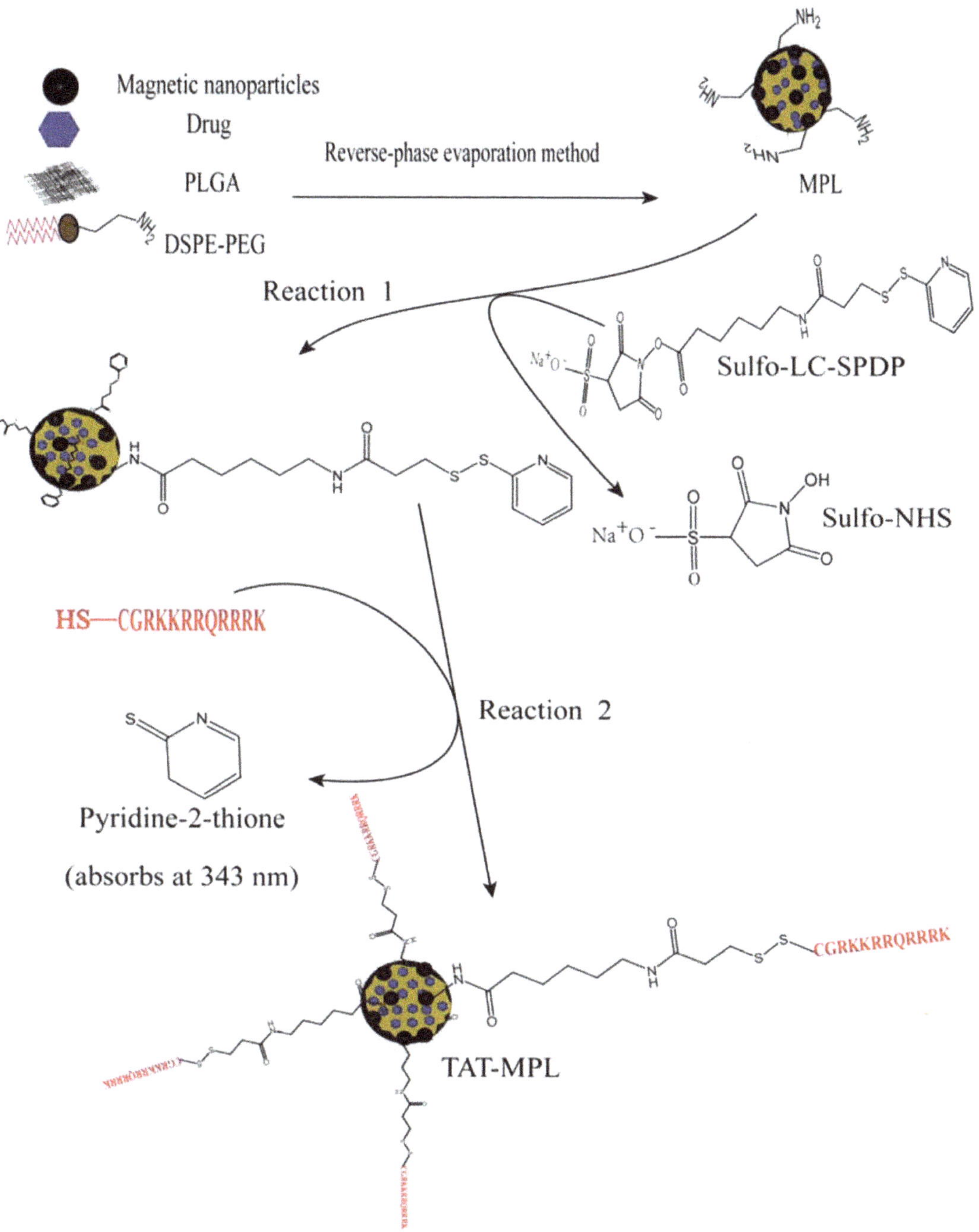

Figure 1. Schematic of the preparation of stealth MPLs and the conjugation of TAT peptide to MPLs.

simple fabrication [24], and have broad applications, including drug delivery and biodetection [25–27]. Monodispersed superparamagnetic magnetite/lipid nanospheres have been studied extensively [28–30]. Compared with conventional stealth liposomes [31,32], the surface of MPLs can be easily modified by groups, including functional amino (-NH_2) headgroups. In this work, we combine magnetic guidance and cell penetrating peptides to improve the delivery of drugs by TAT-conjugated MPLs.

Materials and Methods

Materials

Cholesterol and 1,2-distearoyl-sn-glycero-3-phosphoethanolamine-N-[amino (polyethylene glycol)-2000] (DSPE-PEG2000-NH_2) were purchased from Avanti Polar Lipids (USA). Quantum Dot (QD) were purchased from Wuhan Jiayuan Quantum Dots Co., Ltd (China). TAT-peptide with the sequence CGRKKRRQRRRK was purchased from ShineGene (China). Chitosan (deacetylation >90%, $M_w = 50{,}000$) was supplied by Yuhuan Aoxing (China). Octadecyl quaternized carboxymethyl

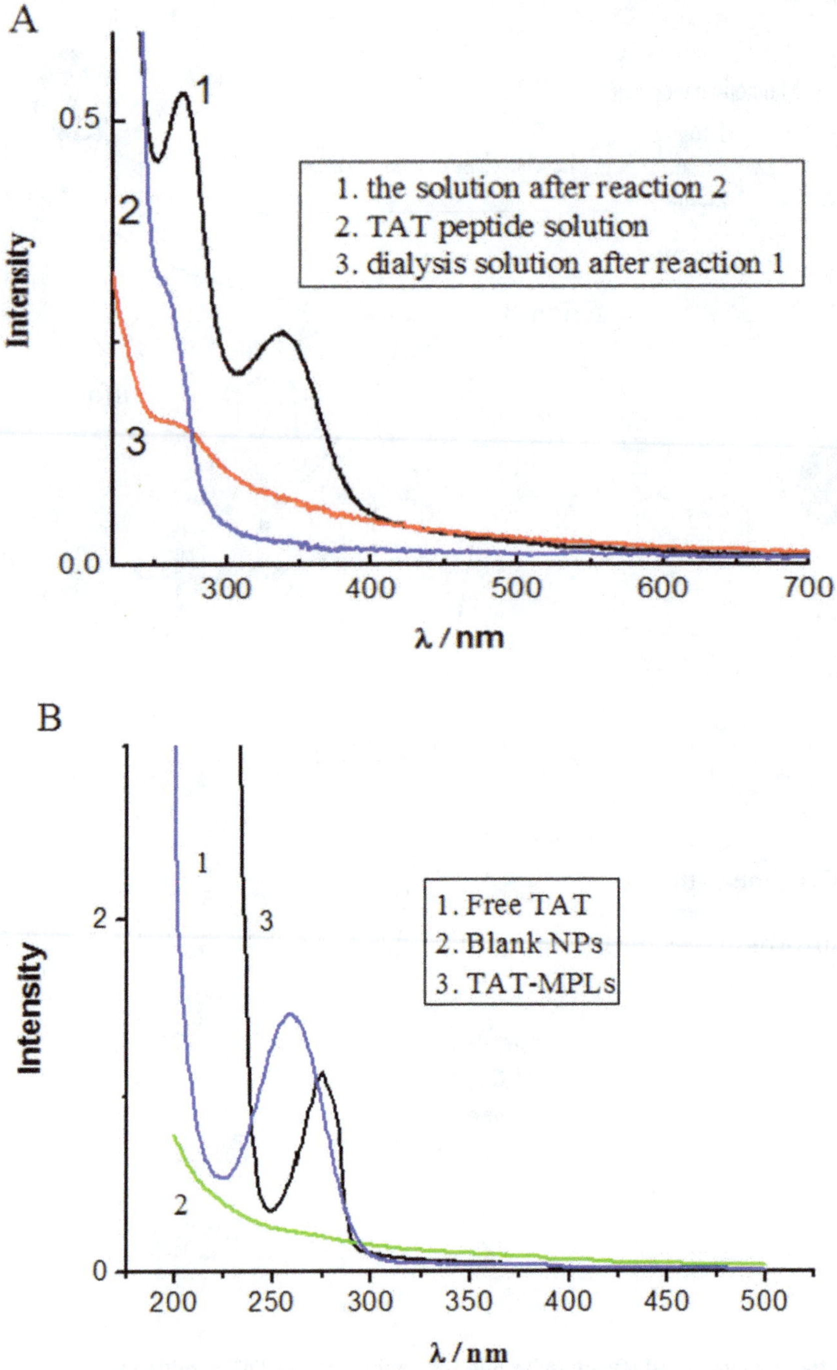

Figure 2. UV/Vis spectra. (A) UV/Vis spectra of the reaction solutions (conjugation of TAT to MPLs). (B) UV/Vis spectra of blank NPs and TAT-MPLs.

chitosan (OQCMC) and hydrophobic magnetic nanoparticles (HMNs) were prepared according to a previously published method [26], [28]. Poly (D,L-lactic-co-glycolic acid) ($M_w = 10,000$, lactic/glycolic acid ratio = 50/50) was purchased from Shandong Key Laboratory of Medical Polymer Material (China). L-α-Phosphatidylethanolamine (DOPE), N-succinimidyl 3-(2-pyridyldithio) propionate (SPDP), 2-iminothiolane, disuccinimidyl suberate (DSS), PD-10 columns were purchased from Sigma-Aldrich (USA). All other chemicals were of reagent grade and were used as received.

Preparation of MPLs

The MPLs were prepared by the reverse-phase evaporation (REV) method. For blank MPLs, PLGA, OQCMC, HMNs, DOPE, and DSPE-PEG-NH_2 (weight ratio = 1:0.2:0.3:0.2:0.2, total weight 30 mg) were dissolved in chloroform (4.0 mL) at room temperature to obtain the organic phase. The aqueous deionized water phase (6.0 mL) was mixed with the organic phase under sonication for 120 s at an output of 100 W. The organic solvents were evaporated on a rotary evaporator to form a gel-like MPL suspension. The MPLs were then separated by using a magnet and

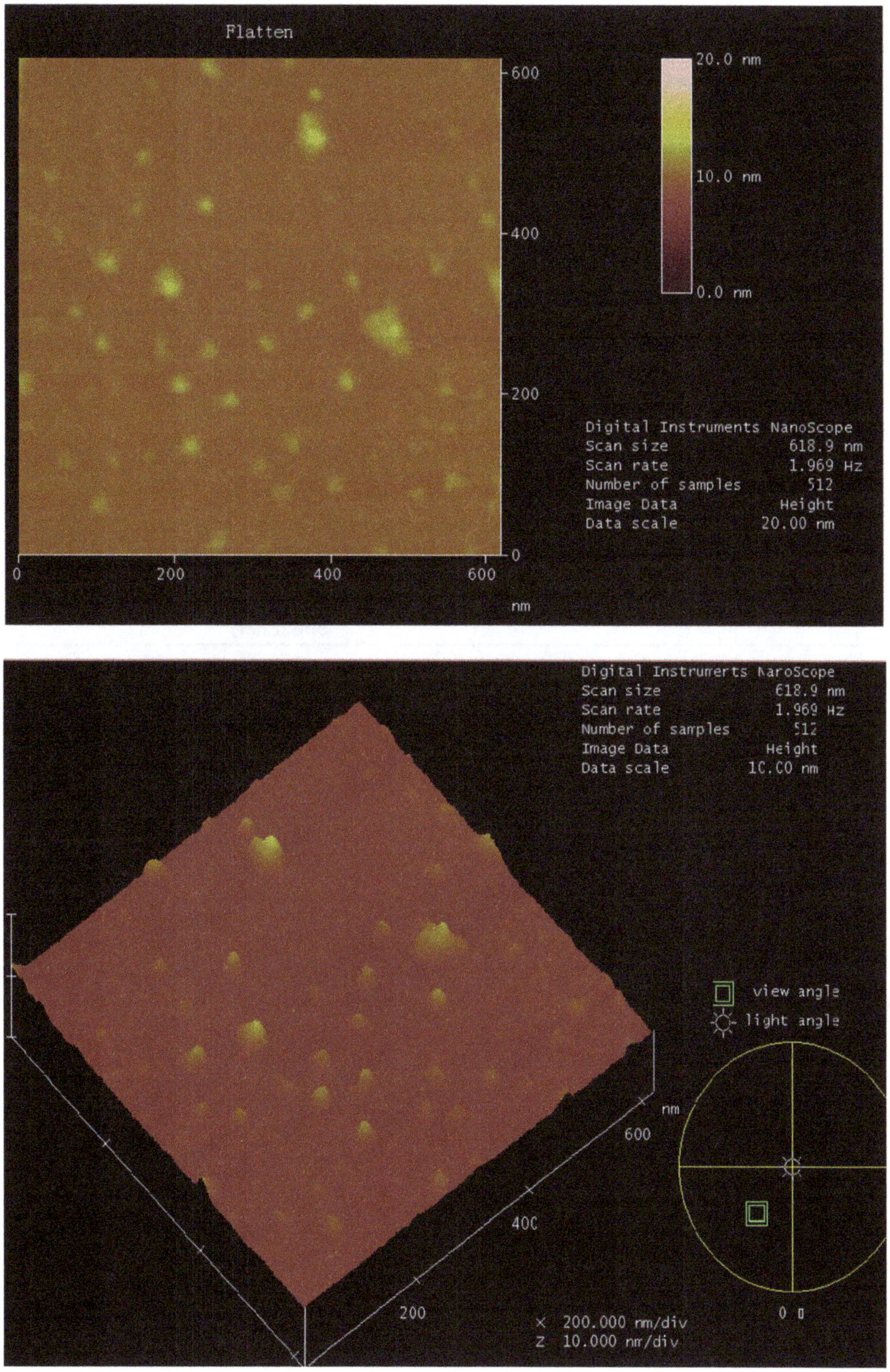

Figure 3. AFM micrographs of TAT-MPLs.

were washed with deionized water for three times. The collected product was freeze-dried and stored at $4^{\circ}C$.

For drug-loaded MPLs, the appropriate drug PLGA, OQCMC, HMNs and DSPE-PEG-NH_2 were dissolved in chloroform. Hesperidin (HES) and naringin (NAR) were soluble in the organic phase whereas glutathione (GSH) was dissolved in aqueous solution. The weight ratio of the drug to PLGA was adjusted according to experimental requirements.

TAT conjugation via a disulfide linkage

The MPLs were reacted with SPDP to install a 2-pyridyldithiol-end group on the surface of the NPs. A 0.1 M phosphate-buffered

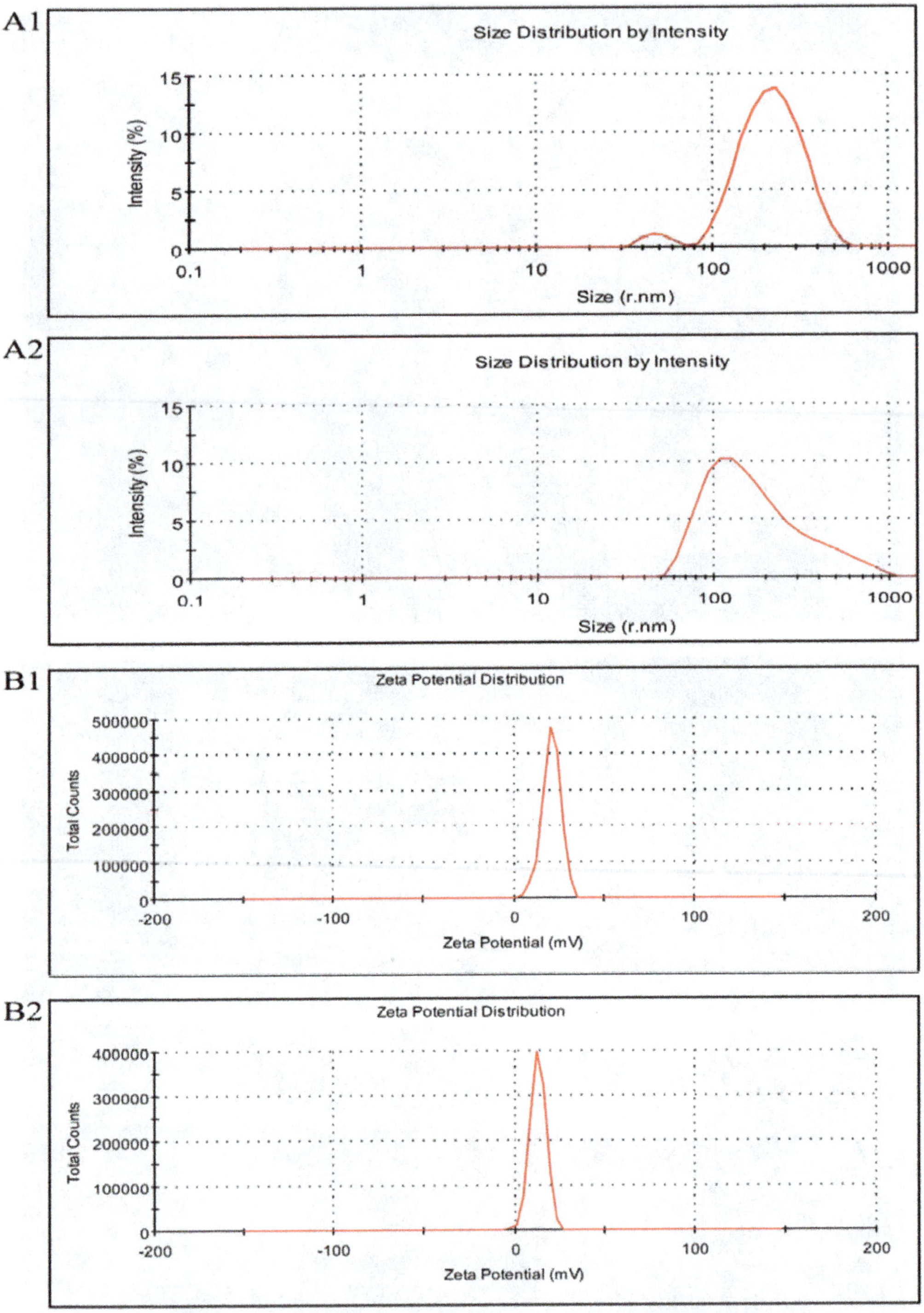

Figure 4. XRD spectrum and Magnetization curve. (A) XRD spectrum of TAT-MPLs. (B) Magnetization curve of Fe_3O_4 ferrofluid (1) and TAT-MPLs (2).

saline (PBS; pH 7.4) solution of MPL (5 mg/mL, 2.0 mL) was added to SPDP (2.0 mg) in DMSO (0.32 mL). The mixture was incubated at room temperature for 60 min. Low molecular weight impurities were dialyzed against 0.1 M PBS for 5 h with a dialysis bag (M_w = 12,000–14,000).

The 2-pyridyl disulfide-conjugated MPL solution was added to a 0.1 M PBS solution of TAT (5 mg/mL, 1.0 mL). The mixture was incubated overnight at 4°C to form a disulfide linkage between the surface of the MPLs and the TAT peptide. The excess TAT peptide was not removed and the TAT-conjugated MPL solution was stored at 4°C. The P2T method was used to verify the conjugation of the 2-pyridyl disulfide groups to the MPLs. The TAT-conjugated MPL solution was separated with a magnet and the supernatant solution was collected. The supernatant (300 µL) was diluted to 3 mL with PBS. UV-Visible Spectrophotometer

Table 1. Physical characterization of TAT-conjugated MPLs.

Formulation	Mean diameter (nm)	Polydispersity (μ/Γ^2)	Zeta potential (mV)
MPLs	102.6±1.3	0.202	20.7±3.62
TAT-MPLs	102.0±0.7	0.304	12.7±1.82
GSH-loaded TAT-MPLs	131.8±11.2	0.556	31.7±4.53
HES-loaded TAT-MPLs	112.9±1.1	0.220	5.39±0.42
NAR-loaded TAT-MPLs	93.1±1.6	0.237	32.8±2.43

was used to measure the absorbance of the MPL samples at 343 nm.

Characterization of MPLs

The particle size of the MPLs in solution was measured by quasielastic laser light scattering with a zeta potential analyzer. The MPL concentration in PBS was 0.3 mg/mL. Each measurement was repeated three times, and an average value was used. The size measurements were performed by multimodal analysis.

The morphologies of MPLs were observed by atomic force microscopy. For the AFM observations, droplets of the samples (approximately 30 μL) were deposited onto freshly cleaved mica and left for 10 min. Images were captured with scan rates between 0.5 and 1 Hz. The magnetic properties of magnetic TAT-MPLs were determined with a vibrating sample magnetometer.

Drug loading efficiency and release *in vitro*

The concentration of the three drugs was determined by UV/Vis spectroscopy at a fixed wavelength. The calibration curve was obtained in the concentration range of 0.5–50 μg/mL and the detection limit was 0.05 μg/mL.

After preparing the drug-loaded MPLs, the solution was centrifuged to remove any unencapsulated drug (4,000 rpm for 10 min). Drug content was determined by calculating the weight of the drug encapsulated in the MPLs.

The drug encapsulation efficiency (EE) and drug loading efficiency (LE) of the process were calculated using the following equation:

$$EE(\%) = \frac{A-B}{A} \times 100,\ LE(\%) = \frac{C}{D} \times 100,$$

where A is the total amount of drug; B is the amount of unencapsulated drug; C is the weight of drug in vesicle; D is the weight of vesicle.

In vitro drug release experiments of drug-loaded MPLs were carried out under shaking at 100 rpm and 37±0.5°C. The drug-loaded samples were enclosed in a dialysis membrane and then incubated in Phosphate buffer saline (10 mL, pH = 7.4). The buffer solution was exchanged completely at regular time points. The amount of drug release was determined by UV-Visible Spectrophotometer at set times, with PBS as a reference.

Cell culture and cytotoxicity studies

Bend.3 cells were grown in Dulbecco Modified Eagle Medium supplemented with 10% (v/v) fetal bovine serum and 1% (v/v) penicillin/streptomycin. The cytotoxicity was evaluated by MTT assays. bEnd.3 cells were seeded at a density of 1×10^4 cells/well in 96-well flat-bottomed microassay plates and incubated for 24 h at 37°C, in a fully humidified atmosphere of 5% CO_2. An increasing amount of drug-loaded MPLs and TAT-MPLs (1–100 μg/mL) were added and incubated for 12 h, 24 h and 48 h at 37°C. MTT saline solution (5 mg/mL, 100 μL/well) was added to the cells and formazan crystals were allowed to form over 3 h, then the crystals were dissolved with DMSO. The absorbance was measured at 490 nm with a Multi-Mode Microplate Reader.

Uptake studies

The uptake and intracellular distribution of QD-loaded fluorescein isothiocyanate (FITC)-TAT-MPLs in bEnd.3 cells were determined qualitatively using confocal fluorescence microscopy (Leica TCS SP8 MP, Leica Micosystems, Germany). bEnd.3 cells were seeded at a density of 8×10^4 cells/well in a 24-well plate with a pre-sterilized cover glass at the bottom and the cells were allowed to attach overnight. The following day, the cells were treated with QD-loaded FITC-MPLs and QD-loaded FITC-TAT-MPLs in the medium at a concentration of 20 μg/mL. At 0.5, 3, and 12 h after treatment, the cells were washed three times with PBS and fixed with 4% (w/w) paraformaldehyde in PBS for 15 min. The cells were counterstained with 4′,6-diamidino-2-phenylindole (DAPI) and rinsed three times. The images were captured with a confocal laser scanning microscope with appropriate filters for the red QD fluorescence (excitation at 560–575 nm and emission at 605 nm), green FITC fluorescence (excitation at 480–495 nm and emission at 525 nm) and blue DAPI fluorescence (excitation at 358 nm and emission at 461 nm). Finally, images captured using red and blue filters were overlain to determine the localization and association of red QD fluorescence in the cytoplast or nucleus, respectively.

Qualitative images and quantification of drug-loaded MPLs internalization

To measure the internalization of QD-loaded TAT-MPLs quantitatively, bEnd.3 cells were cultured on 24-well plates for 24 h to achieve approximately 80% confluence. Free FITC, free QDs, QD-loaded FITC-MPLs, or QD-loaded FITC-TAT-MPLs were then added to the wells. After incubation for 0.5, 3, or 12 h the cells were collected for fluorescence measurements (FITC and QDs). The fluorescence from individual cells was detected with a flow cytometer (FACS Calibur, BD Biosciences, USA). To detect the green FITC fluorescence, excitation was with the 488 nm line of an argon laser, and the emission fluorescence was measured at 525 nm. To detect red QD fluorescence, excitation was with the 570 nm line of an argon laser, and the emission fluorescence was measured at 605 nm.

For quantitative analysis, the uptake of FITC and QDs in bEnd.3 cells was determined by using fluorescence and the bicinchoninic (BCA) method. At the end of the treatment period,

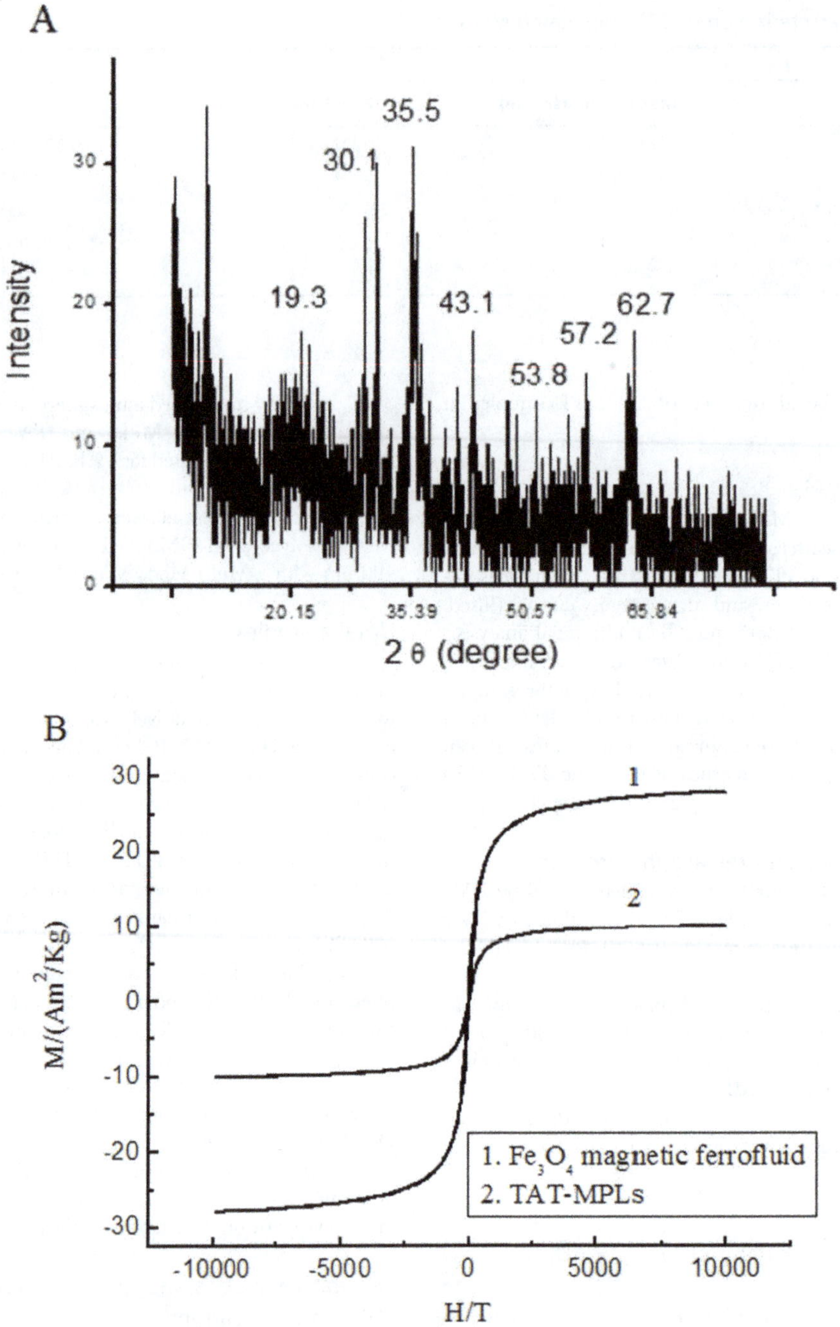

Figure 5. Particle-size-distribution and Zeta potential. (A) Particle-size-distribution based intensity of MPLs (1) and TAT-conjugated MPLs (2) in PBS. (B) Zeta potential of MPLs (1) and TAT-conjugated MPLs (2) in PBS.

the cells were washed three times with PBS (pH 7.4) and then incubated with cell culture lysis reagent (50 μL) for 10 min at 37°C. The protein content of the cell lysate was determined using the Pierce BCA protein assay. Cell lysates were harvested by adding PBS (50 μL, pH 7.4) and shaking at 37°C for 2 h. Samples were centrifuged at 10,000 rpm for 10 min at 4°C. The concentrations of the fluorescent materials (FITC and QDs) in the PBS extract were determined by a microplate spectrophotometer. Data are expressed as the amount of fluorescence material normalized to the total cell protein.

Statistical analysis

All data are expressed as mean±standard error of means. Statistical analyses were performed using Student's T-test. The differences were considered significant for p values$<$0.05.

Results and Discussion

Formulation of magnetic PLGA/lipids NPs

PLGA/lipid complexes have many advantages as delivery vehicles. They combine the properties of liposomes and PLGA and can be modified with molecular targeting factors. Multifunc-

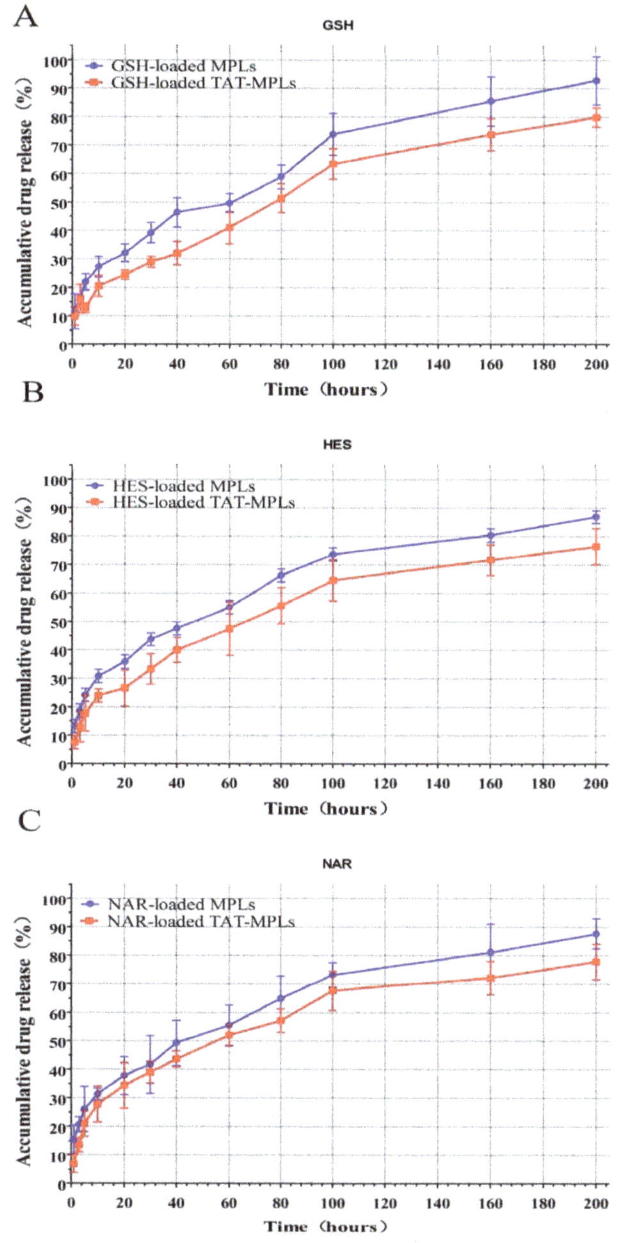

Figure 6. Drug release profiles of the TAT-conjugated MPLs in PBS (pH 7.4) at 37±0.5°C *in vitro*.

tional targeted drug delivery systems, such as magnetic cationic liposomes [30] and PEG- and TAT-conjugated MPLs, can be fabricated from DSPE-PEG or DOPE. Attaching flexible PEG polymers to the liposome surface increases the blood circulation time significantly. These PEG-coated liposomes are referred to as stealth liposomes [31,32]. A schematic illustration of the preparation of stealth TAT-conjugated MPLs is presented in Figure 1. PEGylated MPLs can be assembled by the REV method from DSPE-PEG-NH_2, OQCMC, and DOPE. The DSPE-PEG-NH_2 and OQCMC components of MPLs mean that amine groups are present on the surface of stealth MPLs [33–35]. In this study, SPDP reagents, which are a unique group of amine- and sulfhydryl-reactive heterobifunctional cross-linkers, were used to form amine-to-sulfhydryl cross-links between molecules. Because TAT peptide contains sulfhydryl groups (-SH), the MPLs are modified by the SPDP reagent in reaction 1. Reaction 2 results in the displacement of a pyridine-2-thione group, the concentration of which may be determined by measuring the absorbance at 343 nm.

UV/Vis spectra of the reaction solutions are shown in Figure 2A. An absorbance peak at 343 nm was clearly visible after reaction 2, which confirmed the presence of pyridine-2-thione. In addition, the peak at 343 nm was not observed for the dialyzed solution after reaction 1 and the TAT peptide solution, indicating that pyridine-2-thione must be the product of reaction 2. The results also suggest that amine groups were present on the surface of MPLs. UV/Vis spectroscopy was also used to determine the content of TAT peptide on the MPLs (Figure 2B). Differences were observed in the UV absorption of MPLs and TAT-MPLs. TAT had an absorption peak at 275 nm. The UV spectrum of the TAT-MPLs was similar to that of TAT, although it also contained a bathochromic shift at 277.5 nm, which was attributed to the addition of TAT to the MPLs. These results indicate that the modification of the TAT unit was responsible for the differences between the UV spectra of MPLs and TAT-MPLs.

Characterization of MPLs

The TAT-MPLs generally had irregular spherical shapes (Figure 3) and were about 80 nm in size. The hydrodynamic diameter of TAT-conjugated MPLs was 102.0±0.7 nm, with a corresponding polydispersity index (PDI) of 0.304, which was greater than the AFM diameter because of the hydration of MPLs in aqueous solution. The TAT conjugation decreased the zeta potential of NPs (Figure 4 and Table 1). HES were encapsulated effectively in the TAT-conjugated MPLs, and the drug encapsulation efficiency and loading capacity were above 90% and 10%, respectively. The size of the HES-loaded TAT-conjugated MPLs in PBS solution was 112.9±1.1 nm with a narrow size distribution and a polydispersity index of 0.220 (Table 1). The AFM images also show the spherical shape and homogeneous size distribution of the magnetic NPs.

X-ray powder diffraction analysis (XRD) is a kind of useful method to demonstrate the structure of magnetic nanoparticles. The XRD pattern of TAT-MPLs was detected as illustrated in Figure 5a. The characteristic peaks of Fe_3O_4 ferrofluid are at $2\theta = 30.1°$, 35.5°, 43.1°, 53.7° and 62.7°, which corresponding to crystal face of (220), (311), (400), (422), (511) and (440). The results indicated that TAT-MPLs has the same crystalline structure with Fe_3O_4 ferrofluid. The broad peak in the $2\theta = 15°–25°$ region approve the existence of PLGA polymer. Figure 5b shows the room-temperature magnetization curves of Fe_3O_4 ferrofluid (1) and TAT-MPLs. As shown in the figure, both the samples show a typical superparamagnetic behavior at room temperature without any hysteresis loop. The saturation magnetization value of TAT-MPLs is 10.1 emu/g at 300 K, which is about 36.2% of the magnetization of Fe_3O_4 ferrofluid.

The drug release profiles of TAT-conjugated MPLs showed a high burst release during the first 24 h followed by slower release (Figure 6). During the initial burst release, 20%–40% of the encapsulated drug was released from the TAT-conjugated MPLs. After 8 days, 70%–90% of the total drug was released. The surface conjugation of the TAT-MPLs meant that they had a slower drug release than the MPLs.

Cytotoxicity and growth inhibition of bEnd.3 cells *in vitro*

The cytotoxicity of MPLs and TAT-MPLs in bEnd.3 cells was examined with an MTT assay. Figure 7 shows the cytotoxicity of MPLs and TAT-MPLs at concentrations of less than 100 μg/mL.

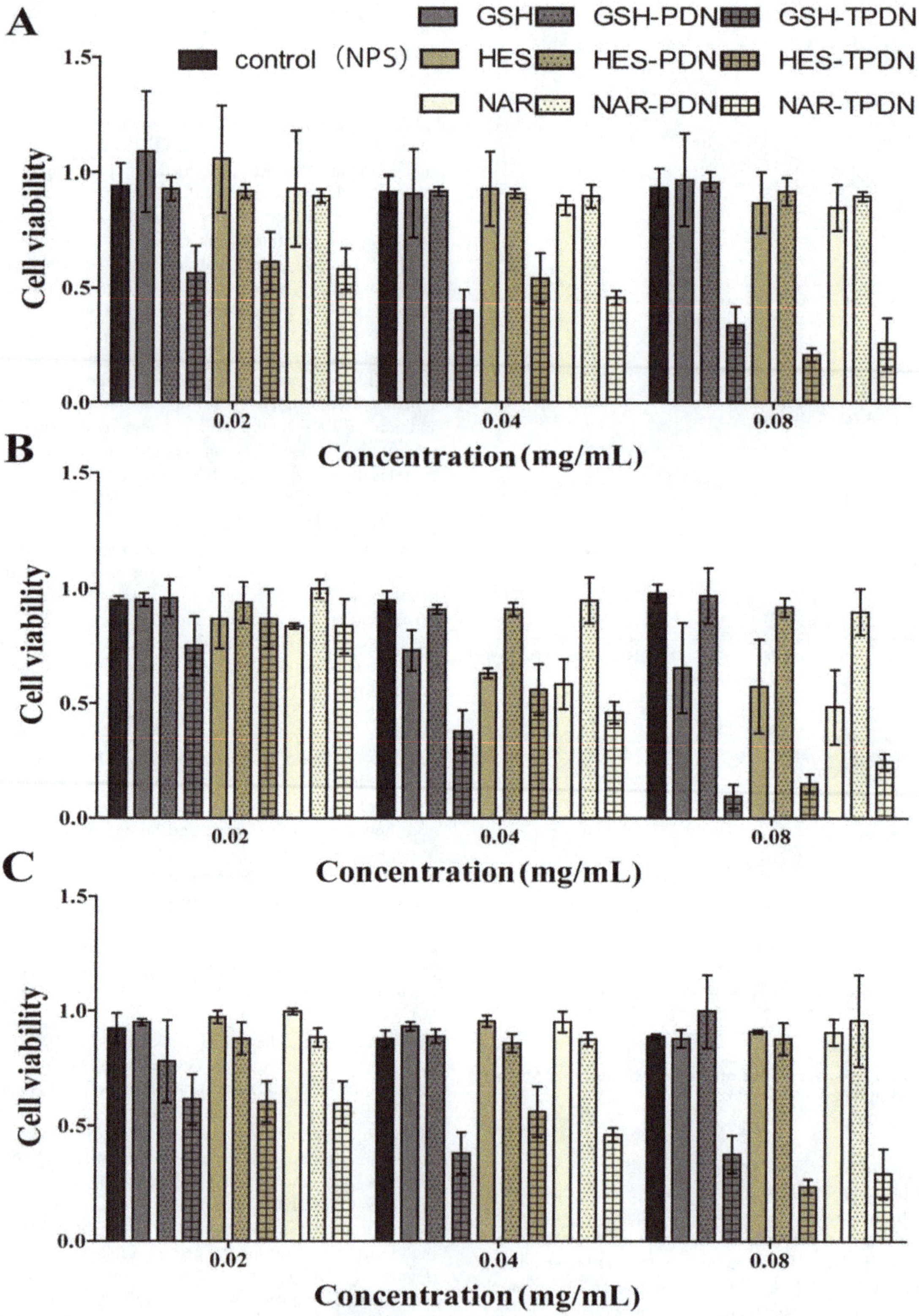

Figure 7. Cytotoxicity of MPLs and drug-loaded TAT-MPLs measured using MTT assays after. (A) 12, (B) 24, and (C) 48 h incubation with bEnd.3 cells. (GSH: glutathione, HES: hesperidin, NAR: naringin).

The bEnd.3 cells treated with MPLs at concentrations of 20.0, 40.0, and 80.0 μg/mL showed good viability (>85%), whereas the cells treated with TAT-MPLs showed poor viability (<75%) after incubation for 12, 24, and 48 h. As the concentration of NPs increased, the drug-loaded TAT-MPLs were more cytoxic than the MPLs. This was because the TAT conjugation delivered a

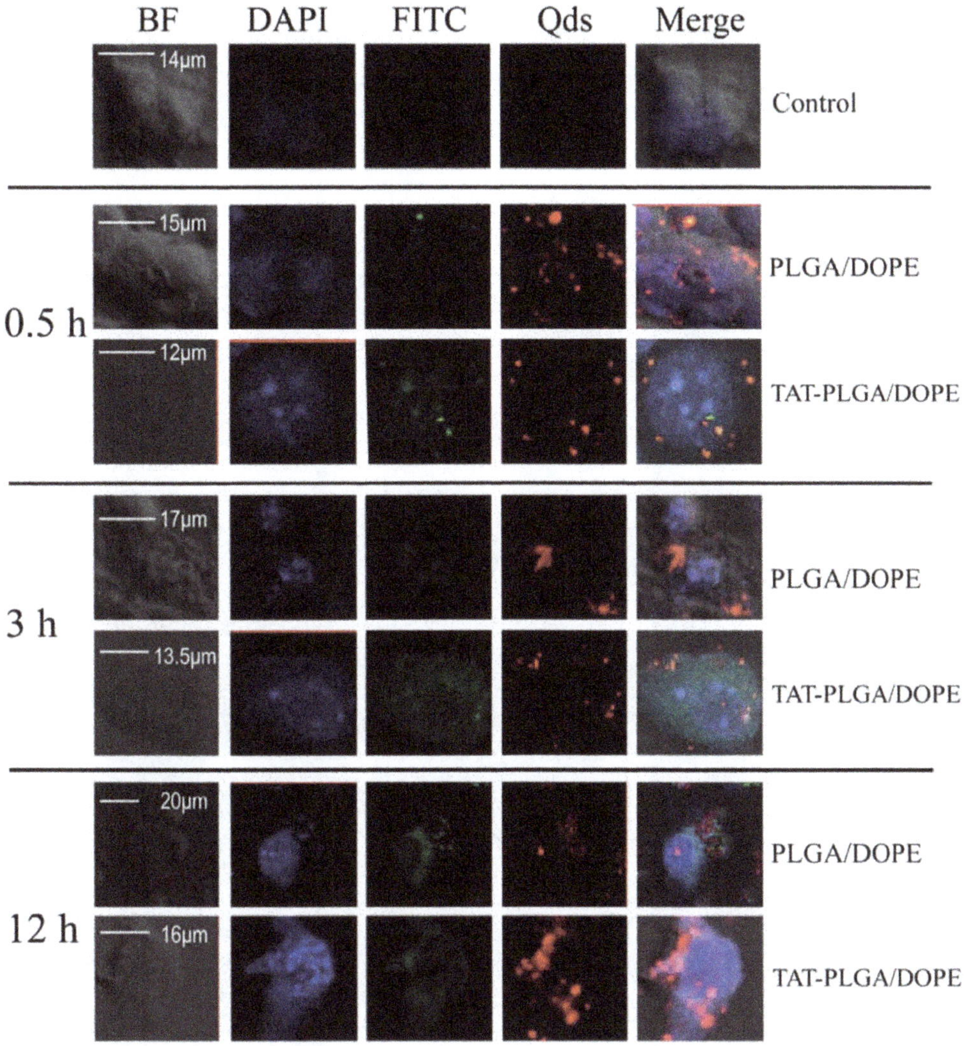

Figure 8. Localization and distribution of QDs encapsulated in TAT-MPLs in bEnd.3 cells. Cells were cultured in FITC-labeled NP-containing medium (1 μM QDs) on a glass-bottomed culture plate for 0.5, 3, and 12 h, treated with DAPI for 5–10 min, and then examined by confocal microscopy.

greater amount of the drugs into cells. Furthermore, the cytotoxicity of the blank TAT-MPLs was low and this was confirmed by observing morphological changes in the cells by microscopy. These results demonstrate that TAT-MPLs has low cellular toxicity and were suitable for use in experimental concentrations.

Figure 7 also shows the growth inhibition of bEnd.3 cells by GSH, HES, and NAR in MPLs, TAT-MPLs, and in solution after 48 h at concentrations of GSH, HES, and NAR from 20 to 80 μg/mL. The cell growth inhibition rate was dose-dependent in all the experiments. At GSH, HES, and NAR concentrations of 20 μg/mL, there was no difference in the growth inhibition of bEnd.3 cells treated with the drug solutions and drug-loaded NPs. As the concentration of the drugs increased, the cytotoxicity of the TAT-MPLs was significantly higher ($P<0.05$ for NPs concentrations of 40 and 80 μg/mL). The cell growth inhibition of the TAT-MPLs was also greater than that of the MPLs without TAT, indicating that a greater number of drug-loaded TAT-MPLs entered the cells because TAT increased the cell membrane penetration.

Intracellular distribution of QD-loaded NPs

To verify whether encapsulating different drugs in the NPs affected their trafficking in tumor cells, we evaluated the intracellular distribution of free FITC/QDs, QD-loaded FITC-MPLs, and QD-loaded FITC-TAT-MPLs in bEnd.3 cells with a nuclear stain. The intracellular trafficking of FITC and QDs was studied by laser confocal microscopy to clarify the mechanism of efficacy of drug-loaded NPs. The QD-loaded FITC-NPs showed a diffuse distribution within the cells, with a significant fraction appearing in the cytoplasm near the cell nucleus at 0.5 h. A significant proportion of QD-loaded FITC-NPs also appeared in the cytoplasm. Therefore, the strong fluorescence of TAT-MPLs in the cytoplasm and cell nucleus demonstrates that they can deliver QDs efficiently to bEnd.3 cells. In addition, the FITC-TAT-MPLs were concentrated in the perinuclear region rather than at the cell periphery at 12 h. QDs were also present in the nuclei of cells treated with FITC-TAT-MPLs at 12 h. (Figure 8).

Interestingly, the cells treated with FITC-TAT-MPLs accumulated QDs in the nucleus, whereas cells treated with FITC-MPLs did not. The nuclear delivery of QDs by TAT-MPLs was greater

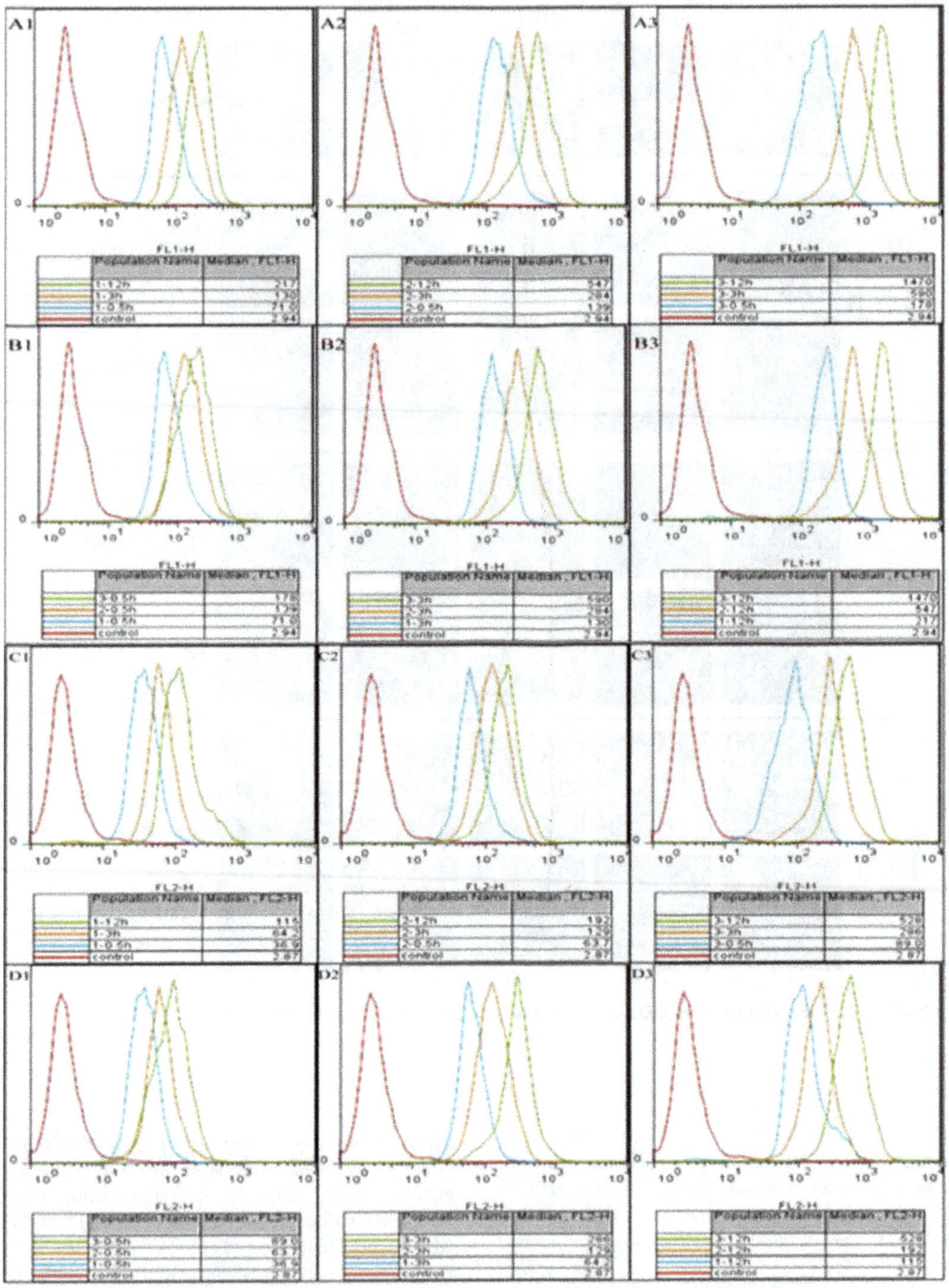

Figure 9. Flow cytometry analysis of bEnd.3 cells. Cells incubated with free FITC and QDs (1), MPLs (2), and TAT-MPLs (3) for 0.5 h, 3 h and 12 h at a NP concentration of 20 μg/mL. The NPs were labeled with FITC. The FITC (A and B) and QD fluorescence intensity (C and D) are shown.

than that by MPLs, which is also consistent with the greater cytotoxicity observed in the MTT assay. These results were further verified by quantitative analysis of accumulation of FITC and QDs.

Quantitative analysis of accumulation in bEnd.3 cells

To determine the efficacy of cellular drug delivery by TAT-MPLs, the cellular accumulation of equivalent doses of FITC and QDs was quantitatively analyzed in bEnd.3 cells. Figure 9 and Figure 10 show that cells treated with QD-loaded TAT-MPLs accumulated higher levels of QDs than those treated with QD-loaded MPLs. Furthermore, bEnd.3 cells treated with TAT-MPLs accumulated a significantly higher level of QDs and FITC than those treated with QDs and FITC in MPLs and in solution ($P< 0.05$) at 3 h and 12 h. Thus, the accumulation of QDs and FITC in bEnd.3 cells is enhanced by TAT conjugation.

Our results show that NPs enhance QDs accumulation considerably in bEnd.3 cells compared with free QDs, and that

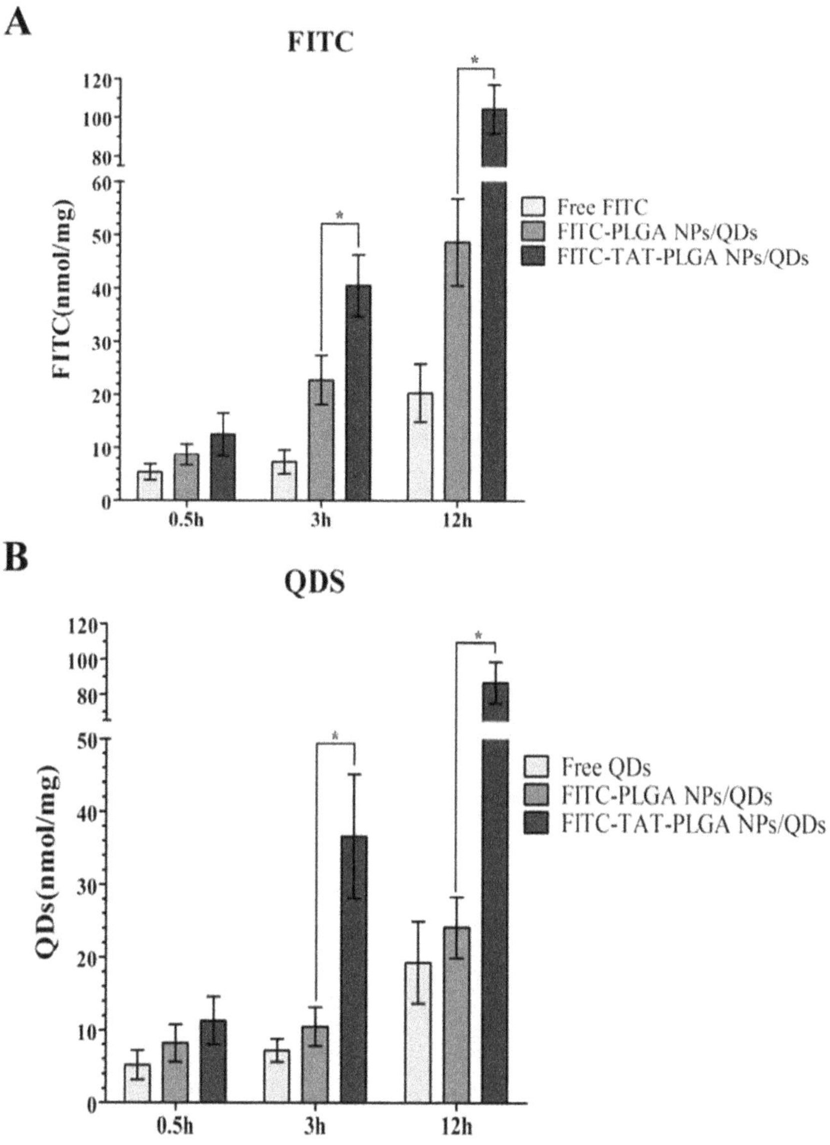

Figure 10. Quantitative analysis of QD-loaded FITC-MPLs and FITC-TAT-MPLs in bEnd.3 cells. Cells were cultured in a 24-well plate for 0.5 h, 3 h and 12 h, lysed, and the FITC and QDs fluorescence were measured by a microplate spectrophotometer to determine FITC (A) and QDs (B) contents in the cells.

TAT-MPLs increase QDs accumulation more efficiently than MPLs. These results were confirmed by laser confocal microscopy. Many studies have shown that the increased level of drug accumulation in cells treated with MPLs contributes to the enhanced therapeutic efficacy of drug-loaded NPs [15]. Thus, our method of fabricating TAT-conjugated magnetic NPs successfully produced TAT-MPLs that may be effective for delivering drugs across the BBB.

Conclusion

Previous studies indicate that there are many applications of magnetic nanoparticles for cells and bacteria [36–38]. In this study, we fabricated TAT-conjugated MPLs from OQCMC, DOPE, and magnetic NPs. The size of the HES-loaded TAT-MPLs in aqueous solution was close to 112.9±1.1 nm with a narrow size distribution with a polydispersity index of 0.220. AFM images showed the TAT-MPLs were spherical and had a homogeneous size distribution. The TAT-MPLs showed very strong fluorescence in the cytoplasm and cell nucleus, and delivered QDs to bEnd.3 cells efficiently. The levels of QDs and FITC that accumulated in bEnd.3 cells were dose- and time-dependent for MPLs and TAT-MPLs. The TAT conjugation of MPLs could significantly enhance the cellular delivery and the therapeutic efficacy of drugs in bEnd.3 cells by penetrating the cell membrane. This may be useful in designing drug-loaded NPs for crossing the BBB and delivering drugs to the brain.

Author Contributions

Conceived and designed the experiments: HZL YJS XRW YFZ. Performed the experiments: KW ZMZ YFZ. Analyzed the data: FZ JW YYF YD LZ KM. Contributed reagents/materials/analysis tools: TTS YS YHL. Wrote the paper: KW.

References

1. Liu L, Guo K, Lu J, Venkatraman SS, Luo D, et al. (2008) Biologically active core/shell nanoparticles self-assembled from cholesterol-terminated PEG-TAT for drug delivery across the blood-brain barrier. Biomaterials 29: 1509–1517.
2. Abbott NJ, Patabendige AA, Dolman DE, Yusof SR, Begley DJ (2010) Structure and function of the blood-brain barrier. Neurobiol Dis 37: 13–25.
3. Andreu A, Fairweather N, Miller AD (2008) Clostridium neurotoxin fragments as potential targeting moieties for liposomal gene delivery to the CNS. Chembiochem 9: 219–231.
4. Aichberger KJ, Herndlhofer S (2007) Liposomal cytarabine for treatment of myeloid central nervous system relapse in chronic myeloid leukaemia occurring during imatinib therapy. Eur J Clin Invest 37: 808–813.
5. Rao KS, Reddy MK, Horning JL, Labhasetwar V (2008) TAT-conjugated nanoparticles for the CNS delivery of anti-HIV drugs. Biomaterials 29: 4429–4438.
6. Mika P, Jere P, Thomas W, Tommy T (2008) Three-step tumor targeting of paclitaxel using biotinylated PLA-PEG nanoparticles and avidin-biotin technology: Formulation development and in vitro anticancer activity. Eur J Pharm Biopharm 70: 66–74.
7. Tiwari SB, Amiji MM (2006) A review of nanocarrier-based CNS delivery systems. Curr Drug Deliv 3: 219–232.
8. Pan BF, Cui DX, Sheng Y (2007) Dendrimer-modified magnetic nanoparticles enhance efficiency of gene delivery system. Cancer Res 67: 8156–8163.
9. Choi KM, Choi SH, Jeon H (2011) Chimeric capsid protein as a nanocarrier for siRNA delivery: stability and cellular uptake of encapsulated siRNA. ACS Nano 5: 8690–8699.
10. Dobson J (2006) Gene therapy progress and prospects: magnetic nanoparticle-based gene delivery. Gene Ther 13: 283–287.
11. Akhtari M, Bragin A, Cohen M (2008) Functionalized magnetonanoparticles for MRI diagnosis and localization in epilepsy. Epilepsia 49: 1419–1430.
12. Lu W, Tan YZ, Hu KL, Jiang XG (2005) Cationic albumin conjugated pegylated nanoparticle with its transcytosis ability and little toxicity against blood-brain barrier. Int J Pharm 295: 247–260.
13. Salman HH, Gamazo C, Agüeros M, Irache JM (2007) Bioadhesive capacity and immunoadjuvant properties of thiamine-coated nanoparticles. Vaccine 25: 8123–8132.
14. Kievit FM, Zhang M (2011) Cancer Nanotheranostics: Improving Imaging and Therapy by Targeted Delivery Across Biological Barriers. Adv Mater 23: H217–247.
15. Chavanpatil MD, Khdair A, Gerard B, Bachmeier C, Miller DW, et al. (2007) Surfactant-polymer nanoparticles overcome P-glycoprotein-mediated drug efflux. Mol Pharm 4: 730–738.
16. Torchilin VP (2008) Cell penetrating peptide-modified pharmaceutical nanocarriers for intracellular drug and gene delivery. Biopolymers 90: 604–610.
17. Lazar AN, Mourtas S, Youssef I, Parizot C, Dauphin A, et al. (2013) Curcumin-conjugated nanoliposomes with high affinity for Aβ deposits: possible applications to Alzheimer disease. Nanomedicine 9: 712–721.
18. Costantino L, Gandolfi F, Tosi G, Rivasi F, Vandelli MA, et al. (2005) Peptide-derivatized biodegradable nanoparticles able to cross the blood-brain barrier. J Control Release 108: 84–96.
19. Schwarze SR, Ho A, Vocero-Akbani A, Dowdy SF (1999) In vivo protein transduction: delivery of a biologically active protein into the mouse. Science 285: 1569–1582.
20. Santra S, Yang H, Stanley JT, Holloway PH, Moudgil BM, et al. (2005) Rapid and effective labeling of brain tissue using TAT-conjugated CdS: Mn/ZnS quantum dots. Chem Commun 25: 3144–3156.
21. Malhotra M, Tomaro-Duchesneau C, Prakash S (2013) Synthesis of TAT peptide-tagged PEGylated chitosan nanoparticles for siRNA delivery targeting neurodegenerative diseases. Biomaterials 34: 1270–1280.
22. Tian XH, Wang ZG, Meng H, Wang YH, Feng W, et al. (2013) Tat peptide-decorated gelatin-siloxane nanoparticles for delivery of CGRP transgene in treatment of cerebral vasospasm. Int J Nanomedicine 8: 865–876.
23. Teixidó M, Giralt E (2008) The role of peptides in blood-brain barrier nanotechnology. J Pept Sci 14: 163–173.
24. Sophie L, Delphine F, Marc P (2008) Magnetic Iron Oxide Nanoparticles: Synthesis, Stabilization, Vectorization, Physicochemical Characterizations, and Biological Applications. Chem Rev 108: 2064–2110.
25. Cui Y, Xu Q, Chow PK, Wang D, Wang CH (2013) Transferrin-conjugated magnetic silica PLGA nanoparticles loaded with doxorubicin and paclitaxel for brain glioma treatment. Biomaterials 34: 8511–8520.
26. Krack M, Hohenberg H, Kornowski A, Lindner P, Weller H, et al. (2008) Nanoparticle-loaded magnetophoretic vesicles. J Am Chem Soc 130: 7315–7320.
27. Liang XF, Wang HJ, Luo H, Tian H, Zhang BB, et al. (2008) Characterization of novel multifunctional cationic polymeric liposomes formed from octadecyl quaternized carboxymethyl chitosan/cholesterol and drug encapsulation. Langmuir 24: 7147–7153.
28. Liang X, Li X, Chang J, Duan Y, Li Z (2013) Properties and Evaluation of Quaternized Chitosan/lipid Cation Polymeric Liposomes for Cancer Targeted Gene Delivery. Langmuir 29: 8683–8693.
29. Zhao AJ, Yao P, Kang CS (2005) Synthesis and characterization of tat-mediated O-CMC magnetic nanoparticles having anticancer function. J Magn Magn Mater 295: 37–43.
30. Liang XF, Wang HJ (2010) Development of monodispersed and functional magnetic nanospheres via simple liposome method. J Nanopart Res 12: 1723–1732.
31. Gabizon AA (2001) Stealth Liposomes and Tumor Targeting: One Step Further in the Quest for the Magic Bullet. Clin Cancer Res 7: 223–225.
32. Garbuzenko O, Barenholz Y, Priev A (2005) Effect of grafted PEG on liposome size and on compressibility and packing of lipid bilayer. Chem Ph Lipids 135: 117–129.
33. Liang X, Tian H, Luo H, Wang H, Chang J (2009) Novel quaternized chitosan and polymeric micelles with cross-linked ionic cores for prolonged release of minocycline. J Biomater Sci Polym Ed 20: 115–131.
34. Yu Z, Schmaltz RM, Bozeman TC, Paul R, Rishel MJ, et al. (2013) Selective tumor cell targeting by the disaccharide moiety of bleomycin. J Am Chem Soc 135: 2883–2886.
35. Yamanouchi D, Wu J, Lazar AN, Kent KC, Chu CC, et al. (2008) Biodegradable arginine-based poly(ester-amide)s as non-viral gene delivery reagents. Biomaterials 29: 3269–3277.
36. Pan Y, Du X, Zhao F, Xu B (2012) Magnetic nanoparticles for the manipulation of proteins and cells. Chem Soc Rev 41: 2912–2942.
37. Shin J, Lee KM, Lee JH, Lee J, Cha M (2014) Magnetic manipulation of bacterial magnetic nanoparticle-loaded neurospheres. Integr Biol (Camb) 6: 532–539.
38. Liu F, Mu J, Wu X, Bhattacharjya S, Yeow EK, et al. (2014) Peptide-perylene diimide functionalized magnetic nano-platforms for fluorescence turn-on detection and clearance of bacterial lipopolysaccharides. Chem Commun (Camb) 50: 6200–6203.

8

Nanodrug-Enhanced Radiofrequency Tumor Ablation: Effect of Micellar or Liposomal Carrier on Drug Delivery and Treatment Efficacy

Marwan Moussa[1], S. Nahum Goldberg[1,2], Gaurav Kumar[1], Rupa R. Sawant[3], Tatyana Levchenko[3], Vladimir P. Torchilin[3], Muneeb Ahmed[1]*

1 Laboratory for Minimally Invasive Tumor Therapies, Department of Radiology, Beth Israel Deaconess Medical Center/Harvard Medical School, Boston, MA, United States of America, **2** Division of Image-guided Therapy and Interventional Oncology, Department of Radiology, Hadassah Hebrew University Medical Center, Jerusalem, Israel, **3** Department of Pharmaceutical Sciences and Center for Pharmaceutical Biotechnology and Nanomedicine, Northeastern University, Boston, MA, United States of America

Abstract

Purpose: To determine the effect of different drug-loaded nanocarriers (micelles and liposomes) on delivery and treatment efficacy for radiofrequency ablation (RFA) combined with nanodrugs.

Materials/Methods: Fischer 344 rats were used (n = 196). First, single subcutaneous R3230 tumors or normal liver underwent RFA followed by immediate administration of IV fluorescent beads (20, 100, and 500 nm), with fluorescent intensity measured at 4–24 hr. Next, to study carrier type on drug efficiency, RFA was combined with micellar (20 nm) or liposomal (100 nm) preparations of doxorubicin (Dox; targeting HIF-1α) or quercetin (Qu; targeting HSP70). Animals received RFA alone, RFA with Lipo-Dox or Mic-Dox (1 mg IV, 15 min post-RFA), and RFA with Lipo-Qu or Mic-Qu given 24 hr pre- or 15 min post-RFA (0.3 mg IV). Tumor coagulation and HIF-1α orHSP70 expression were assessed 24 hr post-RFA. Third, the effect of RFA combined with IV Lipo-Dox, Mic-Dox, Lipo-Qu, or Mic-Qu (15 min post-RFA) compared to RFA alone on tumor growth and animal endpoint survival was evaluated. Finally, drug uptake was compared between RFA/Lipo-Dox and RFA/Mic-Dox at 4–72 hr.

Results: Smaller 20 nm beads had greater deposition and deeper tissue penetration in both tumor (100 nm/500 nm) and liver (100 nm) ($p<0.05$). Mic-Dox and Mic-Qu suppressed periablational HIF-1α or HSP70 rim thickness more than liposomal preparations ($p<0.05$). RFA/Mic-Dox had greater early (4 hr) intratumoral doxorubicin, but RFA/Lipo-Dox had progressively higher intratumoral doxorubicin at 24–72 hr post-RFA ($p<0.04$). No difference in tumor growth and survival was seen between RFA/Lipo-Qu and RFA/Mic-Qu. Yet, RFA/Lipo-Dox led to greater animal endpoint survival compared to RFA/Mic-Dox ($p<0.03$).

Conclusion: With RF ablation, smaller particle micelles have superior penetration and more effective local molecular modulation. However, larger long-circulating liposomal carriers can result in greater intratumoral drug accumulation over time and reduced tumor growth. Accordingly, different carriers provide specific advantages, which should be considered when formulating optimal combination therapies.

Editor: Dominique Heymann, Faculté de médecine de Nantes, France

Funding: This work was supported by grants from the National Cancer Institute, National Institutes of Health, Bethesda, MD (R01CA133114, R01 CA100045, and CCNE 1U54CA151881-01), Harvard Medical Faculty Physicians Faculty Radiology Foundation, and the Israel Science Foundation. The funders had no role in study design, data collection, and analysis, decision to publish, or preparation of the manuscript.

Competing Interests: The authors have declared that no competing interests exist.

* Email: mahmed@bidmc.harvard.edu

Introduction

Radiofrequency ablation (RFA) is now a mainstay treatment for primary and secondary small focal tumors in the liver, lung, kidney, and other organs, with long-term studies demonstrating good outcomes in well-selected patient populations [1,2]. However, challenges to RF ablation of larger tumors remain, including the potential persistence of residual tumor cells within the ablation zone and the surrounding ablative margin despite apparent adequate treatment [3,4]. Therefore, strategies to target residual viable tumor cells and achieve a more complete treatment are being actively pursued. One such strategy has been to combine RF ablation with chemotherapy delivered in liposomal nanocarriers to target partially-injured viable cells in the ablation zone and surrounding periablational rim [5–7]. Early studies demonstrate increased local tumor coagulation, intratumoral drug accumulation, increased animal endpoint survival, and increased tumor coagulation in clinical studies using long-circulating liposomal doxorubicin as an adjuvant to RF [5–9].

Over the last several years, greater mechanistic understanding of the RFA-induced tissue reactions and low-level hyperthermia in the periablational margin has led to refined approaches such as modulating chemotherapy drug payload, composition, and liposomal drug release profile [10–15]. Key examples include the use of liposomal quercetin to eliminate upregulated heat shock proteins and bortezomib to eliminate HIF-1a and thereby increase tumor destruction [14,16]. Yet, limitations persist, either in the form of incomplete modulation of target post-RFA tissue reactions, inadequate spatial and temporal coordination of drug delivery to the periablational rim, or sub-optimal drug release [14,17,18]. Specifically, in the case of liposomal quercitin, although marked reduction in the thickness of the rim of HSP was noted, persistence of more peripheral expression of HSP was seen. This provides ample rationale for further study to uncover the optimal nanocarriers to be used in the setting of ablation.

Most studies have used 100 nm-size liposomal carriers, based upon original combination therapy studies and the long-circulating nature of many of these formulations [12,18]. Yet, within the fields of oncology and pharmacotherapeutics, there is increasing interest in using smaller carriers (micelles and spheroids) to improve intratumoral drug delivery and deeper interstitial penetration on its own, and in combination with low-level generalized hyperthermic treatments [19,20]. However, such carrier alterations will likely affect properties of drug delivery such as kinetics, warranting formal evaluation of potential trade-offs between different outcomes (e.g., delivery, modulation of specified targets, and overall survival).

Along these lines, here, we sought to determine whether or not we could alter the nanodrug formulation to improve the spatial distribution of specific drugs to target relatively "short-acting" processes in a rim further from the ablation zone that were inadequately treated using long-circulating liposomes in prior studies [14,21]. Accordingly, we studied the comparative effects of smaller (20 nm beads or micelles) and larger-sized (100+ nm beads or long-circulating PEG-coated liposomes) particles/carriers: on 1) distribution in the periablational rim using fluorescent beads (to determine the extent to which smaller particles have deeper penetration in periablational inflammatory tissue; 2) suppressing key ablation-induced reactions including pro-angiogenic hypoxia-inducible factor (HIF-1α) and protective heat shock protein (HSP70) production in the periablational rim using targeted drug payloads (doxorubicin/Dox and quercetin/Qu); 3) intratumoral drug accumulation of a target drug payload (doxorubicin); and finally 4) determine whether any of these primary end-points ultimately affected tumor growth rate and animal endpoint survival.

Materials and Methods

Experimental Overview

All animal work was conducted according to relevant national and international guidelines. Approval of the Beth Israel Deaconess Medical Center Institutional Animal Care and Use Committee was obtained prior to the start of this study. The study was performed in four phases. A total of 196 female Fischer 344 rats were used. All drugs were administered intravenously (IV). The following abbreviations are used: liposomal doxorubicin (Lipo-Dox), micellar doxorubicin (Mic-Dox), liposomal quercetin (Lipo-Qu), and micellar quercetin (Mic-Qu).

Phase1. Effect of particle size on distribution in the periablational rim after RF ablation. Studies were performed in two models, representing the tumor and the necessary surrounding normal tissue that must be ablated to achieve an adequate ablation margin [1]. First, 16 single subcutaneous R3230 breast adenocarcinoma tumors were implanted. Animals were randomized to receive RFA combined with color-labeled fluorescent beads of three sizes (20, 100, and 500 nm) given I5 min post-RF (6 animals×2 time points, n = 12) or IV fluorescent beads treatment alone (control tumors; n = 4). Next, the left liver lobes of 16 normal (tumor-free) animals were treated with RF ablation/IV fluorescent beads (20 nm and 100 nm, 15 min post-RFA) (6 animals×2 time points, n = 12) and control IV fluorescent beads alone (control livers; n = 4). Animals were sacrificed at 4 and 24 hr post-treatment, and tissues harvested for histopathologic and fluorescent microscopic analysis and quantification.

Phase 2. Effect of carrier (20 nm micelles vs. 100 nm liposomes) on combination therapy (RF ablation with doxorubicin or quercetin). Seventy single subcutaneous R3230 tumors were divided into the following 7 treatment arms (n = 10 per group): RF alone, RF ablation with liposomal or micellar doxorubicin (both formulations: 1 mg in 0.5 ml, given 15 min post-RFA), and RF ablation with either liposomal or micellar quercetin (each formulation, 0.3 mg in 0.5 ml, given either 24 hr pre- or 15 min post-RFA based upon prior studies using these two time points for liposomal quercetin [14]). Doxorubicin (an HIF-1α inhibitor) and quercetin (an HSP70 inhibitor) were selected as both agents have known suppressive effects on hypoxia and RF ablation-induced heat stress responses, respectively [14,22]. Animals were sacrificed and tumors harvested 24 hr post-RFA. Outcome measures included tumor coagulation and immunohistochemistry (IHC) for HIF-1α and HSP70 (including rim thickness and % cell positivity/high powered field [hpf]).

Phase 3. Effect of nanocarrier on tumor growth and survival after RF ablation. A total of 30 single subcutaneous R3230 tumors were used. Animals were allocated to the following 4 treatment arms: RF ablation with liposomal or micellar doxorubicin (both formulations: 1 mg in 0.5 ml, given 15 min post-RFA; n = 8 each arm), and RF ablation with either liposomal or micellar quercetin (each formulation, 0.3 mg in 0.5 ml) given 15 min post-RFA (n = 7–8 each arm). The administration time for RF/quercetin studies was selected based upon the results of Phase 2. Tumor growth was measured daily and animals were sacrificed at a pre-determined endpoint of 30 mm mean tumor diameter or 60 days survival post-ablation, whichever came first. Outcome measures included tumor growth curves and Kaplan Meier analysis of survival rates.

Phase 4. Effect of nanocarrier on intratumoral drug delivery and retention after RF ablation. Here, 64 paired subcutaneous R3230 tumors were implanted in 32 animals. Animals were allocated to the following treatment arms: RF ablation of one tumor followed by either liposomal doxorubicin or micellar doxorubicin (IV, 1 mg in 0.5 ml, given 15 min post-RFA). The second, paired non-ablated tumor served as in internal control that was exposed to either IV liposomal or micellar doxorubicin alone. Animals were sacrificed at 4 different time points (1–72 hr post-RFA), for a total of 64 tumors (n = 4 treatments×4 time points×4 per group). Ablated and unablated tumors and the left liver lobes were harvested. Outcome measures included gross and histopathologic evaluation for tumor coagulation, and fluorescent quantitative studies for intratumoral doxorubicin

Animal Models

For all experiments and procedures, anesthesia was induced with 0.1 ml intraperitoneal (IP) injection of a mixture of ketamine (100 mg/ml, Ketaject; Phoenix Pharmaceutical, St. Joseph, MO)

and xylazine (50 mg/ml, Bayer, Shawnee Mission, KS). To maintain adequate anesthesia, increments of 0.01 ml were used when necessary. Animals were sacrificed with an overdose of 0.3 ml of the same mixture.

Experiments were performed using two animal tissues. The first is a well-characterized established R3230 mammary adenocarcinoma cell line implanted in female Fisher 344 rats (150±20 g; 14–16 weeks old, Charles River, Wilmington, MA) [5,23]. Tumor implantation, evaluation, and preparation techniques were performed as previously described [5]. Briefly, one tumor was implanted into each animal by slowly injecting 0.3–0.4 mL of tumor suspension into the chest mammary fat pad of each animal via an 18-gauge needle. 1.3–1.5 cm solid non-necrotic tumors were used (18–21 days after implantation), randomized to different treatment arms. For Phase 3, the second (remote) tumor was generated using similar implantation technique, with injection into the abdominal subcutaneous space 3.5– 4 cm distal to the primary site of injection in the chest. The second model was normal liver in Fischer F344 female rats. After anesthesia induction, hair was removed at the incision site and the skin was cleansed with a disinfectant (70% EtOH). A 15 mm incision was made in a subcostal location to expose the left lobe of the liver. After completion of the procedure, the abdomen was closed in layers using 4–5 interrupted sutures. All intravenous injections were administered via IV tail injection, under complete anesthesia.

RF Application

Conventional monopolar RFA was applied by using a 500-kHz RFA generator (model 3E; Radionics, Burlington, Mass), as has been previously described [5]. Briefly, the 1-cm tip of a 21-gauge electrically insulated electrode (SMK electrode; Radionics) was inserted into the center of the tumor or left liver lobe. RF energy was applied for 5 min with generator output titrated to maintain a designated tip temperature (70±2°C, continuous monitoring via a thermocouple in the electrode tip). This standardized method of RF application has been previously demonstrated to provide reproducible volumes of coagulation with use of this conventional RFA system [5,23]. To complete the RF circuit, the animal was placed on a standardized metallic grounding pad (Radionics).

Preparation and administration of adjuvant nanoagents

For fluorescent beads, three commercially available carboxylated fluorescent dyed-polystyrene microspheres were used (FluoSpheres; Invitrogen, Eugene, OR), representing three different sizes/colors: 20 nm/crimson (wavelengths, excitation 625 nm/emission 645 nm), 100 nm/orange (540/560), and 500 nm/yellow-green (505/515), which were best observed using the purple, red, and green microscope color filters, respectively (per the manufacturer). Prior to initiating our experiments, single-colored beads were used as positive controls and examined under all fluorescent filters to ensure absence of any fluorescence bleed-through artifacts.

For liposomal doxorubicin, a commercially available preparation (Doxil; ALZA Pharmaceuticals, Palo Alto, CA) was used. Quercetin-loaded liposomes were prepared such that liposome formulation was identical to Doxil, and as has been described [14].

Doxorubicin-loaded micelles were prepared as described [24]. Briefly, first PEG2000-DSPE micelles were prepared using a lipid film hydration method. The lipid film was formed from a chloroform solution of PEG2000-DSPE by removal of the organic solvent by rotary evaporation followed by freeze-drying. The film was hydrated with 10 mM PBS pH 7.4 at room temperature and mixed using a vortex device for 5 min to give a final lipid concentration of 40 mg/ml. The PEG2000-DSPE micelles were then mixed with equal volume of drug solution (4 mg/ml) and incubated at room temperature for 1 h. Free doxorubicin was separated from the doxorubicin-micelle solutions using Amicon centrifuge filters (MWCO = 30 kDa). The micellar doxorubicin concentration was 2 mg/ml after diluting the micelles with methanol using a Labsystems Multiskan MCC/340 microplate reader (Labsystems and Life Sciences International, UK) at excitation and emission wavelengths of 485 and 590 nm, respectively. The micelle size (hydrodynamic diameter) was measured by dynamic light scattering (DLS) using a N4 Plus Submicron Particle System (Coulter Corporation, Miami, FL, USA) and was found to be 17.0±2.1 nm. The zeta-potential was −21.7±4.3 mV.

Quercetin-loaded micelles were also prepared using a lipid film hydration method. Briefly, 0.6 mg of quercetin (1 mg/mL solution in methanol) was added to polyethylene-glycolphosphatidylethanolamine (PEG2000-PE) solutions in chloroform, and a lipid film was formed in a round-bottomed flask by solvent removal on a rotary evaporator. The lipid film was then rehydrated with 1 mL of phosphate buffered saline (pH 7.4) to obtain final lipid concentration 5 mM. After mixing using a vortex device for 15 min at room temperature, the unincorporated quercetin was removed by filtration of the micelle suspension through 0.2 µm membrane filters. The micellar loading efficiency of quercetin was 100% (as for quercetin-loaded liposomes, 0.6 mg of quercetin was loaded in each administered dose). The micelle size was 17 nm±2.1 nm. The zeta-potential was -21.7±4.3 mV.

Tumor specimen retrieval

For Phases 1–3, tumors were removed from the animal and sectioned perpendicularly to the direction of electrode insertion. Tissue samples were split and processed for gross pathologic assessment of tumor coagulation, and for histopathology, immunohistochemistry, fluorescent microscopy, or doxorubicin quantification, as below.

Confocal microscopy and fluorescent quantification

Tumor sections were flash frozen in optimal cutting temperature (OCT) media, to allow analysis of fluorescence. Tissues were sectioned at a thickness of 5 µm. For each tumor one slide was stained for H&E for gross pathology comparison and slides prepared for confocal fluorescent microscopy were counterstained with DAPI nuclear staining. A Zeiss LSM 510 Inverted Live-Cell Confocal System (Carl Zeiss Microscopy, Thornwood, NY) was used for image acquisition and tiling. In brief, slides were counterstained with Gold anti-fade reagent with DAPI (Life Technologies, Grand Islands, NY) and stored overnight, followed the next day with image acquisition. For each sample, at 10× and 40× magnification, a minimum of 100 fields were imaged and automatically tiled by the microscope software, Ziess LSM image examiner (Carl Zeiss Microscopy). Tiled images allowed subjective assessment and quantification of slices of the tumor section that encompassed the center, periablational rim and tumor edge. Images were then quantified for fluorescence using Volocity 6.0 software (PerkinElmer, Waltham, MA). For each tumor section, the peak values, means and sums of each fluorescent color surface area count were quantified. Where "peak values" represent the area with highest uptake, typically the periablational rim (as confirmed by duplicate H&E slides), "means" represent the average fluorescent surface area count per HPF and the "sums" represent the area under the curve (AUC) or total fluorescent surface area of a certain color in an entire section.

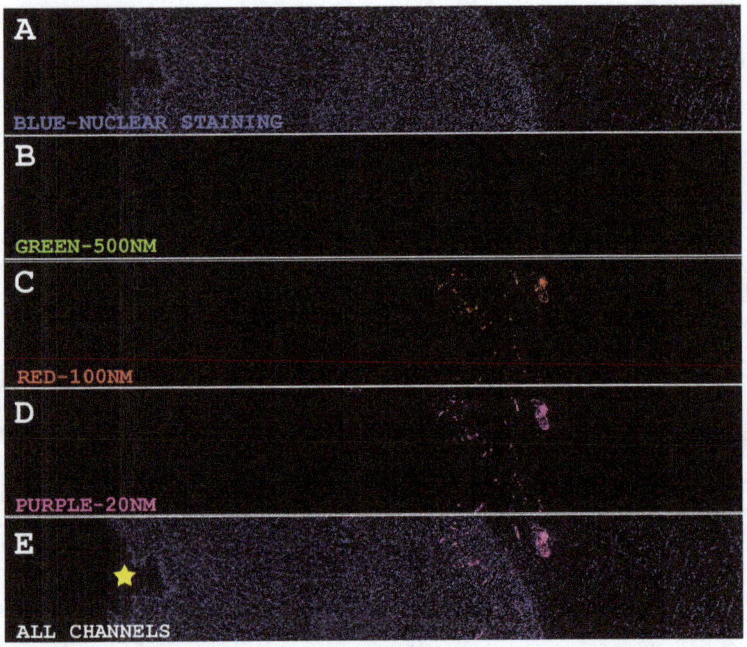

Figure 1. Confocal tiled Imaging for fluorescent surface area quantitation in R3230 tumors sacrificed at 4 hours post RF (10×). R3230 tumors were treated with RF alone, followed by IV injection of equal volumes of 3 fluorescent beads of different colors and sizes (purple 20 nm, red 100 nm, green 500 nm). Quantitation of tiled images of tumor sections (center, periablational rim and tumor margin) demonstrated fluorescent bead accumulation in the periablational rim, with greatest uptake of 20 nm beads (**D**) followed by the 100 nm (**C**) beads followed by the 500 nm beads (**B**) ($p<0.05$, all comparisons).

Gross pathologic evaluation

To assess gross tumor coagulation, one half of each sample was incubated in 50 ml of PBS with 1 mg of 2,3,5-triphenyltetrazolium chloride (TTC, Sigma Aldrich) as has been previously described [5]. Non-viable white tissue, representing the coagulation zone, was identified and measured using manual calibers and recorded.

Immunohistochemical staining

Tumor samples were placed in cassettes containing the central section of tumor. All tissues were fixed in 10% formalin overnight at 4°C, embedded in paraffin, and sectioned at a thickness of 5 μm. Tissues were stained with H&E for gross pathology. For Phase 2, at least 3 samples from each treatment group underwent immunohistochemical staining using previously described tech-

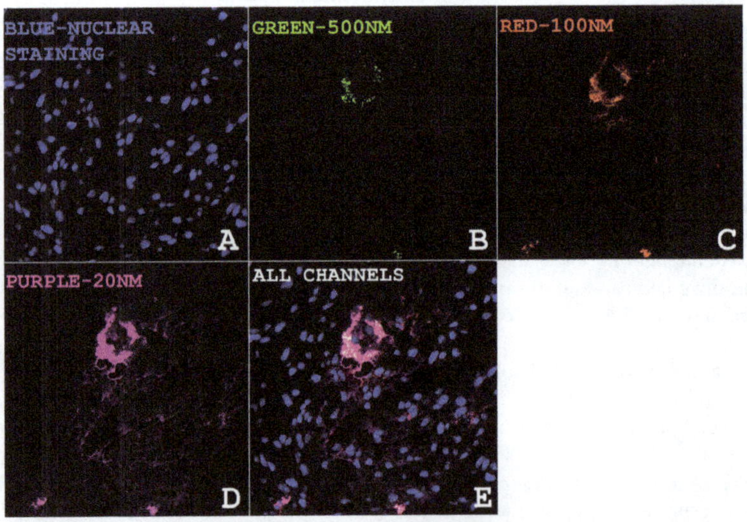

Figure 2. Confocal Imaging of perivascular and interstitial fluorescent bead penetration in the periablational rim 24 hr after RF ablation of R3230 tumors (40×). R3230 tumors were treated with RF alone, followed by IV injection of 3 fluorescent beads of different colors and sizes (purple 20 nm, red 100 nm, green 500 nm). 40× images of the periablational rim reveal deeper penetration of the 20 nm beads into the intracellular spaces beyond the primary site of extravasation, outlining and mapping out the cells they are surrounding (**D,E**), whereas the majority of the 100 nm (**B**) remain confined to the primary site of extravasation. Even less extravasation is seen for the 500 nm beads (**C**).

Table 1. Fluorescence for different sized beads in the periablational rim after RF of R3230 tumors.

Fluorescent Area ± STDV (μm^2) at 4 hr after RF ablation of R3230 tumor	4 hrs post RF				24 hrs post RF			
	20 nm	100 nm	500 nm	P value	20 nm	100 nm	500 nm	P value
Peak uptake	13922±3281	5412±3116	947±347	*,**	5707±1205	2881±1205	1019±46	*,**,***
Total uptake (AUC)	15699±2178	6649±2670	1560±692	*,**,***	15835±3859	5215±182	2930±344	*,**,***
Mean uptake (per HPF)	1445±494	613±254	139±42	**,***	1288±90	783±243	330±71	*,**,***

* p<0.05 when comparing 20 nm values with 100 nm values per single time point.
**p<0.05 when comparing 20 nm values with 500 nm values per single time point.
***p<0.05 when comparing 100 nm values with 500 nm values per single time point.

niques [13,14,21]. Staining was performed using antibodies to HSP70, (Stressgen, Chicago, MI) [25], to detect evidence of HSP production, and HIF-1α (Abcam, Boston, MA) were used to detect the α-subunit of HIF-1.

Specimen slides were imaged at the periablational rim at 10× and 40× magnification and analyzed using a Micromaster I microscope (Fisher Scientific, Pittsburgh, PA) and Micron Imaging Software (Westover Scientific, Inc., Mill Greek, WA) to determine rim thickness and percent (%) cell positivity. Five random high power fields were analyzed for a minimum of 3 specimens for each parameter and scored in a blinded fashion to remove observer bias. As an additional control to insure uniformity of staining, whenever direct comparisons were made, immunohistochemical staining was repeated with all relevant comparison slides stained at the same time. Accuracy of the final data was verified by the senior author, who was blinded to treatment group.

Drug quantification in harvested tissues

Doxorubicin inherent fluorescent properties were used to quantify drug accumulation in tumor and liver samples, as described [5]. In Phase 3, tissue was harvested from the ablated tumor, and remote, untreated tumor and untreated liver as controls. Tissues were weighed, and homogenized in acid alcohol (0.3N HCL, 70% EtOH), and doxorubicin was extracted for 24 hr at 4°C. Doxorubicin extracted from tissue homogenate supernatant samples was quantified by fluorometry with an excitation wavelength of 470 nm and intensity of emission measured at 590 nm and plotted on a standard curve.

Statistical Analysis

The Microsoft Office 2010 Excel software (Microsoft, Redmond, WA) was used for statistical analysis. All data were provided as mean plus or minus SD. Immunohistochemistry results and fluorescence quantification were compared using analysis of variance (ANOVA). Additional post-hoc analysis was performed with paired, two-tailed Student's T-test, if and only if, the analysis of variance achieved statistical significance. A P value of less than 0.05 was considered significant. The Kaplan–Meier method and log-rank test were used for endpoint survival analysis. Given the absence of censoring of our data, one-way analysis of variance was then performed on the survival endpoints for each animal for the comparisons reported. Pair-wise t tests ($p<0.05$; two-tailed test) based on the least square means were subsequently performed only if the overall P values were significant.

Results

Phase 1. Smaller beads (20 nm) have greater deposition and deeper interstitial penetration than larger beads in the post-RFA periablational zone

In R3230 tumors treated with RFA and IV fluorescent beads in animals sacrificed at 4 and 24 hr, greatest deposition was observed in the periablational rim, with peak uptake at 4 hr post-RFA for all sizes of beads. At 4 hr post-RFA, 20 nm beads had the greatest peak, sum and mean of fluorescence deposition, as depicted by fluorescent surface area detected followed by 100 nm beads, with the least uptake seen for 500 nm beads (**TABLE 1**). Similarly at 24 hr post-RFA, 20 nm beads had the greatest deposition as compared to 100 nm and 500 nm beads ($p<0.05$ for all comparisons, **TABLE 1, FIGURE 1, 2**). Similarly, for normal liver we observed greater deposition of smaller beads (20 nm) in the periablational margin compared to larger beads after RF ablation. However, unlike the tumor model, bead deposition peaked later at 24 hr post-RFA (**TABLE 1**).

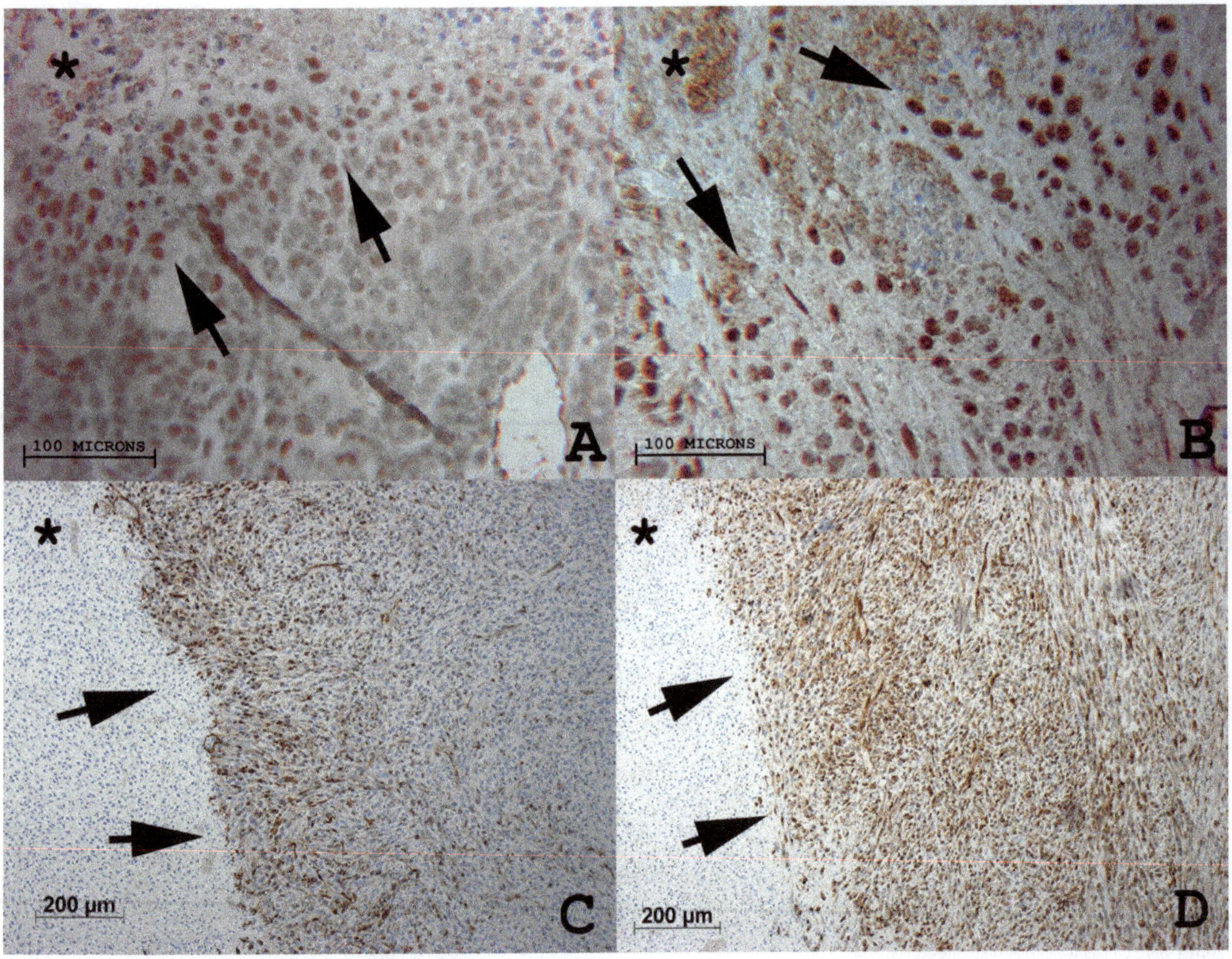

Figure 3. Comparison of micellar and liposomal formulations on modulating local periablational target proteins (HIF-1α and HSP70) 24 hr after RF ablation of R3230 tumor. (**A**) Micellar doxorubicin suppressed periablational HIF-1α expression to a greater degree than (**B**) liposomal doxorubicin 24 hr after RF ablation (40×). Similarly, (**C**) micellar quercetin suppressed ablation-induced periablational HSP70 expression in R3230 tumor at 24 hr compared to (**D**) liposomal quercetin (10×).

Phase 2. Adjuvant micellar Dox/Qu led to greater suppression of stress and hypoxia markers compared to adjuvant liposomal Dox/Qu preparations

RFA combined with Mic-Dox led to greater suppression of HIF-1α expression compared to RFA combined with Lipo-Dox as measured by rim thickness in the periablational rim (45±37 μm vs. 129±68 μm, respectively, $p<0.04$), with equal % cell positivity (14.2±1.1 vs.13.6±2.1, respectively, $p=0.7$) (**TABLE 2, FIGURE 3**). Both adjuvant Mic-Dox and Lipo-Dox therapies resulted in statistically significant reduction of HIF-1α expression as compared to RFA alone groups (210±85 μm and 37.9±4.3% at 24 hr, $p<0.05$ for all comparisons; **TABLE 2, FIGURE 3**).

RFA combined with any quercetin nanopreparation administered at any time point reduced periablational HSP70 expression compared to RFA alone control groups ($p<0.01$ for all comparisons; **TABLE 2**). However, RFA micellar quercetin preparations markedly reduced rim thickness of HSP70 expression compared to RFA combined with liposomal quercetin for both 24 hr pre-RFA and 15 min post-RFA administration (853±157 μm vs. 14888±326 μm and 859±262 μm vs. 2089±569 μm, respectively, $p<0.03$ for all comparisons) (**FIGURE 4**). With regard to timing of adjuvant nanodrug administration, Mic-Qu markedly reduced rim thickness of HSP70 expression equally at both 24 hr pre- and 15 min post-RFA administrations (853±157 μm and 859±262 μm, respectively, p = NS). However, adjuvant Lipo-Qu resulted in the greatest suppression of RFA-induced HSP70 expression when given 24 hr pre-RFA, with significantly less effect on the rim thickness of HSP70 expression when given 15 min post-RFA (14888±326 μm and 2089±569 μm, respectively; $p<0.01$) (**TABLE 2**).

Phase 3. RF ablation combined with long-circulating liposomal nanodrugs led to equal local tumor coagulation and equal or better control of tumor growth and animal endpoint survival compared to micellar nanodrugs

Significantly greater tumor coagulation was achieved in treatment groups combining RFA with any adjuvant nanopreparations of quercetin or doxorubicin, than by RFA alone at 24 hr (all comparisons $p<0.05$, **TABLE 2**). Yet, no statistically significant difference in coagulation was observed based on type of drug or nanopreparation used at 24 hr (**TABLE 2**).

Table 2. Gross and histopathologic outcomes for RFA/nanodrug combinations.

	Coagulation zone (mm)		Marker	Rim thickness (μm)		% Cell Positivity	
	Mean ± SD	P value		Mean ± SD	P value	Mean ± SD	P value
RF alone	7.7±0.6		HSP70	3000±236		80.2±5.6	
			HIF-1α	210±85		43.2±8.2	
RF+Lipo Dox	10.5±0.9	*	HIF-1α	129±68		14.2±3.3	*
RF+Mic Dox	11.3±2.3	*	HIF-1α	45±37	*,**	15.7±4.3	*
RF+LipoQu 15 min post RF	12.4±1.7	*	HSP70	2089±569	*	43.3±7.7	*
RF+MicQu 15 min post RF	11.4±1.5	*	HSP70	859.42±262	*,**	42.8±6.4	*
RF+LipoQu 24 hr pre RF	13.7±2.0	*	HSP70	1488±326	*	38.9±9.4	*
RF+MicQu 24 hr pre RF	13.1±0.9	*	HSP70	853±157	*,**	33.1±11.1	*

* = $p<0.05$ when compared to RF group.
** = $P<0.05$ when compared to adjuvant liposomal drug preparations.

For RFA combined with doxorubicin nanopreparations, the mean endpoint survival for animals treated with RFA/Lipo-Dox was 49.8±9.1 d, including two animals that survived up to the 60 day post-treatment monitoring end-point. This was significantly longer than RFA/Mic-Dox, which had a mean survival of 39.6±8.4 d ($p<0.04$, **FIGURE 5**). By contrast, RFA/Lipo-Qu and RFA/Mic-Qu had similar animal endpoint survival profiles, where RFA/Mic-Qu had a mean survival of 31.1±8.2 d compared to 31.2±9.1 d with RFA/Lipo-Qu ($p = 0.9$, **FIGURE 5**).

Phase 4. Contrasting intratumoral doxorubicin accumulation kinetics for micellar and liposomal preparations after RF ablation

At 1 hr post-RFA, there was minimal doxorubicin detected in tumor samples of either Mic-Dox or Lipo-Dox groups. However, at 4 hr post-RFA, intratumoral doxorubicin levels were approximately 6-fold higher for RFA/Mic-Dox compared to RFA/Lipo-Dox (0.0006±0.0002 μg/g vs. 0.0001±0.000024 μg/g, $p<0.03$). Yet, at the later time points of 24 hr and 72 hr, RFA/Lipo-Dox increased to a much greater degree than micellar doxorubicin concentrations. This resulted in significantly higher levels of intratumoral doxorubicin (approximately 17-fold) for long-circulating liposomal doxorubicin delivery compared to RFA/Mic-Dox ($p<0.01$ for all comparisons, **TABLE 3**). Specifically, at 24 hr post-RFA, doxorubicin levels in the periablational rim were 1.02±0.52 μg/g for RFA/Lipo-Dox compared to only 0.06±0.02 μg/g for RFA/Mic-Dox ($p<0.001$). Similarly, at 72 hr post-RFA, intratumoral doxorubicin levels after RFA/Lipo-Dox were 1.17±0.52 μg/g, compared to RFA/Mic-Dox 0.01±0.02 μg/g ($p<0.001$).

Discussion

There is increasing interest in developing treatment paradigms that combine focal tumor ablation with adjuvant pharmacologic or chemotherapeutic agents to address both challenges with residual viable tumor from incomplete local treatment and difficulties in achieving high concentrations of targeted drug delivery [18,26–28]. Early studies combining RF ablation with a commercially-available liposomal doxorubicin (Doxil) preparation reported increases in local tumor coagulation, periablational drug uptake, and reduced tumor growth in animal studies, and increased tumor destruction in preliminary clinical studies [5,6,8,9]. Subsequent studies have refined the approach, either through modification of the drug payload or using thermosensitive preparations to facilitate intratumoral drug release, though with mixed improvements in treatment efficacy [11–13,17]. While most of these studies have largely used 100 nm sized liposomes as the carrier model, more recent studies on nanoparticle delivery (without ablation) suggest improved carrier and drug penetration with smaller-sized preparations [20,29].

In our current study, smaller-sized particles (20 nm) administered in combination with RF ablation did indeed result in greater and deeper interstitial and perivascular penetration into the periablational rim compared to larger (100 nm and 500 nm) sized particles. Thus, our findings are consistent with uses of smaller-sized carriers to overcome limitations in intratumoral and interstitial drug delivery when using nanoparticles alone or in combination with low-level hyperthermia (40–45°C) applications [29,30]. For example, Tsukioke et al have reported deeper interstitial penetration of micellar doxorubicin into tumor spheroids as compared to liposomal doxorubicin [29]. Yet, our results go well beyond these findings as we achieved a primary goal

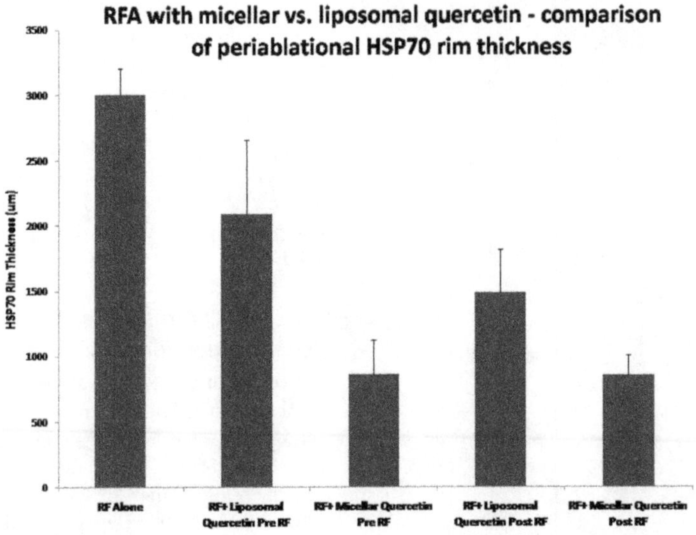

Figure 4. RF ablation combined with micellar quercetin suppresses periablational HSP70 expression more than a liposomal nanocarrier. Interestingly, in addition to the observed superior inhibitory effect of adjuvant micellar quercetin over adjuvant liposomal quercetin, regardless of timing of admininstration (pre-RFA or post-RFA), micellar adjuvant therapy is equally effective when given pre- or post-RFA (853.07 ± 156.59 μm and 859.42 ± 261.51 μm). However, adjuvant liposomal quercetin shows significantly greater HSP70 inhibition when given pre-RFA as compared to tumors treated with liposomal quercetin post-RFA (14888.01 ± 325.53 μm and 2088.58 ± 568.54 μm).

of demonstrating that the greater nanodrug penetration from micellar preparations can be translated into markedly improved modulation/suppression of specifically targeted tissue reactions in the periablational rim. To wit, here ablation-induced expression of both HIF-1α and HSP70 were independently suppressed to a greater degree with micellar nanopreparations compared to their liposomal counterparts in terms of spatial distribution. Specifically, micellar nanodrugs specifically reduced the geographic extent of marker expression (i.e., rim thickness) in the periablational rim, highlighting greater tissue penetration micellar preparations with concurrent greater spatial distribution of the desired biochemical modulation.

While these results are exciting in achieving a primary goal of using refined nanodrug paradigms to target specific cellular reactions, it must be acknowledged that these gains in interstitial penetration and suppression of local tissue reactions do not necessarily translate into improvements in all desired outcome metrics in cancer therapy. Along these lines, in our study micellar preparations had similar or inferior effects on curbing tumor growth and promoting animal survival and likewise micellar preparations did not increase local ablation-induced tumor coagulation compared to liposomal preparations at 24 hr. This reinforces our understanding that local effects of tumor coagulation and periablational proteomic reactions may also not directly translate into reduction in tumor growth and gains in animal endpoint survival outcomes.

To account for the results we observed, we hypothesize that marked, but incomplete reduction of HSP or HIF-1a may be insufficient to induce complete tumor destruction at 24 hr and that, the ability of each drug to increase local coagulation may be susceptible to a threshold effect, with only a certain amount of drug required to target the partially injured remaining cells in the periablational rim. However, other longer-term effects on growth in the remaining untreated tumor may reflect a more complex reality where differences in nanocarrier release and drug uptake that are greater with long-circulating liposomal formulations [31] may very well be of primary importance for overall survival. Indeed, our results are concordant with previously reported findings by Yang et al, where RFA combined with liposomal paclitaxel (an apoptosis enhancer) resulted in greater apoptosis (as measured by caspase 3), yet did not suppress tumor growth to a similar extent as liposomal doxorubicin [13]. Conversely, with increasing evidence that some reactions (such as increased HIF-1α) in the periablational rim may stimulate growth in distant tumor, successful modulation of local tissue reactions may assume increasing clinical relevance as its own endpoint separate from tumor growth [32–34].

Our study adds to the growing body of evidence supporting the notion that it is the variable nanodrug delivery kinetics that are likely to be primarily responsible for the way that different nanopreparations induce better or worse effects on specific outcome metrics [17,35]. For example, while greater intratumoral doxorubicin uptake was observed with micelles compared to liposomes early (4 hr) after RF ablation, liposomes delivered significantly greater doxorubicin to the treated tumor over a longer period of time (24–72 hr post-treatment). Therefore, while micellar preparations had a greater effect on our specific targets (HIF-1α and HSP70), these markers also peak early (4–24 hr post-RFA) and may be more susceptible to early drug delivery. In contrast, if the overall amount of drug delivery to the tumor is the primary goal, then long-circulating liposomal preparations are superior carriers. Greater overall tumor exposure to accumulating doxorubicin may explain the greater animal endpoint survival observed with RFA/liposomal doxorubicin. Along these lines, recently, Andriyanov et al reported corroborating findings when comparing RF ablation combined with conventional long-circulating stealth PEG-ylated liposomal doxorubicin (i.e., Doxil) to fast-releasing 100 nm thermosensitive liposomal doxorubicin (i.e., ThermoDox), in which prolonged slow drug uptake resulted in a greater reduction in long-term tumor growth compared to early flooding of the tumor with intratumoral nanodrug [17]. Indeed, we posit that longer drug circulation, and therefore exposure time, may take on greater importance for processes that are likely to occur over a variable relatively longer time frame in the target

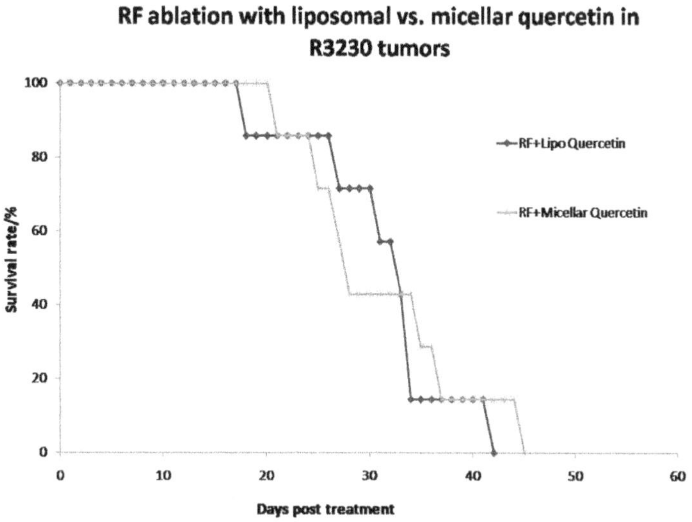

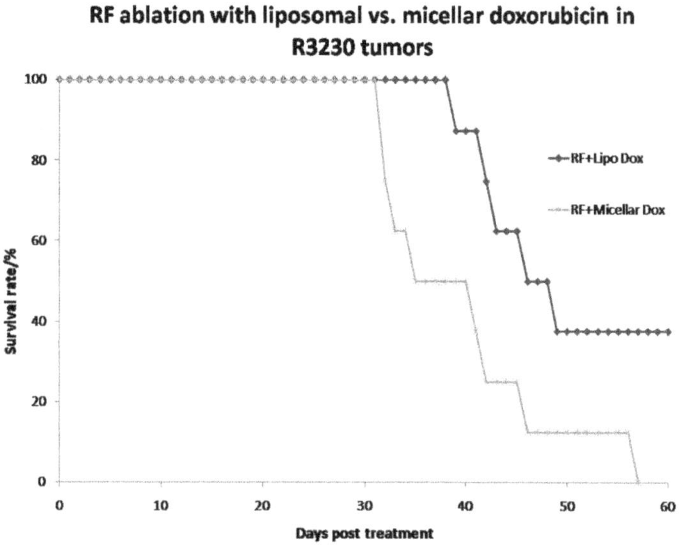

Figure 5. Comparison of animal endpoint survival for micellar and liposomal doxorubicin or quercetin formulations when combined with RF ablation of R3230 tumors. (**A**) RF/Lipo-Dox resulted in the greatest animal survival (49.8±9.1 d), followed by RFA/Mic-Dox (39.6±8.4 d). (**B**) RFA combined with either micellar quercetin or liposomal quercetin resulted in the same mean animal survival (31.1±8.2 d and 31.2±9.1 d, respectively).

Table 3. Periablational intratumoral doxorubicin accumulation for liposomal and micellar nanocarriers combined with RF ablation over time.

Doxorubicin accumulation in RF ablated tumors (μg/g)		
Time post RF	RF+Lipo Dox	RF+Mic Dox
	Mean ± SD	Mean ± SD
1 hour	0.00000081±0.0000003	0.00000007±0.0000001
4 hours	0.0001±0.000024	0.0006±0.000174*
24 hours	1.02±0.517*	0.06±0.024
72 hours	1.17±0.243*	0.01±0.013

* = $p<0.05$ when compared to the other treatment group.

tumor. Specifically, doxorubicin, an intercalating agent, is more effective when cells are in the G2 phase of replication, and cells in and around the ablation zone are likely to enter the G2 phase at variable time points after ablation [36]). Having high concentrations of doxorubicin in the serum when various cells enter this point of the cell cycle over a period of days may well represent the best chance to ensure that efficacious drug concentrations are present when most needed.

Additional potentially useful pharmacologic observations were noted in our study. For quercetin nanopreparations, we also found a wider window of efficacious administration with micellar preparations than may have been expected given the well-known, relatively short (2–3 hr half-life) plasma kinetics for these smaller vehicles [37]. Specifically, we demonstrated equivalent responses and tumor coagulation when micellar quercetin was given between 24 hr pre- to 15 min post-RF ablation compared to the liposomal formulation where optimal HSP70 suppression was observed only when given 24 hr pre-RFA. Thus, our results suggest that intratumoral concentrations are primary over plasma kinetics and that likely very little drug is needed to achieve the desired HSP reduction – provided it is successfully delivered to the desired spatial location. Additionally, we observed variable timing of accumulation for smaller fluorescent bead particles between tumor and normal liver, where peak fluorescence was observed at 24 hr post-RFA in normal liver. This suggests that even with equivalent outcomes, some types of nanocarriers, with ideal therapeutic windows tailored to specific tissues, may offer clinically relevant and practical advantages.

Ultimately, our findings suggest that several different factors need to be considered when developing combination therapy paradigms. Optimal choice of carrier type and drug payload will likely involve both identifying goals of treatment and prioritizing outcome metrics (e.g., local suppression of a specific cytokine such as HIF-1α or control of tumor growth). Tumor and tissue-specific characteristics, and differences in carrier and drug pharmacokinetics will factor into the practical considerations of when to time peri-ablation drug administration. Thus, the choice of nanoparticles should ultimately likely be tailored to achieve specific goals in specific tissues, as optimal carriers may differ depending on whether modulation of local periablational processes or growth suppression of untreated tumor is required.

We acknowledge several limitations with our study. Fluorescent beads were commercially acquired and the number of beads per volume was pre-determined by the manufacturer and was not likely not identical between different particle sizes. Yet, we controlled for the key variable drug concentration in all of our subsequent experiments as the active drug (i.e., 1 mg of doxorubicin loaded in 0.5 ml) was given precedence to the number of particles in the micellar or liposomal vehicle. Thus, as expected, fluorescent beads of a smaller size had a consistently higher concentration than larger-sized beads. Additionally, although the R3230 model used for these studies is a well-characterized tumor model, results demonstrated may be specific to the model and should be interpreted and applied to other scenarios and models with caution, mirroring our call for tailoring nanopreparations to different tumor types and scenarios. Differences also exist in pharmacokinetic profiles between the fluorescent beads and correspondingly sized nanopreparations (i.e., 20 nm beads vs. 20 nm micelles). Therefore, interpretation and correlation of results between fluorescent beads and nanopreparations must be made carefully. Furthermore, in survival studies, we did not include an RFA alone treatment arm, as prior studies have clearly demonstrated a survival benefit for combination therapy arms (liposomal doxorubicin or quercetin) [9,38]. Finally, tumor coagulation for micellar doxorubicin in this study differs from results obtained in an earlier study using a small liposome preparation (~40 nm), where high levels of intratumoral doxorubicin accumulation but smaller amounts of tumor coagulation were reported compared to a 100 nm preparation. Differences in results may represent variable micellar stability due to differences in doxorubicin loading doses [29], and emphasizes that results from experimental and clinical studies using combination paradigms are critically dependent on developing the appropriate nanopreparations for the right application.

In conclusion, when combined with RF ablation, smaller-sized particles have superior deeper tissue penetration and therefore can potentially achieve more effective local molecular modulation of specific post-ablation reactions including heat shock protein and HIF-1α expression, with a wider window of administration as compared to larger (100 nm) particles. However, larger-sized long-circulating particles can result in greater overall long-term intratumoral drug accumulation and reduced tumor growth. Therefore, different nanodrug carriers provide specific advantages, in part based upon size and circulation kinetics, which should be considered when formulating strategies to achieve optimal combination therapies with tumor ablation.

Author Contributions

Conceived and designed the experiments: MA SNG MM TL VPT. Performed the experiments: MM GK RRS. Analyzed the data: MM MA SNG GK. Contributed reagents/materials/analysis tools: MM MA SNG GK RRS TL VPT. Wrote the paper: MM MA SNG GK RRS TL VPT.

References

1. Ahmed M, Brace CL, Lee FT Jr, Goldberg SN (2011) Principles of and advances in percutaneous ablation. Radiology 258: 351–369.
2. Lencioni R, Cioni D, Crocetti L, Franchini C, Pina CD, et al. (2005) Early-stage hepatocellular carcinoma in patients with cirrhosis: long-term results of percutaneous image-guided radiofrequency ablation. Radiology 234: 961–967.
3. Sofocleous CT, Garg SK, Cohen P, Petre EN, Gonen M, et al. (2013) Ki 67 is an Independent Predictive Biomarker of Cancer Specific and Local Recurrence-Free Survival After Lung Tumor Ablation. Ann Surg Oncol.
4. Sofocleous CT, Nascimento RG, Petrovic LM, Klimstra DS, Gonen M, et al. (2008) Histopathologic and immunohistochemical features of tissue adherent to multitined electrodes after RF ablation of liver malignancies can help predict local tumor progression: initial results. Radiology 249: 364–374.
5. Ahmed M, Monsky WE, Girnun G, Lukyanov A, D'Ippolito G, et al. (2003) Radiofrequency thermal ablation sharply increases intratumoral liposomal doxorubicin accumulation and tumor coagulation. Cancer Res 63: 6327–6333.
6. Goldberg SN, Kamel IR, Kruskal JB, Reynolds K, Monsky WL, et al. (2002) Radiofrequency ablation of hepatic tumors: increased tumor destruction with adjuvant liposomal doxorubicin therapy. AJR Am J Roentgenol 179: 93–101.
7. Head HW, Dodd GD 3rd, Bao A, Soundararajan A, Garcia-Rojas X, et al. (2010) Combination radiofrequency ablation and intravenous radiolabeled liposomal Doxorubicin: imaging and quantification of increased drug delivery to tumors. Radiology 255: 405–414.
8. Ahmed M, Goldberg SN (2004) Combination radiofrequency thermal ablation and adjuvant IV liposomal doxorubicin increases tissue coagulation and intratumoural drug accumulation. Int J Hyperthermia 20: 781–802.
9. D'Ippolito G, Ahmed M, Girnun GD, Stuart KE, Kruskal JB, et al. (2003) Percutaneous tumor ablation: reduced tumor growth with combined radio-frequency ablation and liposomal doxorubicin in a rat breast tumor model. Radiology 228: 112–118.
10. Ahmed M, Lukyanov AN, Torchilin V, Tournier H, Schneider AN, et al. (2005) Combined radiofrequency ablation and adjuvant liposomal chemotherapy: effect of chemotherapeutic agent, nanoparticle size, and circulation time. J Vasc Interv Radiol 16: 1365–1371.
11. Poon RT, Borys N (2011) Lyso-thermosensitive liposomal doxorubicin: an adjuvant to increase the cure rate of radiofrequency ablation in liver cancer. Future Oncol 7: 937–945.

12. Wood BJ, Poon RT, Locklin JK, Dreher MR, Ng KK, et al. (2012) Phase I study of heat-deployed liposomal doxorubicin during radiofrequency ablation for hepatic malignancies. J Vasc Interv Radiol 23: 248–255 e247.
13. Yang W, Ahmed M, Elian M, Hady ES, Levchenko TS, et al. (2010) Do Liposomal Apoptotic Enhancers IncreaseTumor Coagulation and End-Point Survival in Percutaneous Radiofrequency Ablation of Tumors in a Rat Tumor Model? Radiology 257: 685–696.
14. Yang W, Ahmed M, Tasawwar B, Levchenko T, Sawant RR, et al. (2011) Radiofrequency ablation combined with liposomal quercetin to increase tumor destruction by modulation of heat shock protein production in a small animal model. Int J Hyperthermia 27: 527–538.
15. Soundararajan A, Dodd GD 3rd, Bao A, Phillips WT, McManus LM, et al. (2011) Chemoradionuclide therapy with 186Re-labeled liposomal doxorubicin in combination with radiofrequency ablation for effective treatment of head and neck cancer in a nude rat tumor xenograft model. Radiology 261: 813–823.
16. Poff JA, Allen CT, Traughber B, Colunga A, Xie J, et al. (2008) Pulsed high-intensity focused ultrasound enhances apoptosis and growth inhibition of squamous cell carcinoma xenografts with proteasome inhibitor bortezomib. Radiology 248: 485–491.
17. Andriyanov AV, Koren E, Barenholz Y, Goldberg SN (2014) Therapeutic efficacy of combining PEGylated liposomal doxorubicin and Radiofrequency (RF) Ablation: Comparison between slow-releasing non thermo-sensitive and fast-releasing drug thermo-sensitive nano-liposomes. Plos One [in press].
18. Ahmed M, Moussa M, Goldberg SN (2012) Synergy in cancer treatment between liposomal chemotherapeutics and thermal ablation. Chem Phys Lipids.
19. Rapoport N (2012) Ultrasound-mediated micellar drug delivery. Int J Hyperthermia 28: 374–385.
20. Perche F, Torchilin VP (2012) Cancer cell spheroids as a model to evaluate chemotherapy protocols. Cancer Biol Ther 13: 1205–1213.
21. Solazzo S, Ahmed M, Schor-Bardach R, Yang W, Girnun G, et al. (2010) Liposomal doxorubicin increases radiofrequency ablation-induced tumor destruction by increasing cellular oxidative and nitrative stress and accelerating apoptotic pathways. Radiology 255: 62–74.
22. Yamazaki Y, Hasebe Y, Egawa K, Nose K, Kunimoto S, et al. (2006) Anthracyclines, small-molecule inhibitors of hypoxia-inducible factor-1 alpha activation. Biol Pharm Bull 29: 1999–2003.
23. Monsky WL, Kruskal JB, Lukyanov AN, Girnun GD, Ahmed M, et al. (2002) Radio-frequency ablation increases intratumoral liposomal doxorubicin accumulation in a rat breast tumor model. Radiology 224: 823–829.
24. Sawant RR, Torchilin VP (2011) Design and synthesis of novel functional lipid-based bioconjugates for drug delivery and other applications. Methods Mol Biol 751: 357–378.
25. Theriault JR, Adachi H, Calderwood SK (2006) Role of scavenger receptors in the binding and internalization of heat shock protein 70. J Immunol 177: 8604–8611.
26. de Smet M, Hijnen NM, Langereis S, Elevelt A, Heijman E, et al. (2013) Magnetic resonance guided high-intensity focused ultrasound mediated hyperthermia improves the intratumoral distribution of temperature-sensitive liposomal doxorubicin. Invest Radiol 48: 395–405.
27. Poon RT, Borys N (2009) Lyso-thermosensitive liposomal doxorubicin: a novel approach to enhance efficacy of thermal ablation of liver cancer. Expert Opin Pharmacother 10: 333–343.
28. Hamano N, Negishi Y, Takatori K, Endo-Takahashi Y, Suzuki R, et al. (2014) Combination of Bubble Liposomes and High-Intensity Focused Ultrasound (HIFU) Enhanced Antitumor Effect by Tumor Ablation. Biol Pharm Bull 37: 174–177.
29. Tsukioka Y, Matsumura Y, Hamaguchi T, Koike H, Moriyasu F, et al. (2002) Pharmaceutical and biomedical differences between micellar doxorubicin (NK911) and liposomal doxorubicin (Doxil). Jpn J Cancer Res 93: 1145–1153.
30. Weissig V, Whiteman KR, Torchilin VP (1998) Accumulation of protein-loaded long-circulating micelles and liposomes in subcutaneous Lewis lung carcinoma in mice. Pharm Res 15: 1552–1556.
31. Goldberg SN, Girnan GD, Lukyanov AN, Ahmed M, Monsky WL, et al. (2002) Percutaneous tumor ablation: increased necrosis with combined radio-frequency ablation and intravenous liposomal doxorubicin in a rat breast tumor model. Radiology 222: 797–804.
32. Kong J, Kong J, Pan B, Ke S, Dong S, et al. (2012) Insufficient radiofrequency ablation promotes angiogenesis of residual hepatocellular carcinoma via HIF-1alpha/VEGFA. PLoS One 7: e37266.
33. Nijkamp MW, van der Bilt JD, de Bruijn MT, Molenaar IQ, Voest EE, et al. (2009) Accelerated perinecrotic outgrowth of colorectal liver metastases following radiofrequency ablation is a hypoxia-driven phenomenon. Ann Surg 249: 814–823.
34. Nikfarjam M, Muralidharan V, Christophi C (2006) Altered growth patterns of colorectal liver metastases after thermal ablation. Surgery 139: 73–81.
35. Gasselhuber A, Dreher MR, Partanen A, Yarmolenko PS, Woods D, et al. (2012) Targeted drug delivery by high intensity focused ultrasound mediated hyperthermia combined with temperature-sensitive liposomes: computational modelling and preliminary in vivovalidation. Int J Hyperthermia 28: 337–348.
36. Potter AJ, Gollahon KA, Palanca BJ, Harbert MJ, Choi YM, et al. (2002) Flow cytometric analysis of the cell cycle phase specificity of DNA damage induced by radiation, hydrogen peroxide and doxorubicin. Carcinogenesis 23: 389–401.
37. Lukyanov AN, Gao Z, Mazzola L, Torchilin VP (2002) Polyethylene glycol-diacyllipid micelles demonstrate increased acculumation in subcutaneous tumors in mice. Pharm Res 19: 1424–1429.
38. Yang W, Ahmed M, Tasawwar B, Levchenko T, Sawant RR, et al. (2012) Combination radiofrequency (RF) ablation and IV liposomal heat shock protein suppression: Reduced tumor growth and increased animal endpoint survival in a small animal tumor model. J Control Release.

9

GDNF-Transfected Macrophages Produce Potent Neuroprotective Effects in Parkinson's Disease Mouse Model

Yuling Zhao[1,2], Matthew J. Haney[1,2], Richa Gupta[1,2], John P. Bohnsack[2], Zhijian He[1,2], Alexander V. Kabanov[1,2,3], Elena V. Batrakova[1,2]*

1 Center for Nanotechnology in Drug Delivery, University of North Carolina at Chapel Hill, Chapel Hill, North Carolina, United States of America, **2** Eshelman School of Pharmacy, University of North Carolina at Chapel Hill, Chapel Hill, North Carolina, United States of America, **3** Department of Chemical Enzymology, Faculty of Chemistry, M.V. Lomonosov Moscow State University, Moscow, Russia

Abstract

The pathobiology of Parkinson's disease (PD) is associated with the loss of dopaminergic neurons in the substantia nigra pars compacta (*SNpc*) projecting to the striatum. Currently, there are no treatments that can halt or reverse the course of PD; only palliative therapies, such as replacement strategies for missing neurotransmitters, exist. Thus, the successful brain delivery of neurotrophic factors that promote neuronal survival and reverse the disease progression is crucial. We demonstrated earlier systemically administered autologous macrophages can deliver nanoformulated antioxidant, catalase, to the *SNpc* providing potent anti-inflammatory effects in PD mouse models. Here we evaluated genetically-modified macrophages for active targeted brain delivery of glial cell-line derived neurotropic factor (GDNF). To capitalize on the beneficial properties afforded by alternatively activated macrophages, transfected with GDNF-encoded *p*DNA cells were further differentiated toward regenerative M2 phenotype. A systemic administration of GDNF-expressing macrophages significantly ameliorated neurodegeneration and neuroinflammation in PD mice. Behavioral studies confirmed neuroprotective effects of the macrophage-based drug delivery system. One of the suggested mechanisms of therapeutic effects is the release of exosomes containing the expressed neurotropic factor followed by the efficient GDNF transfer to target neurons. Such formulations can serve as a new technology based on cell-mediated active delivery of therapeutic proteins that attenuate and reverse progression of PD, and ultimately provide hope for those patients who are already significantly disabled by the disease.

Editor: Tsuneya Ikezu, Boston University School of Medicine, United States of America

Funding: This study was supported by the grants of the US National Institutes of Health 1R01 NS057748 (to EVB), RR021937 and R01 CA116591 (to AVK), US Department of Defense Award No. W81XWH-09-1-0386 (to AVK) and W81XWH11-1-0770 (to AVK), and the Russian Ministry of Science and Education No. 02.740.11.5231 and No. 11.G34.31.0004 (to AVK). The funders had no role in study design, data collection and analysis, decision to publish, or preparation of the manuscript.

Competing Interests: The authors have declared that no competing interests exist.

* Email: batrakov@email.unc.edu

Introduction

An extraordinary goal, such as brain delivery of therapeutic proteins, requires exceptional measures. The blood brain barrier (BBB) is a major obstacle to the successful treatment of many devastating diseases of central nervous system (CNS). Among them are neurodegenerative disorders (PD, Alzheimer's disease, and amyotrophic lateral sclerosis [1–3]), infectious diseases (meningitis, encephalitis, prion disease, and HIV-related dementia [4,5]), stroke [6,7], and lysosomal storage diseases [8,9]. PD is the second most common neurodegenerative disorder of people over 65 year age; 70,000 new cases are registered in US every year. Regrettably, no therapies are currently available that can attenuate disease progression. The use of existing drugs provides only symptomatic relief to patients that are hindered by the development of drug resistance and progressive adverse side effects such as motor complications and dyskinesia [10]. In addition, most current therapies are based on pharmacological replacement of lost striatal dopamine, which only masks or reduces the declining dopaminergic activity in PD patients. Thus, novel therapies are urgently required.

Disease symptoms are characterized by lack of neurotransmitter dopamine due to the loss of dopaminergic neurons located in the nigrostriatal system. A growing body of evidence indicates the usefulness and efficacy of neurotrophic factors for the treatment of PD [11–17]. It has been confirmed that BDNF expression levels are decreased in the *SNpc* of PD patients [18]. Thus, the neurotrophic factors, and in particular GDNF, can promote regeneration of DA neurons and protect these cells from toxic insults [19]. Furthermore, intracranial infusions of GDNF [20,21] and BDNF [22] have been shown to provide protection and restoration of DA neurons in rodent models of PD, and in 1-methyl-4-phenyl-1,2,3,6-tetrahydro-pyridine (MPTP)- or 6-hydroxydopamine (6-OHDA)-lesioned and intact aged primates

[15,17,23–25]. Unfortunately, intracranial infusion is an invasive procedure that carries a high risk of adverse effects. Thus, the development of new drug delivery systems for neurotrophic factors that can be administered systemically is crucial.

The majority of CNS disorders have in common an inflammatory component [26] resulting in the excessive production of reactive oxygen species (ROS) and subsequent neurodegeneration. Immunocytes that include mononuclear phagocytes (dendritic cells, monocytes and macrophages) exhibit an intrinsic homing property of migrating toward the inflammation site *via* the processes known as diapedesis and chemotaxis [27]. Thus, immunocytes are reported to cause BBB breakdown following brain inflammation [28–31] trafficking primarily between adjacent endothelial cells, *i.e.* paracellulary through the junctional complexes [32,33]. Considering that immunocytes readily home to the sites with inflammation, we propose harnessing this natural mechanism, and use macrophages for the active targeted delivery of therapeutic proteins to the brain.

Two approaches are utilized in cell-mediated drug delivery. *First*, host cells are loaded with a drug, usually incorporated into a protective container, and then carry the drug to the disease side. One of the main obstacles of this approach is efficient disintegration of the entrapped foreign particles by monocytes. *Second*, cell-carriers are genetically modified to produce therapeutically active molecules. For example, neurotropic factors, such as glial cell-line derived neurotropic factor (GDNF), neurturin (NTN), or vascular endothelial growth factor (VGEF) produced by transfected neural stem cells (NSC) [34–36] and bone marrow-derived macrophages and microglia [37,38] were used in PD mouse models. In particular, bone marrow stem cells were transduced *ex vivo* with lentivirus expressing a GDNF gene driven by a synthetic macrophage-specific promoter and then transplanted into recipient mice. Macrophage-mediated GDNF delivery dramatically ameliorated PD-related inflammation and neuronal degeneration in *SNpc* [37] resulting in axon regeneration and reversed hypoactivity in mice. Furthermore, transfected NSC were used for delivery of neurotrophic factors [39–43] in Alzheimer's disease mouse model.

Our earlier studies suggest cell-carriers offer distinct advantages over standard drug administration regimens by providing disease-specific homing, sustained on-site drug delivery, and improved therapeutic efficacy [44–52]. Based on our previously developed cell-mediated drug delivery system, present work utilized genetically-modified autologous macrophages for active targeted delivery of GDNF to the inflamed brain. The overall scheme of these investigations is depicted in **Figure 1**. Macrophages were transfected *ex vivo* to produce GDNF, and administered intravenously in mice with PD model. This resulted in significant increases in dopaminergic neurons survival and decreases in inflammation in *SNpc*. Of note, genetically-modified macrophages released exosomes with incorporated GDNF that may facilitate GDNF transport into the target cells and preserve it against degradation.

Exosomes are nanosized vesicles secreted by a variety of cells, in particular, cells of the immune system: dendritic cells [53], macrophages [54], B cells [55], and T cells [56]. These extracellular vesicles were initially thought to be a mechanism for removing unneeded proteins. Recent studies revealed, they are actually specialized in long-distance intercellular communications facilitating transfer of proteins [57], functional mRNAs and microRNAs for subsequent protein expression in target cells [58,59]. To shuttle their cargo, exosomes can attach by a range of surface adhesion proteins and specific vector ligands (tetraspanins, integrins, CD11b and CD18 receptors), and fuse with target cellular membranes delivering their payload [53,60,61]. Indeed, exosomes, comprised of cellular membranes, have an exceptional ability to interact with target cells. Thus, we demonstrated here that exosomes showed an extraordinary ability to abundantly adhere and overflow neuronal cells as was visualized by confocal microscopy. This mechanism may play a significant role in GDNF-mediated protection effects, increasing the blood circulation time, reducing immunogenicity, and facilitation of the protein transfer across the BBB and into target neurons. In addition, the membranotropic properties of GDNF-carrying exosomes may facilitate GDNF binding to GFRα-1 receptors expressed on DA neurons [62]. The present data indicate, intrinsic properties of macrophages can overcome the limitations of current common therapies, alleviate and reverse the symptoms, and may ultimately improve the quality of life of patients with various neurodegenerative disorders.

Materials and Methods

Plasmids

The gWI high expression vectors encoding the reporter gene green fluorescent protein (GFP) (gWIGFP) under control of an optimized human cytomegalovirus (CMV) promoter followed by intron A from the CMV immediate-early (IE) gene were used throughout the study (Gene Therapy Systems, San Diego, CA). Human GDNF cDNA (NM_199234) was provided by OriGene (Rockville, MD). All plasmids are expanded in DH5α E.coli and isolated using Qiagen endotoxin-free plasmid Giga-prep kits (Qiagen, Valencia, CA) according to the supplier's protocol.

Reagents

GenePORTER 3000 transfection agent was purchased from AMS Biotechnology, England). Lipopolysaccharides (LPS), 6-hydroxydopamine (6-OHDA), and Triton X-100 were purchased from Sigma-Aldrich (St. Louis, MO, USA). A lipophilic fluorescent dye, 1,1′-dioctadecyl-3,3,3′,3′-tetramethylindo-carbocyanine perchlorate (DIL), was purchased from Invitrogen (Carlsbad, CA). Interferon gamma (INT-γ), and murine macrophage colony-stimulating factor (MCSF) were purchased from Peprotech Inc (Rocky Hill, NJ).

Cells

Raw 264.7, a mouse macrophage cell line, was purchased from ATCC (cat # TIB-71), and cultured in Dulbecco's Modified Eagle's Media (DMEM) (Invitrogen, Carlsbad, CA, USA) supplemented with 2.5% horse serum and 15% FBS. Neuronal PC12 rat adrenal pheochromocytoma cell line was obtained from ATCC, and cultured in Dulbecco's modified Eagle medium (Hyclone, Utah, USA) supplemented with 10% FBS, and 1% (v/v) of both penicillin and streptomycin. The cells were grown in an incubator with optimal culture conditions of 37°C and 5% CO_2, and the medium was routinely replaced every 2–3 days.

Animals

BALB/C female mice (Charles River Laboratories, USA) eight weeks of age were treated in accordance to the Principles of Animal Care outlined by National Institutes of Health and approved by the Institutional Animal Care and Use Committee of the University of North Carolina at Chapel Hill.

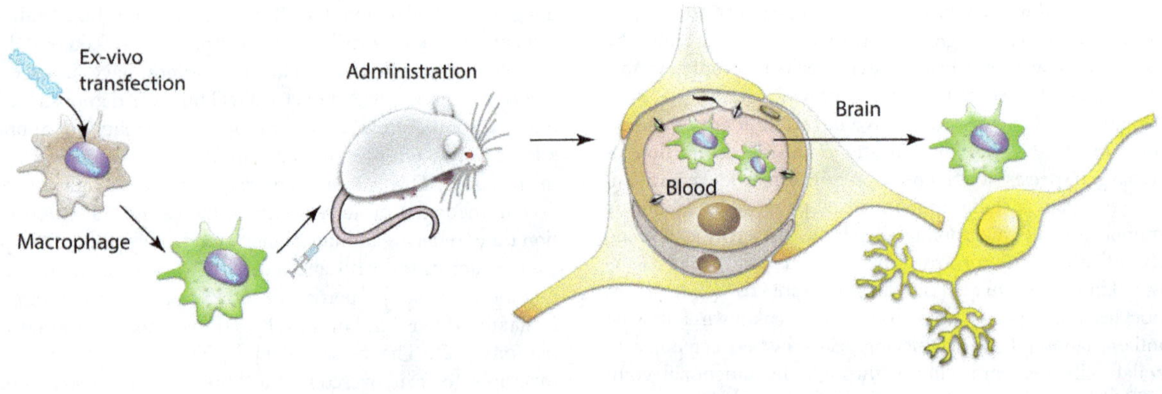

Figure 1. Schematic representation of macrophage-mediated drug delivery approach. Autologous macrophages were transfected with GDNF-encoding *p*DNA *ex vitro* and systemically administered into mice with brain inflammation. Driven by chemotaxis, genetically-modified cell-carriers home the inflamed brain tissues, and deliver the expressed neurotrophic factor to the dopaminergic neurons protecting them from toxic insults. The release of overexpressed GDNF in exosomes protected it against proteases degradation, facilitated the GDNF transfer into target neurons and as a result, improved therapeutic efficacy of this drug formulation.

Transfection of Macrophages with GDNF-encoding *p*DNA and Differentiation toward M2 Regenerative Subtype

Macrophages were incubated with a mixture of 13.6 μg GFP, or GDNF *p*DNA and GenePORTER 3000 in serum free media for four hours. Following incubation, an equal volume of full media containing 20% FBS was added bringing final serum concentration to 10%. To exclude the possibility that cell death explains the release of GDNF and GFP, percentage of live macrophages on the fourth day after transfection was accounted by Fluorescence Activated Cell Sorting (FACS). Transfected cells were collected, washed, stained with Alexa 488 LIVE/DEAD dye according to manufacturer's protocol, and the amount of accumulated LIVE/DEAD dye was assessed. The macrophage transfection efficiency using GenePORTER 3000 reagent was around 40% as determined by FACS for GFP-encoding *p*DNA [48].

To promote specific cell differentiation, Raw 264.7 macrophages were cultured in the presence of: (i) Interleukin 4 (IL-4) (to promote M2 anti-inflammatory subtype); or (ii) Interferon gamma (IFN-γ) and LPS (to obtain M1 pro-inflammatory subtype). For M2 subset differentiation, macrophages were supplemented with IL 4 (20 ng/ml) for 48 hours. For M1 subset differentiation, the cells were cultured in the mixture of IFN-γ (20 ng/ml) and LPS (100 ng/ml) for 48 hours. Following the incubation, media was replaced with a mixture of antibodies to mannose receptor (M2 type marker, anti-CD 206, BD Bioscience, 1 μg/ml), and antibodies to CD86 (M1 type marker, anti-CD 86, BD Bioscience, 2 μg/ml). The cells were incubated with the antibodies for 1 hour, washed, fixed, and examined by confocal microscopy as described below (CD 86, $\lambda = 405$ nm, and CD 206, $\lambda = 647$ nm). An overexpression of specific markers related to M1 or M2 subset of macrophages upon cell differentiation was confirmed by RT-PCR.

Isolation of Exosomes

Conditioned media from genetically-modified Raw 264.7 macrophages grown on T-75 flasks (20×10^6 cells/flask) was collected, and exosomes were isolated using ultra centrifugation [53]. In brief, the culture supernatants were cleared of cell debris and large vesicles by sequential centrifugation at 300×g for 10 min, 1000×g for 20 min, and 10,000×g for 30 min, followed by filtration using 0.2-μm syringe filters. Then, the cleared sample was spun at 100,000×g for 1 hour to pellet the exosomes, and supernatant was collected. The collected exosomes (10^{11}–10^{12} exosomes/flask) were washed twice with PBS. To avoid contamination of the FBS-derived exosomes, FBS was spun at 100,000×g for 2 hours to remove exosomes before use. The recovery of exosomes was estimated by measuring the protein concentration using the Bradford assay and by Nanoparticle Tracking Analysis (NTA). The obtained exosomal fraction was re-suspended in PBS (500 μl, 1 mg/mL total protein), and characterized for size and polydispersity by Dynamic Light Scattering (DLS) and Atomic Force Microscopy (AFM). The obtained exosomal fraction was evaluated for protein content.

Western Blot Analysis

Western blots were utilized to evaluate the presence of GDNF in transfected macrophages as well as in exosomes secreted by GDNF- or empty vector-transfected macrophages. Genetically-modified macrophages and exosomes isolated from the conditioned media were treated with lysis buffer (1% Triton X-100) and protease inhibitors (Sigma) and protein concentration was determined by BCA assay. Samples were mixed with 2×SDS sample buffer, boiled for 5 min and then separated on a precast 4–20% SDS-PAGE gel (BioRad, USA). Proteins were transferred to nitrocellulose membranes and GDNF was visualized with sheep polyclonal antibodies to GDNF (Millipore, AB5252, 1:2000 dilution) and secondary antibodies donkey anti-sheep IgG-HRP (Jackson ImmuneResearch; 1:5000 dilution). To correct for loading differences in cellular lysates and exosomal fractions, the levels of proteins were normalized to constitutively expressed β-actin in cells with goat polyclonal antibodies to β-actin (Abcam, ab8229; 1:500 dilution); and TSG101 in exosomes with goat polyclonal antibodies to TSG101 (Santa Cruz, SC6037; 1:200 dilution). Furthermore, for the characterization of different subtypes of polarized macrophages and released from them exosomes, membranes with corresponding transferred protein bands from macrophages or exosomes were blotted with rabbit polyclonal antibodies to CD63 (Santa Cruz, SC15363; 1:200 dilution), iNOS (Santa Cruz, SC650; 1:200 dilution), Arg1 (Santa Cruz, SC18351; 1:200 dilution) and CD206 (Santa Cruz, SC6037; 1:200 dilution) overnight at 4°C, and incubated with appropriate HRP-conjugated secondary antibodies: goat anti-rabbit IgG-HRP (Santa Cruz, SC2004; 1:2500 dilution), or donkey anti-goat IgG-HRP (Santa Cruz, SC2020; 1:5000 dilution). Membranes were washed and the expression levels were visualized with chemiluminescent substrate (Thermo Scientific) and a FluorChem E imaging

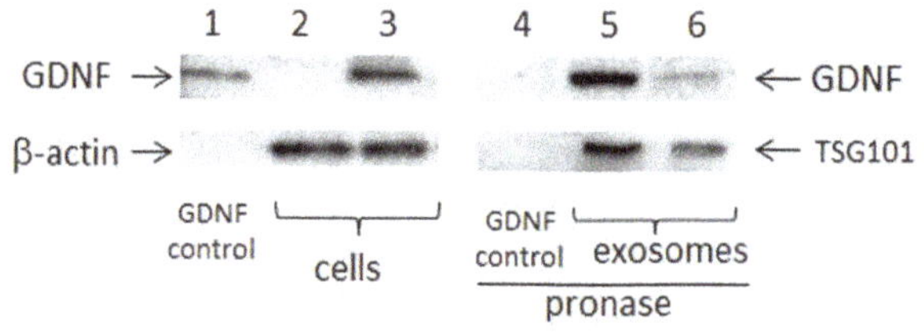

Figure 2. Expression of GDNF by genetically-modified macrophages. Raw 264.7 macrophages were pre-transfected with GDNF-encoding pDNA and GenePorter 3000 reagent for 4 hours. Then, exosomes were collected from concomitant macrophages media for 24 hours, and GDNF levels in cellular lysates (lines 2–3) and in exosomes (lines 5–6) were examined by western blot. Commercially available GDNF (line 1) served as a positive control. Significant amount of GDNF was detected in the cells (line 3) and exosomes released from GDNF-transfected macrophages (line 5), but not in macrophages transfected with empty vector (line 2). Expressed GDNF was protected in exosomes against degradation by pronase (line 5), while control GDNF was degraded at these conditions (line 4). Destruction of exosomes by sonication eliminated their protective effect (line 6). β-actin and TSG101 served as controls for cell lysates and exosomes, respectively.

system (Protein Simple). Specific protein bands were quantitated by densitometry (Bio-Rad Laboratories, Hercules, CA).

RT-PCR analysis

Total RNA of macrophages as well as exosomal RNA was extracted using RNeasy mini kit (Qiagen, CA, USA) according to manufacturer's instructions. Residual genomic DNA of macrophages and exosomes was removed by incubating with Rnase-free DNase set (Qiagen). RNA was analyzed and quantified using nanodrop 2000c (Thermo Scientific, USA). As quality controls of RNA samples purity from contaminating DNA and chaotropic salts was obtained by absorbance Ratio A260/A280 and A260/A230, respectively. RNA (1 μg) isolated from resting and polarized macrophages cells and their respective exosomes was reverse transcribed with Superscript III First-Strand synthesis system for RT-PCR (Invitrogen, CA, USA) according to manufacturer's protocol. To quantify mRNA levels, quantitative reverse transcription PCR was performed using an ABI StepOne Plus Detection System (Applied Biosystems, MA, USA). TaqMan PCR Universal Master Mix and Expression Assays were from Applied Biosystems. Assay IDs: iNOS Mm00440502_m1, CD206 Mm00485148_m1 and CD63 Mm01966817_g1. CD63 was used as exosomal marker and CD11b as macrophage cells marker.

Confocal Microscopy Studies

To visualize exosomal accumulation in target neurons, Raw 264.6 macrophages were transfected with GDNF-encoding DNA, and cultured in exosome-free media for two days. Exosomes were isolated from macrophage conditioned media by ultracentrifugation, and stained with the lipophilic fluorescent dye, DIL (red). PC12 neurons were cultured with DIL-labeled exosomes or PLGA nanoparticles (as a control) for three days, washed with PBS, and stained with phallodin for actin microfilaments (green). The accumulation levels were examined by confocal microscopy.

To track systemically injected macrophages in the inflamed brain, macrophages were transfected with GFP-encoding DNA as described above. For 6-OHDA intoxications, mice were stereotactically injected with 6-OHDA solution (10 μg 6-OHDA in 0.9% NaCL with 0.02% ascorbic acid), flow rate of 0.1 μL/min into the striatum (AP: +0.5; L: −2.0 and DV: −3.0 mm) [52]. Animals with brain inflammation induced were injected with GFP-expressing Raw 264.7 macrophages on day twenty one after intoxication with 6-OHDA *via* the intrajugular vein (*i.v.*). Two days later, animals were sacrificed and perfused as described [52], brains were removed, washed, post-fixed in 10% phosphate-buffered paraformaldehyde, and evaluated by confocal microscopy.

Immunohistochemical and Stereological Analyses

6-OHDA-intoxicated mice were *i.v.* injected with PBS, or GDNF-transfected macrophages, or macrophages transfected with empty vector 48 hours after intoxication. Twenty four days later, animals were sacrificed, perfused; brains were removed, washed, post-fixed, and immunohistochemical analysis was performed in 30 μm thick consecutive coronal brain sections [46]. For detection of microglia activation, tissue sections were incubated with primary monoclonal rat anti mouse anti-CD11b antibodies (AbD Serotec, Raleigh, NC) 1:500 dilution), and secondary biotinylated goat anti-rat antibodies (Vector Laboratories, Burlingame, CA, 1:200 dilution). For the assessment of neuroprotection effect, tyrosine hydroxylase (TH) staining was used to quantitate numbers of dopaminergic neurons [63]. The total number of TH-positive SN neurons and CD11b-positive microglia cells were counted by using the optical fractionator module in StereoInvestigator software (MicroBrightField, Inc., Williston, VT) [46].

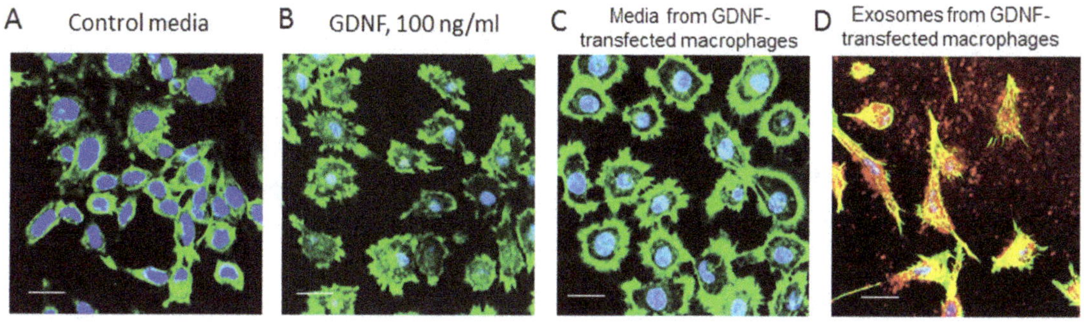

Figure 3. Effect of exosomes released from GDNF-transfected macrophages on the axonal growth in PC12 neurons. PC12 neurons were cultured for 3 days in: (**A**) control media without GDNF; (**B**) in the presence of 100 ng/ml GDNF; or supplemented with (**C**) conditioned media collected from GDNF-transfected macrophages; or (**D**) exosomes isolated from conditioned media released from GDNF-transfected macrophages. Exosomes were fluorescently labeled with lypophilic dye, DIL (red) before the addition to the neurons (**D**). Following incubation, the cells were washed with PBS, and stained with phallodin for actin microfilaments (green). Confocal images revealed the pronounced development of axons upon treatment with media (**C**) and especially exosomes (**D**) released from GDNF-transfected macrophages. The bar: 20 μm.

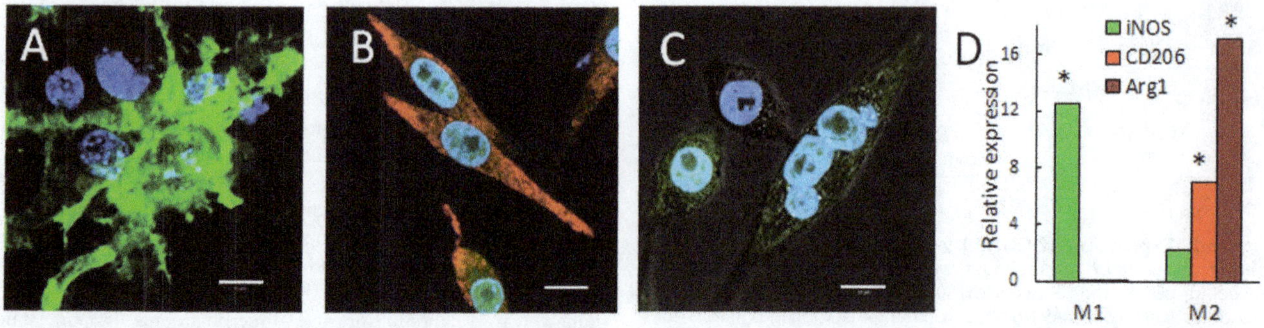

Figure 4. Differentiation of macrophages toward "alternatively" activated M2 subtype. Raw 264.7 macrophages were cultured in the presence of: (**A**) Interferon gamma (IFN-γ) and lipopolysaccharides (LPS) for M1 pro-inflammatory subtype; or (**B**)) Interleukin 4 (IL 4) for M2 anti-inflammatory subtype for two days as described in **Materials and Methods** section. Then, the cells were stained with a mixture of antibodies to CD 86 (green) and mannose receptor CD206 (red) for M1 and M2 phenotype, respectively, and examined by confocal microscopy. Macrophages differentiated in the presence of INF-γ/LPS showed high expression of CD86, but low if any mannose receptor levels indicating classically activated M1 subtype (**A**). In contrast, cells differentiated in the presence of IL-4 showed high expression of mannose receptor, and low expression of CD 86 that is attributed to M2 macrophages (B). Non-differentiated Mo macrophages served as a control (**C**). Bar: 10 μm. RT-PCR studies confirmed statistically significantly elevated levels of inducible Nitric Oxide Synthases (iNOS) mRNA in M1 cells, and high levels of CD206 and Arginase 1 (Arg1) mRNA in M2 macrophages (**D**), compared to Mo macrophages ($p<0.05$).

Behavioral Tests

For the traditional constant speed rotarod test, mice were trained and tested as previously described with slight modifications [64]. 6-OHDA-intoxicated mice were *i.v.* injected with PBS, or GDNF-transfected macrophages 48 hours after intoxication and the latency to fall from the rotarod was determined at three speeds (4, 5, and 7 rpm). Healthy mice *i.c.* injected with PBS were used as a control [65]. For apomorphine test, the animals were injected with apomorphine (0.05 mg / kg, *s.c.*) and rotations were scored every 10 min for 90 min [66].

Statistical Analysis

For the all experiments, data are presented as the mean ±SEM. Tests for significant differences between the groups in *in vitro* experiments investigating transfection of macrophages, as well as in *in vivo* evaluations of therapeutic effects of different drug formulations were performed using a one-way ANOVA with multiple comparisons (Fisher's pairwise comparisons) using GraphPad Prism 5.0 (GraphPad software, San Diego, CA, USA). A standard T-test was performed when only two groups (for example, for the evaluation of expression levels of specific proteins by western blot) were compared. A minimum p value of 0.05 was chosen as the significance level for all tests.

Results

Exosomes secreted from genetically-modified macrophages contaln GDNF

The optimal conditions that provide for high levels and duration of therapeutic proteins expression in macrophages identified previously [48] were used to transfect Raw 264.7 macrophages. Next, exosomes were collected from conditioned macrophages

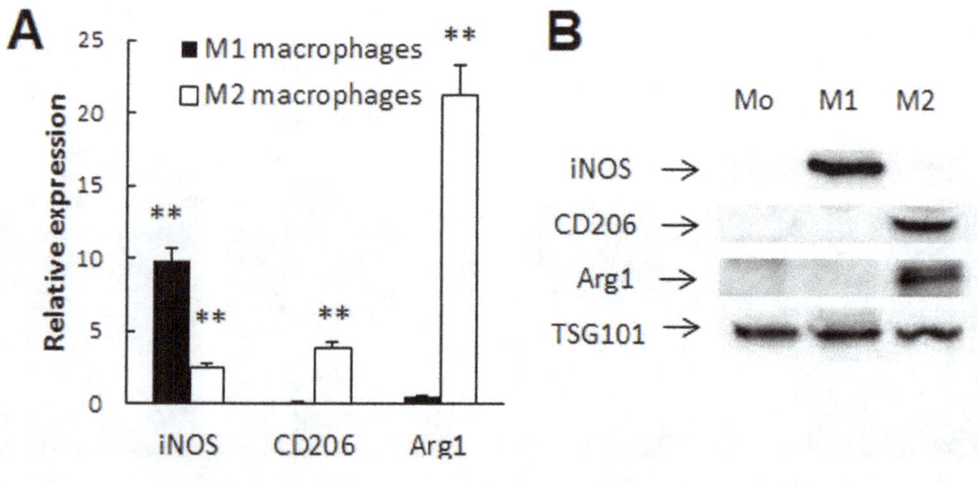

Figure 5. Characterization of exosomes released from differentiated subtypes of macrophages. Exosomes were isolated from conditional media of differentiated macrophages and examined for the presence of specific markers by RP-PCR (**A**) and western blot (**B**). Expression of Arg1 and CD206 mRNA and protein (markers for M2 subtype) was detected in exosomes originated from M2 macrophages, but not in those secreted from M1 macrophages. In contrast, expression of iNOS mRNA and protein was detected in exosomes released from M1 macrophages, but not in those secreted by M2 macrophages. TSG101 was used as house-keeping protein for exosomes. Values are means ±SEM ($N=4$), and $p<0.05$ compared with the expression levels in Mo macrophages.

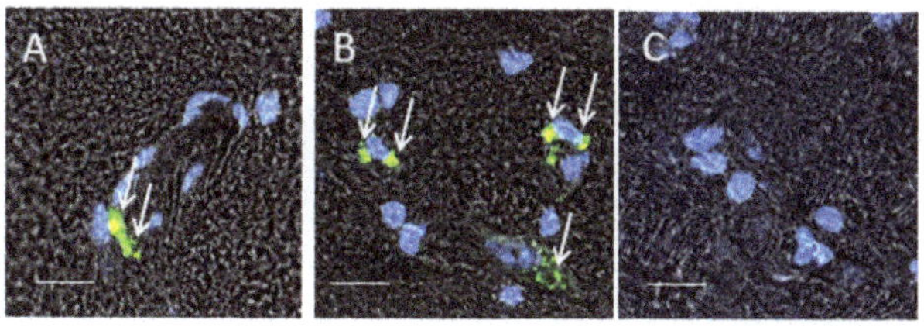

Figure 6. Recruitment of GFP-expressing M2 macrophages to *SNpc* in 6-OHDA-intoxicated mice. Macrophages were transfected with GFP-encoding *p*DNA as described in Materials and Methods section and stained with primary antibodies to CD206, a marker for M2 macrophages, and secondary fluorescently-labeled anti-Mouse-IgG-atto 647N (red). BALB/c mice were *i.c.* intoxicated with 6-OHDA into *SNpc*. Twenty one day later, the animals were *i.v.* injected with GFP-expressing RAW 264.7 macrophages (green, 5×10^6 cells/ mouse in 100 µl). Twenty four hours later mice were sacrificed, and perfused with PBS and 4% PFA. Brains were frozen, sectioned with a cryostat (10 µm thick), and examined by confocal microscopy (60×magnification) (**A, B**). Healthy mice without brain inflammation (with PBS *i.c.* injections) were used as a control group (**C**). Slides were stained with for expression of mannose receptor (CD206 antibodies). Co-localization of GFP-expressing macrophages and CD206 antibodies to mannose receptor manifested in yellow staining (arrows) confirmed presence of significant amounts of the M2 genetically-modified cells in the intoxicated brain endothelial microvesseles (**A**), and parenchyma (**B**). No fluorescence in the healthy brain was found (**C**) indicating that systemically administered Raw 264.7 macrophages did not cross the BBB in the absence of brain inflammation. The bar: 20 µm.

media for 24 hours, and the expression of the encoded protein in the in cellular lysates and exosomes were evaluated by western blot (**Fig. 2**). Significant amounts of GDNF was detected in the cells (line 3) and exosomes released from GDNF-transfected macrophages (line 5), but not in macrophages transfected with empty vector (line 2). Noteworthy, the expressed GDNF was protected in exosomes against degradation by pronase (line 5); while control GDNF was degraded at these conditions (line 4). Destruction of exosomes by sonication eliminated their protective effect against proteases degradation (line 6). The average size for exosomes released from GDNF-transfected macrophages (96.0±9.1 nm) was slightly greater than those released from non-transfected macrophages (90.5±3.4 nm).

Effects of GDNF-transfected Macrophages on axonal growth *in vitro*

A profound therapeutic effect of GDNF released from pre-loaded M2 macrophages in vitro was demonstrated in PC12 neurons that are known to express GDNF receptor (**Fig. 3**). Neurons were cultured for 72 hours in: (**A**) control media without GDNF; (**B**) media supplemented with high concentration of commercially available GDNF (100 ng/ml); (**C**) conditioned media collected from GDNF-transfected macrophages, or (**D**) exosomes isolated from GDNF-transfected macrophages. Following the incubation, the cells were stained with phallodin for actin microfilaments (green) and DAPI for cell nucleus (blue). In parallel, exosomes were stained with a lipophilic fluorescent dye, DID (red). Confocal images revealed the significant axonal growth in neurons cultured with conditioned media from GDNF-preloaded macrophages (**Fig. 3 C**) suggesting GDNF was released from the cell-carriers in a functional state. Noteworthy, treatment of PC12 neurons with exosomes released from pre-transfected macrophages resulted in the drastic increase of neuronal maturation with a pronounced outgrowth of axons and dendrites (**Fig. 3 D**). The effects were greater than those caused by a high dose of commercially-available GDNF (**Fig. 3 B**). It is likely, similar to catalase-transfected macrophages [48], exosomes with incorporated overexpressed neurotropic factor promote GDNF transfer, and secure its efficient accumulation and favorable intracellular localization in target neurons.

Differentiation of Macrophages and Using an Alternatively Activated Neuroregenerative M2 Subtype

To enhance the therapeutic effects of GDNF and avoid the pro-inflammatory neurotoxic effects of classically-activated M1 macrophages [67], Raw 264.7 macrophages were differentiated to M2 regenerative subtype. For this purpose, macrophages were cultured in the presence of Interleukin 4 (IL 4) for M2 subtype; or Interferon gamma (IFN-γ) and lipopolysaccharides (LPS), as a negative control for M1 pro-inflammatory subtype. The obtained subsets of macrophages were characterized by confocal microscopy (**Fig. 4 A–C**) and RT-PCR (**Fig. 4 D**). Mannose receptor (CD206), and Arginase 1 (Arg1) were chosen as principal markers form identifying M2 macrophages subtype. Levels of inducible Nitric Oxide Synthases (iNOS, CD86) were examined as marker of M1 macrophages subtype. Noteworthy, Arg1 and iNOS [68] were demontrated to have anti-inflammatory and pro-inflammatory properties, respectively.

Macrophages differentiated in the presence of INF-γ/LPS demonstrated considerable expression of CD 86, and low, if any, levels of mannose receptor (**Fig. 4 A**) that is indicative for classically activated pro-inflammatory M1 subtype. In contrast, Raw 264.7 macrophages differentiated in the presence of IL-4 showed high expression levels of mannose receptor, and low, if any, expression of CD 86 (**Fig. 4B**) that indicative for "alternatevly activated" anti-inflammatory macrophages. Non-activated Mo macrophages showed low, if any expression of both CD86 and CD206 receptors (**Fig. 4 C**). Noteworthy, the polarization to different macrophages subtypes altered the cells morphology. RT-PCR studies confirmed elevated levels of iNOS mRNA in M1 cells, and high levels of CD206 and Arginase 1 (Arg1) mRNA in M2 macrophages (**Fig. 4 D**).

Next, we hypothesized that exosomal content, at least in part, should reflect the content of parental macrophages. Thus, exosomes released from M2 macrophages may exhibit neuroprotective and regenerative properties by themselves. A presence of Arg1 mRNA and Arg1 protein that indicative for M2 macrophages subtype was evaluated by RT-PCR (**Fig. 5 A**) and western blot analyses (**Fig. 5 B**). The obtained data confirmed exosomes secreted by M2 regenerative macrophages, but not M1 pro-inflammatory macrophages showed high levels of Arg1 and CD206 mRNA and Arg1 protein. In contrast, expression of iNOS mRNA and protein (marker for M1 macrophages) was detected in exosomes released from M1 macrophages, but not in those secreted by M2 macrophages. Noteworthy, although the overall trend of the expression of specific markers in different subtypes macrophages and exosomes is analogous, these levels might not be completely the same, as exosomes should reflect, but not copy the content of parental macrophages they were released from. This approach was utilized further to differentiate the cell-carriers towards the M2 phenotype prior to the infusion to capitalize on the beneficial properties afforded by alternatively activated M2 macrophages in the context of PD, and minimize the potential of the cells converting to the pro-inflammatory M1 subtype.

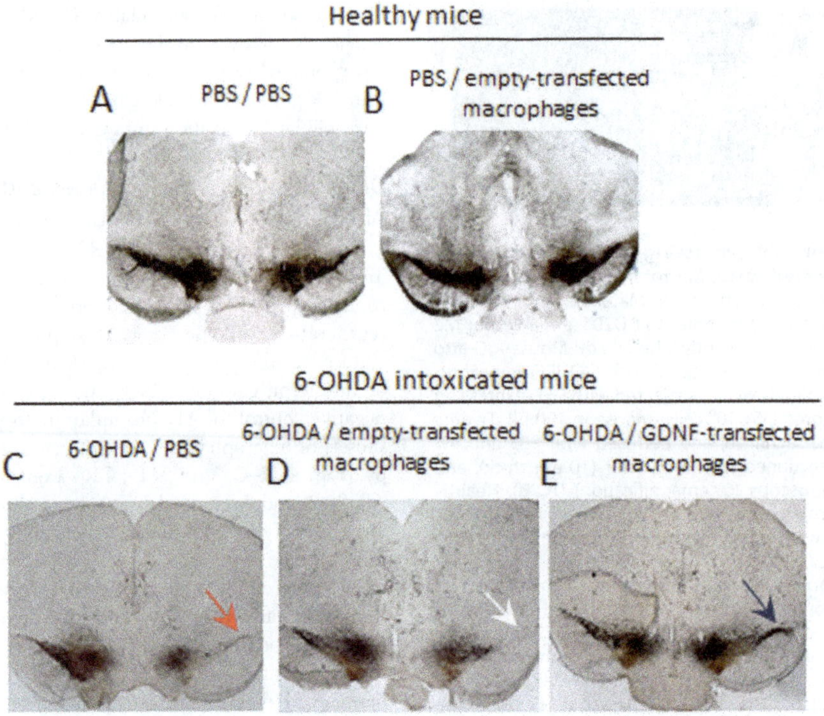

Figure 7. Neuroprotective effects of GDNF-transfected macrophages in PD mouse model. BALB/c mice were *i.c.* injected with 6-OHDA. Forty eight hours later, animals were *i.v.* injected with GDNF-transfected or empty-transfected macrophages, or PBS, and 21 days later they were sacrificed, and mid-brain slides were stained for expression of TH, a marker for dopaminergic neurons. Whereas 6-OHDA treatment caused significant neuronal loss in *SNpc* (red arrow), administration of GDNF-transfected macrophages dramatically increased neuronal survival (blue arrow). Administration of empty-vector transfected macrophages did not affect the number of dopaminergic neurons in healthy mice, and shows mild effect on increased neuronal survival in PD mice (white arrow).

Systemically-administered M2 Macrophages Home Inflamed Brain Tissues and Sustain their Phenotype in Brain Tissues

Raw 264.6 macrophages were transfected with GFP-encoding *p*DNA, and then differentiated to M2 regenerative subtype as described above. BALB/c mice were *i.c.* intoxicated with 6-OHDA into *SNpc*. Twenty one days later (at the pick of inflammation), mice were systemically injected with GFP-expressing macrophages (5×10^6 cells/ mouse in 100 µl). Twenty four hours later, the mice were sacrificed, and perfused with PBS and 4% PFA. Healthy mice without brain inflammation were used as a control group. Brain slides were stained with primary antibodies to CD 206, a marker for mannose receptor attributed to M2 subtype of macrophages. Confocal images of brains sections indicate systemically infused macrophages home the inflamed brain and localize around brain endothelial microvesseles (**Fig. 6 A**), and parenchyma (**Fig. 6 B**). Co-localization of GFP-expressing macrophages (green) and CD206 staining (red) manifested in yellow confirmed, the macrophages sustain their M2 phenotype in the intoxicated brain. No macrophages were found in healthy brain (**Fig. 6 C**) indicating the cells do not cross the BBB in the absence of inflammation.

Macrophage-mediated Neuroprotection in PD mice

A potent neuroprotective effect of GDNF-transfected macrophages was demonstrated in the 6-OHDA-intoxicated mice (**Fig. 7**). GDNF-overexpressing Raw 264.7 macrophages were systemically administered to BALB/c mice with brain inflammation (1×10^6 cells/100 µl) 48 hours after *i.c.* intoxication with 6-OHDA (PD mouse model). Non-intoxicated mice were used as healthy controls. 21 day later, mice were sacrificed, perfused, and the brain slides were stained for tyrosine hydroxylase (TH)-expressing DA neurons. *I.c.* intoxications of 6-OHDA caused substantial neurodegenreation in the *SNpc* (**Fig. 7 C, Table 1)** compared to healthy mice (**Fig. 7 A, Table 1**). Systemic administration of GDNF-transfected macrophages protected DA neurons against 6-OHDA intoxications (**Fig. 7 E, Table 1**). The numbers of TH+ neurons in *SNpc* of 6-OHDA animals treated with GDNF-transfected macrophages were significantly ($p<0.05$) greater than those 6-OHDA intoxicated, and then PBS-injected animals (**Table 1**). Noteworthy, empty-transfected macrophages slightly improved neuronal survival in PD animals, probably due to their regenerative M2 subtype, although this effect was not statistically significant (**Fig. 7D, Table 1**). Indeed, empty-transfected macrophages did not affect neuronal survival in healthy mice (**Fig. 7 B, Table 1**). This signifies that GDNF-transfected macrophages can efficiently protect DA neurons against 6-OHDA-induced intoxication. The therapeutic effect of GDNF-transfected macrophages was also manifested in significant decreases in inflammation and levels of activated microglia in *SNpc* (**Figure 8, Table 1**).

Finally, behavioral tests demonstrated statistically significant improvements in motor functions upon treatment with GDNF-transfected macrophages (**Fig. 9**). Specifically, the loss of dopaminergic input due to the lesion of the left nigro-striatial pathway resulted in number of full-body contralateral rotations induced by a dopaminergic agent, apomorphine (**Fig. 9 A**). In contrast, systemic administration of genetically-modified macrophages to 6-OHDA intoxicated mice drastically ($p<0.005$) reduced number of

Table 1. Effect of GDNF-transfected macrophages on inflammation and neurodegeneration in mice with PD model[a].

Treatment	CD11b+ (cells *per* mm^2)		Total N of neurons [b] $\times 10^3$	
	PBS	6-OHDA	PBS	6-OHDA
PBS	10.1±1.2	90.0±11 (**)[c]	5.9±1.4	2.15±0.3 (**)
GDNF-transfected macrophages	n/a	63.5±5.2 (*)	n/a	3.3±0.6 (*, #)
Empty-transfected macrophages	9.8±1.0	87.0±11.1	5.7±1.5	2.5±0.7

[a]BALB/c mice were *i.c.* injected with 6-OHDA. Forty eight hours later, the animals were *i.v.* injected with various macrophage-based formulations or PBS. A control group was *i.c.* injected with PBS, and then 48 hours later *i.v.* injected with PBS.
[b]Total number of neurons was calculated in ipsilateral hemisphere.
[c]Statistical significance is shown by asterisk: $p<0.05$ (*), and $p<0.005$ (**) compared to mice with *i.c.* PBS injections followed by *i.v.* PBS injections (healthy controls); or $p<0.05$ (#), compared to mice with *i.c.* 6-OHDA injections followed by *i.v.* PBS injections (PD controls). Errors are mean ±SEM, $N=7$.

these rotations on the seventh week following the intoxication in apomorphine test to the levels of the non-intoxicated animals. Furthermore, the motor functions were preserved by systemic administration of GDNF-transfected macrophages in 6-OHDA intoxicated animals at the levels similar to those of control non-intoxicated mice, as demonstrated in rotarod test (**Fig. 9 B**).

Discussion

A long-term objective of these investigations is to develop an active targeted cell-mediated delivery of therapeutic proteins to the brain. We demonstrated here that genetically-modified macrophages can produce therapeutically-active neurotrophic factor, GDNF, and release it in extracellular vesicles, exsosomes. The most important finding of this work is that GDNF-transfected macrophages provide significant neuronal protection in a PD mouse model. Our *in vivo* experiments demonstrated that systemically administered GDNF-expressing macrophages migrate across the BBB towards the inflammation site in large numbers, and provide efficient sustained delivery of their drug payload at the disease site that is consistent with previously reported findings [45–49]. To enforce outcomes of the new formulation, a specific subset of "alternatively activated" (M2) macrophages with regenerative functions was used. Thus, macrophages, polarized to M2 regenerative subtype, represent biologically-active carriers that can promote neuronal regeneration enhancing the therapeutic efficacy of drug formulations.

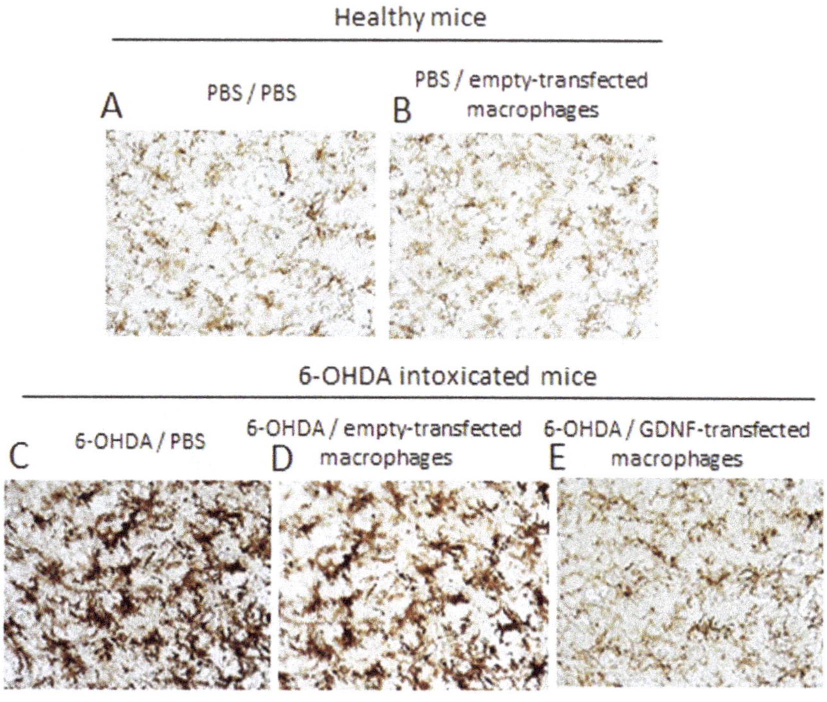

Figure 8. GDNF-transfected macrophages reduce neuro-inflammation in PD mice. BALB/c mice were *i.c.* injected with 6-OHDA. Forty eight hours later, animals were *i.v.* injected with GDNF-transfected or empty-transfected macrophages, or PBS, and 21 days later they were sacrificed, and mid-brain slides were stained for expression of CD11b, a marker for activated microglia. A 6-OHDA-mediated intoxication up-regulated expression of CD11b by microglia within the *SNpc* as exhibited a more amoeboid morphology in 6-OHDA-treated mice compared to ramified microglia in PBS-treated mice. In contrast, treatment of 6-OHDA-intoxicated mice with GDNF-transfected macrophages resulted in the decreased levels of CD11b compared with 6-OHDA-intoxicated control animals. Administration of empty-vector transfected macrophages did not affect the number of dopaminergic neurons in PD or healthy mice.

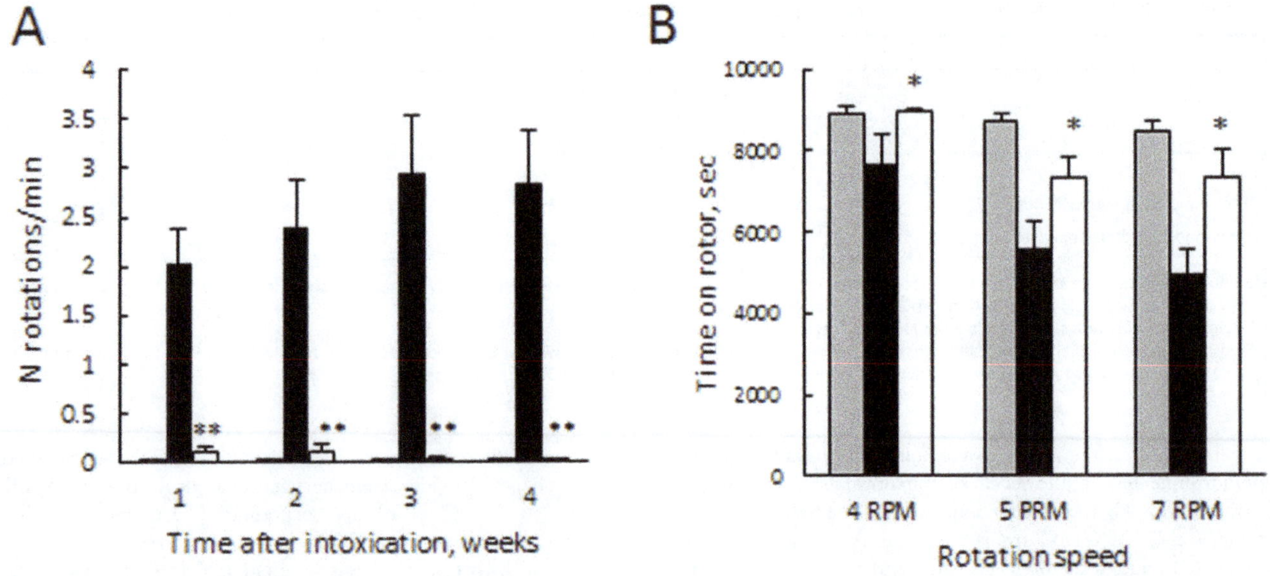

Figure 9. GDNF-transfected macrophages significantly improved motor functions in PD mouse model. 6-OHDA-intoxicated BALB/c mice were ***i.v.*** injected with GDNF-transfected macrophages (white bars), or PBS (black bars) 48 hours after the intoxication. A control group (grey bars) was *i.c.* injected with PBS, and then 48 hours later *i.v.* injected with PBS. Apomorphine (**A**) and rotarod (**B**) tests demonstrated statistically significant improvements in motor functions upon treatment with GDNF-carrying macrophages. Values are means ±SEM ($N=12$), and $p<0.05$ compared with 6-ODHA-intoxicated mice.

The mechanism of the macrophage-mediated drug delivery is not fully understood. Thus, several independent processes may serve to improve GDNF-expressing macrophage therapeutics. In addition to the targeted tissue-specific delivery of therapeutics in macrophages [46,52], drug-carrying macrophages were shown to increase time circulation in the blood, and therefore permit sustained release of the therapeutic protein allowing the drug to enter the brain, independent of carrier cells ("depot effect") [46,52]. Furthermore, we reported earlier that significant catalase transport across the BBB can be attributed to the efficient interaction of exosomes with brain microvessel endothelial cells followed by facilitated protein transfer to the brain [47]. Similar mechanism may be employed in the GDNF transfer from carrier macrophages across the BBB. We demonstrated that exosomes secreted from preloaded with nanoformulated catalase macrophages attach to the plasma membranes, and discharge their cargo into target cells [47]. As a result, the drug-incorporated nanoparticles were transferred from macrophages to adjacent cells, and diffused broadly throughout the recipient cells avoiding degradation in lysosomes. This mechanism enabled the drug to reach different intracellular compartments such as mitochondria, cytoplasm, and endoplasmic reticulum, and produce a powerful therapeutic effects [47]. Indeed, the mechanism of GDNF action differs from catalase neuroprotective effects, as specific binding to GFRα-1 receptors is required in order to accomplish GDNF-mediated neuroprotection. Nevertheless, we hypothesized that the efficient interactions of exosomal carriers with plasma membranes of DA neurons may facilitate GDNF binding to their receptors, and result in the profound therapeutic effect. Unfortunately, at this stage of understanding, we cannot discriminate, which mechanism is the most important for the therapeutic effects of cell-based formulations. A comprehensive examination and detailed understanding of these mechanisms would be of great value in designing strategies for cell-mediated drug delivery.

Several trials human and nonhuman (primate) were initiated to evaluate efficiency of GDNF for PD treatment as well as its off-side effects. Thus, GDNF showed therapeutic promise when injected intracranially through a surgically implanted shunt [69–71]. Although there were significant improvements followed GDNF infusions, some primate subjects revealed damage in the cerebellum found in brain autopsies. This was attributed to the rapid withdrawal from large amounts of GDNF and damaging tissues by the catheter, rather than to the direct GDNF toxic effects [71]. To this end, we believe that cell-mediated GDNF delivery can eliminate these issues, providing continuous targeted GDNF delivery specifically to the inflamed brain areas. Using genetically-modified macrophages as a cell-mediated drug delivery system will target the therapeutic proteins to the brain, prolong drug half-live, and diminish drug immunogenicity. In addition, properly differentiated immune cells accumulating in traumatic, degenerative, ischemic, infectious, and autoimmune lesions of the nervous system might provide a neuroprotective effect, which may further boost the therapeutic effect of cell-mediated drug delivery systems. It is anticipated that these studies will lead to the developing a new technology based on active targeted cell-mediated delivery of therapeutic polypeptides that produce neuroprotection and neuroregeneration in patients with PD.

Acknowledgments

We are grateful to Daria Y. Filonova (Eshelman School of Pharmacy, University of North Carolina at Chapel Hill) for her assistance with graphical abstract.

Author Contributions

Conceived and designed the experiments: MH AVK EVB. Performed the experiments: YZ MH RG JB ZH. Analyzed the data: EVB. Contributed to the writing of the manuscript: EVB.

References

1. Brinton RD (1999) A women's health issue: Alzheimer's disease and strategies for maintaining cognitive health. Int J Fertil Womens Med 44: 174–185.
2. Gozes I (2001) Neuroprotective peptide drug delivery and development: potential new therapeutics. Trends Neurosci 24: 700–705.
3. Kroll RA, Neuwelt EA (1998) Outwitting the blood-brain barrier for therapeutic purposes: osmotic opening and other means. Neurosurgery 42: 1083–1099; discussion 1099–1100.
4. Bachis A, Mocchetti I (2005) Brain-Derived Neurotrophic Factor Is Neuroprotective against Human Immunodeficiency Virus-1 Envelope Proteins. Ann N Y Acad Sci 1053: 247–257.
5. Ying Wang J, Peruzzi F, Lassak A, Del Valle L, Radhakrishnan S, et al. (2003) Neuroprotective effects of IGF-I against TNFalpha-induced neuronal damage in HIV-associated dementia. Virology 305: 66–76.
6. Koliatsos VE, Clatterbuck RE, Nauta HJ, Knusel B, Burton LE, et al. (1991) Human nerve growth factor prevents degeneration of basal forebrain cholinergic neurons in primates. Ann Neurol 30: 831–840.
7. Dogrukol-Ak D, Banks WA, Tuncel N, Tuncel M (2003) Passage of vasoactive intestinal peptide across the blood-brain barrier. Peptides 24: 437–444.
8. Desnick RJ, Schuchman EH (2002) Enzyme replacement and enhancement therapies: lessons from lysosomal disorders. Nat Rev Genet 3: 954–966.
9. Urayama A, Grubb JH, Sly WS, Banks WA (2004) Developmentally regulated mannose 6-phosphate receptor-mediated transport of a lysosomal enzyme across the blood-brain barrier. Proc Natl Acad Sci U S A 101: 12658–12663.
10. Farrer MJ (2006) Genetics of Parkinson disease: paradigm shifts and future prospects. Nat Rev Genet 7: 306–318.
11. Georgievska B, Carlsson T, Lacar B, Winkler C, Kirik D (2004) Dissociation between short-term increased graft survival and long-term functional improvements in Parkinsonian rats overexpressing glial cell line-derived neurotrophic factor. Eur J Neurosci 20: 3121–3130.
12. Hudson J, Granholm AC, Gerhardt GA, Henry MA, Hoffman A, et al. (1995) Glial cell line-derived neurotrophic factor augments midbrain dopaminergic circuits in vivo. Brain Res Bull 36: 425–432.
13. Tomac A, Lindqvist E, Lin LF, Ogren SO, Young D, et al. (1995) Protection and repair of the nigrostriatal dopaminergic system by GDNF in vivo. Nature 373: 335–339.
14. Bilang-Bleuel A, Revah F, Colin P, Locquet I, Robert JJ, et al. (1997) Intrastriatal injection of an adenoviral vector expressing glial-cell-line-derived neurotrophic factor prevents dopaminergic neuron degeneration and behavioral impairment in a rat model of Parkinson disease. Proc Natl Acad Sci U S A 94: 8818–8823.
15. Emborg ME, Moirano J, Raschke J, Bondarenko V, Zufferey R, et al. (2009) Response of aged parkinsonian monkeys to in vivo gene transfer of GDNF. Neurobiol Dis 36: 303–311.
16. Yasuda T, Mochizuki H (2010) Use of growth factors for the treatment of Parkinson's disease. Expert Rev Neurother 10: 915–924.
17. Kells AP, Forsayeth J, Bankiewicz KS (2012) Glial-derived neurotrophic factor gene transfer for Parkinson's disease: Anterograde distribution of AAV2 vectors in the primate brain. Neurobiol Dis 48: 228–235.
18. Mogi M, Togari A, Kondo T, Mizuno Y, Komure O, et al. (1999) Brain-derived growth factor and nerve growth factor concentrations are decreased in the substantia nigra in Parkinson's disease. Neurosci Lett 270: 45–48.
19. Ramaswamy S, Soderstrom KE, Kordower JH (2009) Trophic factors therapy in Parkinson's disease. Prog Brain Res 175: 201–216.
20. Sauer H, Oertel WH (1994) Progressive degeneration of nigrostriatal dopamine neurons following intrastriatal terminal lesions with 6-hydroxydopamine: a combined retrograde tracing and immunocytochemical study in the rat. Neuroscience 59: 401–415.
21. Wang L, Muramatsu S, Lu Y, Ikeguchi K, Fujimoto K, et al. (2002) Delayed delivery of AAV-GDNF prevents nigral neurodegeneration and promotes functional recovery in a rat model of Parkinson's disease. Gene Ther 9: 381–389.
22. Shults CW, Kimber T, Altar CA (1995) BDNF attenuates the effects of intrastriatal injection of 6-hydroxydopamine. Neuroreport 6: 1109–1112.
23. Gash DM, Zhang Z, Ovadia A, Cass WA, Yi A, et al. (1996) Functional recovery in parkinsonian monkeys treated with GDNF. Nature 380: 252–255.
24. Kirik D, Georgievska B, Bjorklund A (2004) Localized striatal delivery of GDNF as a treatment for Parkinson disease. Nat Neurosci 7: 105–110.
25. Grondin R, Cass WA, Zhang Z, Stanford JA, Gash DM, et al. (2003) Glial cell line-derived neurotrophic factor increases stimulus-evoked dopamine release and motor speed in aged rhesus monkeys. J Neurosci 23: 1974–1980.
26. Perry VH, Bell MD, Brown HC, Matyszak MK (1995) Inflammation in the nervous system. Curr Opin Neurobiol 5: 636–641.
27. Kuby J (1994) Immunology; ed. n, editor. New York: Freeman, WH. and Co.
28. Anthony DC, Bolton SJ, Fearn S, Perry VH (1997) Age-related effects of interleukin-1 beta on polymorphonuclear neutrophil-dependent increases in blood-brain barrier permeability in rats. Brain 120 (Pt 3): 435–444.
29. Anthony DC, Blond D, Dempster R, Perry VH (2001) Chemokine targets in acute brain injury and disease. Prog Brain Res 132: 507–524.
30. Blamire AM, Anthony DC, Rajagopalan B, Sibson NR, Perry VH, et al. (2000) Interleukin-1beta -induced changes in blood-brain barrier permeability, apparent diffusion coefficient, and cerebral blood volume in the rat brain: a magnetic resonance study. J Neurosci 20: 8153–8159.
31. Persidsky Y, Ghorpade A, Rasmussen J, Limoges J, Liu XJ, et al. (1999) Microglial and astrocyte chemokines regulate monocyte migration through the blood-brain barrier in human immunodeficiency virus-1 encephalitis. Am J Pathol 155: 1599–1611.
32. Pawlowski NA, Kaplan G, Abraham E, Cohn ZA (1988) The selective binding and transmigration of monocytes through the junctional complexes of human endothelium. J Exp Med 168: 1865–1882.
33. Lossinsky AS, Shivers RR (2004) Structural pathways for macromolecular and cellular transport across the blood-brain barrier during inflammatory conditions. Review. Histol Histopathol 19: 535–564.
34. Akerud P, Canals JM, Snyder EY, Arenas E (2001) Neuroprotection through delivery of glial cell line-derived neurotrophic factor by neural stem cells in a mouse model of Parkinson's disease. J Neurosci 21: 8108–8118.
35. Casper D, Engstrom SJ, Mirchandani GR, Pidel A, Palencia D, et al. (2002) Enhanced vascularization and survival of neural transplants with ex vivo angiogenic gene transfer. Cell Transplant 11: 331–349.
36. Yasuhara T, Shingo T, Muraoka K, Kameda M, Agari T, et al. (2005) Neurorescue effects of VEGF on a rat model of Parkinson's disease. Brain Res 1053: 10–18.
37. Biju K, Zhou Q, Li G, Imam SZ, Roberts JL, et al. (2010) Macrophage-mediated GDNF delivery protects against dopaminergic neurodegeneration: a therapeutic strategy for Parkinson's disease. Mol Ther 18: 1536–1544.
38. Biju KC, Santacruz RA, Chen C, Zhou Q, Yao J, et al. (2013) Bone marrow-derived microglia-based neurturin delivery protects against dopaminergic neurodegeneration in a mouse model of Parkinson's disease. Neurosci Lett 535: 24–29.
39. Martinez-Serrano A, Bjorklund A (1998) Ex vivo nerve growth factor gene transfer to the basal forebrain in presymptomatic middle-aged rats prevents the development of cholinergic neuron atrophy and cognitive impairment during aging. Proc Natl Acad Sci U S A 95: 1858–1863.
40. Martinez-Serrano A, Hantzopoulos PA, Bjorklund A (1996) Ex vivo gene transfer of brain-derived neurotrophic factor to the intact rat forebrain: neurotrophic effects on cholinergic neurons. Eur J Neurosci 8: 727–735.
41. Garcia P, Youssef I, Utvik JK, Florent-Bechard S, Barthelemy V, et al. (2010) Ciliary neurotrophic factor cell-based delivery prevents synaptic impairment and improves memory in mouse models of Alzheimer's disease. J Neurosci 30: 7516–7527.
42. Low WC, Lewis PR, Bunch ST, Dunnett SB, Thomas SR, et al. (1982) Function recovery following neural transplantation of embryonic septal nuclei in adult rats with septohippocampal lesions. Nature 300: 260–262.
43. Pizzo DP, Coufal NG, Lortie MJ, Gage FH, Thal LJ (2006) Regulatable acetylcholine-producing fibroblasts enhance cognitive performance. Mol Ther 13: 175–182.
44. Batrakova EV, Gendelman HE, Kabanov AV (2011) Cell-mediated drug delivery. Expert Opin Drug Deliv 8: 415–433.
45. Batrakova EV, Li S, Reynolds AD, Mosley RL, Bronich TK, et al. (2007) A macrophage-nanozyme delivery system for Parkinson's disease. Bioconjug Chem 18: 1498–1506.
46. Brynskikh AM, Zhao Y, Mosley RL, Li S, Boska MD, et al. (2010) Macrophage delivery of therapeutic nanozymes in a murine model of Parkinson's disease. Nanomedicine (Lond) 5: 379–396.
47. Haney MJ, Suresh P, Zhao Y, Kanmogne GD, Kadiu I, et al. (2012) Blood-borne macrophage-neural cell interactions hitchhike endosome networks for cell-based nanozyme brain delivery. Nanomedicine (Lond) 7: 815–833.
48. Haney MJ, Zhao Y, Harrison EB, Mahajan V, Ahmed S, et al. (2013) Specific Transfection of Inflamed Brain by Macrophages: A New Therapeutic Strategy for Neurodegenerative Diseases. Plos One 8: e61852.
49. Haney MJ, Zhao Y, Li S, Higginbotham SM, Booth SL, et al. (2011) Cell-mediated transfer of catalase nanoparticles from macrophages to brain endothelial, glial and neuronal cells. Nanomedicine (Lond) 6: 1215–1230.
50. Klyachko NL, Haney MJ, Zhao Y, Manickam DS, Mahajan V, et al. (2013) Macrophages offer a paradigm switch for CNS delivery of therapeutic proteins. Nanomedicine (Lond).
51. Zhao Y, Haney MJ, Klyachko NL, Li S, Booth SL, et al. (2011) Polyelectrolyte complex optimization for macrophage delivery of redox enzyme nanoparticles. Nanomedicine (Lond) 6: 25–42.
52. Zhao Y, Haney MJ, Mahajan V, Reiner BC, Dunaevsky A, et al. (2011) Active Targeted Macrophage-mediated Delivery of Catalase to Affected Brain Regions in Models of Parkinson's Disease. J Nanomed Nanotechnol S4.
53. Thery C, Amigorena S, Raposo G, Clayton A (2006) Isolation and characterization of exosomes from cell culture supernatants and biological fluids. Curr Protoc Cell Biol Chapter 3: Unit 3 22.
54. Bhatnagar S, Shinagawa K, Castellino FJ, Schorey JS (2007) Exosomes released from macrophages infected with intracellular pathogens stimulate a proinflammatory response in vitro and in vivo. Blood 110: 3234–3244.
55. Clayton A, Turkes A, Navabi H, Mason MD, Tabi Z (2005) Induction of heat shock proteins in B-cell exosomes. J Cell Sci 118: 3631–3638.
56. Nolte-'t Hoen EN, Buschow SI, Anderton SM, Stoorvogel W, Wauben MH (2009) Activated T cells recruit exosomes secreted by dendritic cells via LFA-1. Blood 113: 1977–1981.

57. Johnstone RM (1992) The Jeanne Manery-Fisher Memorial Lecture 1991. Maturation of reticulocytes: formation of exosomes as a mechanism for shedding membrane proteins. Biochem Cell Biol 70: 179–190.
58. Zomer A, Vendrig T, Hopmans ES, van Eijndhoven M, Middeldorp JM, et al. (2010) Exosomes: Fit to deliver small RNA. Commun Integr Biol 3: 447–450.
59. Valadi H, Ekstrom K, Bossios A, Sjostrand M, Lee JJ, et al. (2007) Exosome-mediated transfer of mRNAs and microRNAs is a novel mechanism of genetic exchange between cells. Nat Cell Biol 9: 654–659.
60. Thery C, Ostrowski M, Segura E (2009) Membrane vesicles as conveyors of immune responses. Nat Rev Immunol 9: 581–593.
61. Rana S, Yue S, Stadel D, Zoller M (2012) Toward tailored exosomes: the exosomal tetraspanin web contributes to target cell selection. Int J Biochem Cell Biol 44: 1574–1584.
62. Eketjall S, Fainzilber M, Murray-Rust J, Ibanez CF (1999) Distinct structural elements in GDNF mediate binding to GFRalpha1 and activation of the GFRalpha1-c-Ret receptor complex. EMBO J 18: 5901–5910.
63. Tieu K, Perier C, Caspersen C, Teismann P, Wu DC, et al. (2003) D-beta-hydroxybutyrate rescues mitochondrial respiration and mitigates features of Parkinson disease. J Clin Invest 112: 892–901.
64. Rozas G, Guerra MJ, Labandeira-Garcia JL (1997) An automated rotarod method for quantitative drug-free evaluation of overall motor deficits in rat models of parkinsonism. Brain Res Brain Res Protoc 2: 75–84.
65. Keshet GI, Tolwani RJ, Trejo A, Kraft P, Doyonnas R, et al. (2007) Increased host neuronal survival and motor function in BMT Parkinsonian mice: involvement of immunosuppression. J Comp Neurol 504: 690–701.
66. Papathanou M, Rose S, McCreary A, Jenner P (2011) Induction and expression of abnormal involuntary movements is related to the duration of dopaminergic stimulation in 6-OHDA-lesioned rats. Eur J Neurosci 33: 2247–2254.
67. Kigerl KA, Gensel JC, Ankeny DP, Alexander JK, Donnelly DJ, et al. (2009) Identification of two distinct macrophage subsets with divergent effects causing either neurotoxicity or regeneration in the injured mouse spinal cord. J Neurosci 29: 13435–13444.
68. Suschek CV, Schnorr O, Kolb-Bachofen V (2004) The role of iNOS in chronic inflammatory processes in vivo: is it damage-promoting, protective, or active at all? Curr Mol Med 4: 763–775.
69. McLeod M, Hong M, Mukhida K, Sadi D, Ulalia R, et al. (2006) Erythropoietin and GDNF enhance ventral mesencephalic fiber outgrowth and capillary proliferation following neural transplantation in a rodent model of Parkinson's disease. Eur J Neurosci 24: 361–370.
70. Slevin JT, Gerhardt GA, Smith CD, Gash DM, Kryscio R, et al. (2005) Improvement of bilateral motor functions in patients with Parkinson disease through the unilateral intraputaminal infusion of glial cell line-derived neurotrophic factor. J Neurosurg 102: 216–222.
71. Nutt JG, Burchiel KJ, Comella CL, Jankovic J, Lang AE, et al. (2003) Randomized, double-blind trial of glial cell line-derived neurotrophic factor (GDNF) in PD. Neurology 60: 69–73.

10

pH-Sensitive Nanomicelles for Controlled and Efficient Drug Delivery to Human Colorectal Carcinoma LoVo Cells

Shi-Ting Feng[¶1], Jingguo Li[¶2], Yanji Luo[¶1], Tinghui Yin[3], Huasong Cai[1], Yong Wang[2], Zhi Dong[1], Xintao Shuai[2], Zi-Ping Li[1]*

1 Department of Radiology, The First Affiliated Hospital, Sun Yat-Sen University, Guangzhou, China, 2 PCFM Lab of Ministry of Education, School of Chemistry and Chemical Engineering, Sun Yat-Sen University, Guangzhou, China, 3 Department of Medical Ultrasonic, The Third Affiliated Hospital of Sun Yat-Sen University, Guangzhou, China

Abstract

Background: The triblock copolymers PEG-P(Asp-DIP)-P(Lys-Ca) (PEALCa) of polyethylene glycol (PEG), poly(N-(N′,N′-diisopropylaminoethyl) aspartamide) (P(Asp-DIP)), and poly (lysine-cholic acid) (P(Lys-Ca)) were synthesized as a pH-sensitive drug delivery system. In neutral aqueous environment such as physiological environment, PEALCa can self-assemble into stable vesicles with a size around 50-60 nm, avoid uptake by the reticuloendothelial system (RES), and encase the drug in the core. However, the PEALCa micelles disassemble and release drug rapidly in acidic environment that resembles lysosomal compartments.

Methodology/Principal Findings: The anticancer drug Paclitaxel (PTX) and hydrophilic superparamagnetic iron oxide (SPIO) were encapsulated inside the core of the PEALCa micelles and used for potential cancer therapy. Drug release study revealed that PTX in the micelles was released faster at pH 5.0 than at pH 7.4. Cell culture studies showed that the PTX-SPIO-PEALCa micelle was effectively internalized by human colon carcinoma cell line (LoVo cells), and PTX could be embedded inside lysosomal compartments. Moreover, the human colorectal carcinoma (CRC) LoVo cells delivery effect was verified *in vivo* by magnetic resonance imaging (MRI) and histology analysis. Consequently effective suppression of CRC LoVo cell growth was evaluated.

Conclusions/Significance: These results indicated that the PTX-SPION-loaded pH-sensitive micelles were a promising MRI-visible drug release system for colorectal cancer therapy.

Editor: Stephanie Filleur, Texas Tech University Health Sciences Center, United States of America

Funding: This work was supported by: 1. National Natural Science Foundation of China (81000626); 2. Zhujiang Scientific and Technological New Star Foundation (2012J2200084); 3. Fundamental Research Funds for the Central Universities (10ykpy11); 4. Natural Science Foundation of Guangdong Province (S2013010016004). The funders had no role in study design, data collection and analysis, decision to publish, or preparation of the manuscript.

Competing Interests: The authors have declared that no competing interests exist.

* Email: liziping163@163.com

¶ These authors contributed equally and are co-first authors on this work.

Introduction

Colorectal carcinoma (CRC) is a malignant disease on the rise. It is the second most common cancer in general and the most common of the gastrointestinal tract cancers [1]. It is currently the second leading cause of death in both female and male patients. Surgical resection is preferred as a curative treatment in early stages of CRC while drug therapy becomes the main preference in advanced or recurrent stages. [2].

In the past decades, a large number of anticancer drugs were identified, although most of them are hydrophobic and poorly soluble in aqeous. Paclitaxel (PTX) is one of the most potent anticancer drugs that can be used in the therapy of several solid tumors. Taxol is one of the formulations of PTX with stratified aqueous solubility and lower toxicity [3,4]. Nevertheless, the clinical use of PTX is limited by high toxicity and low bioavailability [5]. PTX has been found to have side effects including neurotoxicity, hypersensitivity reactions, cardiotoxicity, and nephrotoxicity [6]. Moreover, for PTX, it has been found that the concentration of drug in tumor is rather low. Its use has remained limited due to this unsatisfactory therapeutic efficacy [7]. In comparison, nanoparticles, such as cationic polymers and cationic peptides loaded with anti-tumor drugs, have potential to overcome these shortcomings. These various carriers had been widely studied for targeted tumor therapies. In fact, the release of a drug in plain carriers usually lasts for days or even weeks. Even if effective delivery to tumor tissue and cells is achieved, it is still difficult to achieve an ideal therapeutic effect and reduce the probability of drug resistance [8]. As a result, the amount of released drug is a key for chemotherapeutic agents to efficiently kill the cancer cells and studies involving rapid and adequateh intracellular drug release from nanocarriers are of particular importance at present.

In recent years, nanocarriers with a triggered release mechanism have been developed, such as micelles which could release drugs in response to specific stimuli such as temperature, pH, ultrasound and redox potential, etc [9–12]. Among these carriers, pH-sensitive polymers appears to be the most attractive candidate because the smart delivery systems are stable and can self-assemble in physiological environment (blood, pH = 7.4) but dessembles and releases drug in acidic environments (lysosomal, pH = 5.0), resulting in significantly enhanced anti-tumor efficacy, minimal drug resistance and side effects [13,14].

Meanwhile, magnetic resonance imaging (MRI) techniques have great advantages in monitoring targeting events and therapeutic outcomes noninvasively. MRI-visible nanoparticulate systems have been used for anticancer drug delivery and imaging of cancer [15–17]. Superparamagnetic iron oxide (SPIO), known as a highly efficient T2 contrast agent for MRI, is an ideal small molecular probe. The use of nanocarrier loaded with SPIO can make the vector MRI-visible [16,17]. However, reports on anticancer outcome of stimuli-sensitive SPIO-PTX-loaded polymeric vesicles with a combined feature of intracellular drug release and imaging function are very rare.

In this study, we developed a nano-micelle for anti-tumor drug delivery and intracellular drug release triggered by pH. The polymeric micelle was designed based on polyethylene glycol (PEG), poly (N-(N', N'-diisopropylaminoethyl) aspartamide) (P(Asp-DIP)) and poly (lysine-cholic acid) (P(Lys-Ca)). The copolymer PEG-P(Asp-DIP)-P(Lys-Ca) (PEALCa) can self-assemble into nano-scale vesicles encapsulating PTX and SPIO in aqueous solution at neutral pH, and disassembles in acidic lysosomal compartments resulting in rapid drug release. In order to demonstrate the targeting and therapeutic potential of the vesicle, cell culture experiments of the PTX-SPIO-loaded vesicles against human CRC LoVo cells were conducted. Besides, as an MRI-visible drug delivery system, the intracellular drug release of the vesicles *in vivo* was studied by MRI to validate the efficiency. Our study attempts to explore the transferring efficiency of PTX-PEALCa into tumoral cells and and compare the degree of human CRC LoVo cell growth suppression between PTX-PEALCa with conventional anti-cancer drugs.

Materials and Methods

Materials

PEG-P(Asp-DIP)-P(Lys-Ca) and SPIO-PEG-P(Asp-DIP)-P(Lys-Ca) were provided by School of Chemistry and Chemical Engineering (Fig. 1A, B), Sun Yat-Sen University and the micelles was synthesized as previously reported [18]. LoVo cells from a human CRC cell line were purchased from the Institute of Biochemistry and Cell Biology (Chinese Academy of Sciences, Shanghai, China). Taxol was obtained from Bristol-Myers Squibb Co. (Princeton, NJ, USA), Minimum essential medium (MEM) and fetal bovine serum (FBS) were purchased from Invitrogen Corporation (GIBCO, Carlsbad, CA, USA).

Size and morphology

BI-200 SM dynamic light scattering (DLS) (Brookhaven Instruments Corp., Holtsville, NY, USA) with a 532 nm vertically polarized argon ion laser as the light source, was used to determine the particle size. The measurement was performed at a 90°angle at 25°C and scattered light was collected on a BI-9000AT Digital Autocorrelator (Brookhaven Instruments Corp., Holtsville, NY, USA). The particle size and zeta potential of each sample were measured for five times. Transmission electron microscopy (TEM) images were obtained on a JEOL TEM-2010HR (JEOL Ltd., Japan) operated at 160 kV.

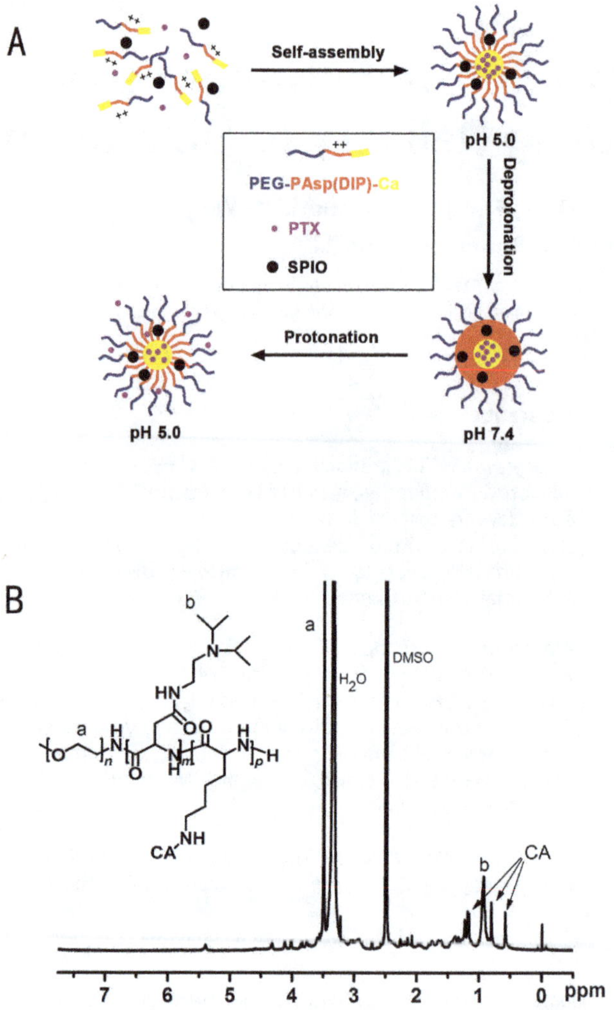

Figure 1. Illustration of PEG-P(Asp-DIP)-P(Lys-Ca):Drawing of pH-tunable drug release (A) and ^{1}H-NMR (300 MHz) spectra of PEG-P(Asp-DIP)-P(Lys-Ca) (B).

Intracellular drug delivery and release efficiency measurements

Delivery efficiency *in vitro*. LoVo cells were seeded in 6-well plates or petri dishes at a density of 1×10^5 cells per well/dish and incubated in 2 mL of MEM containing 10% FBS overnight. 50 µL of FDA-SPIO-PEALCa complex solution was added to each well at a final fluorescein diacetate (FDA, the fluorescent substitute of PTX) concentration of 2 µg/mL. The cells were then incubated with the complex solution for 6 h and finally subjected to flow cytometry analysis and confocal laser scanning microscopic (CLSM) observation to determine the intracellular drug delivery efficiency of FDA-SPIO-PEALCa as a hydrophobic drug vector.

Flow cytometry analysis. After FDA-SPIO-PEALCa (final FDA concentration of 2 µg/mL) was incubated with the LoVo cells for 6 h, cells were trypsinized and washed with phosphate-buffered saline (PBS), resuspended in 0.5 mL of PBS. FDA content was detected by flow cytometry (FACSCalibur, BD Co, USA) using a 488 nm laser for excitation. The green fluorescence emission of FDA was collected through a 525 nm filter. LoVo cells without transfection were used as a control for background calibration. The flow cytometry data were analyzed using the FlowJo software (Version 7.6, Treestar, Inc., San Carlos, CA).

Confocal laser scanning microscopy. The intracellular distribution of hydrophobic green fluorescent FDA was observed on CLSM. Four hours after the incubation with FDA-SPIO-PEALCa, LoVo cells seeded in petri dishes were washed for three times with PBS. To further confirm the intracellular distribution of FDA, the lysosomes and nuclei were stained with red (Lysotracker Red, Molecular Probe, Eugene, OR) and blue (Hoechst 33324, Beyotime Biotech, China) fluorescent dyes, respectively. Cells were observed on a Zeiss LSM 510 META microscope (Carl Zeiss Cl, Ltd, Gottingen, Germany). FDA, Lysotracker Red and Hoechst 33342 were excited at 488 nm, 514 nm and 352 nm respectively, and the corresponding emission wavelengths were 525 nm, 455 nm and 595 nm, respectively.

Drug release at different pH values. The *in vitro* drug release behavior of the micelles was determined using a dynamic dialysis method at 37°C. FDA instead of PTX was encapsulated inside the PEALCa micelle. 50 µL of FDA-PEALCa complex solution was adjusted to pH 5.0 with 1 N HCl or pH 7.4 with PBS at a final FDA concentration of 2µg/mL, then the solution was transferred into a dialysis bag (MWCO: 14000). The bag was then placed into buffered solution (40 mL) at the same pH with gentle shaking of 75 rpm (ZHWY-200B, Shanghai Zhicheng, Shanghai, China). At predetermined time intervals (0.5, 1.0, 4, 18 and 24 h, respectively), the solution outside dialysis bag was removed for UV-Vis analysis and replaced with fresh buffer solution. FDA concentration was calculated based on the absorbance intensity at 430 nm. The cumulative amount of released FDA was calculated against release time for assessment of drug release.

Cytotoxicity and cell apoptosis inducing by PTX-SPIO-PEALCa

Biocompatibility assay. Methyl thiazolyl tetrazolium (MTT) assay was performed to evaluate the cytotoxicity of PEALCa and SPIO-PEALCa complexes. Human (CRC) LoVo cells were cultured in MEM supplemented with 10% FBS and incubated at 37 °C in a humidified atmosphere with 5% CO_2. In MTT assays, the cells were seeded in 96-well plates with the density of 5000 cells/well. Then the cells were incubated in fresh medium with various concentrations of PEALCa or SPIO-PEALCa (0–300 µg/mL) for 24 h. Then the PEALCa- or SPIO-PEALCa-contained MEM was replaced by fresh medium with MTT solution (Sigma, St Louis, MO) at 5 mg/mL and incubated for 4 h; subsequently, 100 µL dimethyl sulfoxide (DMSO) was added to each well to dissolve the formazen after the MTT-contained medium was aspirated. Finally, the absorbance at 494 nm of each well was recorded using the Infinite F200 multimode plate reader (Tecan, Männedorf, Switzerland). Three duplicates were measured for each experimental point.

Cell apoptosis and cytotoxicity detections. Hydrophobic chemotherapeutic drug PTX was simultaneously encapsulated with SPIO in the pH-sensitive PEALCa micelle (PTX-SPIO-PEALCa). To determine the LoVo cell-apoptosis inducing ability and chemotherapeutic efficacy of PTX-SPIO-PEALCa, MTT and terminal deoxynucleotidyl transferase-mediated UTP nick end labeling (TUNEL) assays were performed, respectively.

MTT assays were used to compare the cytotoxicity of the LoVo cells between PTX-SPIO-PEALCa micelles and free Taxol. After seeding at a density of 5000 cells per well in 96-well plates and cultured overnight, the LoVo cells were incubated with PTX-SPIO-PEALCa and Taxol of various PTX concentrations (from 0 µg/mL to 5 µg/mL) for 48 h, respectively. The PTX-containing medium was replaced with 100 µL of fresh MEM containing 0.5 µg/mL MTT (Sigma) and subsequently incubated with the LoVo cells for 4 h. Then the medium in each well was aspirated and replaced by 100 µL of DMSO to dissolve the formazen. Finally, after 5 min gentle agitation of the 96-well plates, the absorbance at 494 nm in each well was detected using the Infinite F200 multimode plate reader.

In TUNEL assay, LoVo cells were seeded at a density of 2.5 × 10^4 per well on coverslips in 6-well plates, normally cultured overnight, and then incubated with PTX-SPIO-PEALCa for 24 h at four PTX concentrations (0, 0.1, 0.5, 1.0 µg/mL). TUNEL assays were carried out using an *in situ* cell death detection kit, peroxidase (POD) (Boehringer Mannheim, Mannheim, Germany) according to the manufacturer's protocol. In brief, cells on coverslips were fixed with freshly prepared 4% paraformaldehyde for 15 minutes (min) at room temperature. After incubated with 0.3% H_2O_2 in methanol for 10 min at room temperature, the LoVo cells were subsequently treated with 0.1% Triton X-100 in 0.1% sodium citrate for 2 min on ice for permeation. The permeabilized cells were incubated with 50 µL of terminal deoxynucleotidyl transferase (TdT) reaction mixture in a humidified chamber for 60 min at 37°C. Then the slides were incubated with 50 µL of anti-fluorescein antibody conjugated with POD for 30 min at 37 °C. Finally, diaminobenzidine (DAB) substrate reacting with apoptotic cells to form the brown staining was defined as the positive signal, while the blue negative signal from hematoxylin was applied to identify the non-apoptotic cells. All samples were observed under optical microscope.

For the quantification analysis of TUNEL assays, we randomly selected three low magnification visions in each sample with ImageJ software, and calculated the number of DAB-positive cells and DAB-negative cells within each one of the vision field. The TUNEL positive rate of tumor cells was calculated using the formula:

$$\begin{aligned} &TUNEL\,positive\,rate \\ &= DAB-P/(DAB-P+DAB-N)\times 100\% \end{aligned} \tag{1}$$

where DAB-P was the number of DAB-positive cells, and DAB-N was the number of DAB-negative cells, and the average value of each group was calculated.

In vivo studies

This study was carried out in strict accordance with the guidance of the Institutional Animal Care and Use Committee (IACUC) of Sun Yat-Sen University (Permit Number:2013 A-038). The use of chloral hydrate were approved by the IACUC as non-pharmaceutical grade and given special exemption by the institutional IACUC, and all efforts were made to minimize suffering.

Human colon carcinoma xenografts model. Human CRC LoVo cells were implanted into the BALB/c nude mice (4–5 weeks) to establish the colorectal carcinoma xenografts models. The mice ($n = 14$) were placed in the stereotactic frame after they were anesthetized with 10% chloral hydrate (400 mg/kg). 1×10^6 LoVo cells were trypsinized, washed for three times with PBS, resuspended in 50 µL of PBS and subcutaneously injected in the right back side of the mice. The tumor-bearing mice and the tumors were monitored every day. In brief, the length (L) and the width (W) of the tumors were measured with caliper. The tumor volume was calculated as following equation [19]:

$$Volume = 0.5 \times L \times W^2 \quad (2)$$

When the volume of tumor reached about 40 mm^3 to 60 mm^3 after 5–7 days, the mice were used for *in vivo* MR imaging and chemotherapy studies.

***In vivo* MR imaging.** As previously reported, most obvious MRI contrast could be achieved at the injection dose of 4.48 μg Fe/g body weight [20]. Therefore, an injection dose of 4.48 μg Fe/g body weight was used to detect tumors by MRI in our study. Two mice were randomly chosen and anesthetized by intraperitoneal injection of 10% chloral hydrate. T2-weighted MRI was performed prior to injection and repeated at 0.5, 1, 1.5 and 2 h after the injection of 10% SPIO-PEALCA (Group 1) at a dose of 4.48 μg Fe/g body weight and 100 μL 10% blank PEALCA (Group 2) intravenously through the tail vein, respectively, on a 3.0 T MRI scanner (Magnetom Avanto; Siemens Healthcare Sector, Erlangen, Germany) with a 5-cm linearly polarized birdcage radio frequency mouse coil. The T2-weighted images were acquired using a fast spin-echo sequence with these parameters: repetition time 2000 ms, echo time 80 ms, FOV 3×3 cm, slice thickness 1.0 mm and flip angle 90°.

Anticancer efficacy studies. In tumor therapeutic experiments, the remaining LoVo tumor-bearing mice were randomly divided into three groups (n = 4 for each group) as Group 1, 2, and 3. In group 1, which was defined as the experimental group, the mice were injected with PTX-SPIO-PEALCa; In Group 2, defined as the experimental control group, the mice were injected with the commercial cremophor-based PTX (Taxol); and in Group 3, defined as the negative control group, the mice was injected with PBS. To demonstrate the tumor targeted PTX delivery efficiency of the pH-sensitive PEALCa micelles compared with commercial PTX preparations, a lower final PTX plasma concentration was used for *in vivo* chemotherapeutic studies. PTX-loaded micelles PTX-SPIO-PEALCa, Taxol and PBS were intravenously injected via tail veins after dilution in normal saline to 100 μL. PTX concentration in both PTX-SPIO-PEALCA group and Taxol group were 1 mg/kg body weight. As the first drug intervention day was defined as day 0, the drug was administrated on day 0, day 2, and day 4. Tumor volumes, living conditions and survival situations in all groups were recorded every two days.

In day 35, mice in all groups were sacrificed and then tumors were collected, fixed in 10% formalin for 24 h and embedded in paraffin. Haematoxylin/eosin (H&E) staining of tumor tissue sections (3 μm) was performed for the observations of cancer tissue morphology in different groups. To better elucidate the anticancer effects and apoptosis inducing ability of the PTX-loaded micelles PTX-SPIO-PEALCa, *in situ* TUNEL assays were carried out on the excised tumor tissue. The TUNEL assays were performed according to the manufacturer's protocol using a FragELTM DNA Fragmentation Detection kid (EMD chemicals Inc, Darmstadt, Germany). Tumor tissue sections were deparaffinized, and permeated using proteinase K (20 μg/mL). After the H_2O_2 aqueous solution (3%) was added to inactivate endogenous peroxidase, the slides were treated with TdT Enzyme at 37 °C for 90 min. The slides were finally incubated with streptavidin-horseradish peroxidase conjugate, during which the DAB reacted with the apoptotic cells to form the brown signal, while non-apoptotic cells were counterstained as blue-green to be distinguished from the apoptotic signal.

Statistical analysis

The tumor size of three groups were presented as mean ± standard deviation and analyzed by the Student's *t*-test (SPSS software, Version 13.0, SPSS Inc.). A two sided *P* value less than 0.05 was considered statistically significant.

Results

Micelle size

The micelle size was about 29 nm before SPIO loading and 54 nm after SPIO loading (Fig. 2 A). TEM images showed that the SPIO-loaded micelles were spherical with an average size of 50 nm (Fig. 2 B).

Intracellular drug delivery and release efficiency measurements

Delivery efficiency *in vitro*. The flow cytometry analysis of LoVo cells was carried out 6 h after the incubation with FDA-SPIO-PEALCa. The green fluorescent positive ratio of LoVo cells was 95.2±3.7%, and that of the negative untreated cells was 4.78±4.6% (Fig. 3A).

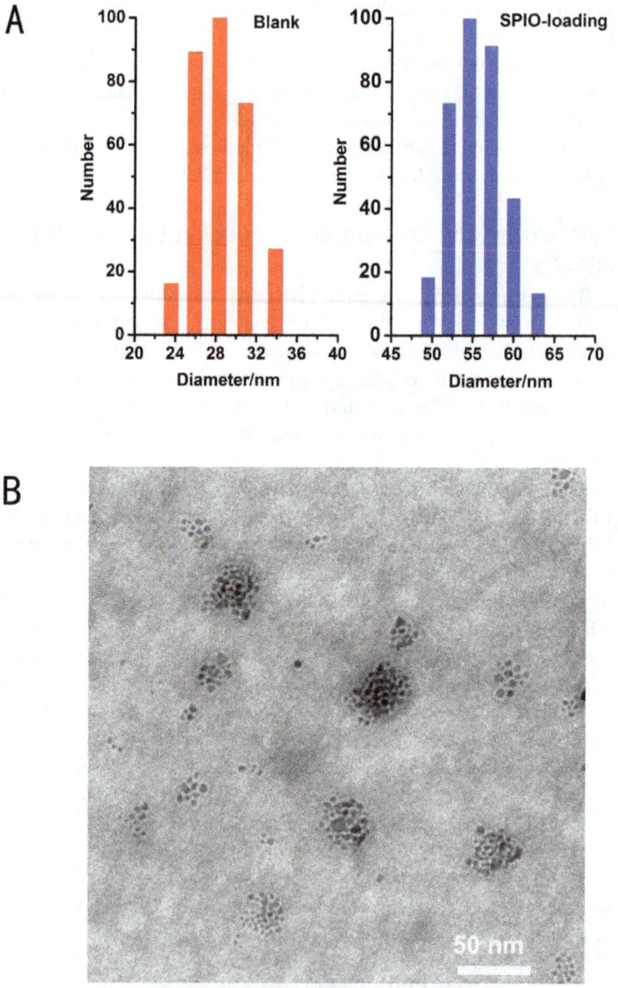

Figure 2. Micelle size measure. Size distribution of PEALCa micelles before and after loading of SPIO(A). Transmission electron microscopy (TEM) image of SPIO-loaded micelle (B). The scale bars represent about 50 nm.

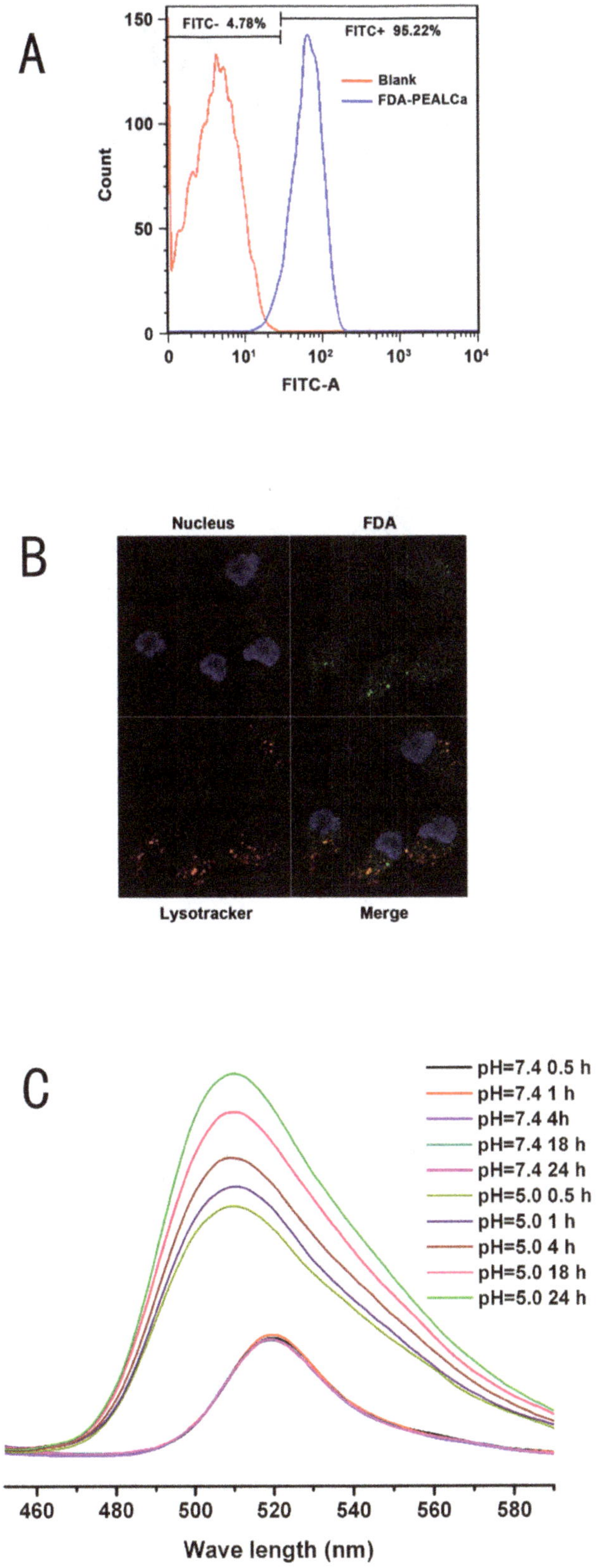

Figure 3. Intracellular drug delivery and release efficiency measurements. Quantitative analysis of FDA-positive LoVo cells by flow cytometry after incubation with FDA-SPIO-PEALCa (A). Confocal laser scanning microscopy (CLSM) images (1000 ×) of LoVo cells after treated with FDA-SPIO-PEALCa (B). The lysosomes and nuclei were stained by red and blue fluorescent probe, respectively. *In vitro* FDA released from PEALCa micelle at 37 °C in HCl (pH 5.0) and PBS (pH 7.4) (C).

The uptake and intracellular distribution of FDA was detected by CLSM observation. To better illustrate the distribution of FDA, the lysosomes and nuclei were stained with red and blue fluorescence as the markers for intracellular localization. Figure 3B showed that after 4 h of incubation with FDA-SPIO-PEALCa, the green fluorescence of FDA was visible both in cytoplasm and nucleus. Especially in red fluorescent lysosomes, higher amount of FDA fluorescence was detected.

Drug release *in vitro*. Drug release test were carried out at pH 5.0 and 7.4, respectively. The result showed that the maximum fluorescence intensity of pH 5.0 at each time interval was higher than that of pH 7.4. Furthermore, fluorescence intensity of pH 7.4 group had no obvious change throughout the experimental time of 24 h (Fig. 3C), implying that micelle structure were stable in neutral condition, with only a small amount of FDA released. In contrast, fluorescence intensity of pH 5.0 significantly increased against time, revealing that FDA release was both time- and pH- dependent.

Cytotoxicity and cell apoptosis inducing by PTX-SPIO-PEALCa

Biocompatibility assay. The cytotoxicity of nano-complexes was evaluated *via* MTT assay. As shown in Figure 4A, the viability of tumor cells incubated in blank micelles decreased gradually. Even at high polymer concentration (300 μg/mL), the viability of LoVo cells remained at a high level (81.0±4.0%). Meanwhile, the pH-sensitive micelles loaded with SPIO also revealed low cytotoxity. All these results illustrated that PEALCa was safe for bio-applications and the presence of SPIO did not increase the cytotoxicity of the copolymers.

Cytotoxicity and apoptosis inducing detections. MTT assay was conducted to further compare the cytotoxicity of the pH-sensitive PTX-SPIO-PEALCa micelles and free Taxol (Fig. 4B). The results revealed that the cell viability decreased along with the increase of PTX concentration. Moreover, under the same PTX concentration, the cell viability of PTX-SPIO-PEALCa micelles was lower than that of the free Taxol. The IC50 value of PTX-SPIO-PEALCa and free Taxol were 1.27 μg/mL and 2.40 μg/mL, respectively. The result of TUNEL assay also confirmed similar phenomenon (Fig. 4C). Quantitative analysis of TUNEL assays revealed that the apoptosis rate induced by PTX-loaded nanoparticles were 0.7±0.5%, 7.4±0.8%, 19.7±1.1% and 48.8±2.3% for 0 μg/mL group, 0.1μg/mL group, 0.5 μg/mL group and 1.0 μ/mL group, respectively.

In vivo studies

MR scanning. To validate the tumor targeting ability of SPIO-PEALCa, two mice bearing LoVo colorectal tumors were randomly chosen in the study. Both mice were injected with blank (group 1) or targeted (group 2) polymers. Prior to injection, both tumors marked with red and blue arrows (Fig. 5A) exhibited hyperintense areas on T2-weighted MRI images. 0.5-1.5 h after injection of blank PEALCa, the signal intensity of tumors showed no obvious drop. However, the T2 signals of the tumors injected with SPIO-PEALCa dropped obviously after 1.5 h of injection. We calculated the Relative T2 value using the formula:

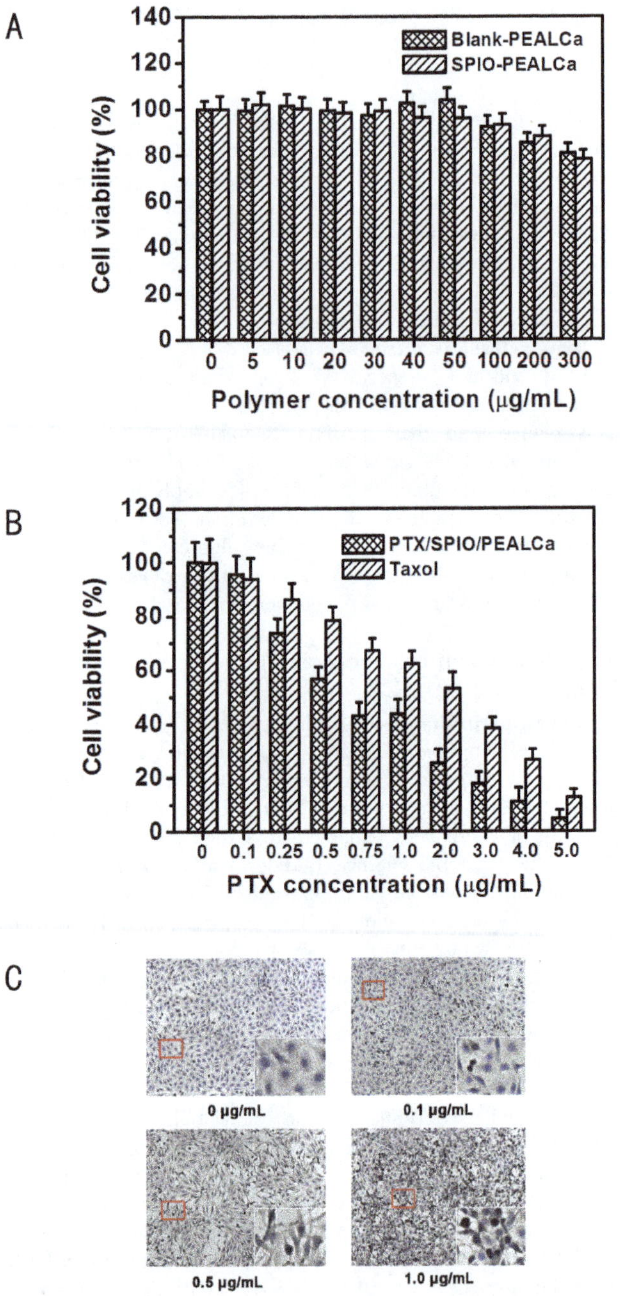

Figure 4. Cytotoxicity and cell apoptosis evaluation. *In vitro* cytotoxicity of various concentrations of PEALCa and SPIO-PEALCa in LoVo cells detected by MTT assay (A). MTT assay of the cytotoxicity of PTX-SPIO-PEALCa and free Taxol with different PTX concentrations (B). LoVo cell apoptosis detected by *TUNEL* assay after PTX-SPIO-PEALCa incubation with different PTX concentrations (50×) (C). Magnified image of the red rectangular represents the representative normal or apoptotic cell.

$$Relative\ T2 = ((T' - T0)/T0) \times 100\% \tag{3}$$

where T′ was the T2 value of the tumor at different time after injection, and T0 was the T2 value prior to injection. (Fig. 5B).

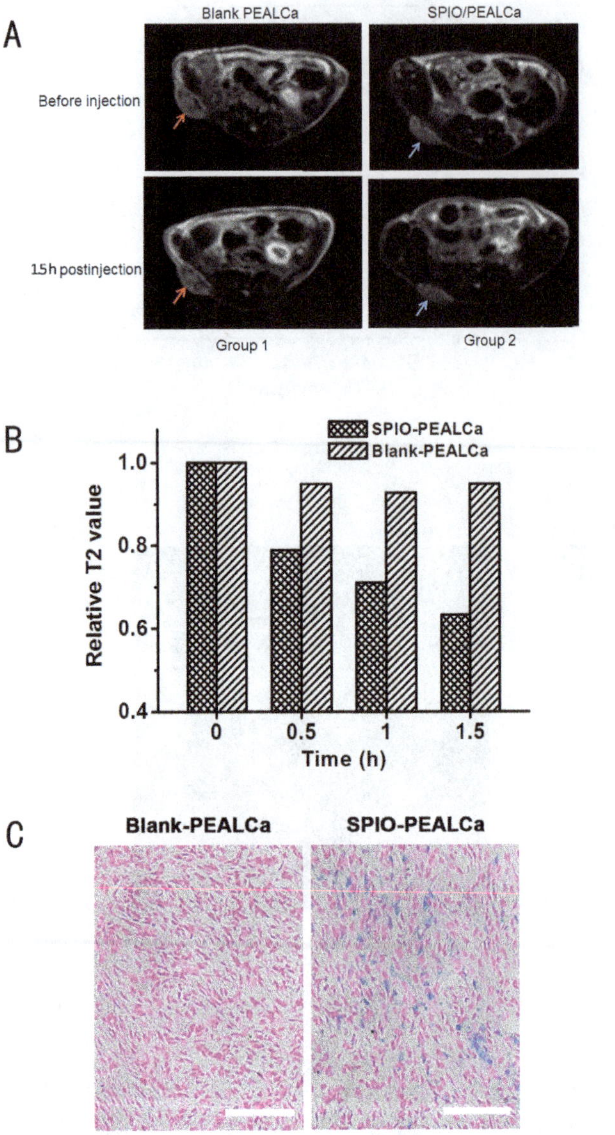

Figure 5. Tumor targeting evaluation *in vivo*. Group 1: mice with LoVo tumors prior and after injection of blank PEALCa; Group 2: mice with LoVo tumors prior and after injection of SPIO-PEALCa (A). The relative T2 value of both groups prior and after injection(B). Prussian blue staining images of the tumor histological sections treated with PTX-PEALCa and PTX-SPIO-PEALCa (200 ×) (C).

Prussian blue staining. The two mice above were then sacrificed for Prussian blue staining of tumor paraffin sections after the SPIO-PEALCa intravenous injection for explanation of the MR signal reduction in tumor tissue. Prussian blue staining in the sections of blank PEALCa group was rare. On the contrary, the sections from SPIO-PEALCa group showed strong Prussian blue staining in large area of the visual field, indicating that high amount of SPIO was delivered into the tumor tissue by the pH-sensitive micellar nanoparticles (Fig. 5C). The results were consistent with the above in vivo MRI image findings.

Anticancer efficacy *in vivo*. To further elucidate the anticancer efficacy of PTX-loaded micelle *in vivo*, the remaining 12 mice were used for tumor apoptosis inducing study. After 35 days of the first treatment, the tumor tissues of 3 groups were paraffin sectioned and stained with H&E to evaluate the histological changes of the tumors. As shown in Figure 6A, more hypercellular and nuclear polymorphism were observed in the H&E stained sections of the PBS negative control group. On the contrary, the morphology of PTX-SPIO-PEALCa group demonstrated more hypocellular, nuclear shrinkage, and the highest level of tumor cell apoptosis and necrosis. The Taxol control group showed medium level of cell density and nuclear atypia. Furthermore, TUNEL assay results confirmed that the TUNEL-positive cells in PTX-SPIO-PEALCa group were significantly higher than the Taxol group, indicating that the tumor apoptosis inducing efficacy of the pH-sensitive micelles was much higher than that of commercial chemotherapeutic agent.

The tumor growth curves also illustrated the therapeutic effects of PTX-loaded micelles in general (Fig. 6B). Tumor volume of the PTX-SPIO-PEALCa group remained in a low level during the whole experimental process, which meant that the tumor growth of the PTX-SPIO-PEALCa group was almost negligible. The averaged tumor volume of the PTX-SPIO-PEALCa group was 65.0±8.4 mm^3 at day 30, which was significantly smaller than the Taxol group of 598.7±77.4 mm^3 and the PBS group of 1050.7±54.4 mm^3 (t = 5.34, P<0.001).

Discussion

PTX is an effective chemotherapeutic agent by stabilizing microtubules and mitotic arrest. It has shown broad-spectrum activity in solid tumors, including colorectal cancer [21,22]. Despite the clinical advantages of PTX, it has a low therapeutic index because of hydrophobic property and serious side effects. As a result, the main challenge in PTX chemotherapy is the development of safe and highly efficient delivery systems that can encapsulate and transfer PTX into cancerous cells with lower systemic toxicity and better anti-tumor efficiency. It is well known that the tumor vasculature has poor architecture due to abnormal basement membrane and fissures between the endothelial cells accompanied with a poor lymphatic drainage system. This state of leaky vasculature causes that particles with size ranging 10 to 100 nm can preferentially accumulate in the tumors and have longer circulation time, unlike the free drugs, which are of much smaller size but may easily deposit in the normal tissue and be cleared by the kidney [23,24]. Notably, TEM observation in our study showed that the PTX-loaded micelles possessed a uniform small size of around 54 nm, which is highly desirable for longer blood circulation time and easier cellular uptake by cancer cells [25,26].

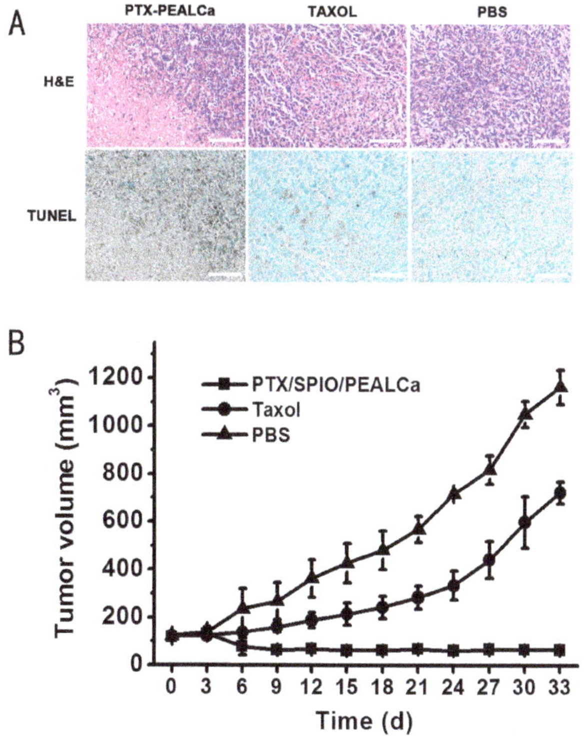

Figure 6. Anticancer efficacy evaluation *in vivo*. Representative haematoxylin and eosin (H&E) and terminal deoxynucleotidyl transferase-mediated UTP nick end labeling (TUNEL) staining images (200 ×) of tumor sections from the mice of different groups(A). Tumor growth curves of the LoVo tumor bearing mice treated with PTX/SPIO/PEALCa, Taxol or PBS (B).

In this study, the PEG-P(Asp-DIP)-P(Lys-Ca) (PEALCa) triblock copolymer was used as an essential component of drug delivery vehicle, and its characteristics under MRI imaging as well as anti-tumor efficay were investigated. Drug release profiles revealed that rate of FDA release from PEALCa micelles was both time- and pH- dependent. In a neutral environment (pH = 7.4), micelle structure was stable and FDA was steadily released from the micelles. Nonetheless, a rapid and much more intensive release of FDA was turned on immediately at acidic environment (pH = 5.0). When the micelle enters cells *via* endocytosis, the experienced pH drops from neutral to as low as 5.5-6.0 in endosomes and 4.5–5.0 in lysosomes and triggers rapid drug release. In micelles, PEG forms an outer corona stabilizing the micelles to avoid uptake of reticuloendothelial system [27,28]. P(Asp-DIP) is a pH-sensitive interlayer that undergoes hydrophobic-hydrophilic transition in the acidic lysosomes of cells [29]. Cholic acid (Ca) forms the micelle core to encapsulate hydrophobic drugs and also contribute to rapid drug release [18,30]. Our results suggested that PEALCa micelle can be used as a nanocarrier of PTX, which can delay drug release and absorption in normal tissue and enhance transportation of the drug to human CRC LoVo cells and improve the anti-tumor efficiency.

MTT assay was used to determine the cytotoxicity of the vectors. With increased polymer concentration, the viability of LoVo cells in the blank and SPIO-loaded micelles decreased gradually. Acceptable cytotoxicity was achieved when polymer concentration remains below 300 µg/mL. It is well known that SPIO is one of the most effective MRI contrast agents and possesses a high biocompatibility and low toxicity [16,17]. The pH-sensitive micelles encapsulated with SPIO also exhibited low cytotoxity. The results revealed that the copolymers had little cytotoxicity to LoVo cells. Moreover, under the same PTX concentration, the cell viability treated with PTX-SPIO-PEALCa micelles was lower than that of free Taxol, which revealed the cytotoxicity of PTX-SPIO-PEALCa micelles was higher than free Taxol. The TUNEL assay clearly demonstrated significantly high levels of apoptosis in LoVo cells as the concentration of targeting polymers increased.

Quantitative flow cytometry results showed that the intracellular delivery of hydrophobic fluorescent dye FDA was highly efficient. The uptake and intracellular distribution of FDA was also detected by CLSM observation, as FDA was visible both in cytoplasm and nucleus, especially in red fluorescent lysosomes, which was consistent with the flow cytometry analysis findings. This assay verified that PEG-P(Asp-DIP)-CA lead to the efficient release of FDA in the LoVo cells.

Encouragingly, the *in vivo* tumor targeting ability of PTX-SPIO-PEALCa was validated by MRI technology. After SPIO-PEALCA or blank PEALCa micelle were administrated through tail intravenous injection in the mice bearing LoVo tumor (right thigh), the tumor signal intensity and relative T2 value of the mouse injected with SPIO-PEALCa had dropped significantly as revealed by MRI scans. However, the mouse injected with blank PEALCa failed to demonstrate such drop in signal intensity or relative T2 value at tumor site. Consistent results were observed by Prussian blue staining, indicating that the hypointensity of the tumor site was due to the intracellular SPIO delivered by PEALCa. Furthermore, the *in vivo* studies revealed a significant delay in tumor growth with PTX-SPIO-PEALCa micelle therapy in mice. All of the above results illustrated that the PEALCa micelle delivered PTX and SPIO into LoVo cells effectively and has assisted an efficient release of PTX, thus promoted the apoptosis of LoVo cells.

In recent years, several representative pH-sensitive polymeric micelles have been reported as potential cancer diagnostics and therapies. A pH-sensitive biodegradable poly (β-amino ester) (PAE) was developed by Langer and coworkers [31]. Fe_3O_4-loaded PEG-b-PAE micelles are stable at 37°C and pH 7.4 but rapidly disassembles at pH below 7.0 [32],resulting in drug release in the extracellular space of tumor (pH= 6.5–7.2) [33] and leading to a reduction of the intracellular release and consequently decreased the therapeutic efficacy of anti-tumor drugs. Poly (L-histidine) (PHis) is another pH-sensitive polymer suitable for cancer therapy with excellent biocompatibility [34]. However, PH is too sensitive to environmental pH, which could affect the stability of the core of the drug carrier. Other potential pH-sensitive polymeric micelles for cancer diagnosis and therapy have been also developed based on pH-sensitive groups, including poly (malic acid) [35], chitosan [36], histidine side groups [37] and so on. In summary, a novel pH-sensitive nanoparticulate vector with PTX delivery and MRI functions was fabricated by entrapping PTX and SPIO into PEALCa micelle. The pH-triggered drug release was found to efficiently amplify the intracellular drug concentration which determined the anticancer outcome. The drug-delivery effect *in vivo* was visualized by MRI technology. The results of this study revealed the great potential of PTX-SPIO-PEALCa micelle as a multifunctional nanomedicine for tumor therapy.

The main limitation for the study is that we only use one CRC cell line (LoVo) to evaluate the efficiency of PEALCa in controlled and efficient drug delivery. Our future study will focus on monitoring the drug transferring of PEALCa and anti-cancer therapeutic efficiency of PTX-PEALCa on larger sample size of animals,other CRC cell lines and other tumors, in order to further validate our findings.

Author Contributions

Conceived and designed the experiments: ZPL XS STF. Performed the experiments: JL YL TY. Analyzed the data: STF TY. Contributed reagents/materials/analysis tools: HC YW ZD. Wrote the paper: STF JL YL.

References

1. Jemal A, Siegel R, Ward E, Hao Y, Xu J, et al. (2009) Cancer statistics. CA Cancer J Clin 59: 225–249.
2. Foersch S, Waldner MJ, Neurath MF (2012) Colitis and colorectal cancer. Dig Dis 30: 469–476.
3. Mi Y, Liu Y, Feng SS (2011) Formulation of Docetaxel by folic acid-conjugated d-alpha-tocopheryl polyethylene glycol succinate 2000 (Vitamin E TPGS(2k)) micelles for targeted and synergistic chemotherapy. Biomaterials 32: 4058–4066.
4. Yang R, Shim WS, Cui FD, Cheng G, Han X, et al. (2009) Enhanced electrostatic interaction between chitosan-modified PLGA nanoparticle and tumor. Int J Pharm 371: 142–147.
5. Panchagnula R (1998) Pharmaceutical aspects of paclitaxel. International Journal of Pharmaceutics 172: 1–15.
6. Mei L, Sun H, Song C (2009) Local delivery of modified paclitaxel-loaded poly(epsilon-caprolactone)/pluronic F68 nanoparticles for long-term inhibition of hyperplasia. J Pharm Sci 98: 2040–2050.
7. Ju C, Sun J, Zi P, Jin X, Zhang C (2013) Thermosensitive micelles-hydrogel hybrid system based on poloxamer 407 for localized delivery of paclitaxel. J Pharm Sci 102: 2707–2717.
8. Wu H, Zhu L, Torchilin VP (2013) pH-sensitive poly(histidine)-PEG/DSPE-PEG co-polymer micelles for cytosolic drug delivery. Biomaterials 34: 1213–1222.
9. Alvarez-Lorenzo C, Concheiro A (2008) Intelligent drug delivery systems: polymeric micelles and hydrogels. Mini Rev Med Chem 8: 1065–1074.
10. Klaikherd A, Nagamani C, Thayumanavan S (2009) Multi-stimuli sensitive amphiphilic block copolymer assemblies. J Am Chem Soc 131: 4830–4838.
11. Sawant RM, Hurley JP, Salmaso S, Kale A, Tolcheva E, et al. (2006) "SMART" drug delivery systems: double-targeted pH-responsive pharmaceutical nanocarriers. Bioconjug Chem 17: 943–949.
12. Torchilin V (2009) Multifunctional and stimuli-sensitive pharmaceutical nanocarriers. Eur J Pharm Biopharm 71: 431–444.
13. Hu YQ, Kim MS, Kim BS, Lee DS (2007) Synthesis and pH-dependent micellization of 2-(diisopropylamino)ethyl methacrylate based amphiphilic diblock copolymers via RAFT polymerization. Polymer 48: 3437–3443.
14. Lee ES, Gao Z, Bae YH (2008) Recent progress in tumor pH targeting nanotechnology. J Control Release 132: 164–170.
15. Khemtong C, Kessinger CW, Ren J, Bey EA, Yang SG, et al. (2009) In vivo off-resonance saturation magnetic resonance imaging of alphavbeta3-targeted superparamagnetic nanoparticles. Cancer Res 69: 1651–1658.
16. Liao C, Sun Q, Liang B, Shen J, Shuai X (2011) Targeting EGFR-overexpressing tumor cells using Cetuximab-immunomicelles loaded with doxorubicin and superparamagnetic iron oxide. Eur J Radiol 80: 699–705.
17. Nasongkla N, Bey E, Ren J, Ai H, Khemtong C, et al. (2006) Multifunctional polymeric micelles as cancer-targeted, MRI-ultrasensitive drug delivery systems. Nano Lett 6: 2427–2430.
18. Wang W, Cheng D, Gong F, Miao X, Shuai X (2012) Design of multifunctional micelle for tumor-targeted intracellular drug release and fluorescent imaging. Adv Mater 24: 115–120.
19. Chen YB, Yan ML, Gong JP, Xia RP, Liu LX, et al. (2007) Establishment of hepatocellular carcinoma multidrug resistant monoclone cell line HepG2/mdr1. Chin Med J (Engl) 120: 703–707.
20. Chen Y, Wang W, Lian G, Qian C, Wang L, et al. (2012) Development of an MRI-visible nonviral vector for siRNA delivery targeting gastric cancer. Int J Nanomedicine 7: 359–368.
21. Hawkins MJ, Soon-Shiong P, Desai N (2008) Protein nanoparticles as drug carriers in clinical medicine. Adv Drug Deliv Rev 60: 876–885.
22. Mo R, Jin X, Li N, Ju C, Sun M, et al. (2011) The mechanism of enhancement on oral absorption of paclitaxel by N-octyl-O-sulfate chitosan micelles. Biomaterials 32: 4609–4620.
23. Byrne JD, Betancourt T, Brannon-Peppas L (2008) Active targeting schemes for nanoparticle systems in cancer therapeutics. Adv Drug Deliv Rev 60: 1615–1626.
24. Ranganathan R, Madanmohan S, Kesavan A, Baskar G, Krishnamoorthy YR, et al. (2012) Nanomedicine: towards development of patient-friendly drug-delivery systems for oncological applications. Int J Nanomedicine 7: 1043–1060.
25. Lee JH, Huh YM, Jun YW, Seo JW, Jang JT, et al. (2007) Artificially engineered magnetic nanoparticles for ultra-sensitive molecular imaging. Nat Med 13: 95–99.
26. Lutz JF, Stiller S, Hoth A, Kaufner L, Pison U, et al. (2006) One-pot synthesis of pegylated ultrasmall iron-oxide nanoparticles and their in vivo evaluation as magnetic resonance imaging contrast agents. Biomacromolecules 7: 3132–3138.
27. Otsuka H, Nagasaki Y, Kataoka K (2003) PEGylated nanoparticles for biological and pharmaceutical applications. Adv Drug Deliv Rev 55: 403–419.
28. Savic R, Luo L, Eisenberg A, Maysinger D (2003) Micellar nanocontainers distribute to defined cytoplasmic organelles. Science 300: 615–618.
29. Dai J, Lin S, Cheng D, Zou S, Shuai X (2011) Interlayer-crosslinked micelle with partially hydrated core showing reduction and pH dual sensitivity for pinpointed intracellular drug release. Angew Chem Int Ed Engl 50: 9404–9408.
30. Luo J, Giguere G, Zhu XX (2009) Asymmetric poly(ethylene glycol) star polymers with a cholic acid core and their aggregation properties. Biomacromolecules 10: 900–906.
31. Lynn DM, Anderson DG, Putnam D, Langer R (2001) Accelerated discovery of synthetic transfection vectors: parallel synthesis and screening of a degradable polymer library. J Am Chem Soc 123: 8155–8156.
32. Gao GH, Im GH, Kim MS, Lee JW, Yang J, et al. (2010) Magnetite-nanoparticle-encapsulated pH-responsive polymeric micelle as an MRI probe for detecting acidic pathologic areas. Small 6: 1201–1204.

33. Yin H, Lee ES, Kim D, Lee KH, Oh KT, et al. (2008) Physicochemical characteristics of pH-sensitive poly(L-histidine)-b-poly(ethylene glycol)/poly(L-lactide)-b-poly(ethylene glycol) mixed micelles. J Control Release 126: 130–138.
34. Lee ES, Shin HJ, Na K, Bae YH (2003) Poly(L-histidine)-PEG block copolymer micelles and pH-induced destabilization. J Control Release 90: 363–374.
35. Yang X, Grailer JJ, Pilla S, Steeber DA, Gong S (2010) Tumor-Targeting, pH-Responsive, and Stable Unimolecular Micelles as Drug Nanocarriers for Targeted Cancer Therapy. Bioconjug Chem 21: 496–504.
36. Liu J, Li H, Jiang X, Zhang C, Ping Q (2010) Novel pH-sensitive chitosan-derived micelles loaded with paclitaxel. Carbohydrate Polymers 82: 432–439.
37. Chang G, Li C, Lu W, Ding J (2010) N-Boc-histidine-capped PLGA-PEG-PLGA as a smart polymer for drug delivery sensitive to tumor extracellular pH. Macromol Biosci 10: 1248–1256.

11

PSMA Ligand Conjugated PCL-PEG Polymeric Micelles Targeted to Prostate Cancer Cells

Jian Jin[1], Bowen Sui[1], Jingxin Gou[2], Jingshuo Liu[1], Xing Tang[2], Hui Xu[2], Yu Zhang[2], Xiangqun Jin[1]*

1 Department of Pharmaceutics, College of Pharmacy Sciences, Jilin University, Changchun, People's Republic of China, 2 Department of Pharmaceutics, Shenyang Pharmaceutical University, Shenyang, People's Republic of China

Abstract

In this content, a small molecular ligand of prostate specific membrane antigen (SMLP) conjugated poly (caprolactone) (PCL)-b-poly (ethylene glycol) (PEG) copolymers with different block lengths were synthesized to construct a satisfactory drug delivery system. Four different docetaxel-loaded polymeric micelles (DTX-PMs) were prepared by dialysis with particle sizes less than 60 nm as characterized by dynamic light scattering (DLS) and transmission electron microscope (TEM). Optimization of the prepared micelles was conducted based on short-term stability and drug-loading content. The results showed that optimized systems were able to remain stable over 7 days. Compared with Taxotere, DTX-PMs with the same ratio of hydrophilic/hydrophobic chain length displayed similar sustained release behaviors. The cytotoxicity of the optimized targeted DTX-PCL$_{12K}$-PEG$_{5K}$-SMLP micelles (DTX-PMs2) and non-targeted DTX-PCL$_{12K}$-mPEG$_{5K}$ micelles (DTX-PMs1) were evaluated by MTT assays using prostate specific membrane antigen (PSMA) positive prostate adenocarcinoma cells (LNCaP). The results showed that the targeted micelles had a much lower IC50 than their non-targeted counterparts (48 h: 0.87$\pm$0.27 vs 13.48$\pm$1.03 μg/ml; 72 h: 0.02$\pm$0.008 vs 1.35$\pm$0.54 μg/ml). *In vitro* cellular uptake of PMs2 showed 5-fold higher fluorescence intensity than that of PMs1 after 4 h incubation. According to these results, the novel nano-sized drug delivery system based on DTX-PCL-PEG-SMLP offers great promise for the treatment of prostatic cancer.

Editor: Gnanasekar Munirathinam, University of Illinois, United States of America

Funding: The authors have no funding or support to report.

Competing Interests: The authors have declared that no competing interests exist.

* Email: jinxq@jlu.edu.cn

Introduction

Polymeric micelles have received considerable attention as promising anticancer drug carriers because of their remarkable advantages, such as small size, narrow size distribution, high biocompatibility, and solubilization of hydrophobic drugs [1,2,3,4,5]. Self-assembled polymeric micelles with core/shell structures enable the system to incorporate poorly water-soluble drugs in the hydrophobic core and protect them from degradation in physiological media [6]. For example, the hydrophobic core of the micelles composed of PCL-PEG offers a reservoir for the incorporation of drugs, while the pegylated shell along with its nanoscopic size guarantees the carrier remain un-recognized by the reticuloendothelial system and undergo a long-circulation period in the blood [7,8,9].

Although polymeric micelles exhibited a number of advantages, one major challenge is their site-specific drug delivery. Ligand-modified polymeric micelle drug delivery systems are capable of site-specific drug delivery. Recently, numerous active targeting delivery systems have been designed by conjugating NPs with ligands that bind specifically to the biomarkers of extracellular domains of cancer cells. PSMA as folate hydrolase I and glutamate carboxypeptidase II, is a well-known transmembrane protein [10] over expressed on prostate cancer epithelial cells [11,12] and has been shown to have great potential for prostatic cancer (PCa) therapy. PSMA has a low expression in normal prostate epithelial cells and benign prostatic hyperplasia. It is also expressed in the neovasculature of most other solid tumors but not in the vasculature of normal tissues [13,14]. All of these characteristics make PSMA an attractive biomarker for the detection, diagnosis, and treatment of PCa [15,16]. A novel small molecular ligand ((S)-2-(3-((S)-5-amino-1-carboxypentyl) ureido) pentanedioic acid, SMLP) binding specifically to PSMA has demonstrated its potential in the treatment of cancer in recent years [17]. The urea-based PSMA inhibitor, SMLP, has a high affinity for PSMA due to strong hydrogen bonding [10]. Hrkach and Langer *et al.* developed ACUPA (PSMA ligand) conjugated DTX NPs composed of PEG-b-PLGA or PEG-b-PLA using a nano-emulsification method to target PSMA and evaluated the anti-tumor efficacy of the NPs *in vitro* and *in vivo* [18]. The excellent potential offered by vehicle-ligand targeting PSMA suggests the necessity in developing more diversified preparation processes and carrier-materials in this field.

In this study,a nano-sized self-assembled drug delivery system based on ligand-conjugated PEG-b-PCL micelles was found to show great promise in the field of targeted drug delivery. Copolymers of PCL and PEG are both well-known biodegradable and biocompatible materials widely used in biomedical field [19,20,21,22,23]. Due to the introduction of glycolic acid (GA) and lactic acid (LA), which disrupted the ordered structure of the molecular chains, PLGA showed low crystallinity. As a result, micelles with cores of PCL which showed higher crystallinity are more stable than those with PLGA cores. Moreover, because PLGA is a random copolymer, it is relatively difficult to control the ratio of GA to LA precisely in large-scale production. However, the ratio of the two monomers is a key factor to influence the property of PLGA [24]. So PCL was used as the core-forming block due to its better stability and ease to produce. PCL-mPEG or PCL-PEG-COOH was synthesized by ring-opening polymerization of ε-caprolactone initiated by mPEG-OH or HOOC-PEG-OH [25,26]. PCL-mPEG and PCL-PEG-SMLP micelles were prepared using DTX as a model drug to examine the cytotoxic effects on LNCaP cells. Also, a schematic illustration of preparation and endocytosis process of DTX-PCL-PEG-SMLP is shown in Figure 1.

Materials and Methods

Materials

L-glutamic acid di-tertbutyl ester hydrochloride and H-Lys(Z)-Ot-Bu hydrochloride were obtained from En lai Biological Technology Co., LTD (Chengdu, People's Republic of China). mPEG-OH (Mw: 2 kDa) and mPEG-OH (Mw: 5 kDa) (Aladdin Agent Co., Shanghai, P R China) and OH-PEG-COOH(Mw: 2 kDa),OH-PEG-COOH(Mw: 5 kDa) (Shanghai Seebio Biological Technology Co., shanghai, P R China) were dehydrated by azeotropic distillation with toluene before use. DTX (Shanghai Sanwei Pharma Ltd, Co, Shanghai, P R China) and the cellulose ester dialysis bag with a molecular cut-off of 7000 Da (Bioscience Ltd, Co, Shanghai, P R China) were used as received. ε-Caprolactone (ε-CL, Aladdin Agent Co., Shanghai, P R China) was dried over CaH_2 at room temperature for 48 h and distilled under reduced pressure. Stannous octoate was purchased from Aladdin Agent Co (Shanghai, P R China). All organic solvents used in the synthesis procedures were purchased from the National Medicine Chemical Reagent Ltd Co (Shanghai, P R China).

The prostate LNCaP and PC3 cell lines were obtained from the Type Culture Collection of the Chinese Academy of Sciences (Shanghai, China). LNCaP Cells were cultured using cell-bind culture bottles (Corning, USA).

Methods

Synthesis of PCL-mPEG (PMs1) and PCL-PEG-SMLP (PMs2) copolymers. Copolymers with a range of block lengths were prepared by ring-opening copolymerization of ε-CL initiated by hydroxyl of PEG. Briefly, a predetermined amount of ε-CL and stannous octoate were added to a reaction vessel containing mPEG-OH or OH-PEG-COOH under a dry argon atmosphere (stannous octoate/ε-CL in 1:1000 molar ratio). Then, the reaction vessel was placed in an oil bath and maintained at 120°C for 24 h. Then the crude copolymers were dissolved in DCM and precipitated in cold diethyl ether to remove the un-reacted monomer and oligomer. Then, the product was filtered and dried to obtain a white precipitate.

PCL_{12k}-PEG_{5k}-COOH (1 g, 0.059 mmol) was dissolved in 5 ml anhydrous tetrahydrofuran (THF) with 1-ethyl-3-[3-dimethylaminopropyl]-carbodiimide hydrochloride (EDC) (57.4 mg, 0.3 mmol, 5 equiv) and N-hydroxysuccinimide (NHS) (27.6 mg, 0.24 mmol, 4 equiv). Then, the solution mixture was stirred at room temperature for over 12 h under argon atmosphere. The PCL_{12k}-PEG_{5k}-NHS copolymer was precipitated in ice-cold diethyl ether to afford a white precipitate which was collected and dried to obtain the desired product as a white powder (yield, 90%). SMLP (300 mg) was dissolved in anhydrous THF (20 ml) to prepare 10 mg/ml (SMLP/THF) aqua. PCL-PEG-NHS (500 mg, 0.03 mmol) and diisopropylethylamine (0.7 ml) were added to 5 ml (SMLP/THF) aqua, and the reaction solution was stirred at room temperature for 20 h under argon. After completion of the reaction, the solution was purified by dialysis for 24 h and dried by lyophilization to obtain a white flocculent powder (yield 90%). The structure of final copolymer was characterized by ^{1}H NMR spectroscopy.

$PCL_{4.8K}$-$mPEG_{2K}$ and $PCL_{4.8k}$-PEG_{2k}-SMLP were prepared using the same method previously stated.

Polymer characterization. The ^{1}H-nuclear magnetic resonance (^{1}H NMR) spectra of all samples were recorded on a Bruker DMX 300 or 600 spectrometer (Billerica, MA). Chemical shifts (δ) were given in ppm using tetramethylsilane as the internal standard. Fourier transform infrared spectroscopy spectra were recorded on a Bruker Tensor 27 spectrometer, and samples were prepared using KBr disks (Scharlau Chemie, Barcelona, Spain).

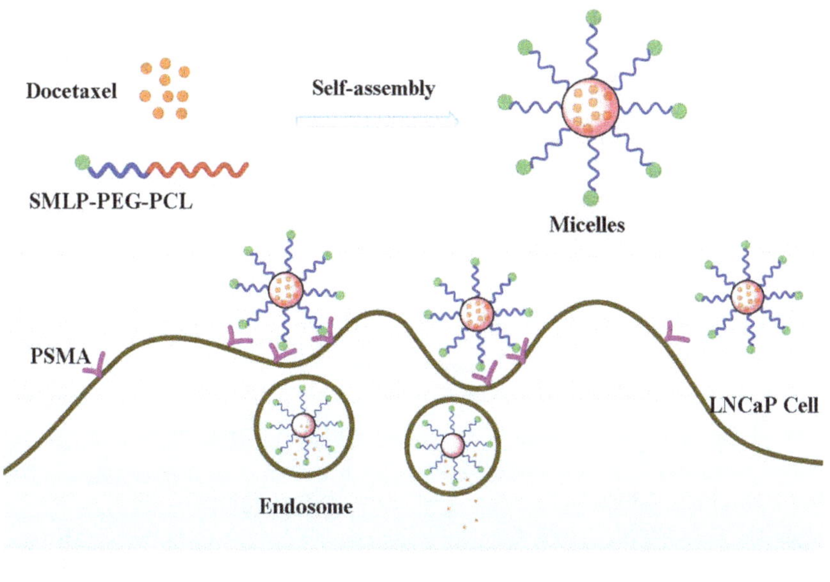

Figure 1. Schematic illustration of DTX-PCL-PEG-SMLP micelles targeted to PSMA.

Gel permeation chromatography (GPC) assay was performed on a Waters 1515 GPC instrument (Waters Corp, Milford, MA) equipped with three styragel columns (Waters Corp; 10^5, 10^4, and 103 Å) in tandem and a 2414 differential refractive index detector. DMF was selected as the eluent at a flow rate of 1.0 ml/min at 35°C. The sample concentrations were approximately 2 mg/ml. The molecular weights were calibrated using polystyrene standards.

Preparation of polymeric micelles. DTX-loaded micelles were prepared by dialysis. First, 7 mg DTX and 50 mg copolymer were completely dissolved in 2 ml THF. Then 4 ml phosphate-buffered saline (PBS; 10 mM, pH 7.4 or 10 mM, pH 5.5) was added drop-wise to the solution under continuous stirring for one hour. Then, THF was removed by dialysis against PBS (10 mM, pH 7.4 or 10 mM, pH 5.5) over 24 h using a cellulose ester dialysis bag (MWCO: 7000 Da). The outer medium was replaced three times (2, 6, and 12 hours). Finally, the mixture was passed through a 0.45 μm filter membrane to remove any precipitants.

Drug-loading content and encapsulation efficiency. To determine the drug-loading content and encapsulation efficiency, 500 μl DTX-loaded micellar solution and 5 ml THF were transferred to a 25 ml volumetric flask, sonicated at 180 W for 10 minutes in an ultrasonic bath, and then diluted with mobile phase. The concentration in the resulting solution was then determined by HPLC. Chromatographic analysis was performed using a Hitachi L-2130 pump and a Hitachi L-2400 UV-Vis detector operated at a wavelength of 230 nm, using a Unitary C18 column (5 μm, 150×4.6 mm). A mobile phase of acetonitrile and water (60/40, v/v) was selected. The flow rate was set at 1 ml/min. The peak area response versus the DTX concentration was linear over the range of 0.5–30 μg/ml ($r^2 = 0.9999$).

The drug-loading content and encapsulation efficiency were calculated from the following equations:

$$\text{Drug loading content} = \frac{\text{Weight of the drug in micelles}}{\text{Weight of the drug in micelles}} \times$$

$$100\,\% + \text{Weight of the copolymers used}$$

$$\text{Encapsulation efficiency} = \frac{\text{Weight of the drug in micelles}}{\text{Weight of the feeding drugs}}$$

$$\times 100\,\%$$

Particle size measurements. The particle size and distribution of micelles were measured by DLS using NICOMP 380 Submicron Particle Sizer (Particle Sizing Systems, Santa Barbara, CA). A laser beam at a wavelength of 632.8 nm was used. The scattering angle was set at 90° when measurements were conducted.

Surface morphology. Samples for TEM observation were prepared by placing a drop of sample solution (2 mg/ml for copolymer) on to a copper grid coated with carbon. Excess solution was wiped away with filter paper. The grid was allowed to dry for a further 15 minutes. Then, the samples were examined using a Hitachi H-600 TEM operated at an accelerating voltage of 100 kV.

***In Vitro* Release.** The *in vitro* DTX release kinetics of drug-loaded micellar solutions or DTX injection (Taxotere, Sanofi-Aventis, Paris, France) containing 300 μg DTX were performed by dialysis diffusion. The drug-loaded micellar solution and free drug solution were placed in the dialysis bags (MWCO: 14000). These bags were immersed in 15 ml PBS pH 7.4 (10 mM) or pH 5.5 (10 mM) containing 0.5% w/v Tween 80. Subsequently, the bottles were placed in a shaking incubator at a shaking speed of 100 rpm under 37°C±0.5°C. All release media were replaced with fresh PBS at predetermined intervals (1 h, 2 h, 4 h, 8 h, 12 h, 24 h, 36 h, 48 h, 60 h, 72 h, 84 h and 96 h) in order to measure the drug concentration. The concentration of DTX was measured by HPLC.

Cell Culture and Cytotoxicity. The prostate LNCaP and PC3 cell lines were cultured in RPMI 1640 medium and Ham's F12K (Invitrogen, USA), supplemented with 10% fetal bovine serum (Hyclone, USA), respectively. The cultures were maintained in a 95% air humidified atmosphere containing 5% CO_2 at 37°C.

MTT assay was conducted to evaluate the cytotoxicity of DTX-PMs1 (nontargeted) and DTX-PMs2 (targeted). LNCaP cells were suspended in culture medium and seeded at 5000 cells/well in 96-well plates for 24 h. Then, dispersed DTX-PMs1, DTX-PMs2, and the DMSO solution of DTX (DSD) containing four drug concentrations (0.1, 1, 10 and 20 μg/ml) in each sample were incubated in LNCaP cells. Finally, the cell viability was determined after 48 h and 72 h using a Microplate Reader (Bio-Rad imark, USA).

The IC50 for each system was then calculated. All assays were conducted with five parallel samples.

Cellular uptake studies. In this study, coumarin 6 was used as a fluorescence probe. Androgen-dependent and androgen-independent prostate cell lines (LNCaP and PC3, respectively) were used. Cellular uptake of targeted and non-targeted PMs (200 μg/ml) carrying coumarin 6 (100 μg/ml) (PMs1 and PMs2, respectively) were conducted on LNCaP and PC3 cell lines to investigate the influence of SMLP conjugation on cellular uptake. The cells were incubated in 96-well plates with micelles for 4 h, washed with cold PBS three times, and then fixed with 70% ethanol for 2 h at −20°C. A competitive inhibition study was also conducted using free SMLP to verify whether the PMs were transported into cells in a SMLP-mediated manner. Free SMLP with three different concentrations (4 μg/ml, 20 μg/ml and 100 μg/ml) was added into the medium together with PMs2, incubated for 4 h, washed thrice with cold PBS and fixed with 70% ethanol for 2 h at −20°C. Cell nuclei were stained with Hoechst 33342.

The cells were examined using an ImageXpress Micro XL Widefield High Content Screening System (ImageXpress Micro XL, Molecular Devices, USA) with MetaXpress Software. The images of the cells were determined by the differential interference contrast channel technique and the images of coumarin 6-loaded PMs and the nuclei of the cells stained by Hoechst 33342 were recorded with the following channels: blue channel (Hoechst 33342) with excitation at 350 nm and green channel (coumarin 6) with excitation at 485 nm. Then, MetaXpress Software was used to quantify the fluorescence intensity per cell.

Statistics. All data were processed using Origin 8.5 software and presented as mean ± SD, and analyzed using Student's *t*-test. Statistical analyses were performed and $P<0.01$ was considered as the level of statistical significance.

Results and Discussion

Synthesis and characterization of PCL-mPEG and PCL-PEG-COOH copolymers

An amphiphilic block copolymer composed of a PCL block as the hydrophobic part and a PEG block as the hydrophilic part was synthesized via ring-opening polymerization using hydroxyl-terminated PEG as a macromolecular initiator.

The molecular weights of the copolymers were calculated from the ^{1}H NMR data by comparing the peak intensities of the methylene protons of PEG with the methylene protons of PCL, as shown in Figure 2E. The ratios of the hydrophobic block to the hydrophilic block were determined from the relative intensities of the PCL proton signal at 2.31 ppm and the PEG proton signal at 3.62 ppm. For GPC analysis, only one peak appeared in the GPC curve (Figure 2A), which means that the ring-opening copolymerization of ε-caprolactone with PEG-OH was complete and all the residues were removed after purification. The polydispersity of the copolymer (Mw/Mn) is outlined in Table 1.

Synthesis and characterization of PCL-PEG-SMLP

Surface functionalization of the copolymer PCL-PEG-COOH with SMLP was achieved under standard amide coupling conditions in the presence of EDC and NHS [27,28]. The coupling efficiency with amine nucleophiles can be increased by the formation of an NHS ester intermediate [29].

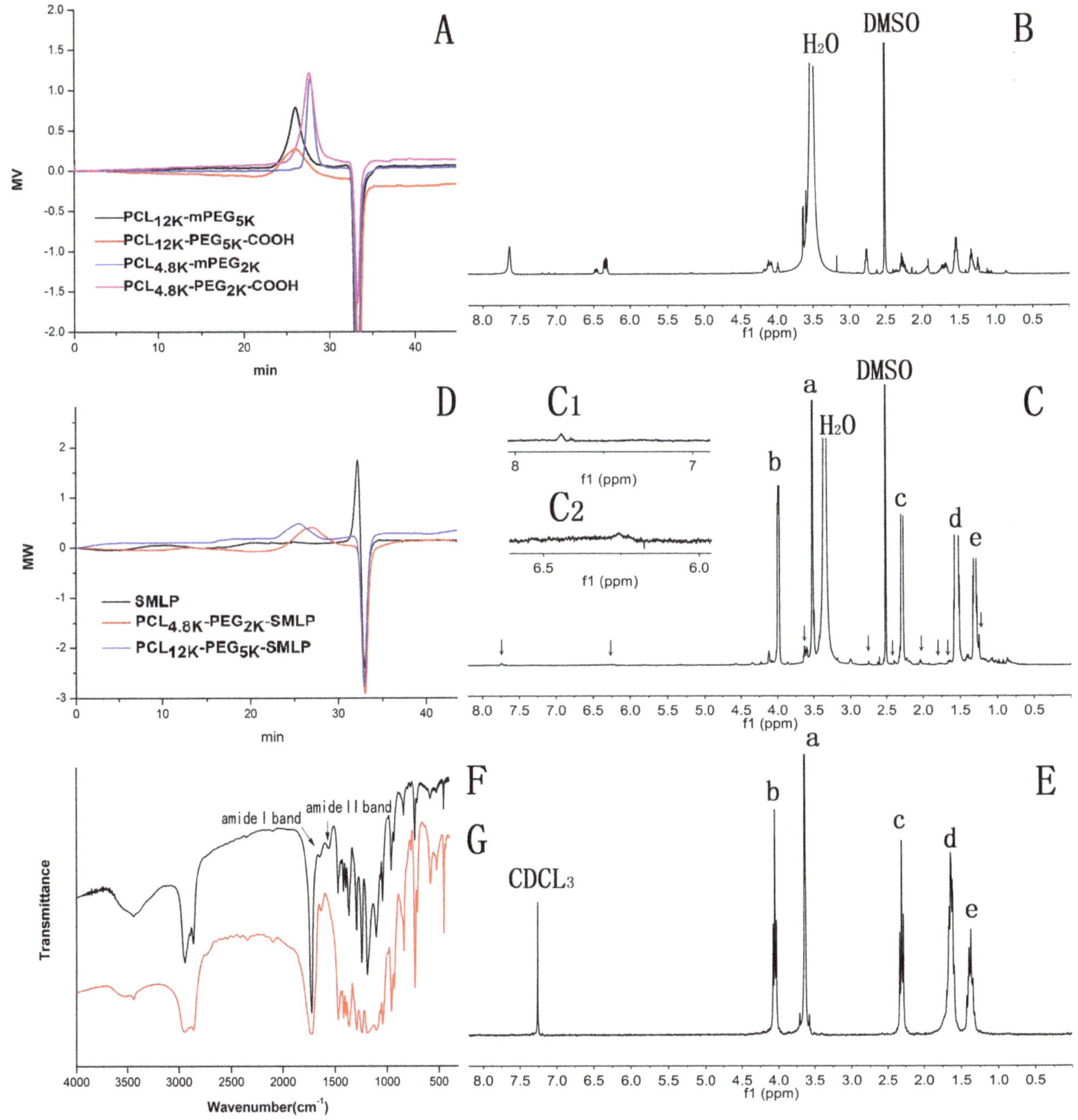

Figure 2. The gel permeation chromatography graphs of four copolymers (A) and SMLP,$PCL_{4.8K}$-PEG_{2K}-SMLP and PCL_{12K}-PEG_{5K}-SMLP (D), the representative ^{1}H NMR spectra of SMLP (B), copolymers PCL_{12K}-PEG_{5K}-SMLP (C) containing SMLP (black arrows) and PCL_{12K}-PEG_{5K}-COOH (E) with the peaks of PCL_{12k}-PEG_{5k} segment (a-e) and Infrared spectra graph of PCL_{12k}-PEG_{5k}-SMLP (F) and PCL_{12K}-PEG_{5K}-COOH (G) copolymers.

Table 1. Characterization data of block copolymers and DTX-PMs.

Polymer	Feed ratio[a] (feed DP)	Final DP[b]	PDI[c]	DTX-PMs	Mean Diameter (nm)	PDI	DLC (%)	EE (%)
PCL_{12K}-$mPEG_{5k}$	110	104	1.08	PCL_{12K}-$mPEG_{5k}$	51.4±1.3	0.038±0.04	8.2±0.3	64.2±2.9
PCL_{12K}-PEG_{5K}-COOH	110	106	1.14	PCL_{12K}-PEG_{5K}-COOH	50.5±1.1	0.044±0.06	8.4±0.2	65.7±1.4
$PCL_{4.8}K$-PEG_{2K}	44	42	1.03	$PCL_{4.8K}$-PEG_{2K}	37.1±0.5	0.038±0.03	7.3±0.3	56.4±2.6
$PCL_{4.8K}$-PEG_{2K}-COOH	44	42	1.07	$PCL_{4.8K}$-PEG_{2K}-COOH	38.6±0.7	0.033±0.02	7.5±0.4	58.0±3.4

(n = 3).
Notes: [a]Calculation of feed ratio by nPCL/nPEG. [b]Degree of polymerization (DP) determined by ^{1}H NMR. [c]Molecular weight polydispersity index (PDI) determined by GPC (Mw/Mn).
Abbreviations: Drug-loading content, DLC; Encapsulation efficiency, EE.

The synthesis of polymer PCL–PEG–SMLP was accomplished by the following method. First, the carboxyl of PCL-PEG-COOH was activated with EDC and NHS to achieve the intermediate PCL-PEG-NHS. Then, the active ester (NHS) of PCL-PEG-NHS was reacted with the amine functional group of the SMLP to obtain the final polymer PCL-PEG-SMLP (Figure 3).

The polymer of PCL_{12k}–PEG_{5k}–SMLP was characterized using FT-IR, as depicted in Figure 2F. The salient peaks shown in Figure 2F at 1671 and 1557 cm^{-1} were attributed to amide band I (carbonyl group) and amide band II (amino group) respectively, while the disappearance of these peaks (Figure 2G) indicated the formation of the amide bond between SMLP and PCL_{12k}-PEG_{5k}-COOH. The structure of the conjugate was further examined by ^{1}H NMR. Figure 2C shows the ^{1}H NMR spectrum of the conjugation of the ligand and copolymer PCL_{12k}-PEG_{5k}-COOH. The characteristic signal appearing at 3.60 ppm (a) was assigned to the PEG unit. The peaks of the PCL units appear at 4.04–4.08 ppm (b), 2.28–2.33 ppm (c), 1.61–1.70 ppm (d) and 1.35–1.43 ppm (e), as shown in Figure 2C. Moreover, the signals at 2.49 ppm and 3.25–3.49 ppm were assigned to the solvent peak (DMSO) and water peak, respectively. According to Figure 2E, there are no SMLP-related signals shown in the ^{1}H NMR spectrum of unconjugated PCL_{12k}-PEG_{5k}-COOH, indicating that there is no interference with SMLP signals shown in Figure 2C.Comparing the peaks of PCL-PEG-SMLP in Figure 2C and the peaks of ligand SMLP in Figure 2B, the chemical shifts were identical. Combing the results of FT-IR and ^{1}H NMR showed that the ligand SMLP had been successfully conjugated to PCL_{12K}-PEG_{5K}-COOH. The purity of ligand conjugated polymers, which is critically related to the *in vitro* performance of the micelles, was verified by gel permeation chromatography. As shown in Figure 2D, no trace of free SMLP was observed in the chromatograms of either PCL_{12K}-PEG_{5K}-SMLP or $PCL_{4.8K}$-PEG_{2K}-SMLP, indicating that the excessive free ligand was completely removed.

Preparation and characterization of micelles

In this work, dialysis was employed to prepare the docetaxel-micelles, leading to the successful preparation of nontargeted [PCL_{12K}-$mPEG_{5k}$ (PMs1), $PCL_{4.8k}$-$mPEG_{2K}$ (PMs3)] and targeted [PCL_{12K}-PEG_{5K}-SMLP (PMs2), $PCL_{4.8K}$-PEG_{2K}-SMLP (PMs4)] micelles. In addition, nanoparticles with diameters larger than 100 nm are more likely to be eliminated by the reticuloendothelial system [30], while their counterparts with diameters less than 100 nm were more likely to accumulate in tumor tissues [31,32].

The average diameters of micelles (PMs1, PMs2, PMs3 and PMs4) prepared by dialysis were 51.4±1.3 nm, 50.5±1.1 nm, 37.1±0.5 nm and 38.6±0.7 nm, respectively. The polydispersity index (PDI) values of the four micelles are shown in Table 1. The DLS graphs of PMs1 and PMs2 are shown in Figure 4 (A, B). The morphology and low PDI of the micelles were further confirmed by TEM imaging. The TEM photograph (Figure 4, A_1 and B2) of PMs1 and PMs2 were in accordance to the results of DLS. The smaller diameters of the PMs obtained from the TEM tests compared with DLS could be ascribed to the shrinkage of the PEG shell induced by water evaporation before TEM measurement [33]. As a result, the diameter given by DLS was bigger than that of TEM due to the hydration of the PEG shell.

To evaluate the maximum drug-loading content and drug-loading efficiency of the four micelles, a simple short-term stability study of the DTX-loaded content was performed and the results are shown in Figure 5. First, excess DTX was added during the preparation of the four DTX-PMs. The over-loaded PMs were

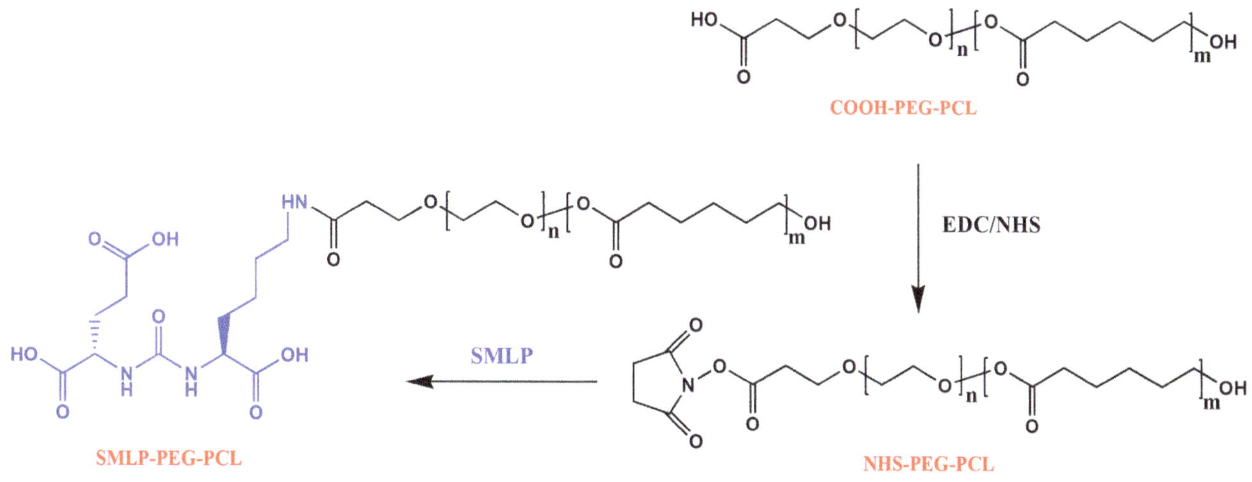

Figure 3. Synthetic representation of the chemical reaction for preparation of PCL-PEG-SMLP copolymer.

kept at room temperature and sampled at predetermined time. Then, the DTX-loading content of the samples was measured by HPLC using the method described. The profile showed that the initial DTX-loading content of the four PMs was 10.4%, 10.8%, 9.6% and 9.8%, respectively. The values of DTX-loading content fell gradually and remained constant after 12 h for PCL_{12k}-PEG_{5k} and 24 h for $PCL_{4.8k}$-PEG_{2k} (Figure 5, circled in squares). The reduction in drug-loading content may be due to the occurrence of phase separation between DTX and PCL. The drug-loading content after a 7 days test period could be deemed as the capacity of PCL for loading DTX. Also, the higher capacity of PMs1 and PMs2 compared with PMs3 and PMs4 could be ascribed to the

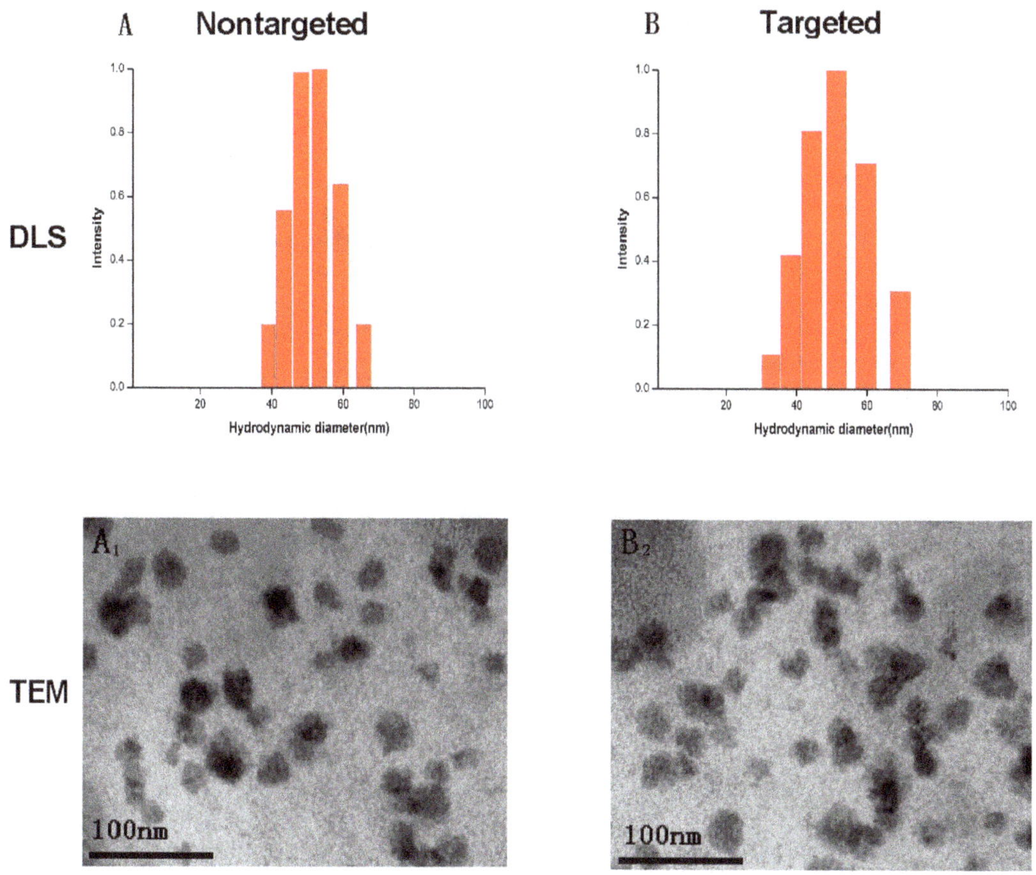

Figure 4. The representative DLS graphs of the DTX-PMs1 (A), and DTX-PMs2 (B), respectively. TEM graphs of DTX-PMs1 (A_1) and DTX-PMs2 (B_2).

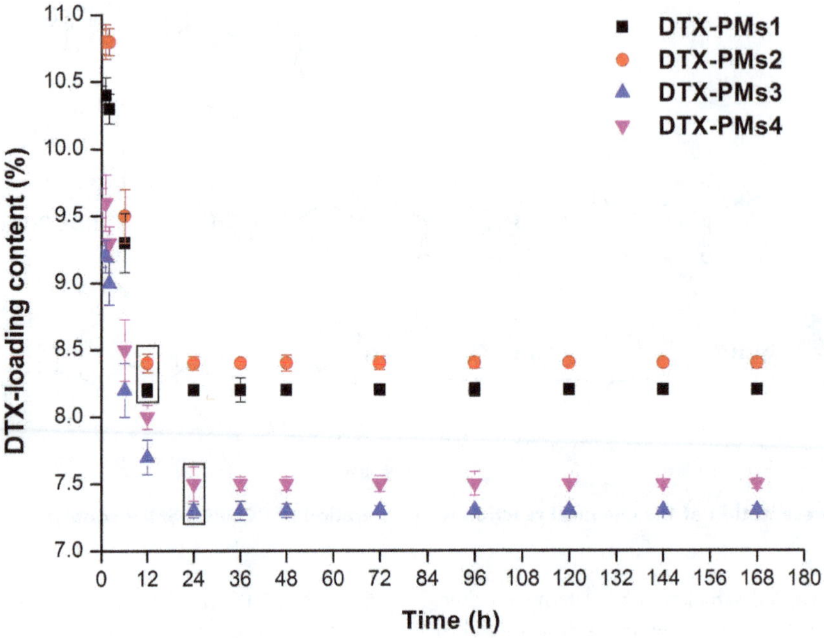

Figure 5. The short-term stability of the DLC of four DTX-PMs stored at room temperature for 7 days. (n = 3).

longer PCL chains of PMs1 and PMs2. With the same ratio of the hydrophilic block length to the hydrophobic block length, the final drug-loading content and encapsulation efficiency of the four PMs are shown in Table 1. These results showed the a good short-term stability of the DTX-loading content, the drug-loading content and efficiency, confirming that the micelles based on PCL_{12K}-PEG_{5K}-SMLP and PCL_{12K}-$mPEG_{5k}$ copolymers were optimal formulations.

In vitro release

The *in vitro* release behavior of four DTX-PMs was investigated by the dialysis diffusion method [34]. The release behavior of Taxotere was used as a control, and the DTX release profiles of the four PMs at pH 7.4 (simulated environment of normal tissues) and pH 5.5 (simulated environment of tumor tissues) are shown in Figure 6. Almost 90% of the DTX was released from Taxotere within 24 h. Unlike Taxotere, all micelles exhibited a fast release of DTX at the initial stage (first 24 h) and a sustained release over the following 72 h. Moreover, the similar release profiles of PMs1 and PMs2 indicated that ligand conjugation did not influence the release pattern.

For the four PMs, because the poly ester structure of PCL is sensitive to acid, the release of DTX from micelles was slower at pH 7.4 than that at pH 5.5. This effect promoted the release of DTX in tumor tissues and in endosomes which are more acidic than blood [35]. The amount of non-released DTX was 20–25%. This proportion of drugs existed in the micellar cores; trapped in precipitations generated by heat and tween 80 induced micellar breakdown and adsorbed on dialysis bag and glassware [36].

Cell cytotoxicity

PSMA is a validated molecular marker overexpressed by LNCaP cells [37,38]. The cytotoxicity enhancing effect of PSMA ligand (SMLP) conjugated DTX-PMs were evaluated by in vitro cytotoxicity experiments using LNCaP and PC3 cells, respectively. The biocompatibility of PCL_{12K}-$mPEG_{5K}$ and PCL_{12K}-PEG_{5K}-SMLP was confirmed by incubating drug-free micelles composed of these two polymers at various concentrations with LNCaP cells and PC3 cells, respectively. The cell viability was not affected over a 72 h incubation period which confirmed the good biocompatibility of these polymers (Figure 7). The results also demonstrated that the cells cannot be interfered in the presence of ligands.

In this study, the DMSO solution of DTX (DSD) was used instead of Taxotere as a positive control because Tween 80 in Taxotere is cytotoxic and this may influence the results [39]. According to the results of the MTT assays (Figure 8), after a 48 h incubation, the cytotoxicity of PMs1 was nearly the same as DSD. However, PMs2 showed a significantly lower LNCaP cell viability at all concentrations. In PC3 cell lines, however, no significant difference was observed in cell viability among DSD, PMs1 and PMs2 (Figure 8). This indicated that ligand conjugation is beneficial in facilitating the cellular uptake of micelles: as PMs1 and PMs2 showed similar release profiles, the decreased cell viability could be ascribed to enhanced intracellular drug accumulation via receptor-mediated endocytosis. After 72 h incubation, both PMs1 and PMs2 showed significant differences from DSD in LNCaP cell line, and PMs2 showed the greatest cytotoxicity. Moreover, significant lower cell viabilities were observed in PC3 cell lines treated with either PMs1 or PMs2 than DSD at drug concentration of 20 μg/ml, which mean that inadequate cellular uptake of micelles could be compensated by increased incubation time and drug concentration. However, there were no significant differences between PMs1 and DSD after 48h incubation for LNCaP cells. This phenomenon confirmed the sustained drug release behavior of DTX from PMs1 *in vitro*.

The cell viability of PMs2 at 20 μg/ml was almost half that of PMs1 for LNCaP cells after either 48 h or 72 h incubation. These data demonstrated that DTX-PMs2 was less effective in enhancing cytotoxicity in PC3 cells, whereas it selectively inhibits proliferation of LNCaP cells. In the other words, these results suggest the high affinity of SMLP for PSMA could enhance the cytotoxicity in LNCaP cells. After 72 h incubation on LNCaP cells with the amount of DTX given at a fixed concentration of 20 μg/ml, the

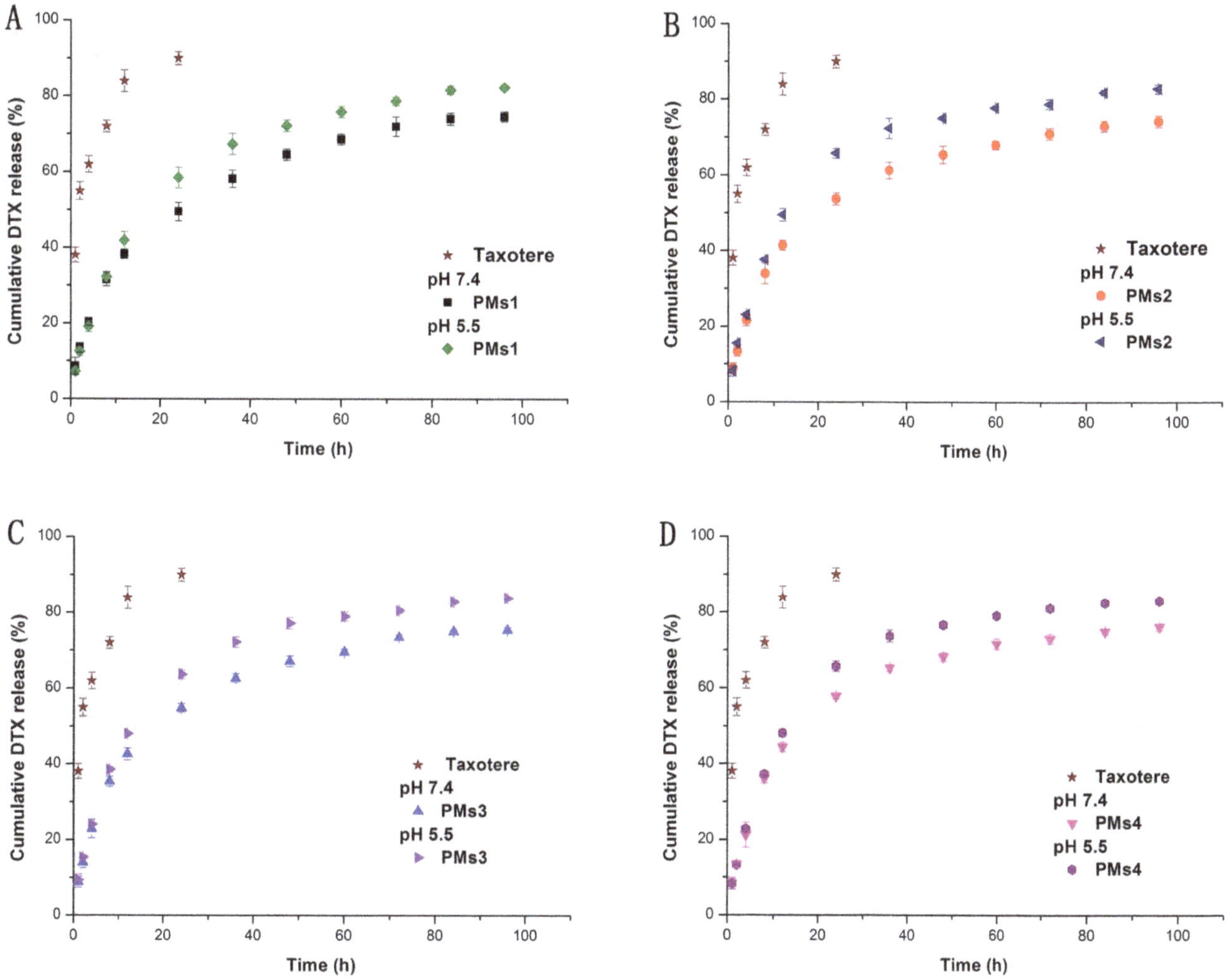

Figure 6. *In vitro* **release profile of DTX from the four types of PMs solution at 37°C in PBS (10 mM, pH 7.4) or PBS(10 mM,pH 5.5), in comparison with Taxotere. (n = 3).**

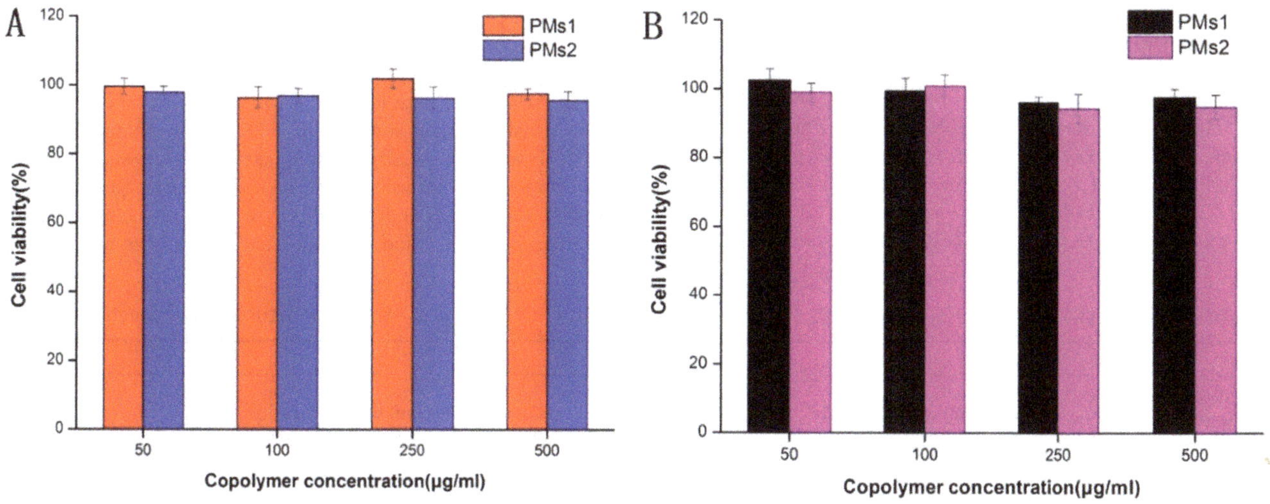

Figure 7. Different concentrations of PMs1 and PMs2 in LNCaP cells (A) and in PC3 cells (B) after incubation for 72 h. (n = 5).

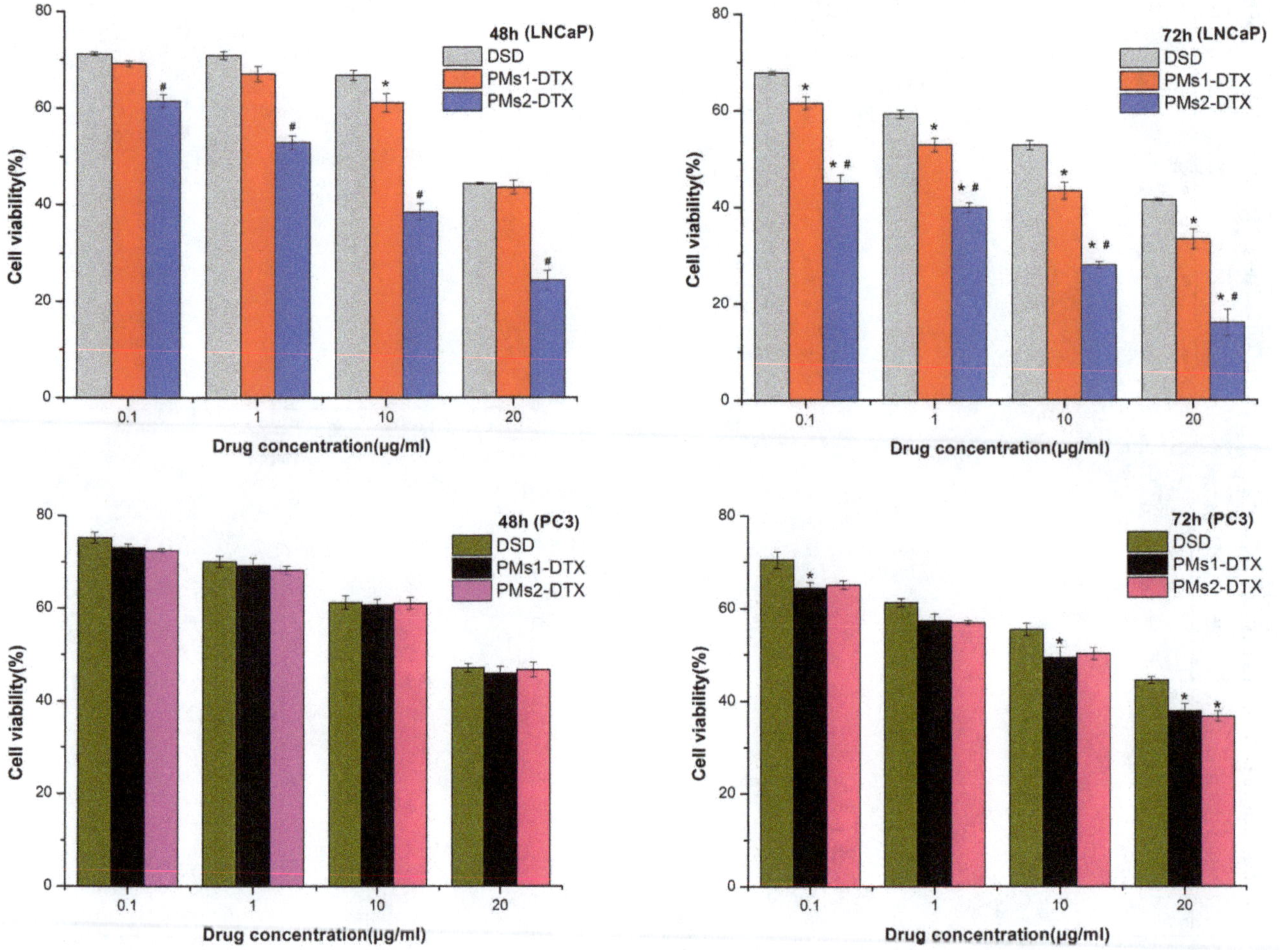

Figure 8. In vitro cytotoxicity determination of different concentrations of DSD, DTX-PMs1 and DTX-PMs2 in LNCaP cells and PC3 cells after incubation for 48 h, 72 h, respectively, using MTT assay. (*) significantly different from DSD; (#) significantly different from PMs1; (n = 5). Note: *P<0.01, #P<0.01.

cell growth inhibition rate of DSD, PMs1 and PMs2 were 58.4%, 67.7% and 83.9%, respectively.

The IC50 for each sample is shown in Table 2. For LNCaP cells, the IC50 of DTX-PMs2 was much lower than that of DTX-PMs1 and DSD after 48 h or 72 h incubation. However, the IC50 of DTX-PMs1 was almost the same as that of DSD after 48 h incubation, but was 5-fold lower after 72 h incubation with LNCaP cells, this further confirmed the compensating effect in cytoxicity of micelles by prolonged incubation time. Although DTX-PMs2 (targeted) exhibited the highest cell-killing efficiency, the DTX-PMs1 also displayed an effect on LNCaP cells. Since the two micelles possessed similar release profiles, the differences in cytotoxicity were related to their different cell-entry ability which was reflected by the differences in affinities to PSMA.

Cellular Uptake

To study the effect of PSMA targeting ligand on the cellular uptake of the PMs, fluorescence microscopy was conducted on LNCaP cells with both targeted (PMs2) and non-targeted (PMs1) micelles labeled with coumarin-6. After 4 h incubation at 37°C, HCSS images of LNCaP cells were taken and shown in Figure 9A. The fluorescence intensity of cells incubated with targeted micelles (PMs2) was significantly higher than that of its non-targeted counterpart (PMs1), and the quantified fluorescence intensity was

Table 2. IC_{50} analysis of DSD, DTX-PMs1 and DTX-PMs2 on LNCaP and PC3 cells after 48 h, 72 h incubation, respectively (n = 5).

Incubation time (h)	IC_{50} values (μg/ml) of LNCaP cells			IC_{50} values (μg/ml) of PC3 cells		
	DSD	DTX-PMs1	DTX-PMs2	DSD	DTX-PMs1	DTX-PMs2
48 h	14.59±2.11	13.48±1.03	0.87±0.27	19.31±3.42	18.65±3.07	19.04±2.81
72 h	7.36±1.51	1.35±0.54	0.02±0.008	11.67±1.98	3.11±0.81	3.02±0.76

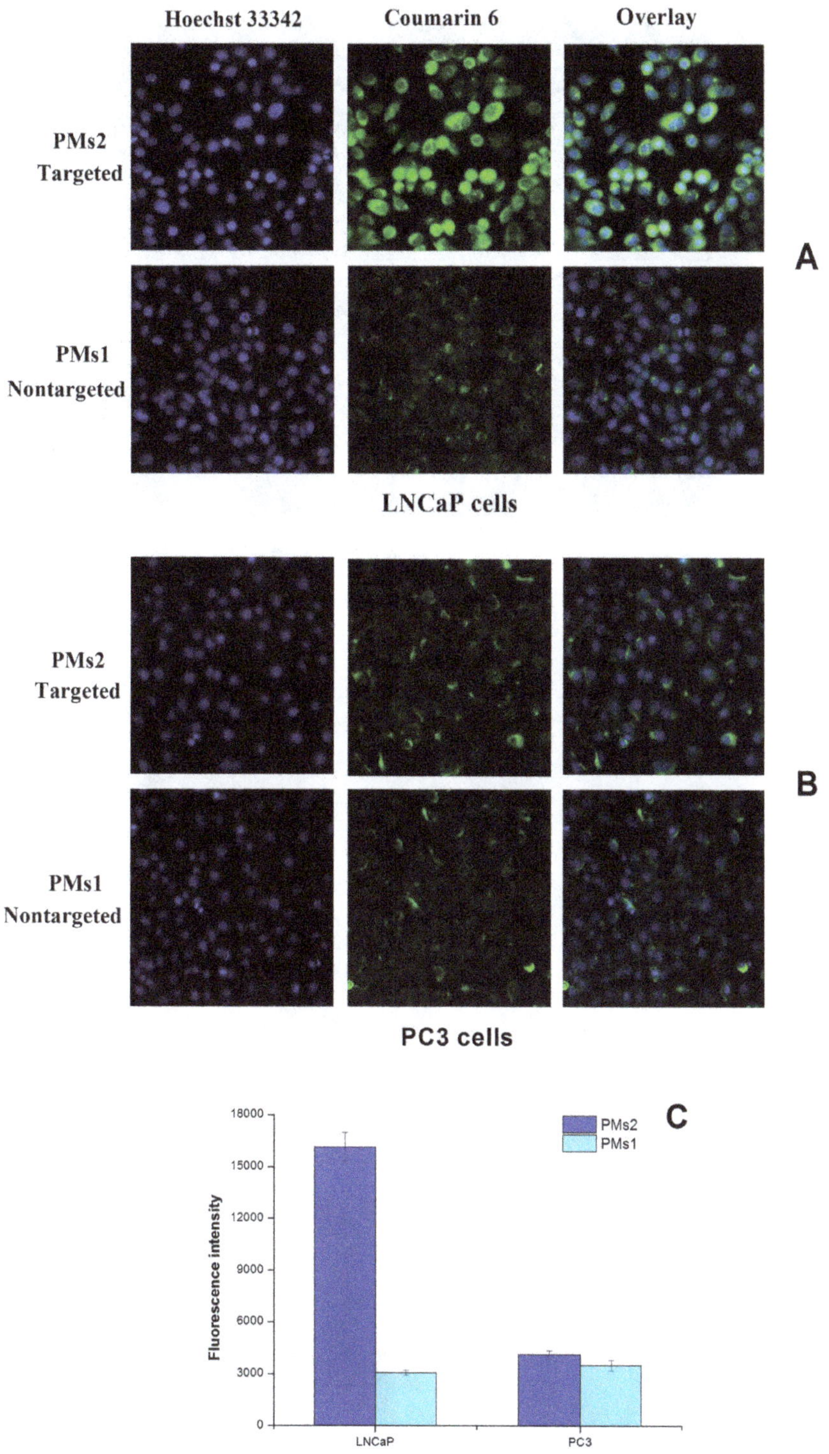

Figure 9. HCSS images of LNCaP (A) and PC3 cells (B) following a 4 h incubation at 37°C with coumarin 6-loaded PMs1 and PMs2, respectively. The cell nuclei were stained with Hoechst 33342 with the blue channel, the coumarin 6-loaded PMs are the green channel. The cellular uptake was visualized by overlaying images displayed by the nuclei channel and the PMs channel. The fluorescence intensity/cell graph of 100 μg/ml coumarin 6-loaded PMs1 and PMs2 with a concentration of 200 μg/ml after 4 h incubation with LNCaP cells and PC3 cells (C).

estimated to be 5-fold (Figure 9C). The capability of SMLP conjugation in enhancing cellular uptake could be reflected in cell viability assays. To further verify the role of SMLP in endocytosis, a ligand competing experiment was conducted. As shown in Figure 8B, addition of free ligands at various concentrations gradually decreased the uptake of PMs2, and the amount of endocytosed micelles reached a similar level to its non-targeted counterpart at high concentration of SMLP (100 μg/ml, Figure 10B), which indicated the presence of free SMLP in the medium inhibited endocytosis of PMs2 by binding to surface

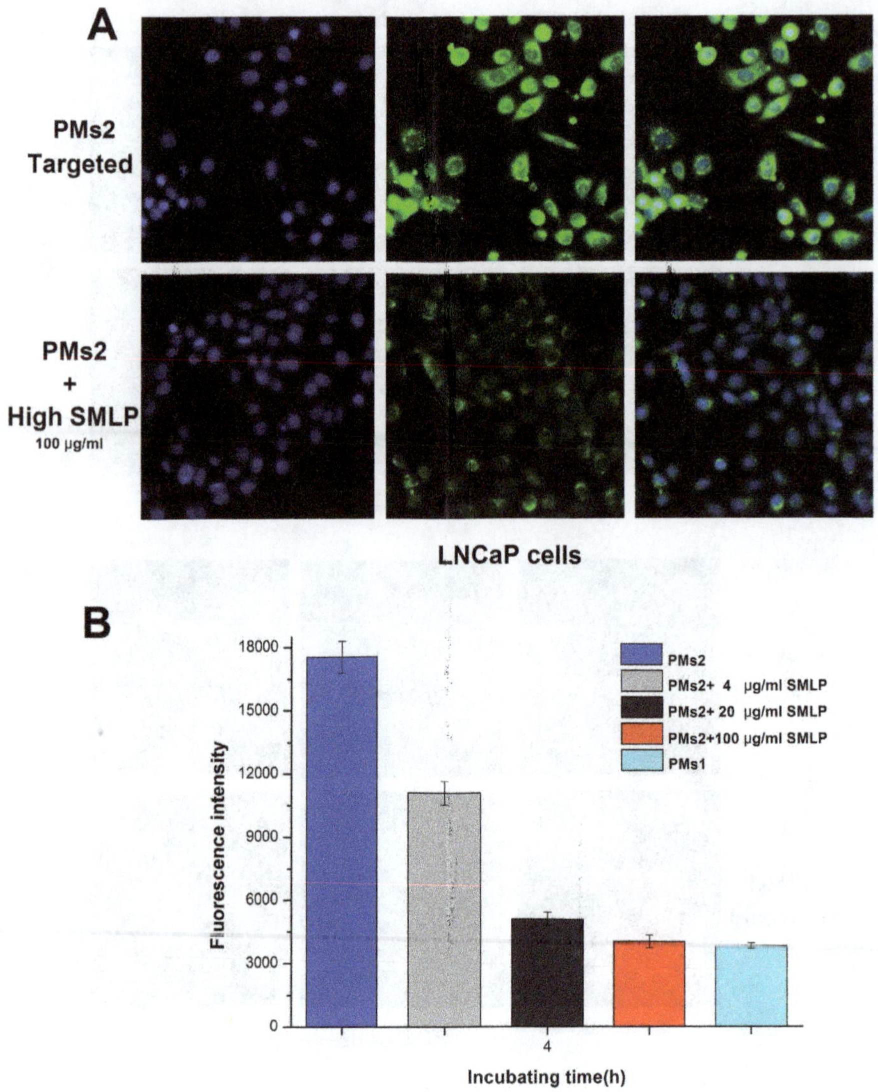

Figure 10. Competitive inhibition analysis of free SMLP (A) and fluorescence intensity/cell on LNCaP cells after 4 h incubation (B).

PSMA in a competitive manner against micelle-conjugated SMLP. To further verify the enhancement of ligand in mediating endocytosis, cellular uptake studies of both preparations with/without SMLP ligand were conducted in PC-3 cell line, which do not express the PSMA protein [40]. As shown in Figure 9 (B and C), targeted- and non-targeted micelles showed similar intracellular fluorescent intensity, which means conjugation of SMLP is a key factor in promoting cellular uptake of prepared micelles in PSMA expressing cells. Also the above results demonstrated that PMs2 was endocytosed into LNCaP cells via multiple routes: part of the micelles was taken up by LNCaP cells in a SMLP-mediated manner, while there were micelles entering cells through other pathways including caveolin-mediated endocytosis or clathrin- and caveolin-independent endocytosis [41] as the cellular uptake of micelles was not completely inhibited by SMLP addition. These results explained the higher cytotoxicity of the targeted micelles (PMs2) in MTT assays and indicated the benefit of PMs with a targeting ligand in prostate cancer therapy.

Conclusions

In this study, a novel self-assembly of DTX-PEG-PCL-SMLP micelles targeting LNCaP cells was developed. With the same hydrophilic/hydrophobic block length ratio, a series of polymeric micelles with diameters less than 60 nm were prepared by dialysis. Stable non-targeted PMs and targeted PMs with constant drug-loading content were obtained by short-term stability assays. Reliable drug loading and sustained releasing behavior were obtained due to removal of the over-loaded drugs. The cytotoxicity experiments demonstrated the advantages in LNCaP cell inhibition with a significant difference of targeted DTX-PMs > non-targeted DTX-PMs > DSD. The fluorescence intensity of coumarin 6-loaded targeted PMs were 5-fold higher than that of non-targeted PMs. Combining the cellular uptake results of both targeted- and non-targeted micelles in LNCaP and PC3 cell lines, the critical role of SMLP conjugation in facilitating micelle uptake in PSMA positive cells was demonstrated. All of these results were ascribed to the ligand targeting of PSMA that guaranteed efficient uptake of micelles composed of DTX-PCL-PEG-SMLP that exhibited highest cytotoxicity on LNCaP cells. In summary, intracellular drug delivery is crucial for the anti-tumor efficacy of poorly-permeable drugs. As shown in this study, DTX-PCL-PEG-SMLP showed remarkable cytotoxicity compared with DMSO solution of DTX. DTX-PCL-mPEG also displayed higher cyotoxicity than DMSO solution of DTX due to enhanced intracellular accumulation via endocytosis of micelles. A more positive effect could be achieved by ligand conjugation that anchored micelles to tumor cells and facilitated cellular uptake. Further investigation into other properties of this drug delivery system, such as pharmacokinetics, *in vivo* antitumor activity and tissue distribution, are still required. Moreover, PCL-PEG-SMLP as a drug carrier is expected to be used in a number of ways for PCa therapy.

Acknowledgments

Dr David B Jack is gratefully thanked for correcting the English in the manuscript.

Author Contributions

Conceived and designed the experiments: XT HX XJ. Performed the experiments: JJ BS JG. Analyzed the data: JJ YZ JL. Contributed reagents/materials/analysis tools: HX XJ. Wrote the paper: JJ XJ.

References

1. Branco MC, Schneider JP (2009) Self-assembling materials for therapeutic delivery. Acta Biomaterialia 5: 817–831.
2. Haag R (2004) Supramolecular drug-delivery systems based on polymeric core-shell architectures. Angew Chem Int Ed Engl 43: 278–282.
3. Huang W, Wang W, Wang P, Tian Q, Zhang C, et al. (2010) Glycyrrhetinic acid-modified poly(ethylene glycol)-b-poly(gamma-benzyl l-glutamate) micelles for liver targeting therapy. Acta Biomater 6: 3927–3935.
4. Saxena V, Hussain MD (2013) Polymeric Mixed Micelles for Delivery of Curcumin to Multidrug Resistant Ovarian Cancer. J Biomed Nanotechnol 9: 1146–1154.
5. Li J, He Z, Yu S, Li S, Ma Q, et al. (2012) Micelles Based on Methoxy Poly(Ethylene Glycol)Cholesterol Conjugate for Controlled and Targeted Drug Delivery of a Poorly Water Soluble Drug. J Biomed Nanotechnol 8: 809–817.
6. Savic R, Eisenberg A, Maysinger D (2006) Block copolymer micelles as delivery vehicles of hydrophobic drugs: micelle-cell interactions. J Drug Target 14: 343–355.
7. Kazunori K, Glenn S K, Masayuki Y, Teruo O, Yasuhisa S (1993) Block copolymer micelles as vehicles for drug delivery. J Control Release 24: 119–132.
8. Gu PF, Xu H, Sui BW, Gou JX, Meng LK, et al. (2012) Polymeric micelles based on poly(ethylene glycol) block poly(racemic amino acids) hybrid polypeptides: conformation-facilitated drug-loading behavior and potential application as effective anticancer drug carriers. Int J Nanomedicine 7: 109–122.
9. Wang Y, Xu H, Liu H, Wang Y, Sun J, et al. (2012) Efficacy and Biodistribution of Tocopheryl Polyethylene Glycol Succinate Noncovalent Functionalized Single Walled Nanotubes Loading Doxorubicin in Sarcoma Bearing Mouse Model. J Biomed Nanotechnol 8: 450–457.
10. Maresca K, Hillier S, Femia F, Keith D, Barone C, et al. (2008) A series of halogenated heterodimeric inhibitors of prostate specific membrane antigen (PSMA) as radiolabeled probes for targeting prostate cancer. J Med Chem 52: 347–357.
11. Murphy GP, Elgamal AAA, Su SL, Bostwick DG, Holmes EH (1998) Current evaluation of the tissue localization and diagnostic utility of prostate specific membrane antigen. Cancer 83: 2259–2269.
12. Israeli RS, Powell CT, Corr JG, Fair WR, Heston WD (1994) Expression of the prostate-specific membrane antigen. Cancer Res 54: 1807–1811.
13. Chang SS, O'Keefe DS, Bacich DJ, Reuter VE, Heston WD, et al. (1999) Prostate-specific membrane antigen is produced in tumor-associated neovasculature. Clin Cancer Res 5: 2674–2681.
14. Ghosh A, Heston WD (2004) Tumor target prostate specific membrane antigen (PSMA) and its regulation in prostate cancer. J Cell Biochem 91: 528–539.
15. Colombatti M, Grasso S, Porzia A, Fracasso G, Scupoli MT, et al. (2009) The Prostate Specific Membrane Antigen Regulates the Expression of IL-6 and CCL5 in Prostate Tumour Cells by Activating the MAPK Pathways1. PloS one 4: e4608.
16. Wolf P, Freudenberg N, Bühler P, Alt K, Schultze-Seemann W, et al. (2010) Three conformational antibodies specific for different PSMA epitopes are promising diagnostic and therapeutic tools for prostate cancer. The Prostate 70: 562–569.
17. Sanna V, Pintus G, Bandiera P, Anedda R, Punzoni S, et al. (2011) Development of polymeric microbubbles targeted to prostate-specific membrane antigen as prototype of novel ultrasound contrast agents. Mol Pharm 8: 748–757.
18. Hrkach J, Von Hoff D, Ali MM, Andrianova E, Auer J, et al. (2012) Preclinical development and clinical translation of a PSMA-targeted docetaxel nanoparticle with a differentiated pharmacological profile. Sci Transl Med 4: 128ra139–128ra139.
19. Bae SJ, Suh JM, Sohn YS, Bae YH, Kim SW, et al. (2005) Thermogelling poly (caprolactone-b-ethylene glycol-b-caprolactone) aqueous solutions. Macromolecules 38: 5260–5265.
20. Chung Y-M, Simmons KL, Gutowska A, Jeong B (2002) Sol-gel transition temperature of PLGA-g-PEG aqueous solutions. Biomacromolecules 3: 511–516.
21. Zamani S, Khoee S (2012) Preparation of core–shell chitosan/PCL-PEG triblock copolymer nanoparticles with ABA and BAB morphologies: Effect of intraparticle interactions on physicochemical properties. Polymer 53: 5723–5736.
22. Liu C, Gong C, Pan Y, Zhang Y, Wang J, et al. (2007) Synthesis and characterization of a thermosensitive hydrogel based on biodegradable amphiphilic PCL-Pluronic (L35)-PCL block copolymers. Colloids and Surfaces A: Physicochem Eng Aspects 302: 430–438.
23. Li J, Li X, Ni X, Wang X, Li H, et al. (2006) Self-assembled supramolecular hydrogels formed by biodegradable PEO-PHB-PEO triblock copolymers and alpha-cyclodextrin for controlled drug delivery. Biomaterials 27: 4132–4140.
24. Gaucher G, Dufresne M-H, Sant VP, Kang N, Maysinger D, et al. (2005) Block copolymer micelles: preparation, characterization and application in drug delivery. J Control Release 109: 169–188.
25. Gou M, Zheng X, Men K, Zhang J, Zheng L, et al. (2009) Poly (ε-caprolactone)/poly (ethylene glycol)/poly (ε-caprolactone) nanoparticles: preparation, characterization, and application in doxorubicin delivery. J Phy Chem B 113: 12928–12933.
26. Qi R, Hu X, Yan L, Chen X, Huang Y, et al. (2011) Synthesis of biodegradable cationic triblock copolymer mPEG-PCL-PLL for siRNA delivery. J Control Release 152: e167–e168.
27. Farokhzad OC, Cheng J, Teply BA, Sherifi I, Jon S, et al. (2006) Targeted nanoparticle-aptamer bioconjugates for cancer chemotherapy in vivo. Proc Natl Acad Sci U S A 103: 6315–6320.
28. Dhar S, Liu Z, Thomale J, Dai H, Lippard SJ (2008) Targeted single-wall carbon nanotube-mediated Pt (IV) prodrug delivery using folate as a homing device. J Am Chem Soc 130: 11467–11476.
29. Hinterwirth H, Lindner W, Lammerhofer M (2012) Bioconjugation of trypsin onto gold nanoparticles: effect of surface chemistry on bioactivity. Anal Chim Acta 733: 90–97.
30. Torchilin V (2011) Tumor delivery of macromolecular drugs based on the EPR effect. Adv Drug Deliv Rev 63: 131–135.
31. Davis ME, Chen ZG, Shin DM (2008) Nanoparticle therapeutics: an emerging treatment modality for cancer. Nat Rev Drug Discov 7: 771–782.
32. Alexis F, Pridgen E, Molnar LK, Farokhzad OC (2008) Factors affecting the clearance and biodistribution of polymeric nanoparticles. Mol Pharm 5: 505–515.
33. Hu Y, Zhang L, Cao Y, Ge H, Jiang X, et al. (2004) Degradation Behavior of Poly(ε-caprolactone)-b-poly(ethylene glycol)-b-poly(ε-caprolactone) Micelles in Aqueous Solution. Biomacromolecules 5: 1756–1762.
34. Nie S, Hsiao WL, Pan W, Yang Z (2011) Thermoreversible Pluronic F127-based hydrogel containing liposomes for the controlled delivery of paclitaxel: in vitro drug release, cell cytotoxicity, and uptake studies. Int J Nanomedicine 6: 151–166.
35. Rofstad EK, Mathiesen B, Kindem K, Galappathi K (2006) Acidic extracellular pH promotes experimental metastasis of human melanoma cells in athymic nude mice. Cancer Res 66: 6699–6707.
36. Samarajeewa S, Shrestha R, Elsabahy M, Karwa A, Li A, et al. (2013) In vitro efficacy of paclitaxel-loaded dual-responsive shell cross-linked polymer nanoparticles having orthogonally degradable disulfide cross-linked corona and polyester core domains. Mol Pharm 10: 1092–1099.
37. Yamamichi F, Matsuoka T, Shigemura K, Kawabata M, Shirakawa T, et al. (2012) Potential establishment of lung metastatic xenograft model of androgen receptor-positive and androgen-independent prostate cancer (C4-2B). Urology 80: 951 e951–957.
38. Denmeade SR, Sokoll LJ, Dalrymple S, Rosen DM, Gady AM, et al. (2003) Dissociation between androgen responsiveness for malignant growth vs. expression of prostate specific differentiation markers PSA, hK2, and PSMA in human prostate cancer models. The Prostate 54: 249–257.
39. Esmaeili F, Dinarvand R, Ghahremani MH, Amini M, Rouhani H, et al. (2009) Docetaxel-albumin conjugates: preparation, in vitro evaluation and biodistribution studies. J Pharm Sci 98: 2718–2730.
40. Farokhzad OC, Jon S, Khademhosseini A, Tran T-NT, LaVan DA, et al. (2004) Nanoparticle-aptamer bioconjugates a new approach for targeting prostate cancer cells. Cancer Res 64: 7668–7672.
41. Conner SD, Schmid SL (2003) Regulated portals of entry into the cell. Nature 422: 37–44.

12

Synthesis, Characterization and In Vitro Study of Biocompatible Cinnamaldehyde Functionalized Magnetite Nanoparticles (CPGF Nps) For Hyperthermia and Drug Delivery Applications in Breast Cancer

Kirtee D. Wani[1], Brijesh S. Kadu[2], Prakash Mansara[1], Preeti Gupta[3], Avinash V. Deore[4], Rajeev C. Chikate[2], Pankaj Poddar[3], Sanjay D. Dhole[4], Ruchika Kaul-Ghanekar[1]*

1 Cell and Translational Research Laboratory, Interactive Research School for Health Affairs (IRSHA), Bharati Vidyapeeth University Medical College Campus, Dhankawadi, Pune, Maharashtra, India, **2** Nanoscience Group, Department of Chemistry, Post-graduate and Research Center, MES Abasaheb Garware College, Pune, Maharashtra, India, **3** Physical and Material Chemistry Division, CSIR-National Chemical Laboratory, Pune, Maharashtra, India, **4** Department of Physics, University of Pune, Pune, Maharashtra, India

Abstract

Cinnamaldehyde, the bioactive component of the spice cinnamon, and its derivatives have been shown to possess anti-cancer activity against various cancer cell lines. However, its hydrophobic nature invites attention for efficient drug delivery systems that would enhance the bioavailability of cinnamaldehyde without affecting its bioactivity. Here, we report the synthesis of stable aqueous suspension of cinnamaldehyde tagged Fe_3O_4 nanoparticles capped with glycine and pluronic polymer (CPGF NPs) for their potential application in drug delivery and hyperthermia in breast cancer. The monodispersed superparamagnetic NPs had an average particulate size of ~20 nm. TGA data revealed the drug payload of ~18%. Compared to the free cinnamaldehyde, CPGF NPs reduced the viability of breast cancer cell lines, MCF7 and MDAMB231, at lower doses of cinnamaldehyde suggesting its increased bioavailability and in turn its therapeutic efficacy in the cells. Interestingly, the NPs were non-toxic to the non-cancerous HEK293 and MCF10A cell lines compared to the free cinnamaldehyde. The novelty of CPGF nanoparticulate system was that it could induce cytotoxicity in both ER/PR positive/Her2 negative (MCF7) and ER/PR negative/Her2 negative (MDAMB231) breast cancer cells, the latter being insensitive to most of the chemotherapeutic drugs. The NPs decreased the growth of the breast cancer cells in a dose-dependent manner and altered their migration through reduction in MMP-2 expression. CPGF NPs also decreased the expression of VEGF, an important oncomarker of tumor angiogenesis. They induced apoptosis in breast cancer cells through loss of mitochondrial membrane potential and activation of caspase-3. Interestingly, upon exposure to the radiofrequency waves, the NPs heated up to 41.6°C within 1 min, suggesting their promise as a magnetic hyperthermia agent. All these findings indicate that CPGF NPs prove to be potential nano-chemotherapeutic agents in breast cancer.

Editor: Alexander V. Ljubimov, Cedars-Sinai Medical Center; UCLA School of Medicine, United States of America

Funding: This work was supported by the Interactive Research School for Health Affairs (IRSHA), Bharati Vidyapeeth University. The funders had no role in study design, data collection and analysis, decision to publish, or preparation of the manuscript.

Competing Interests: The authors have declared that no competing interests exist.

* Email: ruchika.kaulghanekar@gmail.com

Introduction

Breast cancer is the second leading cause of cancer death in women worldwide [1]. The current treatment methods for breast cancer include chemotherapy, radiotherapy, and hormone therapy, which are used alone or in combination [2]. Despite advanced research in diagnostics and therapeutics, the associated side effects [3] as well as the recurrence [4] remain a few inevitable challenges in breast cancer therapy.

Recently, lot of research is being focussed towards the use of herbal medicines to minimize the side effects associated with conventional cancer therapy [5]. Medicinal plants are the valuable sources of anti-cancer bioactives such as curcumin, vinblastine, vincristine, paclitaxel, cinnamaldehyde, capsaicin, wogonin, berberine, artemisinin and so on, which have been shown to suppress and/or prevent cancer [6,7]. However, most of these compounds are hydrophobic in nature and thus show decreased bioavailability [8]. This could be overcome by conjugating these herbal bioactives with biocompatible drug delivery agents that would improve their therapeutic efficacy [9,10].

Cinnamaldehyde, a major bioactive component of the spice cinnamon has been reported to exhibit diverse biological functions including anticancer activity [11,12,13] (Table S1 in File S1). We have also previously reported the anticancer activity of cinnamaldehyde, however, at higher doses [12]. The therapeutic efficacy of cinnamaldehyde is limited due to its low water solubility [14]. This calls attention for drug delivery systems that would not only enhance the drug bioavailability without affecting its bioactivity but would also help in the targeted delivery of cinnamaldehyde at a lower dose.

The superparamagnetic nanoparticles (Fe_3O_4 MNPs) represent one of the most promising biocompatible nanomaterials that can be guided under an external magnetic field for magnetotherapy [15]. Magnetite nanoparticles (Fe_3O_4) have been loaded with different anticancer drugs including doxorubicin, daunorubicin, 5-bromotetrandrine [16,17,18], anti-HER2 immunoliposomes [19] and so on to evaluate their therapeutic potential in breast cancer. MNPs have also been loaded with natural herbal bioactives such as artesunate, silibinin, gambogic acid, tetrandrine, wogonin, curcumin, gallic acid and genistein; and studied for their anticancer efficacy as well as enhancement of bioavailability in cancer cells (Table S2 in File S1). Such studies reveal that the tagged bioactives possess enhanced efficacy than the free drug in terms of MIC and IC_{50} values. MNPs have been widely used for the drug delivery of anticancer agents because of their target specificity and sustained-release properties [15]. The property of target orientation of MNPs helps to reduce the systemic toxicity induced by the chemotherapeutic drugs [20].

In the present report, we have tagged cinnamaldehyde with Fe_3O_4 NPs that had been previously capped with glycine and pluronic polymer (CPGF NPs) to increase its therapeutic efficacy in breast cancer cells. CPGF NPs were initially characterized for their size, morphology, bonding properties and magnetism. They were analyzed for their drug loading and release profiles, stability and biocompatibility. CPGF NPs induced cytotoxicity in breast cancer cell lines at lower doses of cinnamaldehyde compared to the free cinnamaldehyde, thereby showing increased bioavailability in the cells. They also altered the growth kinetics of the cancer cells in a dose-dependent manner. The NPs reduced the migration capability of the cancer cells through reduction in the expression of MMP-2 along with decrease in a pro-angiogenesis marker, VEGF. The NPs also induced apoptosis in breast cancer cells through loss of mitochondrial membrane potential and increase in caspase-3 expression. Moreover, the RF studies indicated the potential of CPGF NPs in hyperthermia applications as well.

Materials and Methods

Chemicals and materials

The chemicals for synthesis, $FeSO_4.7H_2O$, $Fe(NO_3)_3$, NH_4OH, glycine and pluronic F-127, were procured from Merck. Dulbecco's Modified Eagle's Medium (DMEM), penicillin/streptomycin and L-glutamine were obtained from Gibco BRL, CA, USA. Cinnamaldehyde, foetal bovine serum (FBS), 3-(4, 5-dimethylthiazol-2-yl)-2, 5-diphenylthiazolium bromide (MTT), FCCP and JC-1 were procured from Sigma-Aldrich (St. Louis, MO, USA). Neutral red and potassium ferrocyanide were obtained from Sd Fine-Chem. Ltd. Mumbai, India. Antibodies against caspase-3, VEGF and α-tubulin were purchased from Santa Cruz Biotechnology, Inc. (Santa Cruz, CA, USA). All other common reagents were procured from Qualigens fine chemicals (Mumbai, India).

Cell culture

Tissue culture plasticware was purchased from BD Biosciences (CA, USA). MDAMB231, MCF7, MCF10A and HEK 293 were obtained from National Centre for Cell Science (NCCS), Pune. The cells were grown in DMEM supplemented with 2 mM L-glutamine, 100 units/ml of penicillin/streptomycin, and 10% fetal bovine serum (FBS). They were incubated in a humidified 5% CO_2 incubator at 37°C.

Synthesis of iron oxide (F), glycine capped (GF), Glycine and Pluronic stabilized (PGF) and cinnamaldehyde tagged (CPGF) NPs

1. Iron oxide (F) nanoparticle synthesis. Pure iron oxide nanoparticles were synthesized by co-precipitation of ferric and ferrous salts in oxygen free atmosphere at ambient temperature [21]. 100 ml of water containing $FeSO_4.7H_2O$ (0.556 g, 1 mM) and $Fe(NO_3)_3$ (1.636 g, 2 mM) (1:2 molar ratio) was magnetically stirred at 800 rpm under N_2 protection at 80°C for 20 min into a three-necked, round-bottomed flask in a rotamantle (Remi, India). To this solution, 50 ml of 30% ammonia was added slowly by a drop funnel and the speed was increased to 1200 rpm in order to uniformly precipitate magnetic nanoparticles. The colour of the suspension immediately turned black, indicating the formation of magnetite. The resulting solution was stirred for another 20 min followed by rapid cooling to room temperature using an ice bath to prevent further particle growth. The resulting black precipitate was collected with a strong magnet and the supernatant was removed from the precipitate by decantation. The slurry was washed four times with distilled water (DW) to remove excess ammonia and was monitored by a pH drop from 10 to 7. The nanoparticles were re-suspended in 25 ml water and centrifuged at 1000 rpm to remove larger aggregates. These F NPs were characterized and used for biological experiments.

2. Glycine capped iron oxide (GF) nanoparticle synthesis. Similar to the method described above, glycine capped iron oxide nanoparticles were synthesized by co-precipitation of $FeSO_4.7H_2O$ (0.556 g, 1 mM), $Fe(NO_3)_3$ (1.636 g, 2 mM) (1:2 molar ratio) along with glycine (3 g, 0.4 M). The synthesis method and conditions were same as that for bare iron oxide nanoparticles. These GF NPs were characterized and used for biological experiments.

3. Glycine capped pluronic stabilized iron oxide (PGF) nanoparticle synthesis. GF NPs were further coated with pluronic by adding 500 mg pluronic to get a thin coating. The mixture containing $FeSO_4.7H_2O$, $Fe(NO_3)_3$, glycine, ammonia and pluronic was stirred for another 20 min followed by rapid cooling. NPs were washed with DW as described earlier. To ensure complete coating of glycine and pluronic over the nanoparticles, the slurry obtained above was further subjected to sonication for 5 min followed by stirring for 1 h. The NPs were re-suspended in 25 ml water and centrifuged at 1000 rpm to remove larger aggregates. These PGF NPs were characterized and used for biological experiments.

4. Cinnamaldehyde tagged iron oxide (CPGF) nanoparticle synthesis. Briefly, PGF NPs were suspended in 25 ml of absolute ethanol. To this mixture, 0.1 M cinnamaldehyde in 1 ml of ethanol was added and then it was vortexed for 1 h. The solution was magnetically stirred overnight at 900 rpm to complete the reaction. After the magnetic separation, the particles were re-suspended in different grades of ethanol (100%, 70%, 50%) and finally in 25 ml DW. The suspension was centrifuged at 1000 rpm to remove larger aggregates. The final CPGF NPs were used for either biological experiments or were vacuum dried to fine powder that was used for physical characterization.

Physical characterization

The magnetic nanoparticles (F, GF, PGF and CPGF) were vacuum dried to obtain fine powder and used for the physical characterization by X-ray diffraction (XRD), Fourier transform infrared (FTIR) spectroscopy, thermo-gravimetric analysis (TGA), and vibrating sample magnetometry (VSM). Determination of phase purity and identification of NPs was done by XRD using powder diffractometer (Shimadzu, Physics Department, Pune University, Pune) with Cu radiation, operating at 40 kV and 40 mA. For TEM analysis, the colloidal solutions of NPs were ultrasonicated for 15 min. Bonding patterns of all the NPs were studied by FTIR (Shimadzu IR Infinity, Physics department, Pune University, Pune) and the data was acquired between 4000 and 400 cm^{-1}. Percentage of cinnamaldehyde loaded onto the CPGF NPs was evaluated by TGA. The magnetic property of samples was analyzed using a Physical Property Measurement System (PPMS) from Quantum Design Inc., San Diego, California equipped with a 9 Tesla superconducting magnet. Magnetizations versus magnetic field (M–H) measurements were performed by a VSM attachment by using accurate amount of the samples packed inside a plastic sample holder. M–H loops were recorded at a rate of 75 Oe/s in a field sweep from − 10 to 10 kOe at the vibrating frequency of 40 Hz at 300 K. Radiofrequency absorption was carried out with a 20-MHz oscillator at a fixed nominal power of 100 W.

Colloidal stability

The colloidal stability of NPs was analyzed by measuring UV-VIS absorbance. All the NPs of 100 μg/ml concentration were taken either in distilled water (DW) or in phosphate buffer saline (PBS) or in cell culture medium DMEM with or without 10% FBS [22]. Stability of NPs was determined by measuring the absorbance of each solution at 540 nm, as a function of time (t).

Drug release

As-prepared CPGF NPs (50 mg) were put into a 12 kDa cut-off dialysis bag (Sigma-Aldrich, St. Louis, MO, USA) which was immersed into 100 ml of 50 mM sodium acetate buffer having either pH 5.2 or pH 7.4. The whole assembly was stirred for 24 h. The drug release was measured by taking out 1 ml solution at regular intervals of 1, 2, 4 and 24 h and analyzed for UV-VIS absorbance [23] at 290 nm, the absorbance maximum of cinnamaldehyde [24].

Biocompatibility

The Institutional Ethical Committee Bharati Vidyapeeth University Medical College specifically approved this study. Fresh human whole blood (5 ml) was obtained from a healthy donor and centrifuged at 1000 rpm for 15 min to separate RBCs that were washed with saline and diluted to 1:4 ratio. Saline was used as a negative control and distilled water was used as a positive control. Different concentrations of CPGF NPs (0.5, 1, 5 and 10 mg/ml) were mixed with 1:4 diluted blood sample and incubated at 37°C for 30 min. The tubes were centrifuged at 3000 rpm for 5 min, the supernatant was collected and optical density (OD) was determined at 545 nm. The hemolysis rate (HR) was calculated using the mean OD for each group as follows:

$$HR\,(\%) = \frac{OD\ treated - OD\ negative\ control}{OD\ positive\ control - OD\ negative\ control} \times 100$$

The samples were referred [25] to be highly hemocompatibile for HR <5%, hemocompatible for HR <10%, and non-hemocompatible for HR>20%. If HR was less than 5%, the sample would have no hemolytic reaction and thus would be considered as hemocompatibile.

Uptake of CPGF NPs into the breast cancer cells

The internalization of CPGF NPs into the cells was qualitatively evaluated by Prussian blue staining as described previously [26]. MDAMB231 and MCF7 were seeded on coverslips in 6-well plates at a seeding density of 1×10^5 cells/ml. Next day, the cells were treated with CPGF NPs for 24 h. Post treatment, the cells were fixed with 4% paraformaldehyde for 20 min at room temperature. Cells were washed twice with 1X PBS. The coverslips were immersed in Prussian blue stain which was prepared by mixing equal volumes of 20% aqueous solution of HCl and 10% aqueous solution of potassium ferrocyanide [$K_4Fe(CN)_6.3H_2O$] for 20 min. The cells were counterstained with neutral red for 5 min. The stained cells were photographed with Sony DSC-S75 cyber-shot camera under 40X objective.

MTT assay

The effect of CPGF NPs on the viability of MDAMB231, MCF7, MCF10A and HEK 293 was analyzed by using MTT dye [26]. The cells were seeded at 1×10^5 cells/ml density in 96-well plates (Axygen TPP, CA, USA). After 24 h, the cells were incubated with fresh medium containing different concentrations (0–320 μg/ml) of NPs and the plates were further incubated for 24 h. The MTT solution (5 mg/ml) was added to each well, followed by 4 h incubation at 37°C in 5% CO_2 incubator. The intensity of colored formazan derivative was determined by measuring optical density (OD) with the ELISA microplate reader (Biorad, Hercules, CA) at 570 nm ($OD_{570-630\ nm}$). The cell viability was expressed in terms of percentage as

$$\%\ Viability = \frac{Cell\ treated\ with\ CPGF\ NPs}{Untreated\ control\ cells} \times 100$$

Cell growth analysis

Growth kinetics of breast cancer cells was monitored by cell growth assay [27]. MCF7 and MDAMB231 were seeded at a density of 1×10^5 cells/ml in 24-well plates. Next day, the cells were treated with different concentrations (0–5 μg/ml for MDAMB231 and 0–40 μg/ml for MCF7) of CPGF NPs. The cells were harvested and counted for viability using trypan blue dye exclusion method for 24, 48 and 72 h.

Soft agar assay

The assay was performed using the method as reported previously [26]. Briefly, 5×10^3 cells/ml treated with or without different concentrations of CPGF NPs (0–5 μg/ml for MDAMB231 and 0–40 μg/ml for MCF7) were mixed with 0.35% agarose (DNA grade, GIBCO BRL, CA, USA) at 40°C in culture medium. The mixture was poured onto a previously gelled layer of 0.5% agarose in culture medium in 6-well plates and allowed to solidify. After incubation for 10 days in 5% CO_2 incubator at 37°C, the colonies were counted using an Axiovert 200 M microscope (Carl Zeiss, Germany).

Wound healing assay

The migration potential of breast cancer cells was analyzed by the wound healing assay [27]. MDAMB231 and MCF7 cells were plated at a seeding density of 5×10^5 cells/ml in 24-well plates and grown overnight at 37°C in 5% CO_2 incubator. An artificial wound was made with 10 μl micropipette after 6 h serum starvation in control as well as cells treated with different concentrations of CPGF NPs (0–5 μg/ml for MDAMB231 and

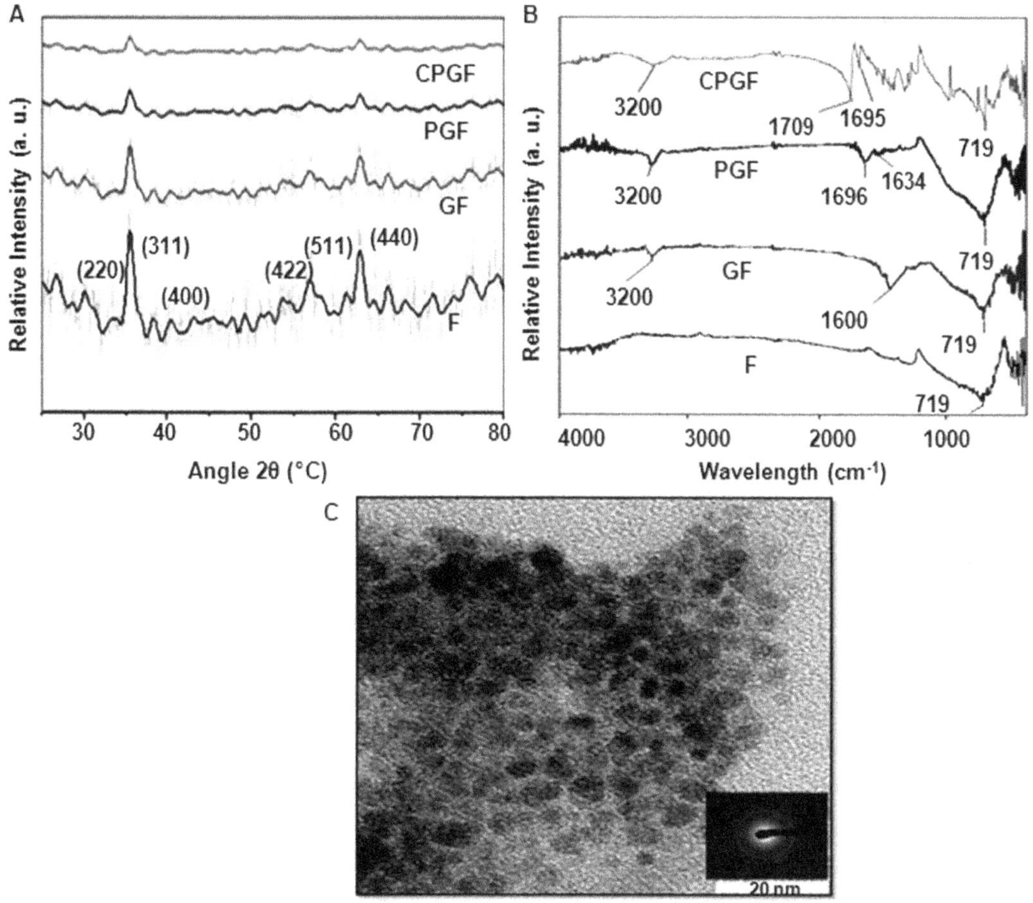

Figure 1. Physical characterization of CPGF NPs. (**A**) XRD patterns of F, GF, PGF and CPGF NPs. (**B**) TEM image with SAED of CPGF NPs. (**C**) FTIR patterns of F, GF, PGF and CPGF NPs.

0–40 μg/ml for MCF7). The cells were incubated for 18 h in a humidified chamber at 37°C and 5% CO_2 atmosphere. Images of migrating cells were obtained by 10X phase objective of an inverted microscope using Sony DSC-S75 cyber-shot camera at 0 and 18 h.

Gelatin zymography

The gelatin zymography was performed to detect the presence of extracellular MMP-2. The conditioned medium of control as well as cells treated with different concentrations of CPGF NPs (0–5 μg/ml for MDAMB231 and 0–40 μg/ml for MCF7) was collected and concentrated [27] in Centricon YM-30 tubes (Millipore, MA). All the samples, containing equal amount of total proteins, were mixed with sample buffer (2% SDS, 25% glycerol, 0.1% bromophenol blue and 60 mM Tris- HCl pH 6.8). The samples were then diluted again with sample buffer in 1:2 ratio. Equal volume of the resulting mixture was then loaded onto 7.5% SDS-polyacrylamide gel containing gelatin (0.5 mg/ml). The gel was washed twice with 0.25% Triton X-100 and incubated overnight in incubation buffer (150 mM NaCl, 100 mM $CaCl_2$, 50 mM Tris-HCl pH 7.5, 1% Triton X-100, 0.02% NaN_3) at 37°C. The gel was stained with staining solution (0.1% Coomassie Brilliant blue R-250 in 40% isopropanol) and destained in 7% acetic acid. Gelatinolytic activity was detected as unstained bands against a blue background. The quantitation of bands in control and treated samples was performed by densitometric analysis using Image J gel analysis tool.

Mitochondrial membrane potential

Both the breast cancer cell lines were seeded at a density of 1×10^5 cells/ml in a black 96-well plate and incubated at 37°C in a CO_2 incubator. Next day, the cells were treated with different concentrations of CPGF NPs (0–5 μg/ml for MDAMB231 and 0–40 μg/ml for MCF7) and were incubated in a CO_2 incubator at 37°C for 24 h. Following day, the medium was removed and the cells were washed with 1X PBS and incubated with 2.5 μg/ml JC-1 staining solution for 1 h in the dark. Fluorescence readings were measured using the Fluostar Omega microplate reader (BMG Labtech) at 520 nm for JC-1 monomers and at 590 nm for JC-1 aggregates.

Immunoblotting

Protein expression was evaluated by western blotting as reported previously [27]. Briefly, the cells were seeded at a density of 5×10^5 cells/ml and treated next day with or without different concentrations of CPGF NPs (0–5 μg/ml for MDAMB231 and 0–40 μg/ml for MCF7). The cells were centrifuged and the pellet was resuspended in 80 μl lysis buffer containing 50 mM Tris (pH 7.4), 5 mM EDTA, 0.5% NP40, 50 mM NaF, 1 mM DTT, 0.1 mM PMSF, 0.5 μg/ml leupeptin (Pro-pure Amersco, Solon, USA), 1 μg/ml pepstatin (Amresco, Solon, USA), 150 mM NaCl,

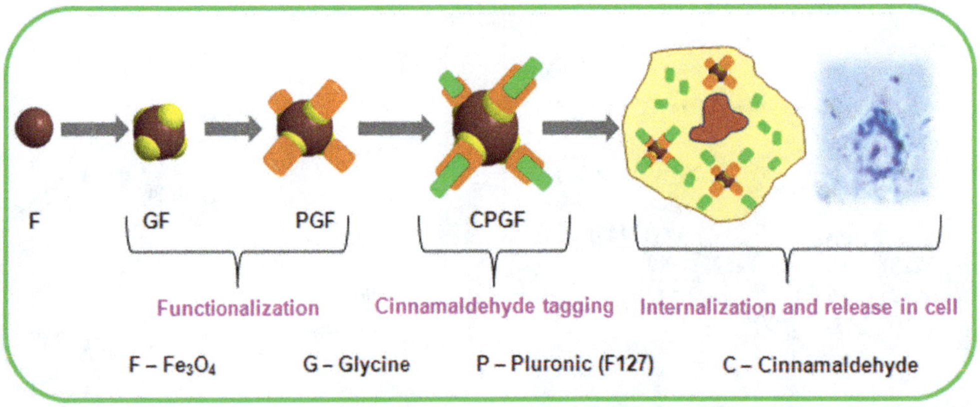

Figure 2. Schematic illustration of synthesis of CPGF NPs and their release in breast cancer cell.

0.5 μg/ml aprotinin (Amersco, Solon, USA) and protease inhibitor cocktail (Roche, Lewes, UK) followed by incubation on ice for 1 h with intermittent mixing. The cell extract was centrifuged for 20 min at 4°C at 12000 rpm to remove the debris. The protein was estimated using Bradford reagent (Biorad Laboratories Inc, CA, USA). Equal amount of protein was loaded onto a 10% SDS-polyacrylamide gel and transferred electrophoretically to Amersham Hybond-P PVDF membrane (GE Healthcare, UK) in sodium phosphate buffer (pH 6.8). The membrane was blocked in 5% BSA in TST and incubated at room temperature for 30 min with rabbit polyclonal primary antibody for VEGF (sc-507) and caspase-3 (sc-7148) whereas mouse

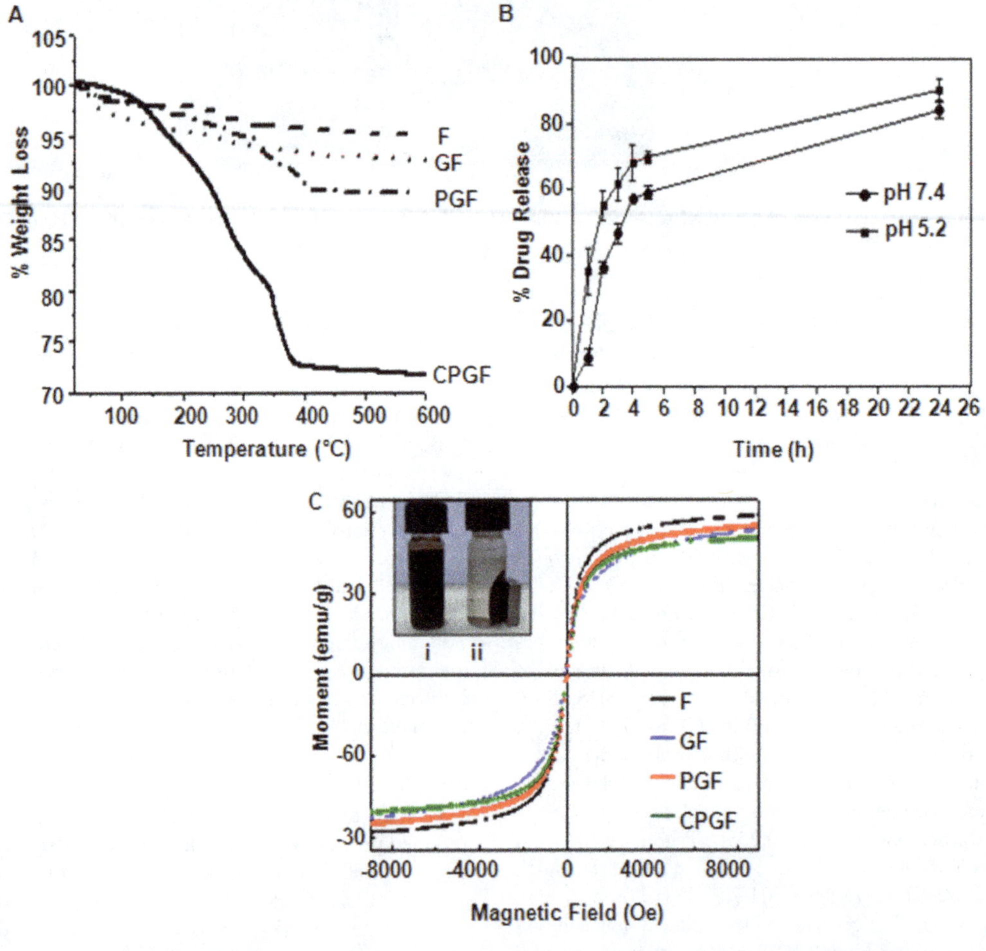

Figure 3. Cinnamaldehyde loading and release profiles along with magnetic behavior of CPGF NPs. (**A**) Thermogravimetric analysis of F, GF, PGF and CPGF NPs. (**B**) Release profile of cinnamaldehyde from CPGF NPs at different pH values at different time points. (**C**) Inset shows uniform suspension of CPGF NPs (i) and (ii) response of the NPs to the externally placed magnet. VSM data shows the magnetic behavior of all the NPs.

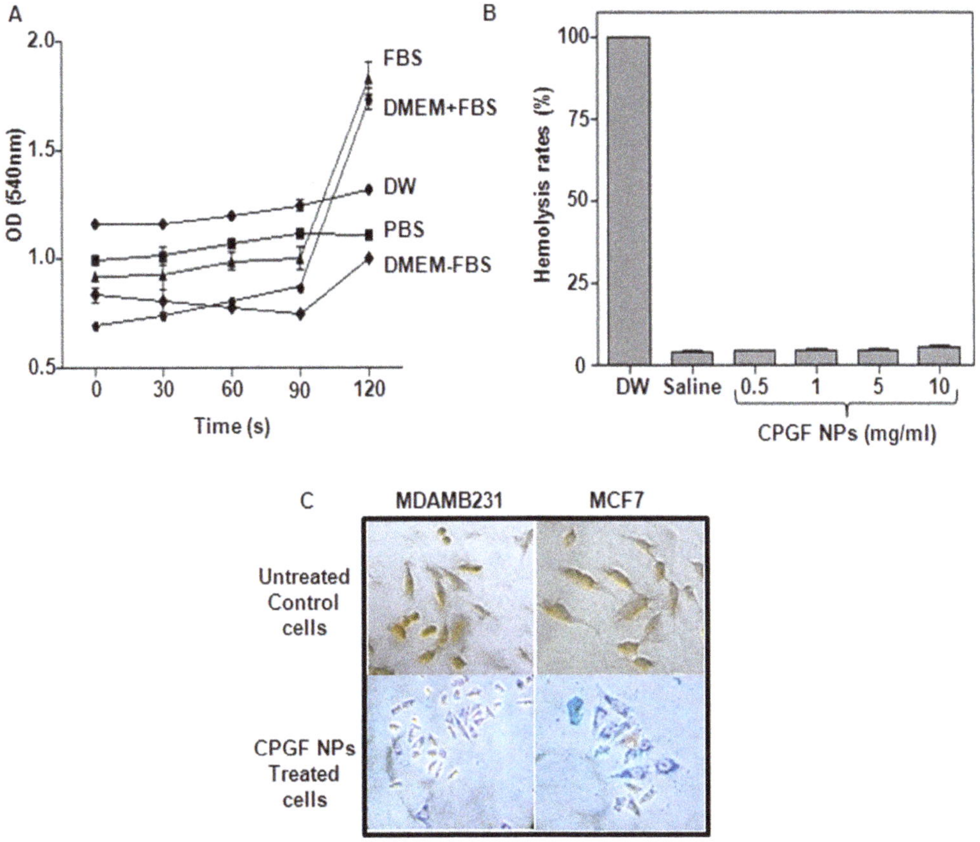

Figure 4. Stability, biocompatibility and uptake of CPGF NPs. (**A**) Stability of CPGF NPs in different solutions was monitored by UV-vis spectroscopy. The data is presented as mean±SD of three independent experiments at $p<0.0001$, indicating statistically significant differences between different solutions. (**B**) Biocompatibility of CPGF NPs performed in freshly prepared human blood. DW and saline were used as positive and negative controls, respectively. The data is presented as mean±SD of three independent experiments at $p<0.001$, indicating statistically significant differences compared to positive control group. (**C**) In vitro uptake of CPGF NPs in MDAMB231 and MCF7, shown by Prussian blue staining, and compared with their respective untreated control cells. The stained cells were photographed with Sony DSC-S75 cyber-shot camera.

monoclonal primary antibody for α- tubulin (sc-5286) (Santacruz, CA, USA), at 1:500 dilutions. The membrane was washed in TST and incubated with respective secondary IgG HRP conjugate at 1:2500 dilution. Proteins were visualized using a chemilluminiscence kit (Amersham ECL Advance western blotting detection kit, GE Healthcare, UK) and densitometric analysis was performed on scanned immunoblot images using the ImageJ (NIH, USA) gel analysis tool.

Statistical analysis

All the experiments were performed in triplicates and repeated thrice. The data has been presented as mean±SD. Statistical analysis was performed with the Graph Pad prism 4 program using one-way ANOVA. The IC_{50} values were calculated by the formula, $Y = 100 \times A1/(X+A1)$, where $A1 = IC_{50}$, Y = response ($Y = 100\%$ when $X = 0$) and X = inhibitory concentration using KyPlot version 2.0 beta 13 (32 bit). The p values used for comparisons were <0.05.

Results and Discussion

Characterization of CPGF NPs

CPGF NPs were characterized by different techniques such as XRD, FTIR, TEM and VSM. Figure 1A indicates powder diffraction patterns of F, GF, PGF and CPGF NPs, which clearly suggest that iron oxide surface was sequentially modified with glycine, pluronic and cinnamaldehyde. These compositions exhibited characteristic magnetite peaks (2θ) at 30.1, 36.2, 42.4, 52.5, 57.5 and 62.2° corresponding to (220), (311), (400), (422), (511) and (440) planes, respectively (JCPDS card no. 01-088-0315), observed for face centered cubic (fcc) lattice structure of iron oxide [26]. It was significant to note that only magnetite phase was formed during the synthesis of all the iron oxide preparations since diffraction peaks corresponding to other phases such as α-Fe_2O_3 (hematite) or γ-Fe_2O_3 (maghamite) were found to be absent. The average crystallite size of all the compositions, as calculated from Scherrer equation, was in the range of 10–20 nm. TEM of CPGF NPs (Figure 1B) showed the particle size to be around 20 nm that had gradually increased from ~5 nm for bare Fe_3O_4 (F) (Figure S1 in File S1) after successive tagging of different moieties onto the NPs. The increase in size of the NPs from F to CPGF corroborated with the observed XRD pattern.

Figure 1C shows the FTIR spectra of F, GF, PGF and CPGF NPs. The basic Fe-O stretch (~719 cm^{-1}) was invariably present in all the compositions, clearly reflecting the capping of organic molecules onto the nanoparticle surface. Upon capping of glycine, a broad peak around 3200 cm^{-1} appeared depicting the presence of hydroxy/amino groups on the surface of Fe_3O_4 NPs. A strong absorption at 1600 cm^{-1} in GF originated from carboxyl stretch of glycine moiety. The capping of glycine to Fe_3O_4 NPs occurred

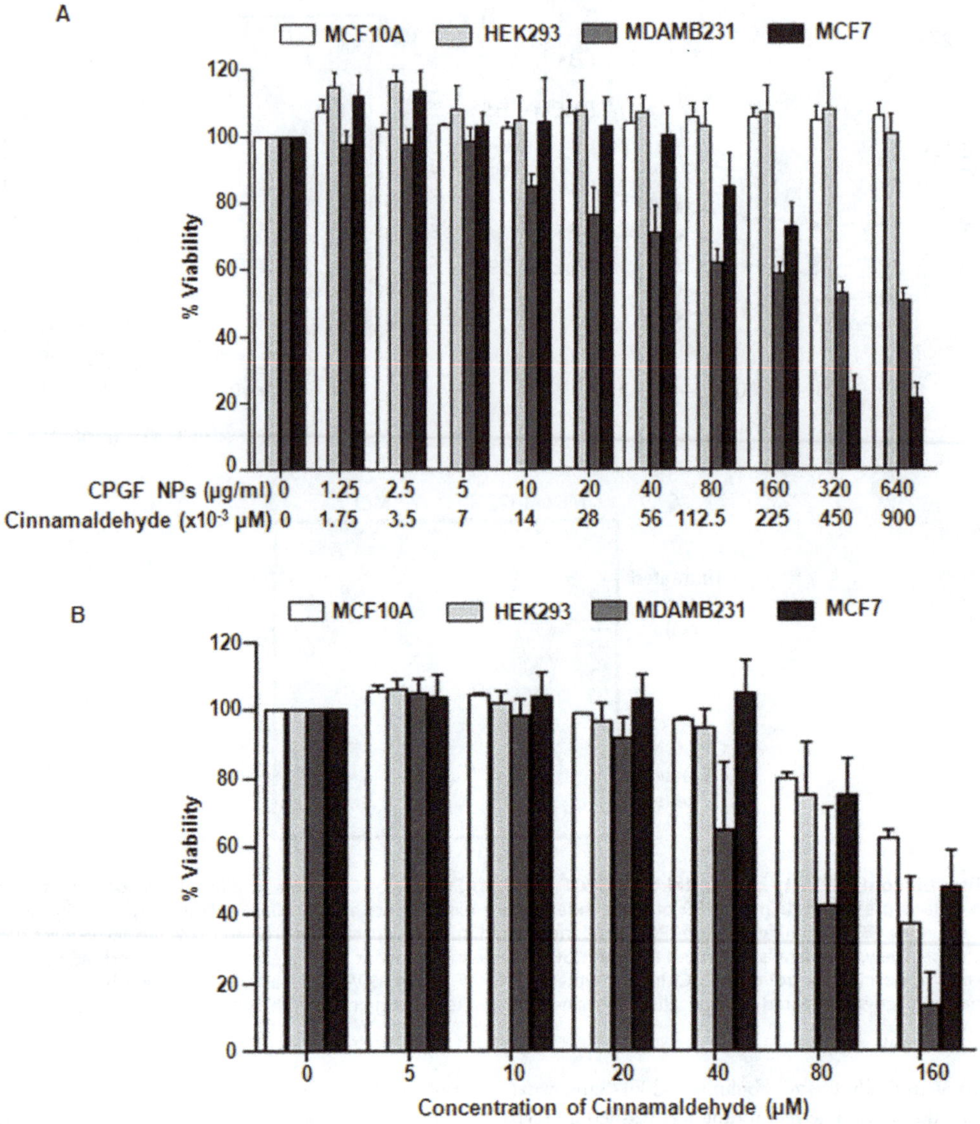

Figure 5. Cytotoxicity analysis of CPGF NPs and cinnamaldehyde. The breast cancer (MDAMB231 and MCF7) and non-cancerous (MCF10A and HEK293) cells were treated with different concentrations of (**A**) CPGF NPs and (**B**) cinnamaldehyde for 24 h and anlayzed for viability by MTT assay. Lower panel of X-axis in (**A**) refers to amount of cinnamaldehyde (μM) present in the corresponding concentrations of CPGF NPs (μg/ml) (as calculated from TGA data). All the data are presented as mean±SD of five independent experiments at $p<0.0001$, indicating statistically significant differences compared to the control untreated group.

due to electrostatic interaction between positively charged Fe_3O_4 and negatively charged glycine. It was interesting to note that, in PGF, signatures at 3200 cm^{-1} and ~1600 cm^{-1} persisted even after the addition of pluronic. The presence of these signatures, though with a reduced intensity, indicated the attachment of pluronic to GF through hydrogen bond. The remarkable shift of –C=C– and –C=O signatures from 1696 cm^{-1} and 1634 cm^{-1} in PGF towards higher energy side at 1709 and 1695 cm^{-1}, respectively, in CPGF, indicated binding of cinnamaldehyde to PGF. Thus, after binding to the hydrophobic end of pluronic, cinnamaldehyde formed a stable electrostatic interaction as is evident from the near merging of the peaks. The FTIR spectra of glycine (G) (Figure S2 in File S1), pluronic (P) (Figure S3 in File S1) and cinnamaldehyde (C) (Figure S4 in File S1) have been given in supplementary information (File S1). Figure 2 depicts the synthesis of CPGF NPs and their release in breast cancer cell. Pluronic F127 has been known to be a versatile polymer for water dispersibility [28]. F127 consists of a hydrophobic (polypropylene, PPO) chain that electrostatically interacts with the hydrophobic cinnamaldehyde whereas the hydrophilic (polyethylene glycol, PEO) end binds to glycine through electrostatic association between –OH end of F127 and $-NH_2$ end of glycine. This generates additional hydrophilicity and stability to the CPGF system.

TGA was performed to quantify the amount of different coatings onto the surface of Fe_3O_4 NPs. Figure 3A shows the stepwise weight loss for all the NPs. Negligible weight loss of ~3.8% in F NPs corresponded to the adsorbed moisture between 100 and 200°C. GF NPs showed weight loss of ~5% starting from 100–300°C that confirmed efficient glycine capping. Due to the addition of pluronic in GF, a two-step weight loss corresponding to ~9.1% was observed in the temperature range of 150–400°C. A pronounced weight loss of ~27.2% was observed in CPGF NPs

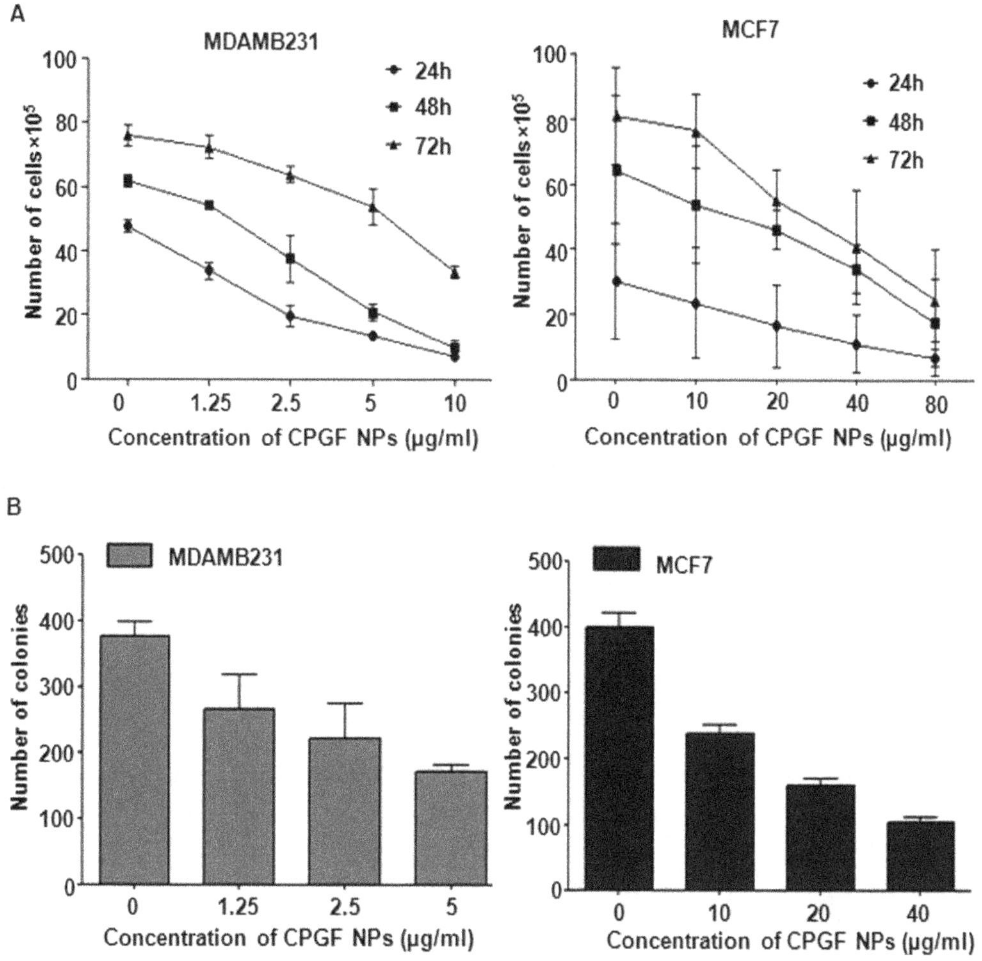

Figure 6. CPGF NPs decrease the growth kinetics of breast cancer cells. (**A**) The NPs decreased the number of cells in MDAMB231 and MCF7, indicated by cell growth assay. Cells were counted from the four quadrants and the average of each has been plotted. The data represents mean±SD of three independent experiments at $p<0.0001$ indicating statistically significant differences compared to the control untreated group. (**B**) Reduction in the number of soft agar colonies was observed in MDAMB231 and MCF7 after treatment with CPGF NPs. Colonies were counted from at least 10 different areas and the average of each has been plotted. The data represents mean±SD of three independent experiments at $p<0.0001$ indicating statistically significant differences compared to the control untreated group.

that occurred in three-steps in the temperature range from 100–400°C. It could be due to the removal of glycine, pluronic and cinnamaldehyde successfully from the CPGF NPs. Thus, the amount of cinnamaldehyde loaded onto the Fe_3O_4 nanoparticles was found to be about 18.1%.

Figure 3B shows release kinetics of cinnamaldehyde in sodium acetate buffer at pH 5.2 and 7.4 that was analyzed by UV-vis spectroscopy. The drug release kinetics of the NPs was studied to analyze the fate of cinnamaldehyde in a) acidic pH, usually present in the tumor microenvironment and b) physiological pH, corresponding to the body fluids [29]. At both pH values, CPGF NPs showed a short burst release of cinnamaldehyde during initial 4 h, followed by a sustained release profile with increased time periods. Due to electrostatic interaction of cinnamaldehyde with PGF system, it could get easily detached from the CPGF NPs resulting into faster release. The rate of release was found to be slightly more at lower pH that could be attributed to ionic interaction of free aldehyde group of cinnamaldehyde with the liberated protons under acidic conditions. The higher rate of payload release in acidic pH is a good indicator of the efficacy of the system to deliver the drug at the tumor site.

The inset of Figure 3C shows uniform suspension of CPGF NPs (i); upon exposure to the external magnet, the NPs got attracted towards the side of the glass vial, leaving behind a clear suspension (ii). Upon removal of the magnetic field, the NPs got re-dispersed into the clear solution, suggesting their magnetic nature. The magnetic properties of CPGF NPs were further analyzed by VSM at 300 K.

Figure 3C depicts the hysteresis loops of F, GF, PGF and CPGF NPs showing zero remanence and coercivity, indicating that the nanoparticles were superparamagnetic in nature. The magnetization reached a saturation point at about 10 kOe, which was found to be strongly dependent upon the organic coating. It is well-known that the saturation magnetization (M_S) decreases with the particle size and also depends on the presence of organic coating on the iron oxide nanoparticles [30]. The M_S value of F NPs was found to be 59.12 emu/g which was less than the reported value of bulk magnetite (92 emu/g) and could be attributed to the small particle size [31]. The M_S value was found to decrease from 59.12 emu/g to 50.97 emu/g (CPGF NPs) with the increase in coatings onto the magnetic core. The NPs capped with glycine (GF) had MS value of 55.7 emu/g that further decreased to

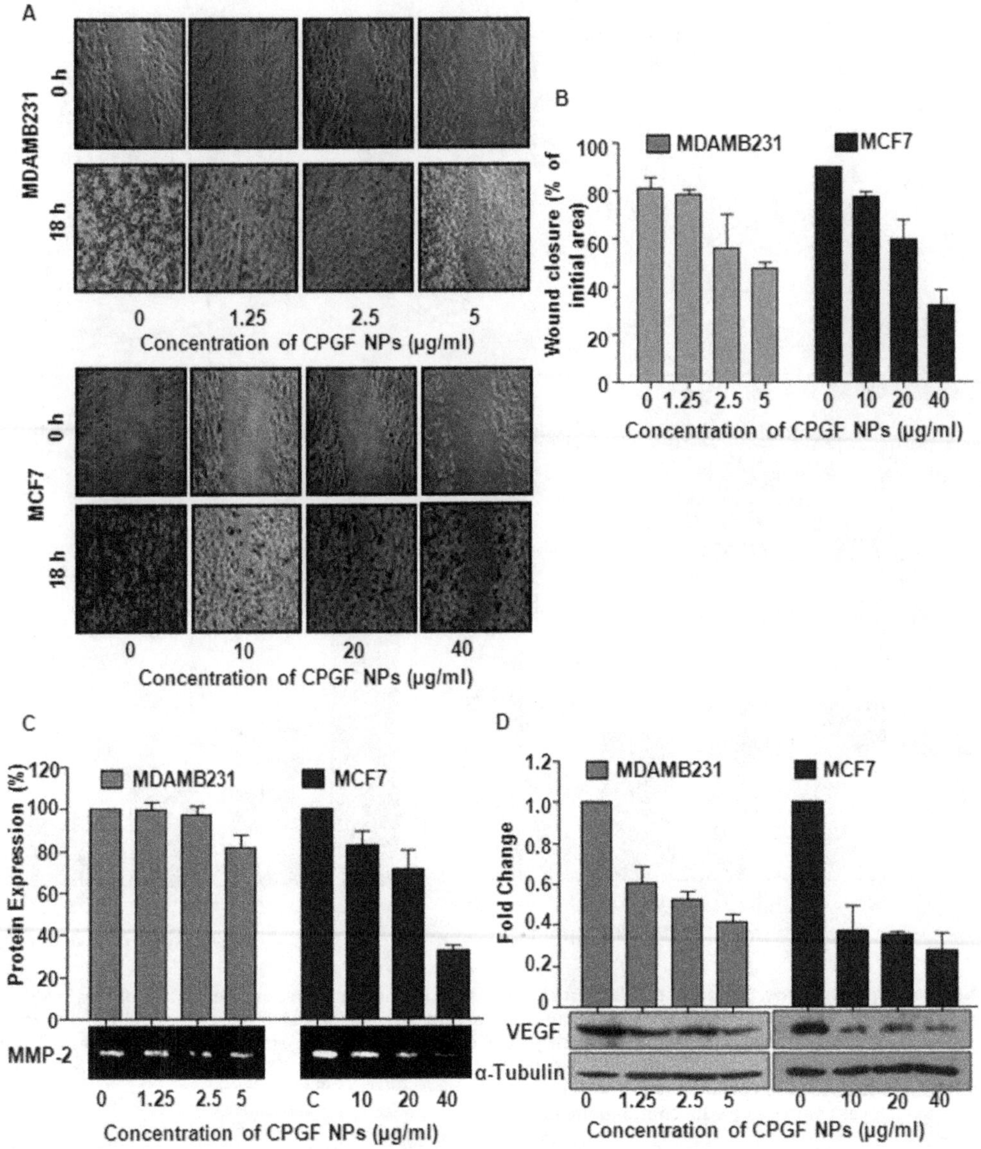

Figure 7. Molecular mechanism underlying anticancer activity of CPGF NPs. CPGF NPs decreased migration and expression of tumor marker proteins in breast cancer cells. (**A**) The NPs reduced migration of MDAMB231 and MCF7 cells. The upper panel of each figure shows the wound made at 0 h and the lower panel shows the migration of cells after 18 h. (**B**) Graphical representation of wound closure in MDAMB231 and MCF7 at 18 h after CPGF NPs treatment. Values are represented as mean±SD of three independent experiments at $p<0.01$ for MDAMB231 and $p<0.0005$ for MCF7, indicating statistically significant differences compared to the untreated control cells. (**C**) Gelatin zymography shows downregulation of MMP-2 expression in MDAMB231 and MCF7 after treatment with CPGF NPs with their corresponding densitometric analysis. The values are represented as mean±SD of three independent experiments at $p<0.001$, indicating statistically significant differences compared to the untreated control cells. (**D**) Western blot analysis shows decrease in VEGF expression in MDAMB231 and MCF7 with their corresponding densitometric analysis. Values are represented as mean±SD of three independent experiments with $p<0.0001$, indicating statistically significant differences compared to the untreated control cells.

53.99 emu/g with an addition of pluronic (PGF) on it. This decrease in the M_S value could be attributed to the presence of non-magnetic coatings onto the surface of Fe_3O_4 NPs. The role of glycine and cinnamaldehyde coating was significant as the decrease in M_S value for these two materials was almost similar. Interestingly, after addition of pluronic, there was no significant difference in M_S value, implying that it played a major role in conjugation of cinnamaldehyde with glycine capped iron oxide NPs.

Stability and biocompatibility studies

Stability and biocompatibility of the NPs are important prerequisites for their application in biological domain. The agglomeration of the NPs was examined in different fluids such as DW, PBS, FBS and DMEM (with or without FBS) by measuring their turbidity at 540 nm (Figure 4A). CPGF NPs showed excellent hydrophilicity and were stable in all the tested solutions for 2 h. Interestingly, the NPs showed high colloidal stability in FBS and DMEM supplemented with FBS (Figure 4A) that could be attributed to the adsorption of negatively charged

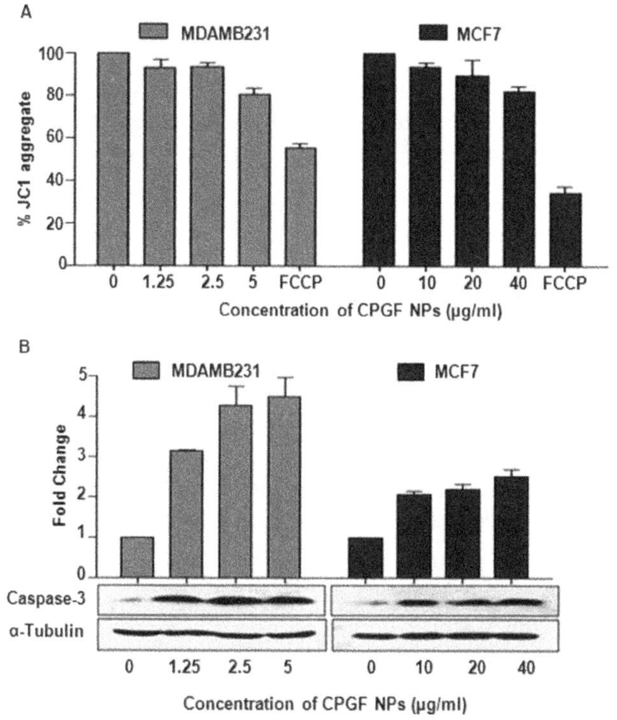

Figure 8. CPGF NPs induce apoptosis in breast cancer cells. (A) CPGF NPs decreased the mitochondrial membrane potential of the breast cancer cell lines as observed by JC-1 staining. The data was analyzed by the MARS data analysis software 2.10R3 (BMG Labtech). All data are presented as means±SD of three independent experiments. $p<0.0001$ indicate statistically significant differences compared to the control untreated group. **(B)** Western blot data shows increase in caspase-3 expressions in both MDAMB231 and MCF7. α-Tubulin was used as a loading control. The histogram depicts densitometric analysis of western blots of caspase-3. Values are represented as mean±SD of three independent experiments. $p<0.001$ indicate statistically significant differences compared to the untreated control cells.

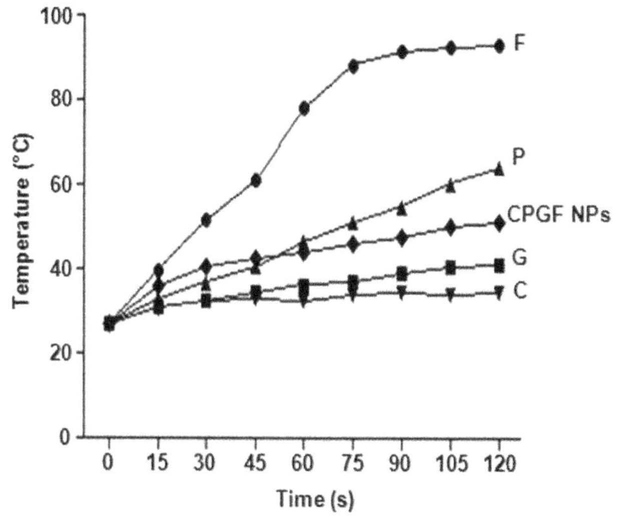

Figure 9. Response of CPGF NPs to the radiofrequency waves for hyperthermia application. CPGF NPs exhibit hyperthermia potential. Response of Fe_3O_4 (F), Glycine (G), Pluronic (P), Cinnamaldehyde (C) and CPGF NPs to the radiofrequency waves have been depicted. The NPs showed a significant rise in the temperature to 41.6°C within a time span of 1 min.

serum proteins onto the Fe_3O_4 core. The NPs were found to be biocompatible with no detectable hemolysis activity (<5%) at concentrations ranging from 0.5–10 mg/ml. Hemolysis rates at 0.5, 1, 5 and 10 mg/ml concentrations of CPGF NPs were found to be 3.36, 3.46, 3.57 and 4.64%, respectively, compared to the DW positive control (100%) and saline negative control (2.91%) (Figure 4B). The uptake of CPGF NPs in the breast cancer cells has been shown in Figure 4C. The blue coloured cytoplasm indicated the presence of Fe^{3+} inside the cells (observed at 40X magnification) whereas the untreated control cells, having no NPs, appeared orange-red in colour. Thus, CPGF NPs depicted a highly stable and biocompatible system.

Growth kinetics of breast cancer cells treated with CPGF NPs

To evaluate whether CPGF system enhanced the bioavailability of cinnamaldehyde in the cancer cells, cytotoxicity assays of the NPs (Figure 5A) as well as F, G and P (Figure S5 in File S1) at different concentrations (0–640 µg/ml), were performed in breast cancer cell lines (MDAMB231 and MCF7). F, G and P were found to be non-toxic to the breast cancer cells (Figure S5 in File S1). However, CPGF NPs (Figure 5A) were found to significantly decrease ($p<0.0001$) the survival of breast cancer cells from 10 and 80 µg/ml concentrations (corresponding to ~0.014 and 0.1 µM concentrations of the cinnamaldehyde, respectively, loaded onto the NPs) in MDAMB231 and MCF7, respectively. Interestingly, the NPs were not toxic to the non-cancerous MCF10A and HEK 293 cells upto 640 µg/ml (containing ~0.9 µM of cinnamaldehyde) (Figure 5A). On the other hand, upon treatment of the cells with different concentrations (0–160 µM) of free cinnamaldehyde (Figure 5B), it induced killing from 40 and 80 µM concentration onwards in MDAMB231 and MCF7, respectively. Such higher concentrations of cinnamaldehyde were also deleterious to the non-cancerous cells, MCF10A and HEK 293. Thus, free cinnamaldehyde was toxic to both the breast cancer as well as the non-cancerous cells at higher doses. However, upon tagging with magnetic nanoparticles, the therapeutic index of cinnamaldehyde was drastically reduced reflecting its increased bioavailability. In MDAMB231 and MCF7 cells, CPGF NPs exhibited IC_{50} of 0.363 and 0.368 µM, respectively (Table S1 in File S1). On the other hand, the free cinnamaldehyde exhibited IC_{50} of 69.81 and 284.7 µM for MDAMB231 and MCF7, respectively. These findings clearly demonstrate that functionalization of MNPs with cinnamaldehyde increased its bioavailability at lower doses, thereby increasing its therapeutic efficacy.

The novelty of CPGF nanoparticulate system was that it exhibited cytotoxicity in both ER/PR positive/Her2 negative (MCF7) and ER/PR negative/Her2 negative (MDAMB231) breast cancer cells, the latter being insensitive to most of the chemotherapeutic drugs [32]. The triple-negative breast cancers (ER/PR^- $Her2^-$) have a more aggressive clinical course than other forms of breast cancer [33]. The lack of ER and PR receptor expression in breast cancer is usually associated with increased visceral metastases, poor prognosis [34,35,36,37] and relatively short relapse-free and overall survival times [33,38,39].Interestingly, compared to MCF7 cells, MDAMB231 showed susceptibility to killing by the NPs at much lower doses (low MIC values) of cinnamaldehyde. It has been reported earlier that 2′-benzoyloxycinnamaldehyde (BCA), a derivative of 2′-hydroxycinnamaldehyde, showed more effective antiproliferation in MDAMB231 than in MCF7 due to increase in the expression of DJ-1 protein in the latter [40]. This protein is known to protect the cancer cells from oxidative stress *via* translocalizing into mitochondria and stabilizing mitochondrial permeability and thus increase in its expression in MCF7 cells could explain their resistance to BCA treatment. The same reason could explain the observed difference in sensitivity of MCF7 and MDAMB231 towards CPGF NPs.

Based on the cytotoxicity data, we used non-killing doses of CPGF NPs, (0–10 μg/ml for MDAMB231 and 0–40 μg/ml for MCF7) for further biological assays. The effect of different concentrations of CPGF NPs was analyzed on the growth of breast cancer cells for 24–72 h. Figure 6A shows a dose-dependent decrease in the growth kinetics of MDAMB231 and MCF7 cells ($p<0.0001$) at 24–72 h. This was supported by a dose-dependent decrease in the number of soft agar colonies in both the cell lines (Figure 6B). Thus CPGF NPs significantly restricted the growth of breast cancer cells in vitro.

Mechanism of anticancer potential of CPGF NPs

Cinnamaldehyde has been reported to control various processes involved in the malignant transformation of cells, such as cell proliferation, invasion and migration that are the key steps in metastasis, one of the major causes of mortality in cancer [41]. To examine the effect of CPGF NPs on cell migration, we performed wound healing assay on confluent monolayers of breast cancer cell lines (Figure 7A). After 18 h, the untreated control cells covered up ~85% of the wound, whereas at 5 and 40 μg/ml concentrations of CPGF NPs, MDAMB231 and MCF7 cells covered up the wound by ~47 and 32%, respectively ($p = 0.0005$) (Figure 7A, B). Thus, the NPs were found to decrease the migration of breast cancer cells in a dose- and time-dependent manner.

MMPs, a family of zinc and calcium-dependent enzymes, are known to degrade extracellular matrix proteins resulting into basement membrane degradation that ultimately leads to metastasis [42]. Since MMP-2 significantly contributes towards the invasive property of the cancer cells, we evaluated its expression in the cells treated with CPGF NPs. The expression of MMP-2 was found to be significantly down-regulated ($p \leq 0.001$) in both MDAMB231 and MCF7 (Figure 7C), thereby suggesting that the NPs inhibited the migration of breast cancer cells through reduction in MMP-2 expression.

VEGF, an oncoprotein responsible for angiogenesis in cancer cells, plays an important role in tumor metastasis by mediating the formation of lymphatic vessels [43]. VEGF and MMP2 proteins have been reported to be positively correlated with each other in various cancers, including breast cancer and have been proposed to be potential tumor markers [44]. VEGF has been known to not only stimulate the proliferation and migration of endothelial cells, but also to activate the inactive pro-MMPs to active MMPs [45]. The latter in turn degrade the vascular basal membrane and ECM proteins, resulting into the migration of endothelial cells and formation of new blood vessels [42]. We found that CPGF NPs significantly down-regulated ($p<0.0001$) the expression of VEGF in both the breast cancer cell lines in a dose-dependent manner compared to the untreated control cells (Figure 7D).

Cinnamaldehyde has been reported to induce apoptosis via caspase-3 activation. Since CPGF NPs altered the growth kinetics of breast cancer cells, we examined the effect of CPGF NPs on the mitochondrial membrane potential of both the breast cancer cell lines. Interestingly, CPGF NPs treatment resulted into the disruption of the mitochondrial membrane potential (Dym) that was observed by a dose-dependent decrease ($p<0.0001$) in red fluorescence intensity, after staining the cells with JC-1 dye (Figure 8A). This was supported by a corresponding increase ($p<0.0001$) in the expression of caspase-3 in cells treated with CPGF NPs as compared to the untreated control cells (Figure 8B). The loss of mitochondrial membrane potential is the hallmark of apoptosis. These results indicated that cinnamaldehyde-Fe_3O_4 induced apoptosis in breast cancer cells through mitochondria dependent pathway.

The mechanistic studies confirmed the potential of CPGF NPs to restrict the growth of breast cancer cells through inhibition of migration, invasion and induction of apoptosis. Therefore, PF127-Glycine-Fe_3O_4 could be an appropriate carrier for hydrophobic agents such as cinnamaldehyde to improve their bioavailability in cancer therapy.

Hyperthermia potential of CPGF NPs

Iron oxide nanoparticles have been used in hyperthermia [46] because of their ability to get heated upto 42–45°C upon exposure to radiation. The magnetite NPs tagged with different anticancer drugs such as doxorubicin [18] or anti-Her2 immunoliposomes [19] have been extensively explored for targeted delivery and hyperthermia in breast cancer. Since CPGF NPs showed enhanced anticancer activity in both ER/PR positive/Her2 negative (MCF7) and ER/PR negative/Her2 negative (MDAMB231) breast cancer cells, we wanted to know whether the NPs had the potential for application in cancer hyperthermia as well. Thus, solutions (10 mg/ml) of F, G, P, C and CPGF NPs in deionized water, were subjected to 20 MHz RF radiation [47] for different time periods (0–150 s), and the temperature rise was monitored (Figure 9). CPGF NPs showed a significant rise in the temperature to 41.6°C within a time span of 1 min. Such rise in temperature upon RF exposure has been reported to be dependent upon the magnetic nature, polar/non-polar nature as well as the concentration of the nanoparticles [48,49]. The results appeared to be quite encouraging since the tumors get ablated at 41.6°C while the normal cells are known to withstand higher temperatures [50].

Conclusions

In summary, cinnamaldehyde, a natural anticancer hydrophobic compound present in *Cinnamomum* sp, was tagged with PF127-Glycine-Fe_3O_4 system that increased its bioavailability and in turn its therapeutic efficacy in breast cancer cells. The resulting CPGF NPs served as a vehicle for targeted delivery of cinnamaldehyde and exhibited anticancer and hyperthermia potential in breast cancer.

Supporting Information

File S1 Supporting Information that includes Table S1, Table S2, and Figure S1 - Figure S5. Cytotoxic studies of cinnamaldehyde and its derivatives (Table S1) as well as those of MNPs loaded with herbal active compounds (Table S2). Physical characterization of F, G, C, P, GF, PGF and CPGF NPs (Figures S1–S4) and cytotoxicity data of F, G and P (Figure S5). Table S1. Cytotoxic studies of cinnamaldehyde and its derivatives. Table S2. Cytotoxic studies of MNPs loaded with herbal active compounds. Figure S1. TEM images of F, GF and PGF NPs. TEM image showed the particle size to be around 5–10 nm for F and GF NPs and ~10–15 nm for PGF NPs. This indicated that the size of the NPs gradually increased from ~5 nm for non-conjugated Fe_3O_4 to ~20 nm for PGF NPs by successive layering of G and P onto the F NPs. Figure S2. FTIR spectra of F, G and GF. Glycine spectrum (G) showed remarkable signatures at ~3200 cm^{-1} for $-NH_2$ or $-OH$ and that for carboxylate stretch at ~1600 cm^{-1}.

The notable difference between Fe_3O_4 spectrum (F) and glycine capped Fe_3O_4 (GF), was the appearance of a strong new signature at 3200 cm^{-1}, along with 1600 cm^{-1}. This indicated that Fe_3O_4 surface was efficiently capped with glycine. Figure S3. FTIR spectra of GF, P and PGF. The appearance of peaks at 3200 cm^{-1} and 1600 cm^{-1} (1696 cm^{-1} in PGF) for both GF and PGF suggested that the hydroxyl/amine and carboxylate functions of G and P are successively loaded onto the Fe_3O_4 NPs. The overall merging of peaks indicated that pluronic possessed similar functional groups as in glycine resulting in similar spectrum of PGF to GF. Figure S4. FTIR spectra of PGF, C and CPGF. Cinnamaldehyde spectrum (C) showed prominent peaks at 1696, 1634, 1140, 960 and 764 cm^{-1} arising due to bonds specified by aldehyde structure. There was an interesting shift of –C = C– and –C = O stretches from 1696 and 1634 cm^{-1} in PGF towards higher energy side at 1709 and 1695 cm^{-1} in CPGF denoting conjugation of cinnamaldehyde with PGF. The invariable presence of other peaks in cinnamaldehyde such as 1140, 960 and 764 cm^{-1} in CPGF spectrum suggested that cinnamaldehyde was electrostatically bound to PGF. Figure S5. Cytotoxicity of F, G and P. The effect of F, G and P on MDAMB231 and MCF7 was analyzed by using MTT dye. The cells were treated with 0–640 μg/ml of F, G and P. Uncoated Fe_3O_4 nanoparticles were non-toxic to all the cell lines which is in accordance with the previously reported data. Both the cell lines showed ≥100% viability post-treatment with glycine and pluronic used to coat Fe_3O_4 nanoparticles. Therefore, these coating materials were non-toxic and safe.

Acknowledgments

We thank our Director, Dr. P. K. Ranjekar for his constant support and encouragement to complete this work.

Author Contributions

Conceived and designed the experiments: RKG. Performed the experiments: KDW BSK PG AVD. Analyzed the data: RKG KDW PM RCC PP SDD. Contributed reagents/materials/analysis tools: RKG RCC PP SDD. Wrote the paper: RKG KDW PM RCC PP.

References

1. Patnaik JL, Byers T, DiGuiseppi C, Dabelea D, Denberg TD (2011) Cardiovascular disease competes with breast cancer as the leading cause of death for older females diagnosed with breast cancer. Breast Cancer Res 13: 1–9.
2. Schott AF, Hayes DF (2012) Defining the benefits of neoadjuvant chemotherapy for breast cancer. J Clin Oncol 30: 1747–1749.
3. Binkley JM, Harris SR, Levangie PK, Pearl M, Guglielmino J, et al. (2012) Patient perspectives on breast cancer treatment side effects and the prospective surveillance model for physical rehabilitation for women with breast cancer. Cancer 118: 2207–2216.
4. Veronesi U, Marubini E, Del Vecchio M, Manzari A, Andreola S, et al. (1995) Local recurrences and distant metastases after conservative breast cancer treatments: partly independent events. J Natl Cancer Inst 87: 19–27.
5. Liao GS, Apaya MK, Shyur LF (2013) Herbal medicine and acupuncture for breast cancer palliative care and adjuvant therapy. Evid Based Complement Alternat Med 2013: 1–17.
6. Yin SY, Wei WC, Jian FY, Yang NS (2013) Therapeutic applications of herbal medicines for cancer patients. Evid Based Complement Alternat Med 2013: 1–15.
7. Ahmed M, Khan MI, Khan MR, Muhammad N, Khan AU, et al. (2013) Role of medicinal plants in oxidative stress and cancer. Open Access Scientific Reports 2: 641.
8. Bhattaram VA, Graefe U, Kohlert C, Veit M, Derendorf H (2002) Pharmacokinetics and bioavailability of herbal medicinal products. Phytomedicine 9: 1–33.
9. Kareparamban JA, Nikam PH, Jadhav AP, Kadam VJ (2012) Phytosome: a novel revolution in herbal drugs. IJRPC 2: 299–310.
10. Bhadoriya SS, Mangal A, Madoriya N, Dixit P (2011) Bioavailability and bioactivity enhancement of herbal drugs by "Nanotechnology": a review. JCPR 8: 1–7.
11. Koppikar SJ, Choudhari AS, Suryavanshi SA, Kumari S, Kaul-Ghanekar R, et al. (2010) Aqueous cinnamon extract (ACE-c) from the bark of *Cinnamomum cassia* causes apoptosis in human cervical cancer cell line (SiHa) through loss of mitochondrial membrane potential. BMC Cancer 10: 210.
12. Singh R, Koppikar SJ, Paul P, Gilda S, Kaul-Ghanekar R, et al. (2009) Comparative analysis of cytotoxic effect of aqueous cinnamon extract from *Cinnamomum zeylanicum* bark with commercial cinnamaldehyde on various cell lines. Pharmaceutical Biology 47: 1174–1179.
13. Kwon BM, Lee SH, Choi SU, Park SH, Lee CO, et al. (1998) Synthesis and in vitro cytotoxicity of cinnamaldehydes to human solid tumor cells. Arch Pharm Res 21: 147–152.
14. Stammati A, Bonsi P, Zucco F, Moezelaar R, Alakomi HL, et al. (1999) Toxicity of selected plant volatiles in microbial and mammalian short-term assays. Food Chem Toxicol 37: 813–823.
15. Jain TK, Morales MA, Sahoo SK, Leslie-Pelecky DL, Labhasetwar V (2005) Iron oxide nanoparticles for sustained delivery of anticancer agents. Mol Pharm 2: 194–205.
16. Ren Y, Zhang H, Chen B, Cheng J, Cai X, et al. (2012) Multifunctional magnetic Fe_3O_4 nanoparticles combined with chemotherapy and hyperthermia to overcome multidrug resistance. Int J Nanomedicine 7: 2261–2269.
17. Aljarrah K, Mhaidat NM, Al-Akhras MH, Aldaher AN, Albiss BA, et al. (2012) Magnetic nanoparticles sensitize MCF-7 breast cancer cells to doxorubicin-induced apoptosis. World journal of surgical oncology 10:62.
18. Sadeghi-Aliabadi H, Mozaffari M, Behdadfar B, Raesizadeh M, Zarkesh-Esfahani H (2013) Preparation and cytotoxic evaluation of magnetite (Fe_3O_4) nanoparticles on breast cancer cells and its combinatory effects with doxorubicin used in hyperthermia. Avicenna J Med Biotech 5: 96–103.
19. Kikumori T, Kobayashi T, Sawaki M, Imai T (2009) Anti-cancer effect of hyperthermia on breast cancer by magnetite nanoparticle-loaded anti-HER2 immunoliposomes. Breast Cancer Res Treat 113: 435–41.
20. Berry CC, Curtis SG (2003) Functionalisation of magnetic nanoparticles for applications in biomedicine. J Phys D: Appl Phys 36: R198–206.
21. Hasany SF, Ahmed I, Rajan J, Rehman A (2012) Systematic review of the preparation techniques of iron oxide magnetic nanoparticles. Nanoscience and Nanotechnology 2: 148–158.
22. Petri-Fink A, Steitz B, Finka A, Salaklang J, Hofmann H (2008) Effect of cell media on polymer coated superparamagnetic iron oxide nanoparticles (SPIONs): colloidal stability, cytotoxicity, and cellular uptake studies. Eur - J Pharm Biopharm 68: 129–137.
23. Akbarzadeh A, Zarghami N, Mikaeili H, Asgari D, Goganian AM, et al. (2012) Synthesis, characterization, and in vitro evaluation of novel polymer-coated magnetic nanoparticles for controlled delivery of doxorubicin. Nanotechnology, Science and Applications 5: 13–25.
24. Williams CH, Lawson J, Colette FR (1988) Oxidation of 3-amino-1-phenylprop-1-enes by monoamine oxidase and their use in a continuous assay of the enzyme. Biochem J 256: 911–915.
25. Shieh DB, Su CH, Chang FY, Wu YN, Su WC, et al. (2006) Aqueous nickel-nitrilotriacetate modified Fe_3O_4–NH_3^+ nanoparticles for protein purification and cell targeting. Nanotechnology 17: 4174–4182.
26. Wani KD, Kitture R, Ahmed A, Choudhari AS, Kaul-Ghanekar R, et al. (2011) Synthesis, characterization and in vitro study of Curcumin-functionalized Citric acid-Capped Magnetic (CCF) Nanoparticles as drug delivery agents in cancer. Journal of Bionanoscience 5: 59–65.
27. Choudhari AS, Suryavanshi SA, Kaul-Ghanekar R (2013) The aqueous extract of *Ficus religiosa* induces cell cycle arrest in human cervical cancer cell lines SiHa (HPV-16 Positive) and apoptosis in HeLa (HPV-18 Positive). PLoS ONE 8: e7012.
28. Gonzales M, Krishnan KM (2007) Phase transfer of highly monodisperse iron oxide nanocrystals with Pluronic F127 for biomedical applications. Journal of Magnetism and Magnetic Materials 311: 59–62.
29. Ganta S, Devalapally H, Shahiwala A, Amiji M (2008) A review of stimuli-responsive nanocarriers for drug and gene delivery. Journal of Controlled Release 126: 187–204.
30. Poddar P, Telem-Shafir T, Fried T, Markovich G (2002) Dipolar interactions in two- and three-dimensional magnetic nanoparticle arrays. Phys Rev B66: 060403.
31. Shafi K, Ulman A, Dyal A, Yan X, Yang N, et al. (2002) Magnetic enhancement of γ-Fe_2O_3 nanoparticles by sonochemical coating. Chem Mater 14: 1778–1787.
32. Paone JF, Abeloff MD, Ettinger DS, Arnold EA, Baker PR (1981) The correlation of estrogen and progesterone receptor levels with response to chemotherapy for advanced carcinoma of the breast. Surg Gynecol Obstet 152: 70–74.
33. Dent R, Hanna WM, Trudeau M, Rawlinson E, Sun P, et al. (2009) Pattern of metastatic spread in triple-negative breast cancer. Breast Cancer Res Treat 115: 423–428.
34. Rose DP, Vona-Davis L (2009) Influence of obesity on breast cancer receptor status and prognosis. Expert Review of Anticancer Therapy 9: 1091–1101.
35. Mauri FA, Maisonneuve P, Caffo O, Veronese S, Aldovini D, et al. (1999) Prognostic value of estrogen receptor status can be improved by combined

evaluation of p53, Bcl2 and PgR expression: an immunohistochemical study on breast carcinoma with long-term follow-up. Int J Oncol 15: 1137–1147.
36. Bentzon N, During M, Rasmussen BB, Mouridsen H, Kroman N (2008) Prognostic effect of estrogen receptor status across age in primary breast cancer. Int J Cancer 122: 1089–94.
37. Clark GM, McGuire WL, Hubay CA, Pearson OH, Marshall JS (1983) Progesterone receptors as a prognostic factor in Stage II breast cancer. N Engl J Med 309: 1343–1347.
38. Dent R, Trudeau M, Pritchard KI, Hanna WM, Kahn HK, et al. (2007) Triple-negative breast cancer: clinical features and patterns of recurrence. Clin Cancer Res 13: 4429–4434.
39. Haffty BG, Yang Q, Reiss M, Kearney T, Higgins SA, et al. (2006) Locoregional relapse and distant metastasis in conservatively managed triple negative early-stage breast cancer. J Clin Oncol 24: 5652–5657.
40. Ismail IA, Kang HS, Lee HJ, Kwon BM, Hong SH (2012) 2'-Benzoyloxycinnamaldehyde-mediated DJ-1 upregulation protects MCF-7 cells from mitochondrial damage. Biol Pharm Bull 35: 895–902.
41. Aggarwal BB, Van Kuiken ME, Iyer LH, Harikumar KB, Sung B (2009) Molecular targets of nutraceuticals derived from dietary spices: potential role in suppression of inflammation and tumorigenesis. Exp Biol Med (Maywood) 234:825–849.
42. Overall CM, López-Otín C (2002) Strategies for MMP inhibition in cancer: Innovations for the post-trial era. Nat Rev Cancer 2:657–672.
43. Hoeben A, Landuyt B, Highley MS, Wildiers H, Van Oosterom AT, et al. (2004) Vascular Endothelial Growth Factor and Angiogenesis. Pharmacol Rev 56:549–580.
44. Quaranta M, Daniele A, Coviello M, Venneri MT, Abbate I, et al. (2007) MMP-2, MMP-9, VEGF and CA 15.3 in breast cancer. Anticancer Res 27: 3593–3600.
45. Unemori EN, Ferrara N, Bauer EA, Amiento EP (1992) Vascular endothelial growth factor induces interstitial collagenase expression in human endothelial cells. J Cell Physiol 153: 557–562.
46. Hilger I, Kaiser WA (2012) Iron oxide-based nanostructures for MRI and magnetic hyperthermia. Nanomedicine (Lond) 7: 1443–1459.
47. Kale SN, Jadhav AD, Verma S, Koppikar SJ, Kaul-Ghanekar R, et al. (2012) Characterization of biocompatible $NiCo_2O_4$ nanoparticles for applications in hyperthermia and drug delivery. Nanomedicine 8: 452–459.
48. Kong G, Braun RD, Dewhirst MW (2000) Hyperthermia enables tumor-specific nanoparticle delivery: Effect of particle size. Cancer Res 60: 4440–4445.
49. Asin L, Ibarra MR, Tres A, Goya GF (2012) Controlled cell death by magnetic hyperthermia: Effects of exposure time, field amplitude, and nanoparticle concentration. Pharmaceutical Research 29:1319–1327.
50. Song CW (1984) Effect of local hyperthermia on blood flow and microenvironment: a review. Cancer Res 44: 4721–4730.

13

Regulation of Action Potential Waveforms by Axonal $GABA_A$ Receptors in Cortical Pyramidal Neurons

Yang Xia[1], Yuan Zhao[2], Mingpo Yang[1], Shaoqun Zeng[2]*, Yousheng Shu[3]*

1 Institute of Neuroscience, State Key Laboratory of Neuroscience, Shanghai Institutes for Biological Sciences, Chinese Academy of Sciences, Shanghai, P. R. China,
2 Britton Chance Center for Biomedical Photonics, Wuhan National Laboratory for Optoelectronics-Huazhong University of Science and Technology, Wuhan, P. R. China,
3 State Key Laboratory of Cognitive Neuroscience and Learning & IDG/McGovern Institute for Brain Research, Center for Collaboration and Innovation in Brain and Learning Sciences, Beijing Normal University, Beijing, P. R. China

Abstract

$GABA_A$ receptors distributed in somatodendritic compartments play critical roles in regulating neuronal activities, including spike timing and firing pattern; however, the properties and functions of $GABA_A$ receptors at the axon are still poorly understood. By recording from the cut end (bleb) of the main axon trunk of layer -5 pyramidal neurons in prefrontal cortical slices, we found that currents evoked by GABA iontophoresis could be blocked by picrotoxin, indicating the expression of $GABA_A$ receptors in axons. Stationary noise analysis revealed that single-channel properties of axonal $GABA_A$ receptors were similar to those of somatic receptors. Perforated patch recording with gramicidin revealed that the reversal potential of the GABA response was more negative than the resting membrane potential at the axon trunk, suggesting that GABA may hyperpolarize the axonal membrane potential. Further experiments demonstrated that the activation of axonal $GABA_A$ receptors regulated the amplitude and duration of action potentials (APs) and decreased the AP-induced Ca^{2+} transients at the axon. Together, our results indicate that the waveform of axonal APs and the downstream Ca^{2+} signals are modulated by axonal $GABA_A$ receptors.

Editor: Fabien Tell, The Research Center of Neurobiology-Neurophysiology of Marseille, France

Funding: This work was funded by the 973 Program (No. 2011CBA00400 YS), the National Natural Science Foundation of China Project (No. 31025012 YS, 81327802 SZ), and the Hundreds of Talents Program (YS) from Chinese Academy of Sciences. The funders had no role in study design, data collection and analysis, decision to publish, or preparation of the manuscript.

Competing Interests: The authors have declared that no competing interests exist.

* Email: yousheng@bnu.edu.cn (YS); sqzeng@hust.edu.cn (SZ)

Introduction

In general, the dendrites and cell body receive and summate synaptic inputs, whereas the axon is responsible for action potential (AP) initiation and propagation. The axon usually functions as a reliable cable conducting APs in all-or-none (digital) mode; however, this long-held view of the axon has recently been challenged Emerging evidences has shown that subthreshold changes in presynaptic membrane potential (V_m) can regulate the amplitude of AP-triggered postsynaptic responses, indicating that neurons also communicate in an analog mode [1,2,3]. This mode of neuronal communication may result from activities of axonal ion channels [4,5] and receptors [6,7] that regulate AP waveforms, presynaptic Ca^{2+} signals and, thus, neurotransmitter release [8,9].

Ionotropic $GABA_A$ receptors are one of the most important components involved in the operation of neural circuits in the central nervous system (CNS) [10]. These ligand-gated receptors are heteropentamers selectively permeable to Cl^- (predominantly) and HCO_3^- [11]. Previous studies demonstrated that somatodendritic $GABA_A$ receptors could regulate neuronal excitability, spike timing and firing pattern [12,13]. Also there were several lines of evidence implicating a role for axonal $GABA_A$ receptors in regulating neuronal activities [14,15].

During development of the vertebrate brain, the effect of $GABA_A$ receptor activation on V_m switches from depolarization to characteristic hyperpolarization. This transition is attributable to a decrease in the concentration of intracellular Cl^- ($[Cl^-]_i$), resulting from changes in the expression level of cation–chloride co-transporters such as NKCCs (Na^+-K^+-$2Cl^-$ co-transporters) and KCCs (K^+-$2Cl^-$ co-transporters) [16]. It has been reported that interneurons exert a hyperpolarizing action along the entire somatodendritic axis and the axon initial segment (AIS) of CA1 hippocampal pyramidal cells [17]. However, GABA release from axo-axonic synapses onto the AIS depolarizes cortical pyramidal cells [15]. In addition, $GABA_A$ receptors on hippocampal mossy fibers could depolarize presynaptic boutons, enhance neurotransmission and facilitate LTP induction [18]. Another study in cerebellar granule cells also showed an increase in spike reliability and release probability after activation of axonal $GABA_A$ receptors [19]. In these studies, noninvasive approaches such as extracellular recording, cell-attached or gramicidin perforated patch recording were employed to maintain the intracellular milieu and reveal the actual function of $GABA_A$ receptors under physiological conditions.

In this study, we performed direct whole-cell recording from axon blebs of layer -5 pyramidal cells to investigate the role of $GABA_A$ receptors located at the main axon trunk in regulating neuronal signaling. Using gramicidin perforated patch recording from axonal blebs (>100 μm away from the soma), we found that the reversal potential of the GABA-mediated response was more negative than the resting V_m of the axon, suggesting that the activation of axonal $GABA_A$ receptors could cause hyperpolarization in distal axons. In addition, we show that the GABA-induced shunting and hyperpolarizing effect can shape AP waveforms and thereby AP-triggered Ca^{2+} signals at the axon.

Materials and Methods

Animals

The care and use of animals complied with the guidelines of the Animal Advisory Committee at the Shanghai Institutes for Biological Sciences. This committee also approved this research. All efforts were made to minimize animal suffering and reduce the number of animals used.

Slice Preparation

Coronal slices from prefrontal cortex were prepared from Sprague-Dawley rats (postnatal day 15–22, male). After sodium pentobarbital (30 mg/kg, i.p.) anesthesia, the animal was euthanized by decapitation. The brain was then dissected out and immersed in the following slicing solution. Slices (350–400 μm in thickness) were cut on a vibroslicer (Leica Instruments) in ice-cold slicing solution containing (in mM): 2.5 KCl, 1.25 NaH_2PO_4, 26 $NaHCO_3$, 2 $MgSO_4$, 2 $CaCl_2$, 25 dextrose, 213 sucrose (315–325 mOsm, pH 7.2–7.3). After slicing, individual slices were then transferred to an incubation chamber filled with normal ACSF similar to the slicing solution but with sucrose replaced by 126 mM NaCl. Slices were then maintained in this chamber at 34.5°C for approximately 1 hour before use. For electrophysiological experiments, slices were placed in a recording chamber and perfused with the normal ACSF (36–36.5°C). All solutions were oxygenated with carbogen gas (95% O_2 and 5% CO_2). Cortical neurons were visualized with an upright infrared differential interference contrast (IR-DIC) microscope (BX51WI; Olympus).

Electrophysiological Recordings

Whole-cell recordings were obtained from both the somata and the axonal blebs of layer -5 regular-spiking pyramidal neurons in prefrontal cortical slices [2,5]. The patch pipettes had open-tip resistances of 3–6 MΩ for somatic and 8–12 MΩ for axonal recordings. In this study, we used five types of intracellular solution (ICS) for different experiments (see below). The low-Cl^- intracellular solution (low-Cl^- ICS) contained (in mM): 140 K gluconate, 3 KCl, 2 $MgCl_2$, 2 Na_2ATP, 10 HEPES, and 0.2 EGTA (280–290 mOsm, pH 7.2 adjusted with KOH). Alexa Fluor 488 (100 μM) and Biocytin (0.2%) were also added to the ICS for visualizing the cell morphology during and after recording. The low-Cl^- ICS was used in most of our experiments unless otherwise stated. The resistance of sharp electrodes for GABA iontophoresis was 30–50 MΩ when filled with 500 mM GABA (pH 3.6). During the experiments, a retention current (−10 nA) was applied to prevent passive leakage of GABA. Currents were sampled at 20 kHz and low-pass filtered at 3 kHz. AP waveforms recorded in current-clamp mode were sampled at 50 kHz and low-pass filtered at 30 kHz.

To exclude the contribution of somatodendritic GABA receptors, we performed recordings from axon blebs isolated from the soma. Isolated axon blebs could be obtained by sweeping a sharp electrode at the border between layer -6and the white matter [20]. We then recorded axonal blebs in the white-matter side. Data collected from blebs that were disconnected from the soma but attached with segments of the axon (usually tens of micrometers) were chosen for analysis. Similarly, Alexa Fluor 488 and Biocytin were added to the ICS to confirm that the blebs were indeed isolated from the soma. CsCl-based ICS containing 2 mM TEA and 145 mM CsCl (replacing K gluconate and KCl in the low-Cl^- ICS) were used in this experiment.

Patch pipette solution for gramicidin perforated patch recording contained (in mM) 140 KCl, 10 NaCl, 10 HEPES (pH = 7.2 adjusted with KOH). Gramicidin was first dissolved in DMSO to prepare a stock solution and then diluted to a final concentration of 10 μg ml^{-1} (soma) or 100 μg ml^{-1} (bleb) in the pipette solution. The gramicidin-containing solution was prepared and sonicated immediately before the experiment. To facilitate the formation of a tight seal, the tip of the pipette was dipped into and filled with a gramicidin-free solution, and then the patch pipette was backfilled with a gramicidin-containing solution. After 10–20 minutes in the cell-attached configuration, the series resistance decreased and stabilized at 100–200 MΩ (soma) or 150–300 MΩ (bleb). The series resistance was monitored during all recording sessions. Alexa Fluor 488 was also added to this pipette solution for monitoring the integrity of perforated recording. The recording was terminated upon rupture of the patch membrane, as indicated by the presence of fluorescence in the recorded cell, a sudden decrease in series resistance or a dramatic change in reversal potential.

In experiments using extracellular stimulation to evoke APs, we placed a concentric electrode at layer 2/3 near the recorded cell and delivered single electrical shocks (0.1–0.3 ms in duration) to the slice. Low-Cl^- ICS, modified -ICS and high-Cl^- ICS were used in these experiments. In the modified -ICS, the concentration of K gluconate and KCl were adjusted to 127 and 16 mM, respectively. For high-Cl^- ICS, they were adjusted to 72 and 71 mM, respectively.

We employed a MultiClamp 700B amplifier (Molecular Devices) for patch-clamp recording and Spike2 software (Cambridge Electronic Design) for data acquisition. The series resistance and capacitance were compensated before and after every experimental protocol. AxoClamp 900A (Molecular Devices) was used for GABA iontophoresis (200 nA, 2–5 ms) and Picospritzer III (Parker Hannifin Corporation) was used for local puffing of baclofen (10–30 psi, 15–20 ms). The V_m shown in the text and figures were not corrected with a liquid junction potential unless otherwise stated.

GABA, Picrotoxin (PTX), baclofen, CGP 35348, muscimol and Biocytin were obtained from Tocris; gramicidin from Sigma; Alexa Fluor 488, Alexa Fluor 594 and OGB-1 from Invitrogen.

Stationary noise analysis

The membrane currents recorded in voltage-clamp mode were sampled at 20 kHz and low-pass filtered at 6 kHz; then, the current traces were used for noise analysis. For stationary noise analysis, currents were first low-pass filtered at 400 Hz using FIR digital filtering and then transformed into AC signals using DC remove with a time constant of 1 s (Spike2 software). From each recording, we chose two segments (20–40 s) of the current trace before and during drug application.

The variance of membrane current σ_i^2 was calculated from the AC signals using the following formula:

$$\sigma_i^2 = \frac{1}{(N-1)} \sum_{k=1}^{N} (i_k - \bar{i})^2$$

where N is the total number of points in each data segments, i_k is the individual data point and $\bar{i}$ is the mean value of the current.

Subtraction of the variance under control condition from those obtained during drug application produced the drug-induced variance. The average conductance of a single channel γ can be calculated from equation $\gamma = \sigma_i^2/(\Delta I \cdot V_D)$, where σ_i^2 is the drug-induced variance, ΔI is the drug-induced change of the membrane current and V_D is the driving force.

Power spectra of current fluctuations were calculated as the average of fast Fourier transform of subsamples of the membrane current. Each subsample lasted for 2 s. Subtraction of baseline values from those obtained during drug application yielded the power spectra of drug-induced fluctuations. In most cases, the drug-induced spectra could be fitted by a double Lorentzian equation of the form

$$S(f) = \sum_{i=1}^{2} S_i(0)/(1 + \left(\frac{f}{f_i}\right)^2)$$

where $S_i(0)$ is the zero frequency asymptote value and f_i is the cut-off frequency of each component. The corresponding time constant τ_i is derived from $\tau_i = 1/(2\pi f_i)$. More details can be found in previous reports [21,22].

In the experiments for stationary noise analysis, in addition to using the CsCl-based ICS described above, we also added 3 mM 4-AP, 100 μM DL-AP5, 20 μM CNQX, 100 μM CGP 35348, 100 μM $CdCl_2$ and 1 μM TTX to the bath solution to minimize the baseline noise and contribution from receptors other than $GABA_A$ receptors.

Two-photon laser-scanning microscopy

Two-photon imaging was conducted on a custom-built random scanning two-photon microscope [23]. An 840-nm femtosecond laser beam (pulse width of approximately 140 fs and repetitive rate of 80 MHz) was generated by a mode-locked Ti:sapphire laser (Chameleon Vision II, Coherent) and directed into a custom-made scanner head. A pair of perpendicular acousto-optic deflectors (AODs, DTSXY-400, AA optoelectronic, France) was employed for random-access scanning. The laser beam was then relayed through a dichroic mirror (DM665) into an upright microscope (BX61WI, Olympus) equipped with a 40× water-immersion objective. The average laser power on the sample was generally 10–20 mW. Emitted green and red fluorescence were simultaneously collected by photomultiplier tubes (H7422-40, Hamamatsu). Imaging was controlled by a LabVIEW-based program on a PC with a PCI-6259 card (National Instruments, NI, USA) for communications and a PCI-6111 card (NI) for data acquisition.

For two-photon imaging, neurons were patched with the normal ICS without EGTA but with 200 μM Oregon Green Bapta-1 (OGB-1) and 50 μM Alexa Fluor 594. Ca^{2+} transients induced by APs were monitored at an acquisition rate of approximately 1 kHz in most cases, and represented as average (10 traces, 100-points moving average) time courses of ΔF/F. To synchronize the imaging and patch clamp recording, a 5-V TTL pulse was sent from the MultiClamp 700B amplifier to the PCI-6259 card.

To examine the role of axonal $GABA_A$ receptors in regulating AP-induced Ca^{2+} transients, GABA was applied through iontophoresis using sharp electrodes. For visualizing the pipette tip and estimating the distance between the tip and the axon trunk, we also added 50 μM Alexa Fluor 594 to the pipette solution.

DAB staining

After recording, slices were transferred to 4% paraformaldehyde (PFA) in 0.1 M PB and kept in this fixative overnight. DAB staining was performed for visualization of the morphology of recorded neurons and measurement of the axon length.

Statistical analysis

Values are presented as the mean ± s.e.m. Excel (Microsoft) and OriginPro 8 (OriginLab Corporation) were used for statistical analysis. Student's t-test was used for statistic examination. Differences were considered to be statistically significant with $P<0.05$.

Results

$GABA_A$ receptors are located in axon blebs and trunks

Previous studies have revealed the presence of GABA receptors at specific locations of the axon, including presynaptic terminals and the AIS [15,24]. To examine whether these receptors are also expressed at the main axon trunk of layer -5 pyramidal neurons in prefrontal cortex, we performed whole-cell recordings from axon blebs, the resealed cut ends of axons formed during slicing, and applied GABA locally to the axon via iontophoresis using sharp electrodes (Figure 1A).

Because GABA is positively charged at pH 3.6, we applied a retention current of −10 nA to prevent passive leakage of GABA but extruded GABA by delivering positive current pulses (200 nA, 2–5 ms in duration). These pulses could evoke an outward current at the axon bleb recorded with a low-Cl^- pipette solution (7 mM $[Cl^-]_i$, holding potential: −50 mV). In contrast, no response could be observed when we applied negative current pulses (Figure 1A, inset). We next measured the diffusion distance of GABA by placing the iontophoresis electrode lateral to the recorded axon bleb with varying distance. The peak amplitude of GABA-induced currents (I_{GABA}) decreased progressively with increasing distance between the bleb and the tip of iontophoresis electrode. For 5-ms pulses (200 nA), GABA responses could hardly be detected if the distance was greater than 25 μm (Figure 1B). The retention current (−10 nA) applied to the iontophoresis electrode and the limited diffusion distance suggested that GABA did not spread widely and therefore did not activate dendritic receptors. However, GABA responses could be reliably obtained if the iontophoresis was performed near the axon trunk. As shown in Figure 1C, application of GABA at a lateral site *b* that was 25 μm away from the bleb could not induce any response; in contrast, at the site *c* (approximately 50 μm away from the bleb) we could observe GABA responses similar to those at the recorded bleb (site *a*). These results indicate the presence of GABA receptors at both the bleb and the main axon trunk. The filtering effect of the axon cable could be observed when we performed whole-cell recordings at the somata and applied GABA to the axon blebs with various distance from the somata (Figure S1). As expected, the rising slope of GABA-induced currents decreased but the decay time course increased with increasing distance between the soma and the axon bleb.

Application of GABA can activate both $GABA_A$ and $GABA_B$ receptors. Activation of $GABA_A$ receptors mainly induces a Cl^- conductance, whereas activation of $GABA_B$ receptors induces a K^+ conductance. To examine the contribution of these receptors to axonal GABA responses, we measured the reversal potential of GABA-induced currents (E_{GABA}) by holding the V_m at different levels (−100 to −40 mV, Figure 2A). The average reversal potential was −78.2±0.8 mV (n = 12, corrected with a liquid junction potential of 15.4 mV), similar to the calculated equilibrium potential of Cl^- (−78.3 mV) using the Nernst equation. Consistent with these results, bath application of 25 μM picrotoxin (PTX), a $GABA_A$ receptor antagonist, could abolish the GABA-induced

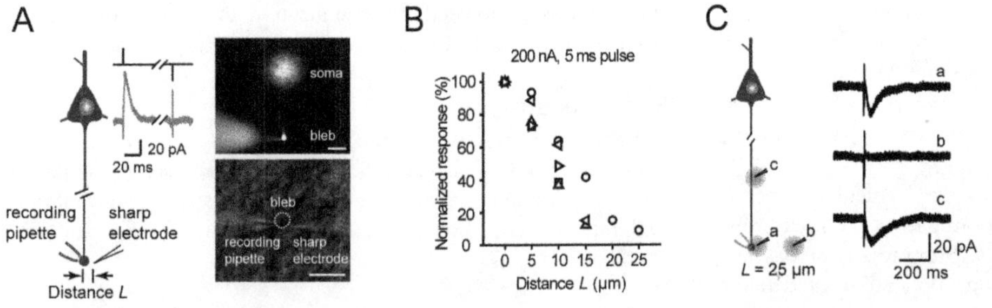

Figure 1. GABA receptors are located at axon bleb and trunk. A, Left, schematic diagram of bleb recording and GABA iontophoresis in a pyramidal neuron. Positive (but not negative) pulses could induce current responses. $V_{hold} = -50$ mV; iontophoresis pulses: 200 nA, 5 ms; retention current: −10 nA. Right, whole-cell recording from an axon bleb (top, fluorescence image; bottom, DIC image). Scale bar: 20 μm. The sharp electrode was used for GABA iontophoresis. Alexa Fluor 488 was added to the patch pipette solution so that the recording pipette was visible. B, Plot of the normalized GABA response as a function of the distance between the bleb and the tip of the iontophoresis electrode. Different symbols indicate different cells. The measurement of distance *L* is shown in the schematic diagram in panel A (indicated by arrows). C, GABA-induced responses could be observed when GABA was applied to the bleb (site *a*) or the main axon trunk (site *c*). The distance between sites *a* and *c* was approximately 50 μm, whereas that between *a* and *b* was approximately 25 μm. $V_{hold} = -80$ mV; iontophoresis pulses: 200 nA, 5 ms.

current recorded at the axon bleb (reduced to 11.3±3.7% of control, n = 6, Figure 2B). These results indicate that GABA responses at the axon are mediated by $GABA_A$ receptors.

We next applied baclofen, a $GABA_B$ receptor agonist, to further address whether $GABA_B$ receptors were expressed at the axon trunk. Consistent with previous findings [25], local puff application of 200 μM baclofen at the soma induced a current with a reversal potential of −102.1±1.1 mV (n = 13, corrected with a liquid junction potential of 15.4 mV. Figure 2C), which was close to the calculated equilibrium potential of K^+ (−107.8 mV). However, we observed no significant changes in the baseline currents (holding potential: −100 to −50 mV) after the application of baclofen to the axon bleb (Figure 2C). Consistent with these results, the $GABA_A$ receptor antagonist PTX but not the $GABA_B$ receptor antagonist CGP 35348 could block the currents evoked by iontophoresis of GABA at the axon (Figure 2D). Together, these results show that $GABA_A$ but likely not $GABA_B$ receptors (at least not $GABA_B$-coupled potassium channels) are expressed along the axon.

The GABA receptors at the AIS can be activated upon GABA release from the axo-axonic synapses [26,27]. Considering the lack

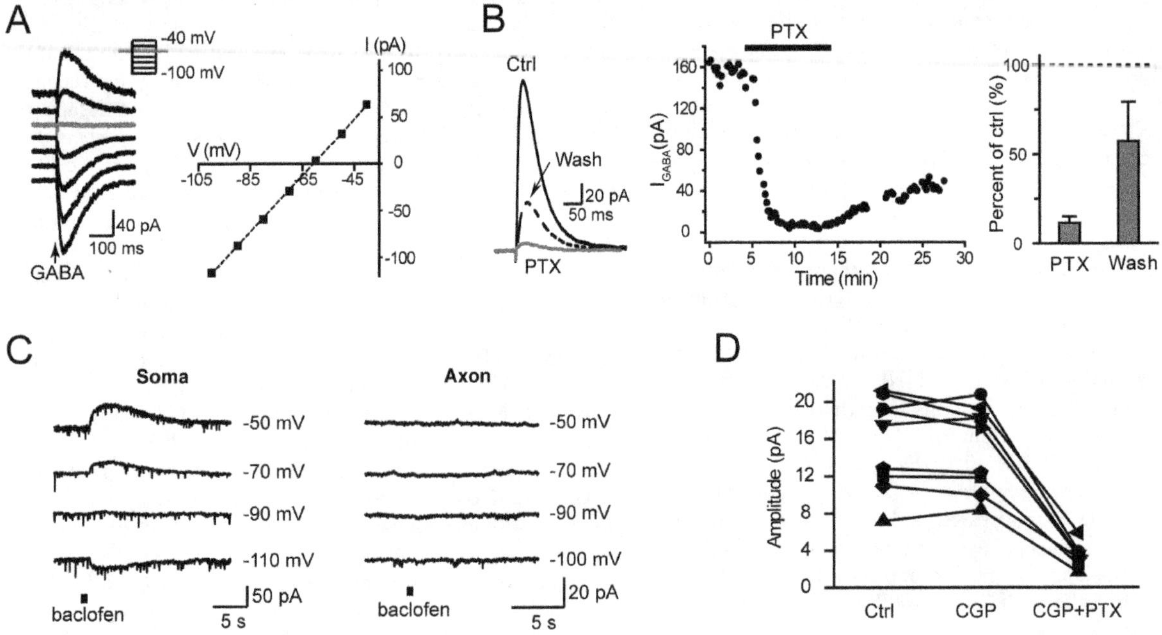

Figure 2. The presence of $GABA_A$ (but likely not $GABA_B$) receptors in the axon. A, Reversal potential of GABA responses (I_{GABA}) in the axon bleb. Left, representative currents induced by GABA application at different holding potentials (from −100 to −40 mV). At −60 mV (near reversal potential), GABA application induced no obvious change in baseline current (gray). Right, I-V curve of the GABA-induced responses shown on the left. B, I_{GABA} could be blocked by $GABA_A$ receptor blocker PTX. Left, example traces before (black), during (gray) and after (Wash, dashed line) the bath application of PTX (25 μM). $V_{hold} = -50$ mV, GABA was applied via iontophoresis. Middle, time course of the effect of PTX. Right, group data showing the change of I_{GABA} during (n = 6) and after (n = 3) PTX application. The dashed line indicates 100% of control. C, Left, currents evoked by puffing baclofen (200 μM), a $GABA_B$ receptor agonist, to the soma (16 psi, 15 ms). Right, no response was observed when baclofen was applied to the axon trunk (16 psi, 20 ms). D, Group data showing that GABA-induced currents at the axon blebs could not be blocked by the $GABA_B$ receptor antagonist CGP 35348 (100 μM); however, PTX could diminish these responses. Different symbols indicate different cells.

of direct evidence of GABAergic synapses at the axon trunk, we speculated that these axonal $GABA_A$ receptors may be activated by ambient GABA. To exclude the contribution of somatodendritic GABA receptors, we performed the following experiments in isolated axon blebs that were disconnected from the soma but with axon segments attached (see the Methods section, Figure 3A). In the presence of the $GABA_A$ receptor agonist muscimol (5 μM), we observed an increase in outward holding current ($\Delta I = 14.8 \pm 4.3$ pA, n = 11; low-Cl^- ICS) at a holding potential of 10 mV. Again, 100 μM PTX could block this effect (Figure 3B). At a holding potential of −70 mV, we also observed a decrease in the inward holding current after the application of PTX ($\Delta I = -5.8 \pm 2.3$ pA, n = 6; CsCl ICS), even without the presence of muscimol (Figure 3C). These results suggest that ambient GABA (mimicked by a low concentration of muscimol) can activate axonal $GABA_A$ receptors.

Next, we investigated the average conductance γ and the open time constant τ of these axonal receptors by using noise analysis (see the Methods section). Membrane current responses to 5 μM muscimol were recorded at isolated blebs, and the variance σ_i^2 and cut-off frequency f_c could be then obtained (Figure 3D, E, F). In most cases, the power spectral density plots of membrane current fluctuations could be well fitted by a double Lorentzian function and yielded two f_c values and consequently two τ values. The γ, τ_1, and τ_2 values for axonal $GABA_A$ receptors activated by 5 μM muscimol were 23.4 ± 1.6 pS, 45.7 ± 3.0 ms and 8.2 ± 0.9 ms, respectively (n = 10). All values were quite similar to those obtained from somatic $GABA_A$ receptors by using nucleated patch recording (23.5 ± 1.2 pS, 45.1 ± 6.0 ms and 7.0 ± 0.6 ms, n = 9). These results show no significant difference in single-channel properties between axonal and somatic $GABA_A$ upon activation by a low concentration of muscimol.

Axonal $GABA_A$ receptors hyperpolarize the axon

Activation of $GABA_A$ receptors in the somatodendritic compartments hyperpolarizes the V_m and thus inhibits and structures neuronal activities [14]. However, different results were observed for axonal $GABA_A$ receptors in different subcellular locations and brain regions, such as the AIS of hippocampal [17] and neocortical pyramidal neurons [15], the axon trunk of cerebellar granule cells [19] and axon terminals of hippocampal mossy fibers [18].

In our experiment, we used noninvasive gramicidin perforated patch recording to examine the reversal potential of GABA responses (E_{GABA}) under physiological conditions. Because gramicidin-formed holes are not permeable to Cl^-, the intracellular Cl^- gradient is not perturbed during this type of perforated patch recording. Because we added Alexa Fluor 488 to the pipette solution, rupture of the membrane would result in the presence of fluorescence in the recorded cell or bleb (Figure 4A). In these experiments, we used a high-Cl^- pipette solution, and rupture of the membrane would also lead to a dramatic change in E_{GABA} (Figure 4B). These results revealed that E_{GABA} at the distal axonal bleb (>100 μm apart from the soma) was -67.3 ± 1.5 mV (n = 14), significantly more positive than that at the soma (-79.0 ± 2.3 mV, n = 13. $p < 0.01$, two-sample t-test). However, both values were more negative (hyperpolarizing) than the respective local resting V_m (RMP) (Figure 4C). In distal axons, the RMP and E_{GABA} were -61.0 ± 2.1 mV and -67.2 ± 1.6 mV (n = 13. P = 0.02, paired t-test), respectively. Similar results were obtained when we

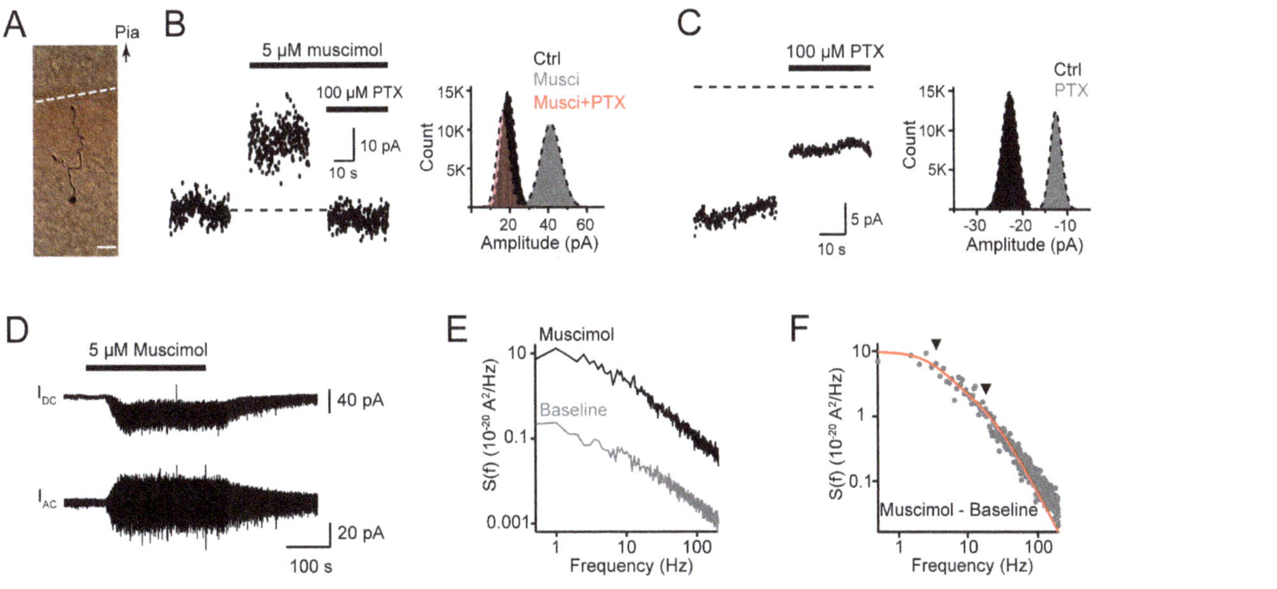

Figure 3. Properties of axonal $GABA_A$ receptors. A, DAB staining of an isolated axon bleb. The axon bleb was mechanically isolated from the main axon trunk before recording (see the Methods section). Arrow indicates the direction of the pia. Dashed line indicates the cut. Scale bar: 20 μm. B, Left, an example trace showing an increase in outward holding current after bath application of 5 μM muscimol ($V_{hold} = 10$ mV) and the blockade of this increase by 100 μM PTX. The dashed line indicates the baseline holding current. The mean values of I_{hold} for "Ctrl", "Musci" and "Musci + PTX" group were 19.8, 41.4 and 16.9 pA, respectively. Right, histograms of the membrane currents shown on the left. The best-fit curves (dashed lines) were single Gaussian distributions. Axon blebs were recorded with patch pipettes filled with a low-Cl^- ICS (7 mM $[Cl^-]_i$). C, Left, an example trace showing a decrease in inward holding current after bath application of 100 μM PTX ($V_{hold} = -70$ mV). The mean values of I_{hold} for "Ctrl" and "PTX" group were −22.8 and −12.5 pA, respectively. Right, histograms of the membrane currents shown on the left. Patch pipettes were filled with CsCl-based ICS (149 mM $[Cl^-]_i$). D, Current traces recorded in an isolated bleb. $V_{hold} = -60$ mV, CsCl-based ICS was used. Top, the actual current response; bottom, current trace with DC Remove. E, Power spectral density plots of membrane current fluctuations in control and muscimol-treated conditions (same data as in D). F, Subtraction of the power spectral density in the control from that with muscimol treatment (same data from D and E). The red line was the fitting curve of double Lorentzian functions. Cut-off frequencies (f_c) of the two components (arrowheads) were 3.5 and 18.1 Hz.

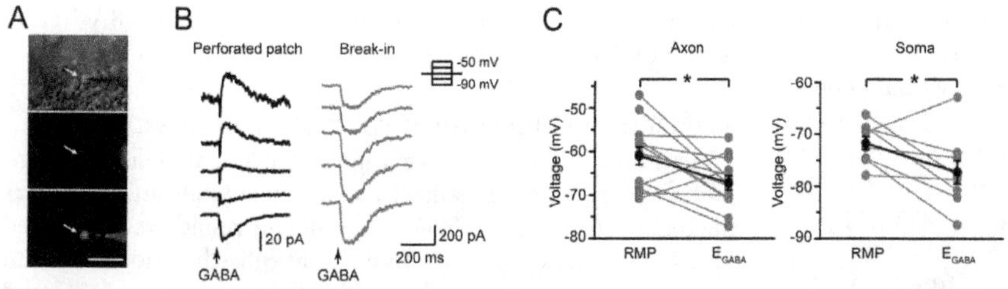

Figure 4. Reversal potential of GABA responses (E_{GABA}) is more negative than the local RMP. A, Gramicidin perforated patch recording from an axon bleb. Arrow indicates the recorded bleb. Top, DIC image of the recording; middle, fluorescence image (unlabeled bleb); bottom, fluorescence image (labeled bleb, indicating rupture of patch membrane). Scale bar: 50 μm. B, Example traces showing GABA responses at different holding potentials (from −90 to −50 mV) before (black) and after the break-in (membrane rupture, gray). C, Comparison of E_{GABA} and RMP. Note that E_{GABA} at both the soma and the distal axon bleb were more hyperpolarized than their local RMP. *, P<0.05, paired t-test.

performed perforated patch recording at the soma (RMP: −71.7±1.2 mV; E_{GABA}: −77.3±2.3 mV, n = 9. P = 0.03, paired t-test). Together, these results suggest that GABA functions as an inhibitory transmitter (hyperpolarizing the axon) at V_m levels more positive than the RMP.

Axonal $GABA_A$ receptors regulate AP waveform

We next investigate the role of axonal $GABA_A$ receptors in regulating orthodromically propagating APs along the axon. APs were evoked by extracellular stimulation with a concentric electrode and AP waveforms were monitored at the bleb. Three types of intracellular solutions (ICS) were employed in this experiment, they were low-Cl^- ICS (7 mM $[Cl^-]_i$), modified ICS (20 mM $[Cl^-]_i$) and high-Cl^- ICS (75 mM $[Cl^-]_i$), respectively.

Based on the results that activation of axonal $GABA_A$ receptors may hyperpolarize the axon, we speculated that the $[Cl^-]_i$ in the distal axon trunk should be low. We therefore used the low-Cl^- ICS first and found that the waveform of the evoked AP could be modulated by GABA applied to the axon bleb (Figure 5A). When the V_m was maintained at approximately −50 mV in current-clamp mode, GABA application at the bleb could cause hyperpolarization (−2.4±0.6 mV, ranging from −1.0 to −5.5 mV, n = 7). Although the amplitude showed no significant change (99.0±2.8% of control, P = 0.81, 41.3 vs. 41.0 mV, n = 7), the half-widths of APs were significantly decreased to 91.4±3.2% (P = 0.04, 1.4 vs. 1.3 ms, n = 7) of the control (black plots, Figure 5B., paired t-test). Then, we clamped the V_m of the bleb to a more hyperpolarized level at approximately −65 mV, application of GABA to the axon caused depolarization (3.4±1.1 mV, ranging from 1.0 to 8.0 mV, n = 6). Interestingly, both the AP amplitude and the AP half-width were significantly reduced (gray, Figure 5B). These values were decreased to 91.5±2.6% (P = 0.03, 78.9 vs. 72.1 mV) and 92.6±2.5% (P = 0.04, paired t-test, 0.94 vs. 0.87 ms) of the control, respectively. Together, our results indicate that GABA application at the axon reduces AP duration whether it hyperpolarizes or depolarizes the V_m, presumably resulting from a shunting effect of the GABA-induced conductance.

It has been reported that axo-axonal chandelier cells innervate the AIS of postsynaptic pyramidal cells and induce depolarizing responses, due to a high $[Cl^-]_i$ at this strategic location (AP initiation site). Therefore, we increased the $[Cl^-]_i$ from 7 to 20 mM (modified ICS) to mimic conditions of relatively high $[Cl^-]_i$ at AIS, depolarizing E_{GABA} to −48.0±0.5 mV (n = 19, corrected with a liquid junction potential of 14 mV). Although GABA iontophoresis at the bleb caused a larger depolarization (8.0±0.9 mV, ranging from 5.3 to 13.6 mV, n = 8), the amplitude and the half-width of APs decreased to 77.9±2.9% and 93.5±0.9% of control (P<0.001), respectively (Figure 5C). Bath application of PTX (25–50 μM) could block these GABA-induced depolarization and AP waveform changes (Figure 5D). Again, application of baclofen at the bleb caused no significant change in either the amplitude (P = 0.18) or the half-width (P = 0.22, paired t-test. n = 5) of AP waveforms. These results further support the shunting effect of $GABA_A$ receptors on AP waveform at the axon.

Further increasing the $[Cl^-]_i$ in the pipette solution to 75 mM (high-Cl^- ICS; reversal potential: −10.8±0.6 mV, corrected with a liquid junction potential of 9 mV, n = 17) produced larger depolarization and even facilitated the generation of APs. As shown in Figure 5E, GABA iontophoresis could evoke a large depolarization and sometimes even generate APs (arrow). Again, this GABA response also showed an inhibitory effect on the AP waveform when the orthodromic AP was evoked during GABA application (asterisk, Figure 5E). The dramatic decrease in AP amplitude resulted from an increase in membrane conductance (shunting effect) and a decrease in Na^+ channel availability (depolarization-induced inactivation). Interestingly, GABA-evoked depolarization could not promote the initiation of APs even when the strength of extracellular stimulation was very close to the threshold (data not shown).

Together, these results indicate that the waveforms of orthodromically propagating APs at the axon can be modulated by axonal $GABA_A$ receptors. Activation of these receptors mainly showed a shunting effect on AP waveforms regardless of the polarity of GABA-induced V_m changes.

Propagation of GABA-induced hyperpolarization along the axon

The shunting effect induced by increased conductance may occur only at the location where the receptors were activated; however, it remains unclear whether GABA-induced V_m changes at remote locations could influence AP initiation and propagation. To address this question, we performed simultaneous recordings from the soma and the bleb with low-Cl^- ICS, and then applied GABA through iontophoresis to the axon trunk to investigate its role in regulating AP generation (Figure 6A).

GABA application to the axon trunk could result in V_m hyperpolarization or depolarization (with low-Cl^- ICS), depending on the V_m when GABA was applied. These V_m changes could propagate to the soma and the recorded bleb (Figure 6B). Because E_{GABA} at the axon was more negative than the RMP (Figure 4), GABA receptor activation could hyperpolarize the axon. Given that the voltage fluctuations could propagate along the main axon with a length constant of hundreds of micrometers [2], V_m hyperpolarization could spread along the axon trunk and even reach the presynaptic terminals. Activation of axonal GABA

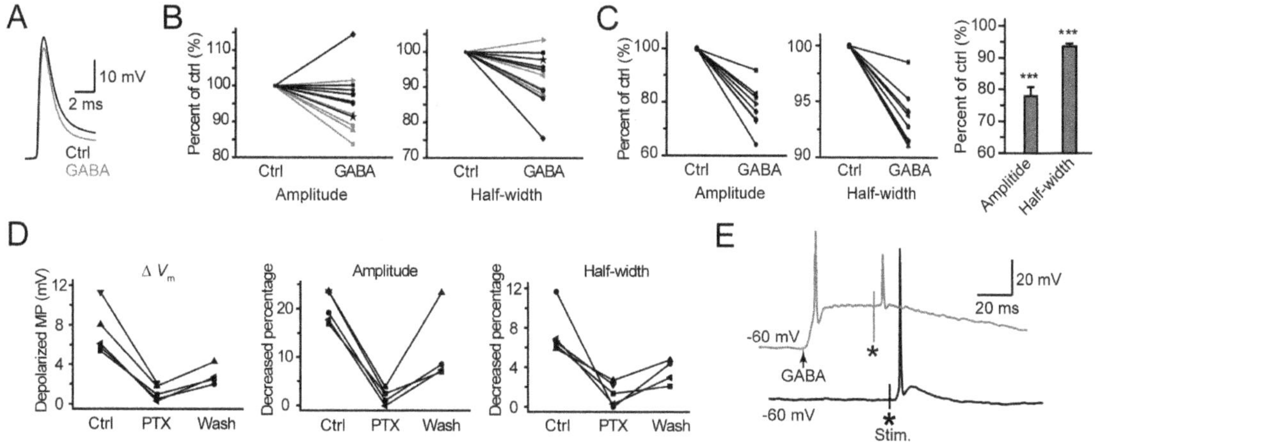

Figure 5. Activation of axonal GABA$_A$ receptors shapes the AP waveform. A, Example traces showing the change in AP waveform after GABA iontophoresis to the axon bleb. V_m change was −3.9 mV in this bleb. The amplitude and the half-width of APs decreased to 95.6% and 86.8% of the control, respectively. B, Group data showing that activation of axonal GABA$_A$ receptors shaped AP waveforms by regulating the amplitude and the half-width. Note that the recordings were performed under current-clamp and that the V_m could be manipulated by DC current injection. Black, GABA responses were hyperpolarizing; gray, depolarizing. The blebs were recorded with low-Cl$^-$ ICS (7 mM [Cl$^-$]$_i$). C, Increasing [Cl$^-$]$_i$ depolarized the V_m but still showed a shunting effect on AP waveforms. Amplitude and half-width were significantly reduced. Modified ICS (20 mM [Cl$^-$]$_i$) was used for these recordings. ***, P<0.001, paired t-test. D, Bath application of PTX could block the GABA-induced V_m depolarization and its shunting effect on AP waveform. Modified ICS was used. E, Example traces showing that GABA application caused a shunting effect on APs evoked by electric shocks (asterisks), although GABA itself could evoke an AP (arrow). High-Cl$^-$ ICS (75 mM [Cl$^-$]$_i$) was used here.

receptors at the main trunk could increase the amplitude (by 3.2±0.7%, n = 7. P<0.01) but did not produce a significant change in AP half-width (decreased by 2.2±1.4%, n = 7. P = 0.15). This phenomenon was similar to the AP waveform changes caused by hyperpolarization induced by negative current injection (amplitude: by 4.7±2.0%, P = 0.04; half-width: by 3.4±0.7%, P = 0.04; n = 5. Figure 6C). Therefore, activation of remote axonal GABA receptors could also regulate the waveform of propagating APs by hyperpolarizing the membrane potential.

We next injected step currents (100–500 pA, 500 ms) at the soma to evoke a train of APs, and corresponding APs could be observed at the bleb. As shown in Figure 6D, we observed a failure of AP initiation for weak somatic stimulation (gray, 100–200 pA, n = 3) and a decrease in firing frequency for strong stimulation (black, 400–500 pA, n = 5) when GABA was applied to the distal axon trunk (>100 μm apart from the soma). In contrast, when GABA was delivered at the AIS, substantial hyperpolarization (recording with pipettes filled with Low-Cl$^-$ ICS) and failure of AP initiation could be observed during both weak and strong current stimulation (200 and 400 pA, n = 7), presumably due to the strategic function of AIS for AP initiation. Iontophoresis of GABA to the main trunk could cause a decrease in the instantaneous firing frequency at the distal axon bleb (Figure 6E). The mean frequency of APs evoked by step current injection (400–500 pA) dropped from 24.7±2.0 to 20.1±2.3 Hz (P<0.01, paired t-test. n = 5) immediately after GABA application (Figure 6E). These results indicate a role for axonal GABA$_A$ receptors in regulating AP generation and firing frequency.

Regulation of AP-induced Ca^{2+} transients by axonal GABA$_A$ receptors

Previous studies revealed that changes in AP waveforms could regulate the amount of Ca^{2+} entry, leading to changes in neurotransmitter release [28,29]. We therefore speculated that AP waveform changes induced by the activation of axonal GABA$_A$ receptors could also regulate intracellular Ca^{2+} levels in the axon and the consequent neurotransmitter release.

We performed two-photon Ca^{2+} imaging to investigate whether AP-induced Ca^{2+} transients at the axon were subject to modulation by iontophoresis of GABA. As shown in Figure 7A, a layer −5 pyramidal neuron was filled with Alexa Fluor 594 (50 μM) and the Ca^{2+} indicator OGB-1 (200 μM) through the whole-cell patch pipette. Several regions of interest (ROIs) were selected for optical recording. We observed a decrease in Ca^{2+} transients in the axon (ROI 1 and 2, Figure 7A) after GABA application; however, the Ca^{2+} signals at the soma, which was remote from the GABA iontophoresis site, were not affected. In this particular cell, the distance between the iontophoresis site and ROI 1, ROI 2 and the soma were 36, 21 and 127 μm, respectively. The direction of bath flow was always from the soma to the axon, and the GABA application site was defined as 0. The distances between the application site and downstream or upstream ROIs were shown as positive or negative values, respectively. Group data from 13 cells showed that local GABA application decreased the Ca^{2+} transients induced by single APs by 14.1±1.4% at the axonal segments (ranging from −39 to 55 μm, n = 68 ROIs) that were close to the iontophoresis site (Figure 7B); no significant change was observed in 9 ROIs with distances longer than −40 μm. In contrast, Ca^{2+} transients at the soma showed no significant decrease (P = 0.84) after GABA application at a distance>100 μm from the soma. Significant reduction (P< 0.01) in Ca^{2+} transients was detected only when the distance between the soma and GABA application site was less than 100 μm (Figure 7B).

Similarly, axonal Ca^{2+} transients evoked by a train of 3 APs at 100 Hz were also significantly decreased by local GABA application (by 10.9±1.2%, axonal segments ranging from −59 to 59 μm, n = 61 ROIs of 9 cells. Figure 7C); no significant change was observed in 7 ROIs with distance greater than −60 μm. Bath application of PTX could block the GABA-induced decrease in Ca^{2+} transients evoked by either single APs (n = 11 ROIs of 3 cells) or bursts of 3 APs (n = 25 ROIs of 6 cells), indicating a role for axonal GABA$_A$ receptors in modulating local Ca^{2+} signals (Figure 7D).

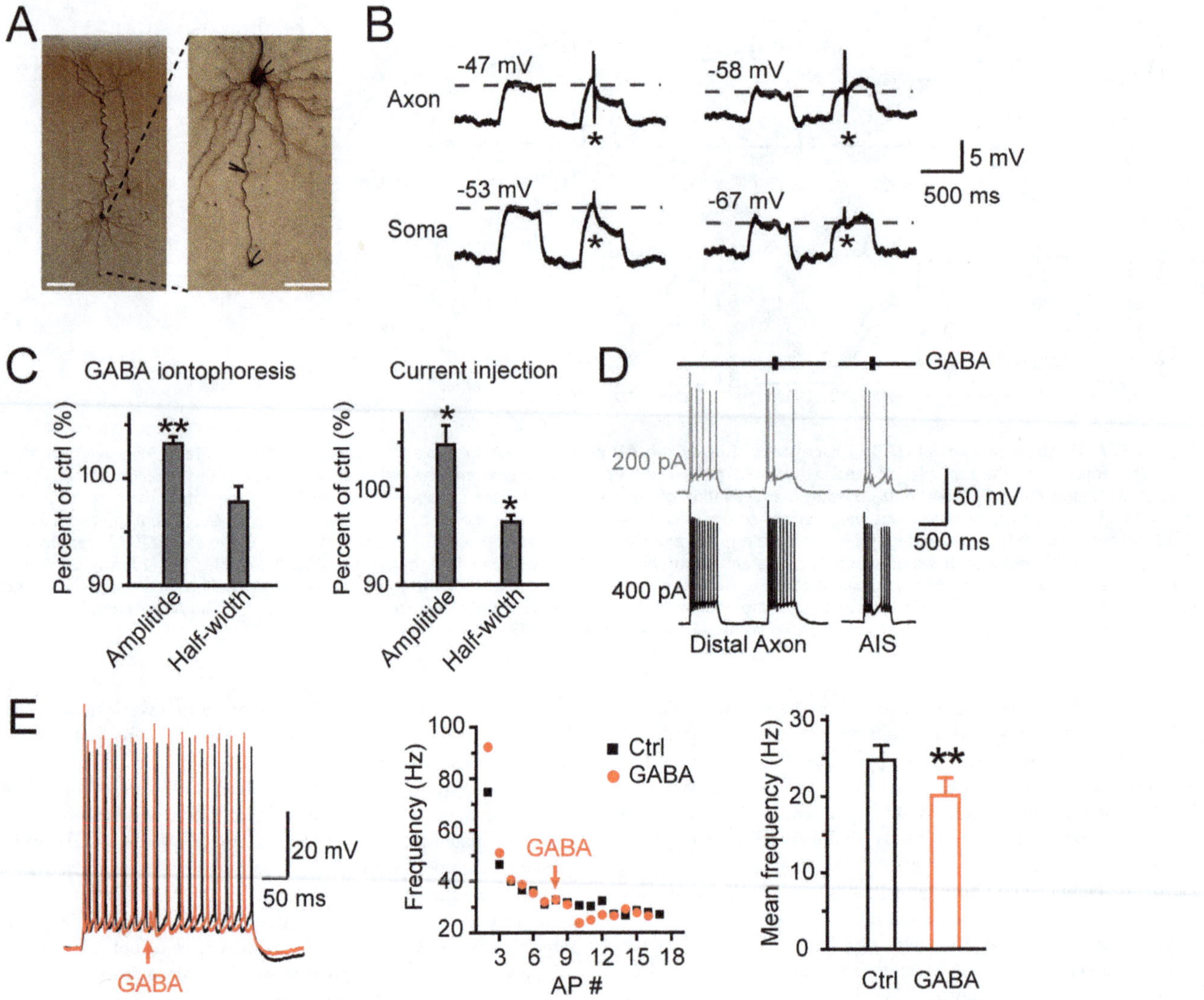

Figure 6. Propagation of GABA-induced hyperpolarization at the axon regulates AP generation. A, DAB staining of recorded neurons. Simultaneous recording from the soma and axon bleb were performed in a pyramidal neuron (left), and GABA was applied to the axon trunk (right). The axon length was 239 μm in this case. The distance between the iontophoresis site and the soma was 117 μm. Scale bar: 100 μm (left); 50 μm (right). B, The sign of the effect of GABA (hyperpolarization or depolarization) depended on the V_m. Top, traces were taken from the bleb. Bottom, traces were the corresponding responses at the soma. The V_m was clamped through somatic DC current injection. Asterisk indicates application of GABA to the main trunk. C, Left, application of GABA to the axon increased the amplitude but decreased the half-width of propagating APs. GABA iontophoresis hyperpolarized the V_m by 2.3±0.4 mV (n = 7). Right, similar results were obtained when V_m was hyperpolarized by 2.8±0.3 mV (n = 5) through DC current injection. *, P<0.05; **, P<0.01, paired t-test. D, Example traces showing activation of axonal $GABA_A$ receptors reduced firing probability and frequency. The distances between the iontophoresis site and the soma were 100 μm (distal axon) and 18 μm (AIS). E, Left, repetitive firing recorded at an axon bleb induced by 400 pA DC current injection at the soma before (black) and after (red) GABA application to the axon trunk. The arrow indicates GABA iontophoresis. Middle, instantaneous firing frequency of APs decreased after GABA application (same data as shown in the left). Right, group data showing a decrease in the mean frequency of APs after GABA iontophoresis at the axon trunk. **, P<0.01, paired t-test. Low-Cl^- ICS was used in these experiments.

Discussion

In this study, we found that $GABA_A$ receptors were expressed at the main axon trunks of layer – 5 pyramidal neurons and that activation of these receptors mainly hyperpolarized local V_m under physiological conditions. Importantly, we also show that waveforms of propagating APs could be shaped by either GABA-induced shunting or hyperpolarizing effects. Consistent with these results, AP-induced Ca^{2+} transients were substantially reduced by GABA application to the axon trunk, suggesting an important role for axonal $GABA_A$ receptors in regulating the output signal of pyramidal neurons.

Previous studies revealed the expression of $GABA_A$ receptors at presynaptic axons [24,30,31,32,33,34]. Those axonal $GABA_A$ receptors have been described as localizing in various brain regions including the spinal cord, brainstem, the cerebellum, the hippocampus and the cortex. Due to difficulties in recording from thin axons with diameter less than 1 μm [35], the properties and function of axonal GABA receptors have received much less attention than somatodendritic receptors. At the axon, GABA receptors distributed in some special axonal compartments such as the AIS (thicker than the main axon) and axon terminals (e.g., hippocampal mossy fiber boutons and midbrain calyx of Held)

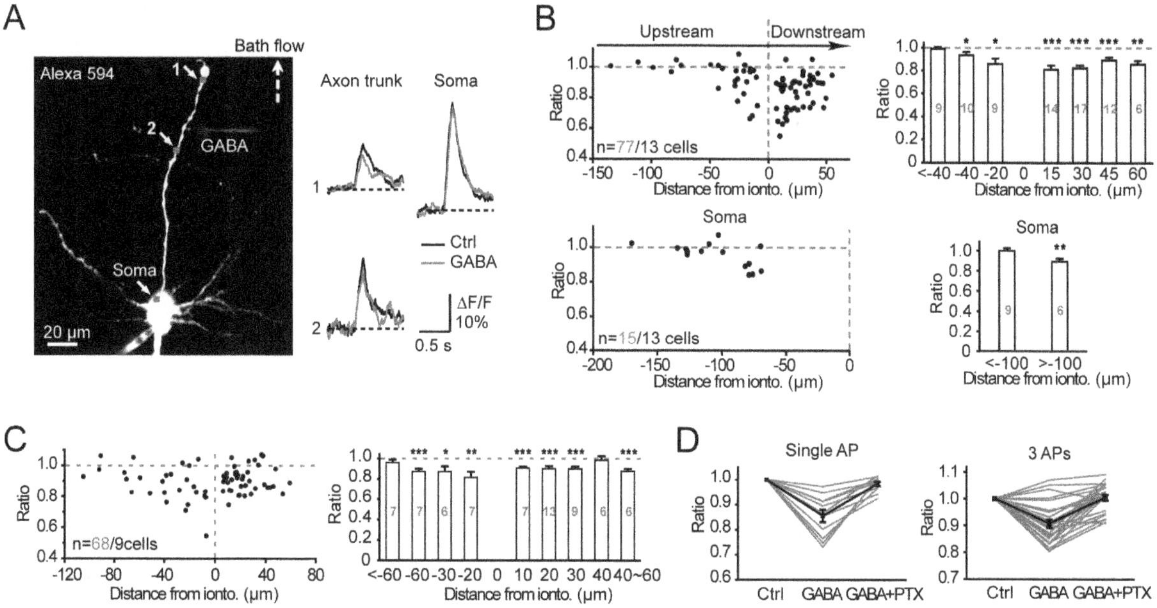

Figure 7. Activation of axonal GABA$_A$ receptors decreases AP-induced Ca^{2+} transients. A, Left, projection of 2-photon fluorescence images of a recorded pyramidal neuron filled with Alexa Fluor 594 (50 μM) and OGB-1 (200 μM). The dashed arrow indicates the direction of bath flow. Right, iontophoresis of GABA at the axon trunk (labeled by "GABA" in the left image) decreased Ca^{2+} transients evoked by single APs at nearby locations (ROI 1 and 2) but showed no effect on somatic transients. B, Group data showing the effect of GABA on single-AP-triggered Ca^{2+} transients. The results are presented as the ratio of the Ca^{2+} signal amplitude for "GABA" to "Ctrl." Top, data collected from the axon trunk (n = 13 axons). Bottom, data collected from the soma. The site for GABA iontophoresis was defined as 0. If the ROI was located downstream from the iontophoresis site, the sign of the distance was positive; otherwise it was assigned a negative sign. *, P<0.05; **, P<0.01; ***, P<0.001, paired t-test. C, Group data showing the effect of GABA on Ca^{2+} transients induced by 3 APs (100 Hz). Data were collected from the axon trunk (n = 9 axons). D, PTX blocked GABA-induced decrease in Ca^{2+} transients. Gray, individual cells; black, average data.

have been studied. In this study, by using the bleb recording method [2], we could directly examine the properties of ion channels and transmitter receptors located in the axon trunk. A previous study using high-Cl$^-$ ICS (approximately 140 mM) revealed that pairing GABA iontophoresis with antidromic axonal stimulation could substantially decrease spike failures [36]. Here, we employed multiple types of ICS with varying Cl$^-$ concentrations and showed the existence of GABA$_A$ receptors at the distal axon of layer –5 pyramidal neuron in prefrontal cortex. In addition, both that previous study and our findings revealed no presence of glutamate receptors at the axon, which is different from the pattern found in CA3 pyramidal neurons [7].

There is still debate regarding whether activation of axonal GABA$_A$ receptors induces hyperpolarization or depolarization. To address this question, one must know the difference between the RMP and E_{GABA} at the axon. With a variety of noninvasive recording methods performed on axon including the AIS [15,37], axon trunk [19] and presynaptic terminals [18], previous studies showed that axonal E_{GABA} was more depolarized than RMP so GABA responses increased neuron excitability. However, the unitary field potential recordings performed on hippocampal CA1 pyramidal cells suggested that activation of axo-axonic synapses induces hyperpolarizing responses [17]. In our experiments, we found that E_{GABA} in the distal axon trunk (beyond the AIS) is more hyperpolarized than the local RMP (–67 vs. –61 mV). Unlike some of the reports mentioned above, our findings suggest that GABA can induce hyperpolarization at distal axonal segments. Because E_{GABA} is mainly determined by $[Cl^-]_i$, the conflicting results could be explained by different $[Cl^-]_i$. A higher $[Cl^-]_i$ can result in a more depolarized E_{GABA}. The $[Cl^-]_i$ varies across developmental stages and brain regions. Even within the same brain region, it has also been reported that the response induced by GABA can be cell-type specific [38,39,40]. At one extreme, the GABA-mediated response in the suprachiasmatic nucleus is excitatory during the day but inhibitory during the night [41]. Various cation-chloride co-transporters play pivotal roles in maintaining intracellular chloride homeostasis [42,43]. The Na^+-K^+-$2Cl^-$ co-transporters (NKCCs) account for Cl$^-$ accumulation, whereas K^+-$2Cl^-$ co-transporters (KCCs) account for Cl$^-$ extrusion. In retina, the expression pattern of cation-chloride co-transporters shows specificity in cell type and subcellular locations [44]. In cortex, the co-operation of NKCC1 and KCC2 results in a relatively high $[Cl^-]_i$ in AIS and therefore depolarizes E_{GABA} [15,37]. The distribution pattern and function of these co-transporters at the axon trunk remains to be further examined.

However, hyperpolarization and depolarization cannot simply be considered as inhibitory and excitatory, respectively. Under some circumstances, presynaptic depolarization mediated by axonal GABA$_A$ receptors results in activation of voltage-gated Ca^{2+} channels, even causing AP initiation [45]. In other cases, presynaptic inhibition occurs because of inactivation of Na$^+$ and/or Ca^{2+} channels. GABA-induced depolarization may reduce the amplitude of APs and cause a decrease in Ca^{2+} influx [24,46]. Furthermore, opening of GABA$_A$ receptor channels will introduce a leaky conductance during generation of APs and propagation of postsynaptic potentials whether the GABA response is depolarizing or hyperpolarizing [47,48]. The actual effect of GABA also depends on the precision of the timing and location [49,50]. Therefore, the shunting inhibition together with V_m changes must be taken into account in analyses of the effect of GABA. In our study, GABA-mediated inhibition is associated with both hyperpolarization and shunting under physiological conditions. By increasing the $[Cl^-]_i$ to a high level (75 mM), GABA application itself can evoke APs if the depolarizing response overcomes the shunting conductance and reaches the threshold for AP generation (Fig. 5E).

The concentration of GABA in the synaptic cleft can reach a millimolar level [51,52] and the ambient GABA concentration varies from nanomolar to a few micromolar [53,54]. $GABA_A$ receptors located in the distal axon trunk can be activated by a low concentration of muscimol (5 μM). Additionally, the change of holding current in the presence of PTX was consistent with previous findings [55,56]. These results suggest that axonal $GABA_A$ receptors have high affinity to GABA and can be tonically activated. Before entering the white matter, the axon segments (approximately 400 μm in length) of layer –5 pyramidal neurons in prefrontal cortex are not myelinated [57]. These axon segments may be subcellular candidates for the modulation of neuronal output signals. We have recently shown that at these unmyelinated axons K^+ currents and AP waveforms are subject to dopaminergic modulation [58]. At the direct activation site, the GABA-induced shunting effect can regulate the AP waveform by decreasing the amplitude and the half-width. Beyond this site, GABA-induced hyperpolarization can propagate for hundreds of micrometers and decrease the AP width in contrast to the action of subthreshold depolarization [2,59]. Consistent with previous findings showing a linear dependence of Ca^{2+} influx on AP half-width [28,60], our Ca^{2+} imaging results show a decrease in AP-induced Ca^{2+} transients after GABA application to the axon.

In summary, we show the existence of $GABA_A$ receptors at the axon trunk of cortical pyramidal neurons. Activation of these receptors shortens propagating APs and decrease AP-induced Ca^{2+} entry by shunting and/or hyperpolarization. GABA-induced changes in axonal AP waveforms may represent a new mechanism for GABAergic modulation of synaptic transmission in the cortex.

Supporting Information

Figure S1 Filtering effect of the axon cable on GABA-induced currents. A, Example recording at the soma with GABA iontophoresis at the axon bleb. The red line indicates the linear fit of the rising phase, the rising slope can be derived from this fit. The red dashed line is an exponential fit of the decay phase, the decay time course can be then obtained. In this experiment, whole-cell recording was achieved at the soma with low-Cl^- ICS (V_{hold} = –40 mV) while GABA was applied at the axon bleb via iontophoresis (200 nA, 5 ms). B, Left, a plot of the rising slope of the GABA-induced currents as a function of the distance between the bleb and the soma (distance *L*, n = 29). Right, the pooled data shown on the left were divided into three subgroups according to the distance *L*. The rising slope of each group was 6.0±0.7 (n = 6), 2.0±0.4 (n = 15), 0.9±0.3 (n = 8), respectively. C, Left, a plot of the decay time course as a function of the distance *L* (n = 29). Right, the decay time course of each subgroup was 168.4±47.6 (n = 6), 216.6±34.1 (n = 15), 305.8±88.2 (n = 8), respectively.

Author Contributions

Conceived and designed the experiments: SZ YS. Performed the experiments: YX YZ. Analyzed the data: YX YZ MY. Contributed reagents/materials/analysis tools: YX YZ MY. Contributed to the writing of the manuscript: YX YS.

References

1. Alle H, Geiger JR (2006) Combined analog and action potential coding in hippocampal mossy fibers. Science 311: 1290–1293.
2. Shu Y, Hasenstaub A, Duque A, Yu Y, McCormick DA (2006) Modulation of intracortical synaptic potentials by presynaptic somatic membrane potential. Nature 441: 761–765.
3. Christie JM, Jahr CE (2008) Dendritic NMDA receptors activate axonal calcium channels. Neuron 60: 298–307.
4. Kole MH, Letzkus JJ, Stuart GJ (2007) Axon initial segment Kv1 channels control axonal action potential waveform and synaptic efficacy. Neuron 55: 633–647.
5. Shu Y, Yu Y, Yang J, McCormick DA (2007) Selective control of cortical axonal spikes by a slowly inactivating K+ current. Proc Natl Acad Sci U S A 104: 11453–11458.
6. Turecek R, Trussell LO (2001) Presynaptic glycine receptors enhance transmitter release at a mammalian central synapse. Nature 411: 587–590.
7. Sasaki T, Matsuki N, Ikegaya Y (2011) Action-potential modulation during axonal conduction. Science 331: 599–601.
8. Engelman HS, MacDermott AB (2004) Presynaptic ionotropic receptors and control of transmitter release. Nat Rev Neurosci 5: 135–145.
9. Zucker RS, Regehr WG (2002) Short-term synaptic plasticity. Annu Rev Physiol 64: 355–405.
10. Moss SJ, Smart TG (2001) Constructing inhibitory synapses. Nat Rev Neurosci 2: 240–250.
11. Farrant M, Kaila K (2007) The cellular, molecular and ionic basis of GABA(A) receptor signalling. Prog Brain Res 160: 59–87.
12. Miles R, Toth K, Gulyas AI, Hajos N, Freund TF (1996) Differences between somatic and dendritic inhibition in the hippocampus. Neuron 16: 815–823.
13. Pouille F, Scanziani M (2001) Enforcement of temporal fidelity in pyramidal cells by somatic feed-forward inhibition. Science 293: 1159–1163.
14. Somogyi P, Klausberger T (2005) Defined types of cortical interneurone structure space and spike timing in the hippocampus. J Physiol 562: 9–26.
15. Szabadics J, Varga C, Molnar G, Olah S, Barzo P, et al. (2006) Excitatory effect of GABAergic axo-axonic cells in cortical microcircuits. Science 311: 233–235.
16. Ben-Ari Y (2002) Excitatory actions of gaba during development: the nature of the nurture. Nat Rev Neurosci 3: 728–739.
17. Glickfeld LL, Roberts JD, Somogyi P, Scanziani M (2009) Interneurons hyperpolarize pyramidal cells along their entire somatodendritic axis. Nat Neurosci 12: 21–23.
18. Ruiz A, Campanac E, Scott RS, Rusakov DA, Kullmann DM (2010) Presynaptic GABAA receptors enhance transmission and LTP induction at hippocampal mossy fiber synapses. Nat Neurosci 13: 431–438.
19. Pugh JR, Jahr CE (2011) Axonal GABAA receptors increase cerebellar granule cell excitability and synaptic activity. J Neurosci 31: 565–574.
20. Hu W, Shu Y (2012) Axonal bleb recording. Neurosci Bull 28: 342–350.
21. Barker JL, McBurney RN, MacDonald JF (1982) Fluctuation analysis of neutral amino acid responses in cultured mouse spinal neurones. J Physiol 322: 365–387.
22. Neher E, Stevens CF (1977) Conductance fluctuations and ionic pores in membranes. Annu Rev Biophys Bioeng 6: 345–381.
23. Lv XH, Zhan C, Zeng SQ, Chen WR, Luo QM (2006) Construction of multiphoton laser scanning microscope based on dual-axis acousto-optic deflector. Rev Sci Instrum 77.
24. Ruiz A, Fabian-Fine R, Scott R, Walker MC, Rusakov DA, et al. (2003) GABAA receptors at hippocampal mossy fibers. Neuron 39: 961–973.
25. Howe JR, Sutor B, Zieglgansberger W (1987) Baclofen reduces post-synaptic potentials of rat cortical neurones by an action other than its hyperpolarizing action. J Physiol 384: 539–569.
26. Freund TF, Buzsaki G (1996) Interneurons of the hippocampus. Hippocampus 6: 347–470.
27. Somogyi P, Tamas G, Lujan R, Buhl EH (1998) Salient features of synaptic organisation in the cerebral cortex. Brain Res Brain Res Rev 26: 113–135.
28. Geiger JR, Jonas P (2000) Dynamic control of presynaptic Ca(2+) inflow by fast-inactivating K(+) channels in hippocampal mossy fiber boutons. Neuron 28: 927–939.
29. Augustine GJ (1990) Regulation of transmitter release at the squid giant synapse by presynaptic delayed rectifier potassium current. J Physiol 431: 343–364.
30. Trigo FF, Marty A, Stell BM (2008) Axonal GABAA receptors. Eur J Neurosci 28: 841–848.
31. Eccles JC, Eccles RM, Magni F (1961) Central inhibitory action attributable to presynaptic depolarization produced by muscle afferent volleys. J Physiol 159: 147–166.
32. Turecek R, Trussell LO (2002) Reciprocal developmental regulation of presynaptic ionotropic receptors. Proc Natl Acad Sci U S A 99: 13884–13889.
33. Pouzat C, Marty A (1999) Somatic recording of GABAergic autoreceptor current in cerebellar stellate and basket cells. J Neurosci 19: 1675–1690.
34. Tachibana M, Kaneko A (1987) gamma-Aminobutyric acid exerts a local inhibitory action on the axon terminal of bipolar cells: evidence for negative feedback from amacrine cells. Proc Natl Acad Sci U S A 84: 3501–3505.

35. Debanne D (2004) Information processing in the axon. Nat Rev Neurosci 5: 304–316.
36. Christie JM, Jahr CE (2009) Selective expression of ligand-gated ion channels in L5 pyramidal cell axons. J Neurosci 29: 11441–11450.
37. Khirug S, Yamada J, Afzalov R, Voipio J, Khiroug L, et al. (2008) GABAergic depolarization of the axon initial segment in cortical principal neurons is caused by the Na-K-2Cl cotransporter NKCC1. J Neurosci 28: 4635–4639.
38. Golding NL, Oertel D (1996) Context-dependent synaptic action of glycinergic and GABAergic inputs in the dorsal cochlear nucleus. J Neurosci 16: 2208–2219.
39. Martina M, Royer S, Pare D (2001) Cell-type-specific GABA responses and chloride homeostasis in the cortex and amygdala. J Neurophysiol 86: 2887–2895.
40. Chavas J, Marty A (2003) Coexistence of excitatory and inhibitory GABA synapses in the cerebellar interneuron network. J Neurosci 23: 2019–2031.
41. Wagner S, Castel M, Gainer H, Yarom Y (1997) GABA in the mammalian suprachiasmatic nucleus and its role in diurnal rhythmicity. Nature 387: 598–603.
42. Payne JA, Rivera C, Voipio J, Kaila K (2003) Cation-chloride co-transporters in neuronal communication, development and trauma. Trends Neurosci 26: 199–206.
43. Ben-Ari Y, Gaiarsa JL, Tyzio R, Khazipov R (2007) GABA: a pioneer transmitter that excites immature neurons and generates primitive oscillations. Physiol Rev 87: 1215–1284.
44. Vardi N, Zhang LL, Payne JA, Sterling P (2000) Evidence that different cation chloride cotransporters in retinal neurons allow opposite responses to GABA. J Neurosci 20: 7657–7663.
45. Kullmann DM, Ruiz A, Rusakov DM, Scott R, Semyanov A, et al. (2005) Presynaptic, extrasynaptic and axonal GABAA receptors in the CNS: where and why? Prog Biophys Mol Biol 87: 33–46.
46. Rudomin P, Schmidt RF (1999) Presynaptic inhibition in the vertebrate spinal cord revisited. Exp Brain Res 129: 1–37.
47. Cattaert D, El Manira A (1999) Shunting versus inactivation: analysis of presynaptic inhibitory mechanisms in primary afferents of the crayfish. J Neurosci 19: 6079–6089.
48. Segev I (1990) Computer study of presynaptic inhibition controlling the spread of action potentials into axonal terminals. J Neurophysiol 63: 987–998.
49. Chiang PH, Wu PY, Kuo TW, Liu YC, Chan CF, et al. (2012) GABA is depolarizing in hippocampal dentate granule cells of the adolescent and adult rats. J Neurosci 32: 62–67.
50. Gulledge AT, Stuart GJ (2003) Excitatory actions of GABA in the cortex. Neuron 37: 299–309.
51. Mody I, De Koninck Y, Otis TS, Soltesz I (1994) Bridging the cleft at GABA synapses in the brain. Trends Neurosci 17: 517–525.
52. Mozrzymas JW (2004) Dynamism of GABA(A) receptor activation shapes the "personality" of inhibitory synapses. Neuropharmacology 47: 945–960.
53. Santhakumar V, Hanchar HJ, Wallner M, Olsen RW, Otis TS (2006) Contributions of the GABAA receptor alpha6 subunit to phasic and tonic inhibition revealed by a naturally occurring polymorphism in the alpha6 gene. J Neurosci 26: 3357–3364.
54. Cavelier P, Hamann M, Rossi D, Mobbs P, Attwell D (2005) Tonic excitation and inhibition of neurons: ambient transmitter sources and computational consequences. Prog Biophys Mol Biol 87: 3–16.
55. Semyanov A, Walker MC, Kullmann DM, Silver RA (2004) Tonically active GABA A receptors: modulating gain and maintaining the tone. Trends Neurosci 27: 262–269.
56. Farrant M, Nusser Z (2005) Variations on an inhibitory theme: phasic and tonic activation of GABA(A) receptors. Nat Rev Neurosci 6: 215–229.
57. Shu Y, Duque A, Yu Y, Haider B, McCormick DA (2007) Properties of action-potential initiation in neocortical pyramidal cells: evidence from whole cell axon recordings. J Neurophysiol 97: 746–760.
58. Yang J, Ye M, Tian C, Yang M, Wang Y, et al. (2013) Dopaminergic modulation of axonal potassium channels and action potential waveform in pyramidal neurons of prefrontal cortex. J Physiol 591: 3233–3251.
59. Alle H, Geiger JR (2008) Analog signalling in mammalian cortical axons. Curr Opin Neurobiol. 2008/09/20 ed. 314–320.
60. Bischofberger J, Geiger JR, Jonas P (2002) Timing and efficacy of Ca2+ channel activation in hippocampal mossy fiber boutons. J Neurosci 22: 10593–10602.

14

Enhanced Cellular Uptake of Albumin-Based Lyophilisomes when Functionalized with Cell-Penetrating Peptide TAT in HeLa Cells

Etienne van Bracht[1], Luuk R. M. Versteegden[1], Sarah Stolle[1¤a], Wouter P. R. Verdurmen[1¤b], Rob Woestenenk[2], René Raavé[1], Theo Hafmans[1], Egbert Oosterwijk[3], Roland Brock[1], Toin H. van Kuppevelt[1], Willeke F. Daamen[1]*

1 Department of Biochemistry, Radboud Institute for Molecular Life Sciences, Radboud university medical centre, Geert Grooteplein 28, 6525 GA, Nijmegen, The Netherlands, **2** Department of Laboratory Medicine, Laboratory of Hematology, Radboud university medical centre, Geert Grooteplein 8, 6525 GA, Nijmegen, The Netherlands, **3** Department of Urology, Radboud Institute for Molecular Life Sciences, Radboud university medical centre, Geert Grooteplein 28, 6525 GA, Nijmegen, The Netherlands

Abstract

Lyophilisomes are a novel class of biodegradable proteinaceous nano/micrometer capsules with potential use as drug delivery carrier. Cell-penetrating peptides (CPPs) including the TAT peptide have been successfully implemented for intracellular delivery of a broad variety of cargos including various nanoparticulate pharmaceutical carriers. In the present study, lyophilisomes were modified using CPPs in order to achieve enhanced cellular uptake. Lyophilisomes were prepared by a freezing, annealing, and lyophilization method and a cystein-elongated TAT peptide was conjugated to the lyophilisomes using a heterobifunctional linker. Fluorescent-activated cell sorting (FACS) was utilized to acquire a lyophilisome population with a particle diameter smaller than 1000 nm. Cultured HeLa, OVCAR-3, Caco-2 and SKOV-3 cells were exposed to unmodified lyophilisomes and TAT-conjugated lyophilisomes and examined with FACS. HeLa cells were investigated in more detail using a trypan blue quenching assay, confocal microscopy, and transmission electron microscopy. TAT-conjugation strongly increased binding and cellular uptake of lyophilisomes in a time-dependent manner *in vitro*, as assessed by FACS. These results were confirmed by confocal microscopy. Transmission electron microscopy indicated rapid cellular uptake of TAT-conjugated lyophilisomes via phagocytosis and/or macropinocytosis. In conclusion, TAT-peptides conjugated to albumin-based lyophilisomes are able to enhance cellular uptake of lyophilisomes in HeLa cells.

Editor: Maxim Antopolsky, University of Helsinki, Finland

Funding: The research project was funded by the Radboud university medical centre. The funders had no role in study design, data collection and analysis, decision to publish, or preparation of the manuscript.

Competing Interests: The authors have declared that no competing interests exist.

* Email: Willeke.Daamen@radboudumc.nl

¤a Current address: Department of Pediatrics, Center for Liver, Digestive and Metabolic Disease, University Medical Center Groningen, Hanzeplein 1, 9713 GZ Groningen, The Netherlands
¤b Current address: Department of Biochemistry, University of Zurich, Winterthurerstrasse 190, 8057 Zurich, Switzerland

Introduction

An innovative strategy in cancer therapy utilizes drug delivery carriers to increase the therapeutic effect of anti-tumor drugs. The role of drug delivery carriers in this context is to improve pharmacokinetics and dynamics by protecting the drug from degradation [1–3]. Contemporary drug delivery systems include nanoparticulate systems loaded with anti-tumor drug and conjugates directly coupled to the drug. The unique property of nanoparticle carriers is their ability to encapsulate and deliver a high dose of anti-tumor drugs, including poorly soluble drugs, and to exploit the enhanced permeability and retention (EPR) effect for tumor targeting [4]. Because of these favorable characteristics, there has been intense interest in the development of nanoparticulate drug delivery systems.

Nanoparticles currently investigated for cancer therapeutic applications include liposomes, polymersomes, dendrimers, micelles, carbon nanotubes, nanoconjugates and (protein-based) nanospheres or capsules [5–7]. Among the available potential drug carrier systems, protein-based nanoparticles are particularly interesting as they hold certain advantages such as good stability during storage, non-toxicity, biocompatibility, and biodegradability *in vivo* [8,9]. Recently we showed that lyophilisomes, a novel class of proteinaceous biodegradable hollow nano/micrometer capsules, show potential as a drug delivery capsule [10,11]. Lyophilisomes can be prepared from a large variety of water-soluble macromolecules including proteins (*e.g.* albumin and elastin) but also polysaccharides (*e.g.* heparin). In fact, virtually any biomolecule can be incorporated into the wall/lumen of the capsule, resulting in a highly flexible carrier system with multiple applications. We previously demonstrated that enzymes introduced in the capsule's wall and in the lumen are bioactive and able to convert a substrate [10]. Furthermore, lyophilisomes have been efficiently loaded with doxorubicin resulting in tumor cell elimination *in vitro* [11]. In order to obtain a selective drug delivery system, lyophilisomes have also been modified with antibodies, resulting in specific targeting of the cell of interest *in vitro* [12]. Due to these properties, lyophilisomes can be deployed for the design of multifunctional targeting systems.

Lyophilisomes were prepared from albumin. Albumin is an attractive macromolecular carrier that has been shown to be non-toxic, non-immunogenic, biodegradable to produce innocuous degradation products, and easy to purify [13]. It is thus a suitable candidate for nanoparticle preparation, as demonstrated by FDA-approved products such as Abraxane [14,15] and Albunex [16,17].

Since delivery of nanocarriers is generally based on passive accumulation in pathological tissues, they do not efficiently deliver their cargo to specific cells. When drug delivery carriers arrive at the tumor site, they have to cross the plasma membrane in order to deliver the drug into the cell. The plasma membrane, however, prevent proteins, peptides, and nanoparticulate drug carriers from entering the cell in the absence of an active transport mechanism [18]. Cell-penetrating peptides (CPPs) have been successfully used to deliver a large variety of cargos to the cell interior including proteins [19], peptides [20], nucleic acids [21] and pharmaceutical nanocarriers [22–24]. CPPs are short peptides consisting of up to 30 amino acids that are able to translocate across the cellular membrane [25]. When CPPs are conjugated to drug delivery carriers, efficient cellular uptake of the carriers can be achieved [26]. A representative CPP is the TAT peptide, derived from the TAT protein (trans-activation transcriptional activator) of the human immunodeficiency virus type 1 (HIV-1) [27,28]. The TAT peptide consists of 11 amino acids with the sequence YGRKKRRQRRR. The abundance of lysine and arginine residues makes it highly positively charged, important for the interaction with the plasma membrane. In this study, the TAT peptide was conjugated to lyophilisomes to investigate whether CPPs are able to enhance cellular uptake of lyophilisomes.

Materials and Methods

Bovine serum albumin was purchased from PAA Laboratories (Linz, Austria). FITC-conjugated bovine albumin was purchased from Sigma Aldrich (Steinheim, Germany). Sulfo-GMBS (sulfo-*N*-[γ-maleimidobutyryloxy]sulfosuccinimide ester) was purchased from Pierce Biotechnology (Rockford, IL, USA). Glutaraldehyde and formaldehyde were obtained from Merck (Darmstadt, Germany). Cysteine functionalized TAT peptide (C-Ahx-YGRKKRRQRRR) was purchased from EMC Microcollections GmbH (Tübingen, Germany), in which Ahx = aminohexanoic acid linker.

Preparation of lyophilisomes

Lyophilisomes were prepared from albumin as described previously [11]. Briefly, droplets of a solution of 0.25% (w/v) bovine serum albumin (BSA) in 0.01 M acetic acid were frozen in liquid nitrogen (−196°C). The frozen albumin preparation was incubated at −10 to −20°C for 3 h (annealing step), and subsequently lyophilized. This procedure results in hollow nano/micro spheres ("lyophilisomes"). In order to visualize the lyophilisomes, FITC-conjugated albumin was added to non-labeled albumin (1:10) in the starting solution. To obtain stabilized lyophilisomes, they were vapor crosslinked with glutaraldehyde and formaldehyde. Generally we prepare 40 ml of a 0.25% BSA solution, which corresponds to 100 mg albumin (2.5 mg/ml). The final lyophilisome population was centrifuged three or four times at low speed (60×*g*; Thermo, Heraeus Fresco 17; Newport Pagnell, Great Britain) to remove large lyophilisomes and sheet-like structures, until no pellet was observed. After this procedure, about 30% of the original weight of lyophilisomes remained. Lyophilisomes (1 mg/ml) were stored in 0.1% (v/v) Tween-20 (Sigma Aldrich, Steinheim, Germany) in phosphate buffered saline (PBS-T, pH 7.4).

Conjugation of cell-penetrating peptide to lyophilisomes

A schematic representation of the conjugation reactions is depicted in figure 1.

Reaction 1. Activation of lyophilisomes. To obtain maleimide-activated lyophilisomes, 1 mg lyophilisomes were resuspended in 1 ml PBS-T and incubated overnight with 31 µl of 10 mM sulfo-GMBS in PBS-T (pH 8.0) at 4°C on a rotator (36 rpm, "Assistant" Rotating mixer, Karl Hecht, Sondheim, Germany), resulting in a 20:1 molar ratio of sulfo-GMBS:albumin. Excess sulfo-GMBS was removed by centrifugation (5 min, 17,000×*g*, 4°C) with three washing steps in PBS-T (pH 6.5).

Reaction 2. Conjugation of TAT peptide to lyophilisomes. For the coupling reaction, 1 ml of 1 mg/ml sulfhydryl-reactive lyophilisomes in 0.1% PBS-T was centrifuged and conjugated in 1 ml of cysteine functionalized TAT peptide (100 µM; C-Ahx-YGRKKRRQRRR) in 0.1% PBS-T (pH 6.5). Non-coupled TAT peptides were removed by centrifugation, using three washing steps in 0.1% PBS-T (pH 7.4). TAT-conjugated lyophilisomes were stored at 4°C in the dark.

Sorting of lyophilisomes by fluorescence-activated cell sorting

Fluorescence-activated cell sorting (FACS) was applied to select for small lyophilisomes (<1,000 nm) using a Coulter Epics Elite flow cytometer (BeckmanCoulter, Miami, FL, USA). Only small FITC-positive lyophilisomes were sorted (for settings, see section "Lyophilisomes sorted by fluorescence-activated cell sorting"). To achieve high sensitivity, gain was set at 20.

Particle size measurements by qNano

The qNano (Izon, Science Ltd., Burnside, New Zealand) was used to measure particle size distribution of lyophilisomes [11,29]. To ensure a continuous flow of particles, a pore size of 600–2000 nm was used. Data were analyzed with Izon Control Suite 2.1 software.

Cell culture

HeLa (ACC 57, DSMZ, Braunschweig, Germany) and OVCAR-3 (#HTB-161, ATCC, LGC Standards GmbH, Wesel, Germany) cells were cultured in RPMI 1640 GlutaMAX medium Gibco (Karlsruhe, Germany) supplemented with 10% (v/v) fetal calf serum (FCS; PAA Laboratories, Pasching, Austria). Caco-2 cells (#HTB-37, ATCC) and SKOV-3 cells (#HTB-77, ATCC) were cultured in DMEM 1640 GlutaMAX medium Gibco supplemented with 20% (v/v) and 10% (v/v/) fetal calf serum, respectively. Cells were cultured in a humidified atmosphere with 5% CO_2 at 37°C. Subconfluent cells were dissociated with 0.05% trypsin (w/v) in 0.02% ethylenediaminetetraacetic acid (EDTA) (w/v) in PBS (PAA Laboratories) and were maintained as proliferating cultures.

For FACS, cells were stained with the plasma membrane dye PKH26 (Sigma Aldrich, Missouri, USA) [30,31]. One million cells were incubated in 2 µM PKH26 dye in 500 µl buffer (according to

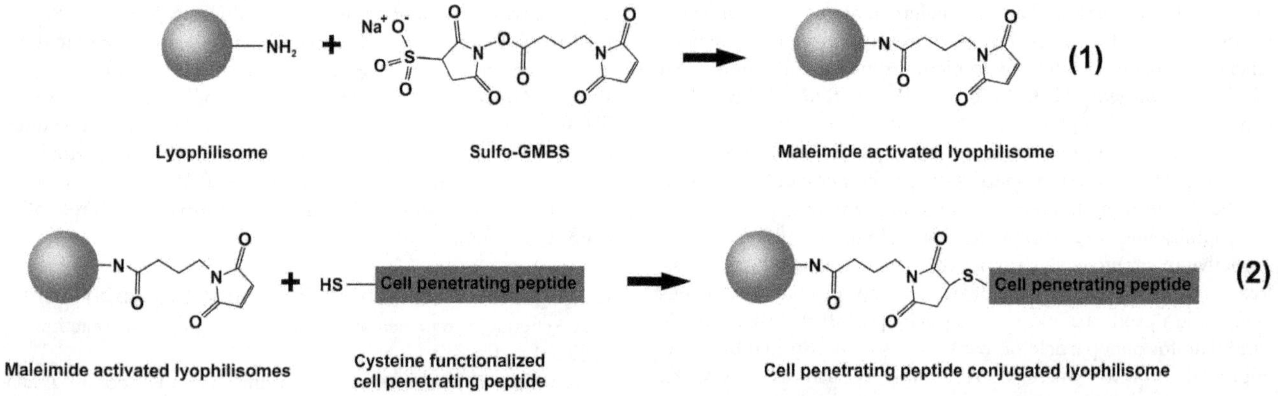

Figure 1. Schematic illustration of the conjugation of the cell-penetrating peptide (CPP) TAT to lyophilisomes. (1) Primary amine groups of lyophilisomes react with Sulfo-GMBS introducing reactive maleimide groups. (2) CPPs (cysteine-functionalized TAT-peptides; C-Ahx-YGRKKRRQRRR) are conjugated to maleimide-conjugated lyophilisomes, resulting in stable CPP-conjugated lyophilisomes. Sulfo-GMBS = sulfo-*N*-[γ-maleimidobutyryloxy]sulfo succinimide ester; Ahx = aminohexanoic acid; TAT = trans-activating transcriptional activator.

manufacturer's protocol) for 5 min. To stop the staining reaction, 500 µl FCS was added and incubated for 5 min. Subsequently, cells were washed three times with culture medium.

Cellular binding and internalization of lyophilisomes with and without TAT peptide

To determine whether the TAT peptide can promote the binding and internalization of lyophilisomes with HeLa, OVCAR-3, Caco-2 and SKOV-3 cells were seeded in a 24-well plate (30,000 cells/well in 1 ml medium). Cells were left to adhere overnight and subsequently incubated for 1 h with unsorted lyophilisomes with and without TAT peptide conjugated to them (25 µg/ml). After incubation, cells were washed three times with PBS to remove unbound lyophilisomes and harvested with enzyme-free EDTA solution (PAA Laboratories). Finally, cells were resuspended in 0.2% BSA in PBS and analyzed by FACS (FACSCalibur Becton Dickinson, Breda, Netherlands). Using the appropriate positive and negative controls FACS settings were adjusted. When lyophilisomes did not bind to cells, lyophilisomes were depicted at a fluorescent signal of 10^1 or below and cells were regarded negative. When lyophilisomes did bind to cells, they showed a fluorescent signal higher than 10^1. Data were analyzed by FlowJo software (Version 9.4, Treestar, Ashland, OR, USA).

Internalization studies of lyophilisomes by cells

FACS. In order to discriminate between attached and internalized lyophilisomes, a FITC quenching trypan blue assay was used [32–34]. Quenching of FITC signal occurs because trypan blue absorbs the light emitted by FITC-labeled lyophilisomes after excitation. The FITC signal of *internalized* lyophilisomes however, is not quenched since trypan blue cannot pass the plasma membrane. The fluorescence remaining after trypan blue quenching must therefore result from internalized lyophilisomes, as only extracellular fluorescence of FITC-lyophilisomes is quenched.

To investigate the cellular uptake of lyophilisomes, PKH26 stained HeLa cells were seeded in a 24-well plate (30,000 cells/well) and left to adhere overnight. Cells were incubated with 500,000 FACS-sorted lyophilisomes with and without TAT peptide for 1 and 4 h. After incubation, cells were washed three times with 0.2% (w/v) BSA in PBS, dissociated with enzyme-free EDTA dissociation buffer, resuspended in 1 ml culture medium and transferred to an eppendorf tube. Subsequently, cells were washed three times with 0.2% BSA-PBS by centrifugation (3 min, room temperature, 100 ×g) and incubated with 0.5% (w/v) trypan blue for 10 min and washed three times with 0.2% BSA-PBS. Cells were analyzed by FACSCalibur flowcytometry. Data were analyzed by FlowJo Software.

Confocal microscopy. To visualize cellular uptake of lyophilisomes, confocal microscopy was performed on living cells. HeLa cells were seeded in an 8-well microscopy chamber (Nunc; 30,000 cells/well) and left to adhere overnight. Cells were incubated with sorted lyophilisomes with and without TAT peptide using 0.8 and 3.5 million lyophilisomes in 200 µl per sample for 4 h in RPMI medium containing 10% FCS at 37°C. As a control, medium without lyophilisomes was used. After incubation, cells were washed three times, incubated for 5 min with CellMask Orange (5 µg/ml) to visualize the plasma membranes and then washed again, all with the same medium. Cells were kept at 37°C on a temperature controlled microscope stage and living cells were imaged immediately with a Leica SP5 confocal microscope (Leica Microsystems, Mannheim, Germany). FITC was excited at 488 nm and emission was collected between 500–550 nm. CellMask orange was excited at 561 nm and emission was collected between 570–650 nm. Images were recorded sequentially using Leica Application Suite Software (Advanced Fluorescence Lite, 2.3.0. build 5131).

Transmission electron microscopy. Cells incubated with lyophilisomes with and without TAT peptide as described in the Materials and Methods section "*FACS*" were embedded in 1.5% (w/v) agarose, fixed in 2% (v/v) glutaraldehyde in 0.1 M phosphate buffer (pH 7.4), post-fixed with 1% (w/v) osmium tetroxide, dehydrated in an ascending series of ethanol, and embedded in Epon 812. Ultrathin sections (60 nm) were cut and picked up on Formvar-coated grids, post-stained with lead citrate and uranyl acetate, and examined with a JEOL 1010 transmission electron microscope (Tokyo, Japan).

Statistical Analysis

Data are presented as mean with standard deviation. Data of Results section "*Cellular binding and internalization of lyophilisomes with and without TAT peptide*" were analyzed using two-tailed Student's *t*-tests. Data of Results section "*Trypan blue assay and FACS*" were analyzed using two-way Anova Bonferroni post-hoc tests. All statistical analyses were performed in Graphpad

Prism 5.0 (Graphpad, San Diego, CA, USA). P values<0.05 were considered significant.

Results

Conjugation of TAT peptide to lyophilisomes

To probe the possibility of using CPP for enhanced intracellular delivery, lyophilisomes were modified with a cysteine-functionalized TAT peptide using the heterobifunctional linker sulfo-GMBS (Fig. 1). The succinimidyl ester functionality is conjugated to primary amine groups on the lyophilisome while the maleimide functionality is used for conjugation to the free thiol of the cysteine residue coupled to the TAT peptide.

Cellular binding and internalization of lyophilisomes with and without TAT peptide

To address the presence of the TAT peptide on TAT-conjugated lyophilisomes, unmodified lyophilisomes and TAT-conjugated lyophilisomes were administered to HeLa, OVCAR-3, Caco-2 and OVCAR-3 cells. Using standard FACS as a functional assay, it is not possible to discriminate between cellular attachment and internalization. Instead, the total of cell binding and internalization is measured (Fig. 2). For HeLa cells, TAT-conjugated lyophilisomes showed an about 8-fold increase in lyophilisome-positive cells compared to lyophilisomes without the TAT peptide (86±3% and 12±4% lyophilisome-positive cells for TAT-conjugated and unmodified lyophilisomes, respectively. OVCAR-3 and Caco-2 cells showed about a 5-fold increase in lyophilisome-positive cells compared to lyophilisomes without the TAT peptide (lyophilisome-positive cells: 97±3% and 19±3% for OVCAR-3; 87±3% and 16±8% for Caco-2) for TAT-conjugated and unmodified lyophilisomes, respectively. SKOV-3 cells gave a high background value when incubated with lyophilisomes without TAT (67±20%), but still showed a 1.6 fold statistically significant increase with the presence of TAT peptide (95±10%).

Lyophilisomes sorted by fluorescence-activated cell sorting

When using lyophilisomes for tumor targeting, lyophilisomal size is an important parameter. The initial lyophilisome population included sizes up to 2.8 µm (Fig. 3a). To obtain a more monodisperse capsule population, lyophilisomes were sorted by FACS. Lyophilisomes were separated based on forward scatter and FITC fluorescence (FL1 channel; Fig. 3c). To verify the procedure, a rerun of sorted lyophilisomes was performed (Fig. 3d). Using this methodology, larger lyophilisomes as well as sheet-like structures (confirmed by scanning electron microscope) were separated from small lyophilisomes. These results were substantiated by qNano size analysis using a lyophilisome preparation before (Fig. 3a) and after (Fig. 3b) sorting (approximately 90% below 1 µm). Measurements using the qNano consisted of 200–250 particles. The size distribution contained multiple peaks that can be explained by the low number of particles. Due to the limitations of the qNano instrument particles smaller than 600 nm could not be reliably detected which overestimates the average size of the lyophilisomes. Pilot experiments with a smaller qNano pore (200–800 nm) revealed the presence of lyophilisomes below 600 nm (results not shown), but larger lyophilisomes in the preparation frequently blocked this pore.

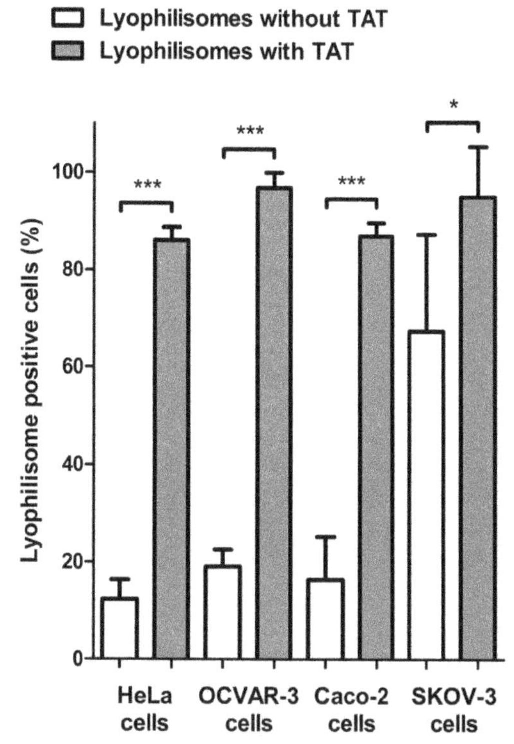

Figure 2. Cellular binding and internalization of unmodified lyophilisomes and TAT-conjugated lyophilisomes. HeLa, OVCAR-3, Caco-2 and SKOV-3 cells incubated with TAT-conjugated and unmodified lyophilisomes resulted in 86±3% and 12±4%, 87±3% and 16±8%, 97±3% and 19±3%, and 95±10% and 67±20% lyophilisome-positive cells, respectively. TAT = trans-activating transcriptional activator. *p<0.01 ***p<0.0001.

Cellular uptake of TAT-conjugated lyophilisomes

Trypan blue assay and FACS. To determine the internalization efficiency of sorted lyophilisomes with and without TAT peptide, a trypan blue quenching assay was used in order to distinguish between internalized and non-internalized (but plasma membrane-associated) lyophilisomes. This assay is based on the quenching of fluorescence of FITC-labeled lyophilisomes by the vital stain trypan blue (which does not penetrate plasma membranes). To validate that trypan blue also quenches fluorescence of FITC labeled lyophilisomes, lyophilisomes were incubated with trypan blue in the absence of cells and evaluated by FACS (Fig. 4). Lyophilisomes that were not incubated with trypan blue showed a mean fluorescence intensity of 1339±252. Lyophilisomes incubated in a 0.5% trypan blue solution gave a mean fluorescent intensity of 85±31, corresponding to a quenching efficacy of 94±2% (Fig. 4b). After one, two and three washings after the trypan blue incubation, the measured mean fluorescence was 161±25, 176±22, and 192±19 or 88±1%, 87±1% and 85±1% quenching efficacy, respectively. This indicates that trypan blue was not easily washed out of the lyophilisomes and fluorescence remained quenched. This is important as three washings steps were used prior to FACS analysis.

To investigate whether TAT peptides can enhance internalization of sorted lyophilisomes, the trypan blue quenching assay was performed in the presence of HeLa cells (Fig. 5). Cells were incubated with 500,000 sorted lyophilisomes with and without TAT peptide. Incubation for 1 h with TAT-conjugated lyophili-

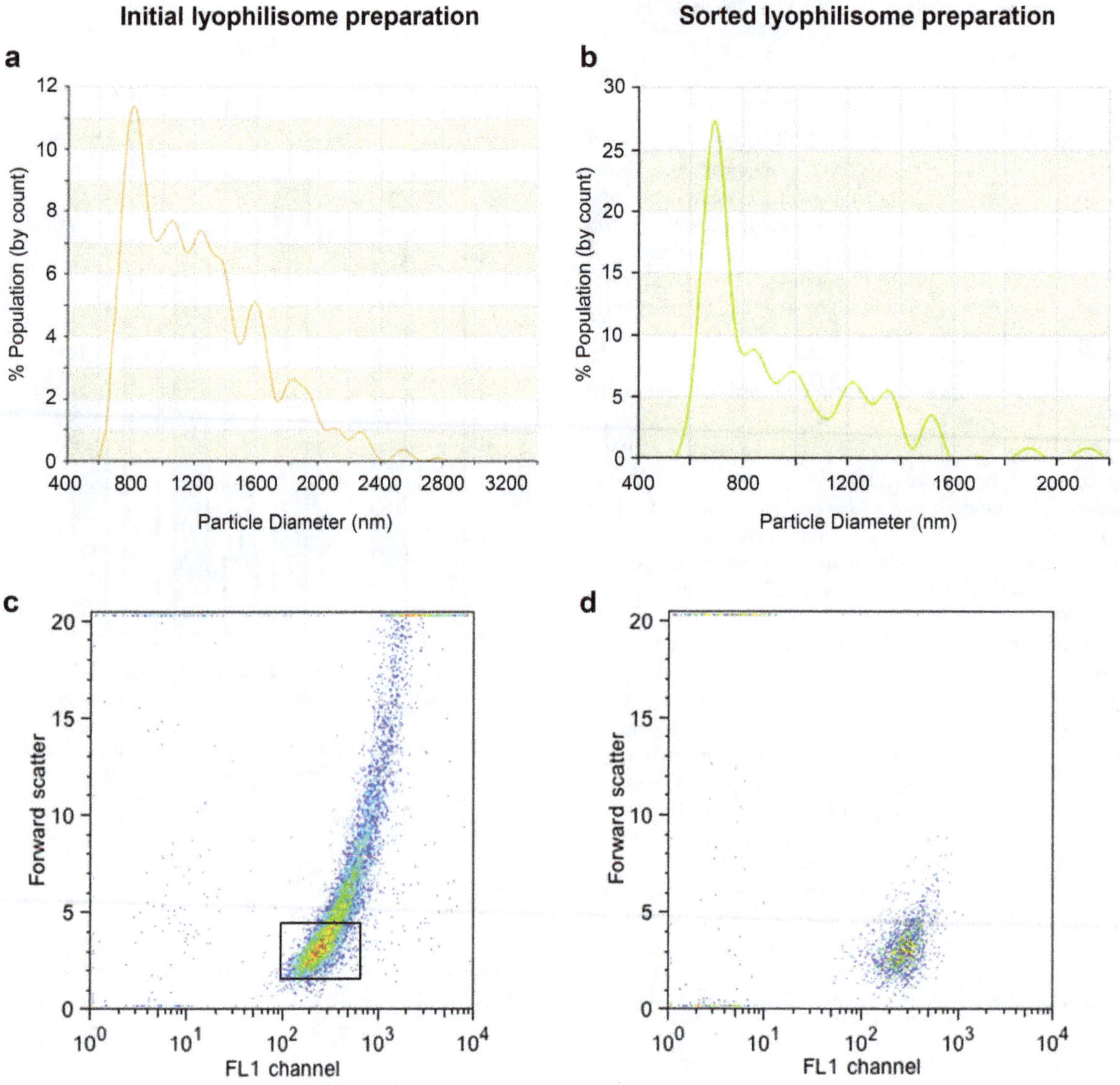

Figure 3. Sorting of lyophilisomes by fluorescence-activated cell sorting. a/b) A representative size distribution of the initial lyophilisome population (a) and sorted lyophilisomes (b) is depicted, showing smaller lyophilisomes after sorting. Note the difference in x and y axes. c) Initial lyophilisome population depicted in a FACS dot plot with forward (size)/FITC-positive lyophilisome (FL1 channel) scatter where gated FITC-positive lyophilisomes were sorted. d) After sorting, the scatter showed merely small lyophilisomes, as large lyophilisomes were removed.

somes resulted in many lyophilisome-positive cells (67±3%) and moderate cellular uptake (25%±1). In contrast, unmodified lyophilisomes showed few lyophilisome-positive cells (6±5%) and almost no internalization (1±1%). Interestingly, when lyophilisomes were incubated for 4 h, the number of lyophilisome-positive cells of TAT-conjugated lyophilisomes remained high (79±8%) and cellular uptake strongly increased (59±14%), whereas unmodified lyophilisomes still showed a moderate number of lyophilisome-positive cells (17±8%) and little internalization (7±2%).

Confocal microscopy. Internalization of TAT-conjugated lyophilisomes in HeLa cells was visualized by confocal microscopy (Fig. 6). After 4 h of incubation, TAT-conjugated lyophilisomes showed extensive uptake for both low (0.8 million/200 μl) and high (3.5 million/200 μl) numbers of lyophilisomes (Fig. 6c/g). Almost no internalization was observed when HeLa cells were incubated with unmodified lyophilisomes (Fig. 6a/e). The corresponding bright field images showed that lyophilisomes did not lead to detectable morphological changes of the cells (Fig. 6b/d/f/h).

Transmission electron microscopy. In order to investigate the binding and uptake of TAT-conjugated lyophilisomes in HeLa cells in detail, TEM was used (Fig. 7). When unmodified lyophilisomes were added to HeLa cells, no binding or uptake was observed and the plasma membrane appeared largely unruffled (Fig. 7a). However, when TAT-conjugated lyophilisomes were added, multiple stages of internalization could be distinguished, including attachment and internalization (Fig. 7b/c). Initially, TAT-conjugated lyophilisomes bound to HeLa cells and initiated membrane ruffling (Fig. 7b). Subsequently, capsules were internalized (Fig. 7c). Furthermore, initial signs of degradation of lyophilisomes could be observed, as degradation products were visible (black arrows; Fig. 7d).

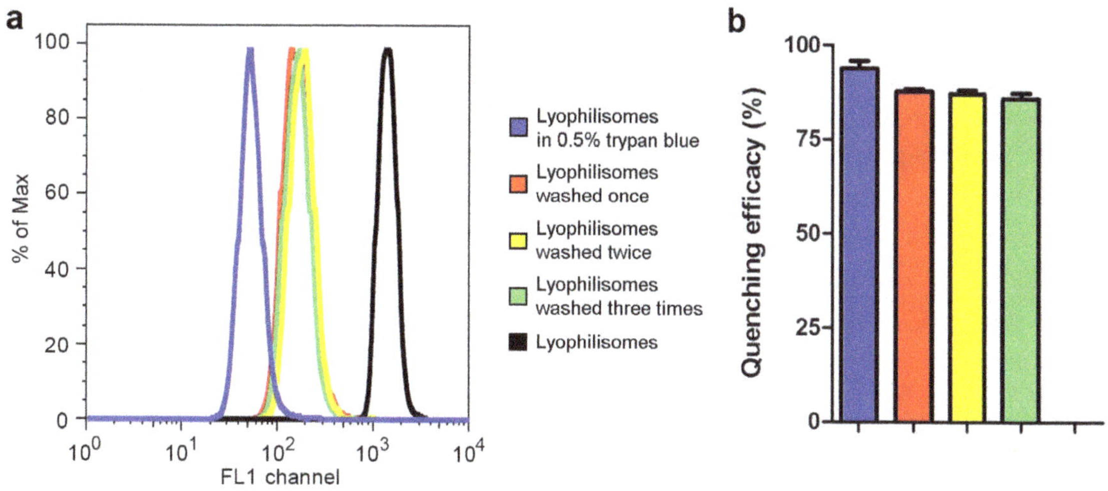

Figure 4. Quenching of FITC fluorescent lyophilisomes by trypan blue in the absence of cells. Results show decreased fluorescence (a) and efficient quenching (b) up to three washings steps of FITC fluorescent lyophilisomes by trypan blue.

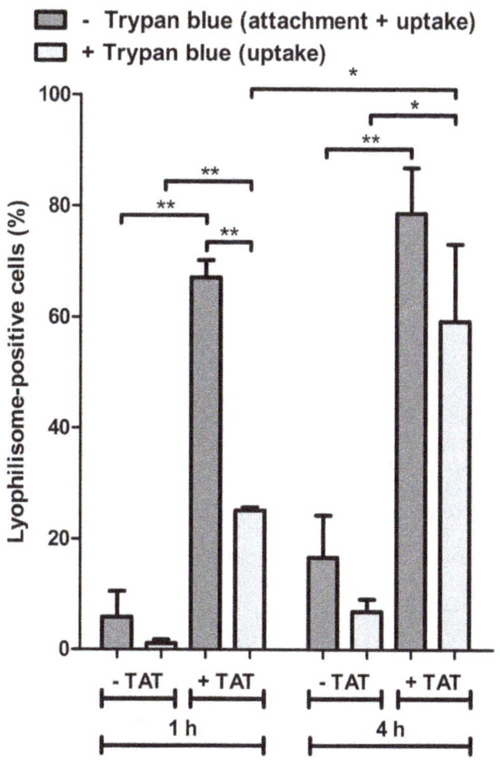

Figure 5. Internalization of lyophilisomes with and without TAT peptide into HeLa cells. FACS showed a large number of lyophilisome-positive cells for TAT-conjugated lyophilisomes after 1 h (67±3%) without trypan blue and a cellular uptake of 25±1% with trypan blue. Values for lyophilisomes without TAT peptide were low. When lyophilisomes were incubated for 4 h, TAT-conjugated lyophilisomes conserved the large number of lyophilisome-positive cells (79±8%) with an increased internalization of 59±14%, while unmodified lyophilisomes still showed few lyophilisome-positive cells and little cellular uptake. *$p<0.01$ **$p<0.001$. CPP = cell penetrating peptide; TAT = trans-activating transcriptional activator.

Discussion

Our laboratory previously demonstrated that lyophilisomes show potential as a drug delivery system [11,12]. To further optimize these biocapsules, we studied the effect of TAT-functionalization on the *in vitro* internalization of lyophilisomes. Intracellular delivery of therapeutic molecules is one of the key problems in drug delivery. Many pharmaceutical compounds have to be delivered intracellularly to exert their therapeutic action [22]. CPPs have been shown to act as a powerful transport vector for inducing the cellular uptake of a large variety of cargos [18]. At present, pharmaceutical nanocarriers are much in focus for their capacity to increase the stability of administered drugs, improve their concentration at their site-of-action and decrease undesired side effects. Various studies report increased uptake and specific delivery to intracellular organelles when conjugating CPPs to drug delivery systems, thereby increasing the efficiency of nanocarriers as drug delivery systems [35–37].

As previously reported, lyophilisomes range in size from 100 up to 3,000 nm in diameter [11]. In this study, we demonstrated that using FACS, small lyophilisomes could be sorted out of the initial population, narrowing the size distribution.

In the present study, FACS was used to investigate the total cell binding and internalization of (TAT-conjugated) lyophilisomes in HeLa, OVCAR-3, Caco-2, and SKOV-3 cells. To investigate the cellular uptake and subcellular distribution of (TAT-conjugated) lyophilisomes in HeLa cells in more detail, confocal microscopy, and TEM were utilized. FACS demonstrated a high number of lyophilisome-positive cells when incubated with TAT-conjugated lyophilisomes compared to unmodified lyophilisomes. This may be explained by interaction of the TAT peptide with negatively charged sulfated glycans at the cell surface, such as heparan sulphate [38,39]. Only SKOV-3 cells showed a high background when incubated with unmodified lyophilisomes, which has been shown for other drug carriers added to this cell line [40].

To discriminate between internalization and attachment, a trypan blue quenching assay was applied on HeLa cells incubated with lyophilisomes. This assay showed that cellular uptake was enhanced when TAT peptides were conjugated to lyophilisomes. The degree of internalization may even have been underestimated as our capsules are likely to enter the acidic lysosomes in the cell [41] and since FITC fluorescein is virtually non-fluorescent below

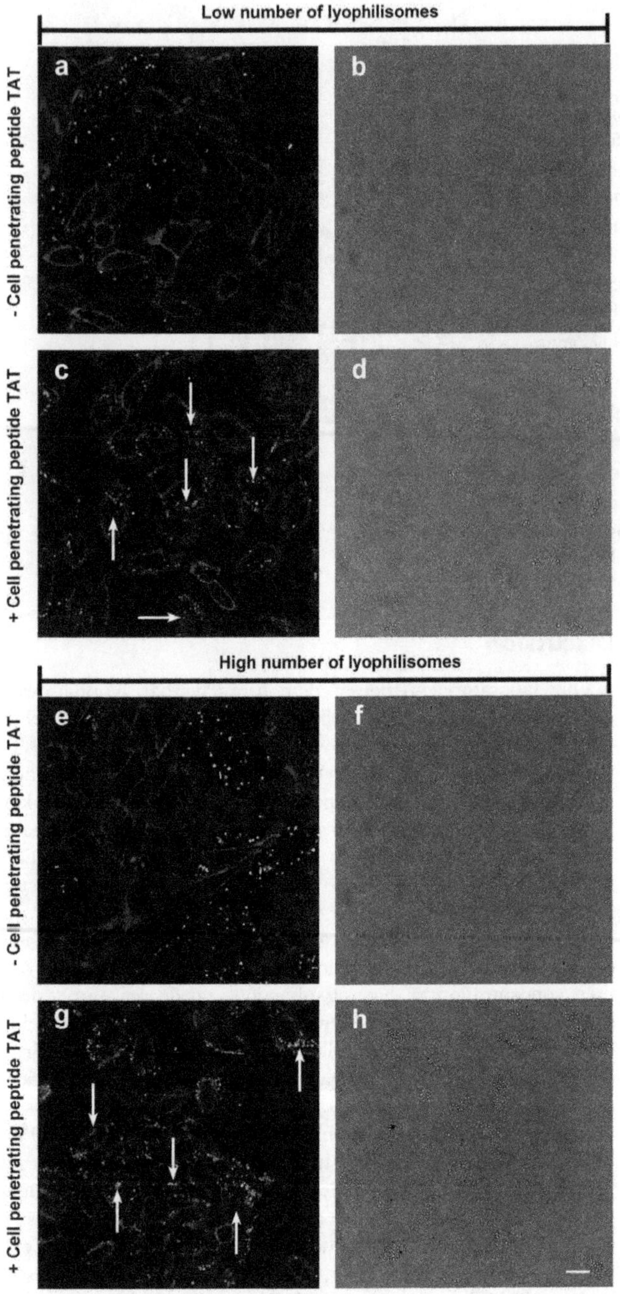

Figure 6. Internalization of lyophilisomes without and with TAT peptide by HeLa cells. Lyophilisomes without and with TAT peptide were administered to 30,000 HeLa cells using two dosages (0.8 million/500 μl (a-d) and 3.5 million/500 μl (e-h). Cells incubated with lyophilisomes without TAT peptide had internalized few lyophilisomes (a/e), whereas TAT-conjugated lyophilisomes showed high cellular uptake for almost all cells (c/g). Green fluorescence corresponds to lyophilisomes and red fluorescence (CellMask orange) visualizes the plasma membrane. Bright field images (b/d/f/h) show normal morphology of the cells. Scale bar represents 20 μm. TAT = trans-activating transcriptional activator.

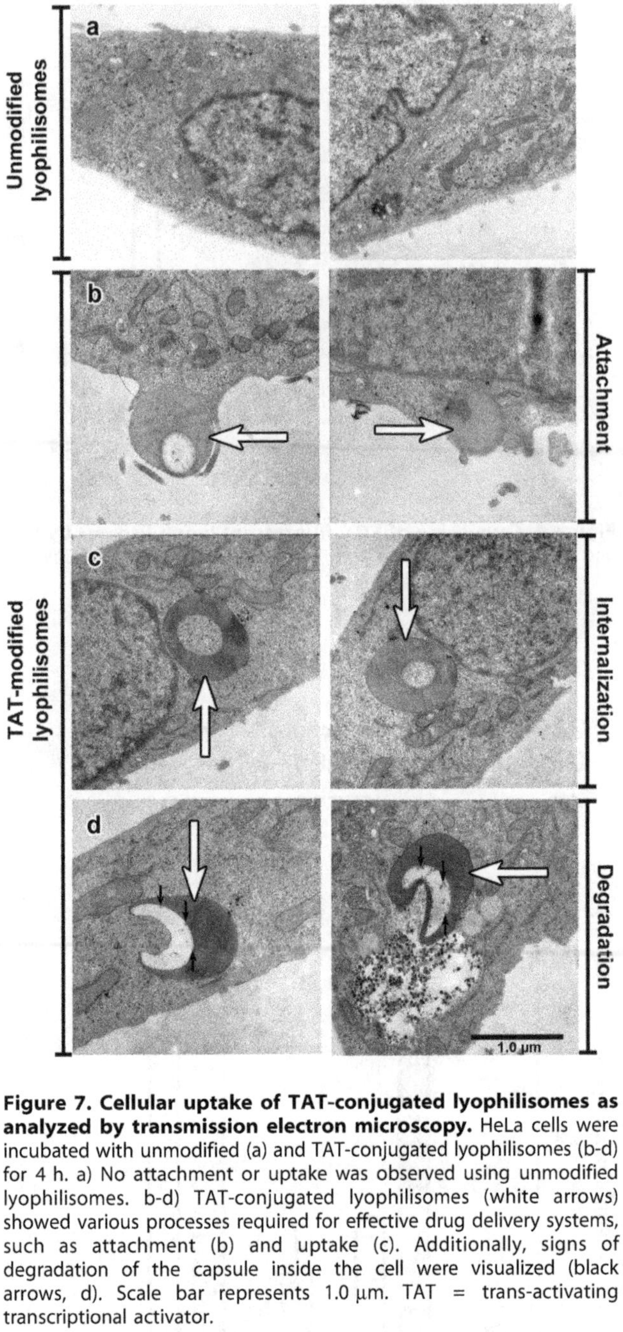

Figure 7. Cellular uptake of TAT-conjugated lyophilisomes as analyzed by transmission electron microscopy. HeLa cells were incubated with unmodified (a) and TAT-conjugated lyophilisomes (b-d) for 4 h. a) No attachment or uptake was observed using unmodified lyophilisomes. b-d) TAT-conjugated lyophilisomes (white arrows) showed various processes required for effective drug delivery systems, such as attachment (b) and uptake (c). Additionally, signs of degradation of the capsule inside the cell were visualized (black arrows, d). Scale bar represents 1.0 μm. TAT = trans-activating transcriptional activator.

pH 5 [42]. The trypan blue assay also demonstrated that cellular uptake of TAT-conjugated lyophilisomes increased over time. After 1 h, 25±1% of the cells internalized TAT-conjugated lyophilisomes, whereas 59±14% of cells had done so after an incubation period of 4 h. We most likely added too little lyophilisomes in the trypan blue internalization study to achieve lyophilisome internalization of all available cells. This is supported by confocal microscopy, which revealed that almost all cells internalized at least one lyophilisome when administering more lyophilisomes. TEM images showed different stages of cellular uptake (attachment and internalization) of TAT-conjugated lyophilisomes. The results strongly suggest that TAT-conjugated lyophilisomes are internalized by phagocytosis and/or macropinocytosis, as intensive plasma membrane ruffling was observed during uptake. This suggestion would be in line with the particle size of lyophilisomes [43]. However, lyophilisomes smaller than 200 nm, could still be internalized by one of the mechanisms of endocytosis.

If we compare our findings to other studies, the increased internalization efficiency compared to unmodified particles is within the range of reported values for TAT peptides conjugated to cargos such as liposomes [44,45]. However, it is difficult to compare internalization for different kinds of nanoparticles, since different cell types and different amounts and sizes of nanoparticles are used for *in vitro* experiments, *e.g.* the larger the particle the more time it takes to establish internalization [46].

The ability of CPPs to enhance cellular uptake non-specifically and receptor-independently provides the opportunity to target diverse cell types with a variety of carriers. In literature, it has been observed that next to HeLa, OVCAR-3, Caco-2 and SKOV-3 cells, the TAT peptide can enter other tumor cells, for instance bladder cancer (HTB-9, MBT2), breast cancer (SK-BR-3, MCF7), and other colon cancer (C26) cells [45,47]. However, their non-specificity presents a significant challenge in systemically administered applications for targeted delivery, as it requires precise control of CPP presentation only at the target site to prevent toxicity [48]. To overcome this problem, several approaches are being investigated to activate CPPs only at the target site. Stimulus-responsive materials may be used for this purpose, as they may provide triggered changes in material properties that allow spatially focused presentation of CPPs in response to intrinsic disease characteristics (*e.g.* abundantly present extracellular matrix proteases) or locally applied extrinsic cues (*e.g.* apply heat or light at a specific location) [49].

As demonstrated in this study, TAT peptides can enhance cellular uptake when conjugated to lyophilisomes. In previous *in vitro* studies, lyophilisomes were loaded with anti-tumor drugs, *e.g.* doxorubicin and curcumin, which could eliminate tumor cells. Antibodies were conjugated to lyophilisomes resulting in specific binding to target cells [11,12]. To probe the possibility of using lyophilisomes for the treatment of cancer, active targeting with specific antibodies and enhanced cellular uptake with CPPs can be combined with the drug delivery properties of lyophilisomes, thereby creating a potential powerful tool for drug delivery.

Conclusion

In the present study, albumin-based lyophilisomes were functionalized with TAT peptides to obtain a drug delivery system with enhanced cellular uptake. Lyophilisomes modified with TAT peptides efficiently bound to HeLa, OVCAR-3, Caco-2 and SKOV-3 cells. Additional cellular uptake studies were performed to verify that TAT-conjugated lyophilisomes were internalized in HeLa cells after binding. TAT-conjugated lyophilisomes may present a novel delivery system to ensure faster and higher cellular uptake of anti-tumor drugs to cancer cells.

Author Contributions

Conceived and designed the experiments: EB EO RB THK WFD. Performed the experiments: EB LRMV SS WPRV RW RR TH. Analyzed the data: EB LRMV SS RR TH THK WFD. Contributed reagents/materials/analysis tools: EB WPRV RW TH. Wrote the paper: EB EO RB THK WFD.

References

1. Davis ME, Chen ZG, Shin DM (2008) Nanoparticle therapeutics: an emerging treatment modality for cancer. Nat Rev Drug Discov 7: 771–782.
2. Haley B, Frenkel E (2008) Nanoparticles for drug delivery in cancer treatment. Urol Oncol 26: 57–64.
3. Danhier F, Ansorena E, Silva JM, Coco R, Le BA, et al. (2012) PLGA-based nanoparticles: an overview of biomedical applications. J Control Release 161: 505–522.
4. Torchilin V (2011) Tumor delivery of macromolecular drugs based on the EPR effect. Adv Drug Deliv Rev 63: 131–135.
5. Cho K, Wang X, Nie S, Chen ZG, Shin DM (2008) Therapeutic nanoparticles for drug delivery in cancer. Clin Cancer Res 14: 1310–1316.
6. Byrne JD, Betancourt T, Brannon-Peppas L (2008) Active targeting schemes for nanoparticle systems in cancer therapeutics. Adv Drug Deliv Rev 60: 1615–1626.
7. De Jong WH, Borm PJ (2008) Drug delivery and nanoparticles:applications and hazards. Int J Nanomedicine 3: 133–149.
8. Langer K, Balthasar S, Vogel V, Dinauer N, von Briesen H, et al. (2003) Optimization of the preparation process for human serum albumin (HSA) nanoparticles. Int J Pharm 257: 169–180.
9. Elzoghby AO, Samy WM, Elgindy NA (2012) Protein-based nanocarriers as promising drug and gene delivery systems. J Control Release.
10. Daamen WF, Geutjes PJ, Nillesen STM, Van Moerkerk HTB, Wismans R, et al. (2007) Lyophilisomes: A new type of (bio)capsules. Adv Mater 19: 673–677.
11. van Bracht E, Raave R, Verdurmen WP, Wismans RG, Geutjes PJ, et al. (2012) Lyophilisomes as a new generation of drug delivery capsules. Int J Pharm 439: 127–135.
12. van Bracht E, Stolle S, Hafmans TG, Boerman OC, Oosterwijk E, et al. (2014) Specific targeting of tumor cells by lyophilisomes functionalized with antibodies. Eur J Pharm Biopharm.
13. Elzoghby AO, Samy WM, Elgindy NA (2011) Albumin-based nanoparticles as potential controlled release drug delivery systems. J Control Release.
14. Ibrahim NK, Desai N, Legha S, Soon-Shiong P, Theriault RL, et al. (2002) Phase I and pharmacokinetic study of ABI-007, a Cremophor-free, protein-stabilized, nanoparticle formulation of paclitaxel. Clin Cancer Res 8: 1038–1044.
15. Ibrahim NK, Samuels B, Page R, Doval D, Patel KM, et al. (2005) Multicenter phase II trial of ABI-007, an albumin-bound paclitaxel, in women with metastatic breast cancer. J Clin Oncol 23: 6019–6026.
16. Feinstein SB, Cheirif J, Ten Cate FJ, Silverman PR, Heidenreich PA, et al. (1990) Safety and efficacy of a new transpulmonary ultrasound contrast agent: initial multicenter clinical results. J Am Coll Cardiol 16: 316–324.
17. Geny B, Mettauer B, Muan B, Bischoff P, Epailly E, et al. (1993) Safety and efficacy of a new transpulmonary echo contrast agent in echocardiographic studies in patients. J Am Coll Cardiol 22: 1193–1198.
18. Koren E, Torchilin VP (2012) Cell-penetrating peptides: breaking through to the other side. Trends Mol Med 18: 385–393.
19. Wadia JS, Dowdy SF (2005) Transmembrane delivery of protein and peptide drugs by TAT-mediated transduction in the treatment of cancer. Adv Drug Deliv Rev 57: 579–596.
20. Massodi I, Bidwell GL, III, Raucher D (2005) Evaluation of cell penetrating peptides fused to elastin-like polypeptide for drug delivery. J Control Release 108: 396–408.
21. Striab-Fisher A, Sergueev D, Fisher M, Shaw BR, Juliano RL (2002) Conjugates of antisense oligonucleotides with the Tat and antennapedia cell-penetrating peptides: effects on cellular uptake, binding to target sequences, and biologic actions. Pharm Res 19: 744–754.
22. Torchilin VP (2008) Cell penetrating peptide-modified pharmaceutical nanocarriers for intracellular drug and gene delivery. Biopolymers 90: 604–610.
23. Qin Y, Chen H, Zhang Q, Wang X, Yuan W, et al. (2011) Liposome formulated with TAT-modified cholesterol for improving brain delivery and therapeutic efficacy on brain glioma in animals. Int J Pharm 420: 304–312.
24. Sawant RR, Torchilin VP (2009) Enhanced cytotoxicity of TATp-bearing paclitaxel-loaded micelles in vitro and in vivo. Int J Pharm 374: 114–118.
25. Patel LN, Zaro JL, Shen WC (2007) Cell penetrating peptides: intracellular pathways and pharmaceutical perspectives. Pharm Res 24: 1977–1992.
26. Chugh A, Eudes F, Shim YS (2010) Cell-penetrating peptides: Nanocarrier for macromolecule delivery in living cells. IUBMB Life 62: 183–193.
27. Frankel AD (1992) Activation of HIV transcription by Tat. Curr Opin Genet Dev 2: 293–298.
28. Vives E, Brodin P, Lebleu B (1997) A truncated HIV-1 Tat protein basic domain rapidly translocates through the plasma membrane and accumulates in the cell nucleus. J Biol Chem 272: 16010–16017.
29. Garza-Licudine E, Deo D, Yu S, Uz-Zaman A, Dunbar WB (2010) Portable nanoparticle quantization using a resizable nanopore instrument - the IZON qNano. Conf Proc IEEE Eng Med Biol Soc 2010: 5736–5739.
30. Tario JD, Jr., Gray BD, Wallace SS, Muirhead KA, Ohlsson-Wilhelm BM, et al. (2007) Novel lipophilic tracking dyes for monitoring cell proliferation. Immunol Invest 36: 861–885.
31. Wallace PK, Tario JD Jr., Fisher JL, Wallace SS, Ernstoff MS, et al. (2008) Tracking antigen-driven responses by flow cytometry: monitoring proliferation by dye dilution. Cytometry A 73: 1019–1034.
32. Nuutila J, Lilius EM (2005) Flow cytometric quantitative determination of ingestion by phagocytes needs the distinguishing of overlapping populations of binding and ingesting cells. Cytometry A 65: 93–102.
33. Ramarao N, Meyer TF (2001) Helicobacter pylori resists phagocytosis by macrophages: quantitative assessment by confocal microscopy and fluorescence-activated cell sorting. Infect Immun 69: 2604–2611.

34. Orr G, Panther DJ, Cassens KJ, Phillips JL, Tarasevich BJ, et al. (2009) Syndecan-1 mediates the coupling of positively charged submicrometer amorphous silica particles with actin filaments across the alveolar epithelial cell membrane. Toxicol Appl Pharmacol 236: 210–220.
35. Oh E, Delehanty JB, Sapsford KE, Susumu K, Goswami R, et al. (2011) Cellular uptake and fate of PEGylated gold nanoparticles is dependent on both cell-penetration peptides and particle size. ACS Nano 5: 6434–6448.
36. Xia H, Gao X, Gu G, Liu Z, Hu Q, et al. (2012) Penetratin-functionalized PEG-PLA nanoparticles for brain drug delivery. Int J Pharm.
37. Liu BR, Li JF, Lu SW, Leel HJ, Huang YW, et al. (2010) Cellular internalization of quantum dots noncovalently conjugated with arginine-rich cell-penetrating peptides. J Nanosci Nanotechnol 10: 6534–6543.
38. Tyagi M, Rusnati M, Presta M, Giacca M (2001) Internalization of HIV-1 tat requires cell surface heparan sulfate proteoglycans. J Biol Chem 276: 3254–3261.
39. Gump JM, Dowdy SF (2007) TAT transduction: the molecular mechanism and therapeutic prospects. Trends Mol Med 13: 443–448.
40. Lei T, Srinivasan S, Tang Y, Manchanda R, Nagesetti A, et al. (2011) Comparing cellular uptake and cytotoxicity of targeted drug carriers in cancer cell lines with different drug resistance mechanisms. Nanomedicine 7: 324–332.
41. Vieira OV, Botelho RJ, Grinstein S (2002) Phagosome maturation: aging gracefully. Biochem J 366: 689–704.
42. Geisow MJ (1984) Fluorescein conjugates as indicators of subcellular pH. A critical evaluation. Exp Cell Res 150: 29–35.
43. Brandhonneur N, Chevanne F, Vie V, Frisch B, Primault R, et al. (2009) Specific and non-specific phagocytosis of ligand-grafted PLGA microspheres by macrophages. Eur J Pharm Sci 36: 474–485.
44. Gupta B, Levchenko TS, Torchilin VP (2005) Intracellular delivery of large molecules and small particles by cell-penetrating proteins and peptides. Adv Drug Deliv Rev 57: 637–651.
45. Tseng YL, Liu JJ, Hong RL (2002) Translocation of liposomes into cancer cells by cell-penetrating peptides penetratin and tat: a kinetic and efficacy study. Mol Pharmacol 62: 864–872.
46. Wang J, Byrne JD, Napier ME, Desimone JM (2011) More effective nanomedicines through particle design. Small 7: 1919–1931.
47. Fretz MM, Koning GA, Mastrobattista E, Jiskoot W, Storm G (2004) OVCAR-3 cells internalize TAT-peptide modified liposomes by endocytosis. Biochim Biophys Acta 1665: 48–56.
48. Aguilera TA, Olson ES, Timmers MM, Jiang T, Tsien RY (2009) Systemic in vivo distribution of activatable cell penetrating peptides is superior to that of cell penetrating peptides. Integr Biol (Camb) 1: 371–381.
49. MacEwan SR, Chilkoti A (2013) Harnessing the power of cell-penetrating peptides: activatable carriers for targeting systemic delivery of cancer therapeutics and imaging agents. Wiley Interdiscip Rev Nanomed Nanobiotechnol 5: 31–48.

15

Supply-Side Barriers to Maternity-Care in India: A Facility-Based Analysis

Santosh Kumar[1,2]*, **Emily Dansereau**[2]

1 Department of Economics & International Business, Sam Houston State University, Huntsville, Texas, United States of America, **2** Institute for Health Metrics and Evaluation, University of Washington, Seattle, Washington, United States of America

Abstract

Background: Health facilities in many low- and middle-income countries face several types of barriers in delivering quality health services. Availability of resources at the facility may significantly affect the volume and quality of services provided. This study investigates the effect of supply-side determinants of maternity-care provision in India.

Methods: Health facility data from the District-Level Household Survey collected in 2007–2008 were analyzed to explore the effects of supply-side factors on the volume of delivery care provided at Indian health facilities. A negative binomial regression model was applied to the data due to the count and over-dispersion property of the outcome variable (number of deliveries performed at the facility).

Results: Availability of a labor room (Incidence Rate Ratio [IRR]: 1.81; 95% Confidence Interval [CI]: 1.68–1.95) and facility opening hours (IRR: 1.43; CI: 1.35–1.51) were the most significant predictors of the volume of delivery care at the health facilities. Medical and paramedical staff were found to be positively associated with institutional deliveries. The volume of deliveries was also higher if adequate beds, essential obstetric drugs, medical equipment, electricity, and communication infrastructures were available at the facility. Findings were robust to the inclusion of facility's catchment area population and district-level education, health insurance coverage, religion, wealth, and fertility. Separate analyses were performed for facilities with and without a labor room and results were qualitatively similar across these two types of facilities.

Conclusions: Our study highlights the importance of supply-side barriers to maternity-care India. To meet Millennium Development Goals 4 and 5, policymakers should make additional investments in improving the availability of medical drugs and equipment at primary health centers (PHCs) in India.

Editor: Waldemar A. Carlo, University of Alabama at Birmingham, United States of America

Funding: This project was funded by the Disease Control Priorities Network grant to the Institute for Health Metrics and Evaluation from the Bill & Melinda Gates Foundation. The funders had no role in study design, data collection and analysis, decision to publish, or preparation of the manuscript.

Competing Interests: The authors have declared that no competing interests exist.

* Email: skumar@shsu.edu

Background

Policymakers in many developing countries are grappling with low utilization of health services and poor health outcomes, with India as no exception. The World Bank estimates that India is one of the highest ranked countries in the world for malnourishment among young children, child mortality, maternal mortality, and other pregnancy-related complications [1]. India contributes to one-fifth of the global burden of absolute maternal deaths despite experiencing a sustained decline in maternal mortality in the last two decades [2]. The recent improvement in the maternal mortality ratio has been supported by the Government of India's efforts to improve financial and geographic access to care, including the establishment of a wide network of public health facilities and implementation of a variety of outreach and incentive-based programs [3]. In particular, the establishment of the National Rural Health Mission (NRHM), by the government of India, in April 2005 expanded the network of public health facilities to many poor and disadvantaged households in rural areas [4]. However, the utilization of public health facilities is abysmally low and is marked by substantial heterogeneity across regions and socio-demographic groups [5]. In spite of a special focus on maternal and child health issues, the institutional delivery rate is less than 60% in 170 districts [6]. Increasing institutional delivery rates has been a key strategy for achieving Millennium Development Goal 5 of reducing maternal mortality, and was named by the World Health Organization as the "single most important factor in preventing maternal death" [7].

Given that the provision of health services is strongly related to improved population health, it is of paramount importance to understand the many factors that affect both the utilization and provision of health care. These factors operate on both the demand and supply side [8], which can be explained in a multi-level framework described by previous studies. The framework identifies three levels of barriers: the community and household level, the health service delivery level, and the health sector policy and strategic management level [9]. At the community and household level, the use of health services is limited by physical, financial, and social barriers, which are also known as demand-side barriers. Income, distance to the health facility, and socioeconomic characteristics influence the use of healthcare by Indian households [10–12]. Supply side barriers operate at the service delivery level. They are characteristics of the health system that exist outside the control of potential health service users and hinder uptake by individuals, households, or the community [13,14]. Finally, both supply and demand side barriers can be addressed at the policy and strategic management level, where policy makers require reliable information to make informed decisions.

Previous studies have identified numerous demand-side factors as important barriers to healthcare utilization in developing countries, but surprisingly few have truly addressed the supply-side barriers [15]. While many studies have described severe shortages of essential supplies, medications, and human resources across countries including India, there is a gap in knowledge as to how these observed supply-side bottlenecks affect service provision [16,17]. The few existing studies addressing how supply-side barriers affect uptake of reproductive health services have found large but inconsistent effects, urging further research. A study in Egypt found that facility quality variables were more influential in the uptake of intrauterine devices at public health facilities than demographic or geographic characteristics [18]. A similar study in Uganda identified several infrastructural and service characteristics, including running water, electricity, and staff accommodations, to be strongly associated with increased deliveries [19]. However, in a study conducted in South Africa, few facility characteristics were found to be associated with contraceptive adoption, though human resource availability was correlated with choice of contraception methods [20].

Quantifying how the availability of doctors, drugs, medical equipment, infrastructure, and staff training affects the provision of health services is of tremendous policy relevance because the government controls and distributes the resources to equip its health facilities, and because of its potential interactions with demand-side factors. In recent years, many countries have abolished user fees or provided financial incentives for seeking maternity-care, but whether health facilities are adequately equipped with the resources to meet the increased demand due to these policy measures is not well understood. For instance, an evaluation of the Indian conditional cash transfer program for pregnant women, Janani Suraksha Yojana (JSY), found that while the volume of deliveries increased, facilities also faced shortages of drugs and equipment [21]. An equally important question is to what extent the alleviation of these constraints would result in improved utilization of health services, and how these constraints should be prioritized. Using a large cross-sectional facility-level dataset, this study contributes to the research on supply-side factors by assessing the effect of facility-level indicators on the volume of deliveries conducted at public health facilities in India.

Methodology

1. Health care system in India

The Indian public healthcare delivery system operates at four hierarchical levels: sub-centers (SC), primary health centers (PHC), community health centers (CHC), and district hospitals (DH). SC is the lowest level of the health system while DH is the highest level. Each district has one DH, which is well-equipped to handle complicated cases. At the next level, CHCs are the most endowed in terms of medical staff and equipment, followed by PHCs, and subsequently SCs, which are the peripheral contact point between the primary health care system and the community. In terms of coverage, CHCs serve a population of 80,000 to 120,000; PHCs cater to a population of 30,000, and SCs look after the needs of approximately 5,000 [22]. We focus our study on PHCs because they are a crucial component of care as the first point of contact between an individual and a qualified public-sector doctor, particularly for rural populations. Furthermore, in many states, PHCs have recorded a four-fold increase in in-facility deliveries, while other public and private health clinics have showed a decline since the implementation of the NRHM and JSY in 2005–2006 [23]. Therefore, we set out to perform the analysis only on the sample of PHCs.

At the time of data collection in 2007–08, a PHC was expected to have one medical officer and 16 paramedical and other staff, and to act as a referral unit for five to six SCs. In terms of infrastructure, PHCs are stipulated to have four to six inpatient beds. The activities of the PHCs involve curative, preventive, and promotional health care. PHCs are expected to be equipped to provide 24/7 normal and assisted deliveries, ante-natal care, post-natal care, newborn care, family planning, and full child immunizations [22].

2. Study hypotheses

The analytical approach in this study was developed to assess the relationship between supply-side barriers and provision of institutional delivery services in India. We hypothesized that facilities with adequate resources will perform a greater number of deliveries, vaccinate more children, and treat more illness. In this study, we specifically examined how the availability of health personnel, medical equipment, drugs, and other infrastructure, such as electricity and water, affected the volume of delivery at the PHCs in India.

3. Data source

We used health facility data from the third wave of the District Level Households Survey (DLHS-3) in India, collected during 2007–2008. The DLHS data are publicly available from the International Institute for Population Sciences, Mumbai [22]. The health facility survey in DLHS-3 collected information on resources available at the facilities and the volume of services delivered. In total, 18,068 sub-centers, 8,619 primary health centers, 4,162 community health centers, and 594 district hospitals were surveyed. We used information from the sample of 8,619 PHCs to assess the association between infrastructure availability and delivery of maternity-care. The PHC facility survey collected information on infrastructure availability (number of beds, rooms etc.), health personnel, medical equipment, availability of drugs, and existence of quality and training measures. Of the 8,619 PHCs surveyed, 95% were in rural areas. Per the DLHS-3 report, 76% of the PHCs had a medical officer, and less than a quarter (24%) had a female medical officer [11]. The sampled PHCs in the DLHS-3 survey reported serving an average population of 49,193 against the population norm of 30,000 in the plain areas [22].

4. Dependent variable

The main dependent variable analyzed in this study is the number of deliveries performed in each facility in the month before the survey. This is a count variable ranging from zero to 414 deliveries. About 27% of the facilities reported performing no deliveries in the prior month. The average number of deliveries per facility was 21.

5. Facility and district-level covariates/predictor variables

We included several covariates (Table 1) as predictors of the volume of facility-based deliveries, which are potentially important bottlenecks for provision of maternity-care. We divided these

Table 1. Definition and descriptive statistics of variables, n = 8227.

	Variable	Definitions	Mean/ percent	SD	Min	Max
	Dependent variable					
1	PHC Delivery	Count variable indicating number of deliveries performed at the primary health center in the month before the survey	20.83	42.81	0	414
	Independent Variables					
2	Doctor	Continuous variable that indicates the number of types of doctors/medical officers at the facility	1.49	0.88	0	4
3	Paramedic staffs	Continuous variable that indicates the number of paramedic staff at the facility	4.02	1.71	0	7
4	Availability of obstetric drug	Binary variable, coded as one if essential obstetric care drugs are available	62%	0.49	0	1
5	Availability of adequate number of beds	Binary variable, coded as one if the facility has more than minimum number of beds (4). Each PHC is mandated to have at least 4 beds.	68%	0.47	0	1
6	Availability of labor room	Binary variable, coded as one if labor room is available at the facility for delivery purpose	69%	0.46	0	1
7	Availability of obstetric and new-born equipment	Number of obstetric-care equipment available at the facility	1.28	1.07	0	4
8	Availability of communication infrastructure	Number of communication equipment, such as computer, telephone, internet, vehicle etc. available at the facility	1.50	1.14	0	6
9	Opening hours	Whether facility is opened 24 hours	53%	0.50	0	1
10	Electricity	Binary variable, coded as one if the facility has access to regular power supply/generators/invertors	62%	0.49	0	1
11	Rural	Facility location, rural is coded as one	95%	0.22	0	1
12	Rogi Kalyan Samiti (RKS)	Establishment of RKS at the facility is coded as one	75%	0.43	0	1
13	Staff training	Binary variable, coded as one if facility's staffs were trained in BEmOC or Skilled Birth Delivery	31%	0.46	0	1
14	Years of schooling	Continuous variable indicating the average years of school completed by adults over age 18 in the district	5.38	1.44	1.57	9.53
15	Percent in lowest wealth quintile	Percent of households in the district categorized as being in the lowest wealth quintile, based on assets	19%	0.17	0	85
16	Percent insured	Percent of households in the district with any member covered by a health scheme or health insurance	5%	0.07	0	49
17	Percent Hindu	Percent of households in the district where the head of household is Hindu	82%	0.22	0.001	100
18	Fertility rate	Average live births per person-year among ever married women, between January 1 2004 and date of data collection (2008)	0.09	0.03	0.01	0.20
19	Log catchment population	Natural log of the catchment population reported by the PHC	10.31	0.95	1.95	13.44

bottlenecks into six categories: (a) health personnel, (b) drug availability, (c) medical equipment availability, (d) infrastructure, (e) quality, and (f) demographic variables.

The DLHS-3 records human resources as a binary indicator for each type of position filled. We included a count variable for the number of types of medical officers at the PHC (male medical officer, female medical officer, AYUSH medical officer, contractual medical officer), and a separate variable which included the number of paramedical position types filled (staff nurse, pharmacist, female health worker, male health assistant, lab technicians, auxiliary nurse midwife, and additional staff nurse). To capture the availability of drugs at the health facilities, we used a binary variable from the survey that indicates if essential obstetric care drugs were available at the time of the survey. To measure the availability of medical equipment, we created a continuous index which measured the availability of delivery-specific equipment at the facility. The index ranged from 0 to 4, with facilities receiving 1 point for having each of the following items: normal delivery kit, equipment for assisted vacuum delivery, equipment for assisted forceps delivery, and equipment for manual vacuum aspiration. We also included a binary indicator for the availability of an adequate number of beds. Since the government of India set a norm of four to six beds per PHC, we defined four beds as an adequate number [24]. The general infrastructure variables included a count of the types of communication and transport equipment available (internet, telephone, computer, NIC terminal, and vehicles), whether the facility was open 24 hours per day, and whether the facility had access to electricity and/or a generator. Two additional variables were also included to capture facility quality and to explore if high quality facilities were more likely to produce higher volume of service. The first variable was establishment of Rogi Kalyan Samiti (RKS), also known as a Patient Welfare Committee, which is a facility-based management structure that aims to provide quality health care services by engaging the local population in the decision-making process. Secondly, an indicator of staff quality was captured by a binary indicator of Basic Emergency and Obstetric Care (BEmOC) or Skilled Birth Attendance (SBA) training received by staff in five years before the survey.

Though the focus of this study is to assess the effect of supply-side factors on maternity-care, we also included variables that might affect the demand for health services, such as socioeconomic, demographic, and geographic factors. In all models, we included the log of the facility's reported catchment area and a district-level fertility indicator as the most basic controls for demand. The district-level annual fertility rate for 2004–2008 was calculated among 15–49 year old women using the DLHS-3 ever married women questionnaire. Additional district-level demographic controls (included in only the final model) were calculated using the DLHS-3 household questionnaire. This included the average years of education among those over age 18; the percentage of households in the lowest wealth quintile (as defined by an asset score calculated by DLHS-3); the percentage of households with any member covered under a health plan or insurance; and the percentage of households where the head of household was Hindu. Sample weights were applied for all district-level calculations.

6. Statistical analysis

We used a negative binomial regression model to examine the association between the availability of resources at the health facility and the volume of deliveries. The negative binomial regression model is commonly used when the dependent variable is non-negative count data [25,26]. We ruled out a Poisson regression model because of its strict assumption that the dependent variable has the same mean and variance $\mu_{ig} = \exp(X_{ig} \beta_g)$. The distribution of institutional deliveries in our dataset clearly exhibited over-dispersion, with a mean of 21 and a variance of 1832. A Poisson regression model would produce inefficient estimates in this case. Therefore, we preferred a negative binomial model over a Poisson model because it does not require the assumption of equality of the conditional mean and variance, and allows for unmeasured characteristics that generate over-dispersion in the count data [27].

We estimated the following negative binomial regression model:

$$Y_{fd} = \beta_0 + \beta_1 X_1 + \beta_2 X_2 + \beta_3 X_3 + \dots\dots\dots + \beta_k X_k + (\sigma_d) + \epsilon_{fd} \quad (1)$$

where Y represents the outcome variable, the number of deliveries performed at the facility in the previous month, at the facility f in district d, and X_n represents the facility and district-level demographic factors affecting this outcome. σ_d is the random effect that varies at the district level ($Z_d \sim N(0, \sigma_d)$). The random intercept σ_d captures the effect of latent district-specific (time-invariant) covariates that cause some districts to have facilities that produce a greater volume of services than others, such as fewer private clinics or socio-demographic characteristics of the population that potentially affect the demand for facility-based delivery. We used Stata (version 13.0) for the analysis.

Results

After excluding facilities with missing information on the variables used in this study, our analytical sample comprises 8,227 PHCs with approximately 200,000 births recorded in the month prior to the survey.

Table 1 displays the definitions and summary statistics for the dependent and independent variables. In row 1, the sample mean and standard deviation of the dependent variable are reported. The mean of the dependent variable, the number of deliveries, is significantly different from the variance justifying the choice of a negative binomial model over a Poisson model, since the dependent variable is widely dispersed. The summary statistics for the independent variables convey the landscape of resource availability. On average, facilities had 1.49 of the 4 medical officer types, and four types of paramedical staff. Nearly 62% of the PHCs had the essential obstetric care drugs, 68% had an adequate number of beds, and 69% of facilities had a separate labor room to provide delivery services to women. Having a separate labor room was neither sufficient nor necessary for conducting deliveries; 44% of facilities without a delivery room still reported a delivery in the last month. Conversely, 36% of facilities without any deliveries had a separate labor room. Slightly less than half of the PHCs (47%) provided services 24 hours per day, despite the guideline that PHCs should be open at all hours of the day. Approximately 62% had a regular supply of electricity available. Nearly all the facilities were rural (95%) and 75% of them had established RKS or a Patient Welfare Committee. While exploring the quality of staff, data suggested that only 31% of the facilities had personnel that were trained either in BEmOC or SBA. There was substantial variation in the district-level demographic characteristics. The percent of households in the lowest wealth quintile ranged from 0 to 85%, and the average years of schooling ranged from less than 2 to over 9 (mean 5.38 years). On average, 5% of households in a district included an individual covered by insurance, but the figure was as high as 49% in one district. Hinduism was the dominant religion in most districts (85% of households on average), but ranged from 0 to 100%.

The results from the negative binomial regression model are reported in Tables 2 and 3. Both tables report the incidence rate ratios (IRR) and 95% confidence interval (CI). An IRR greater than 1 implies that an increase in the independent variable is associated with an increase in the outcome variable and vice versa. Variables are grouped under the six previously described categories: health personnel, drug availability, equipment, infrastructure, facility quality, and district-level socio-demographic composition. In the first four columns of Table 2, groups of variables are included individually, controlling only for the catchment area's population and fertility rate. In column 5, we included all facility resource variables together. Results in column 1 highlight the importance of health personnel. A greater availability of medical and paramedical staff is statistically associated with an increase in the incidence rate of delivery by 1.08 [95% CI: 1.02–1.12] and 1.18 [95% CI: 1.14–1.21], respectively. Results from the other separate models indicate that the delivery rate is higher if essential obstetric drugs and medical equipment are available in the clinics, and increases substantially with the presence of a labor room (IRR: 1.89 [95% CI: 1.68–2.12]), adequate beds (IRR: 1.45 [95% CI: 1.29–1.63]), and 24 hours of operation (IRR: 1.65 [95% CI: 1.56–1.80]). Access to electricity and availability of communication infrastructures are also significantly associated with a higher volume of delivery. Column 5 shows that upon including all predictors in one model, the magnitudes of the effects are reduced, but the significance is maintained. The exception is the number of medical staff, which becomes insignificant. In this combined model, the facility predictors with the largest coefficients are availability of labor room (IRR: 1.53 [95% CI: 1.37–1.72]) and facility opening hours (IRR: 1.39 [95% CI: 1.28–1.52]). Fertility rate and population size

Table 2. Facility-level determinants of institutional deliveries in India.

	Outcome: Number of deliveries performed at the facility									
	Incidence Rate Ratios (IRR) (95% CI)									
	(1)		(2)		(3)		(4)		(5)	
Health Personnel										
Number of medical staffs	1.086**	[1.020,1.156]							1.028	[0.973,1.085]
Number of paramedic staffs	1.177**	[1.142,1.214]							1.075**	[1.042,1.108]
Drug Availability										
Essential obstetric drugs			1.499**	[1.356,1.657]					1.139**	[1.033,1.255]
Equipment										
Adequate beds					1.454**	[1.293,1.636]			1.196**	[1.075,1.331]
Availability of labor room					1.887**	[1.678,2.122]			1.533**	[1.369,1.717]
Adequate obstetric equipment					1.178**	[1.124,1.235]			1.080**	[1.035,1.128]
Infrastructure										
Communication infrastructure (phone, computer, internet)							1.357**	[1.300,1.416]	1.257**	[1.204,1.313]
Facility open 24 hours							1.651**	[1.516,1.799]	1.392**	[1.275,1.518]
Access to electricity/generator/invertor							1.293**	[1.179,1.418]	1.172**	[1.060,1.295]
Log catchment population	1.654**	[1.525,1.794]	1.699**	[1.523,1.895]	1.653**	[1.517,1.801]	1.546**	[1.447,1.651]	1.503**	[1.405,1.607]
Fertility rate	1.162**	[1.107,1.220]	1.126**	[1.067,1.188]	1.144**	[1.087,1.205]	1.148**	[1.095,1.204]	1.220**	[1.161,1.282]

(**p<0.001).

Table 3. Facility-level determinants of institutional deliveries in India.

	Outcome: Number of deliveries performed at the facility							
	Incidence Rate Ratios (IRR) (95% CI)							
	(1)		(2)		(3)		(4)	
Health Personnel								
Number of medical staffs	1.028	[0.973,1.085]	1.014	[0.962,1.069]	1.033*	[1.002,1.064]	1.046**	[1.014,1.078]
Number of paramedic staffs	1.075**	[1.042,1.108]	1.071**	[1.039,1.105]	1.054**	[1.036,1.072]	1.058**	[1.039,1.076]
Drug Availability								
Essential obstetric drugs	1.139**	[1.033,1.255]	1.147**	[1.042,1.261]	1.184**	[1.120,1.251]	1.169**	[1.107,1.235]
Equipment								
Adequate beds	1.196**	[1.075,1.331]	1.204**	[1.083,1.338]	1.247**	[1.168,1.331]	1.245**	[1.167,1.329]
Availability of labor room	1.533**	[1.369,1.717]	1.535**	[1.373,1.716]	1.854**	[1.724,1.994]	1.811**	[1.684,1.946]
Adequate obstetric equipment	1.080**	[1.035,1.128]	1.076**	[1.032,1.122]	1.097**	[1.072,1.122]	1.092**	[1.067,1.116]
Infrastructure								
Communication infrastructure (phone, computer, internet)	1.257**	[1.204,1.313]	1.257**	[1.205,1.312]	1.076**	[1.049,1.103]	1.076**	[1.049,1.104]
Facility open 24 hours	1.392**	[1.275,1.518]	1.379**	[1.266,1.503]	1.435**	[1.358,1.515]	1.429**	[1.353,1.509]
Access to electricity/generator/invertor	1.172**	[1.060,1.295]	1.161**	[1.050,1.284]	1.085**	[1.024,1.150]	1.117**	[1.053,1.183]
Quality variables								
Rogi Kalyan Samiti (RKS)			0.981	[0.875,1.099]	1.052	[0.989,1.120]	1.060	[0.996,1.127]
Staff training			1.123*	[1.026,1.228]	1.045	[0.994,1.098]	1.052*	[1.001,1.105]
Rural			0.773*	[0.633,0.945]	0.891*	[0.811,0.979]	0.880**	[0.801,0.966]
Average years of school among adults							0.844**	[0.817,0.872]
% population in lowest wealth quintile							0.472**	[0.356,0.624]
% population insured							1.03	[0.632,1.678]
% Hindu population							1.354**	[1.139,1.610]
log catchment population	1.503**	[1.405,1.607]	1.502**	[1.409,1.602]	1.144**	[1.108,1.181]	1.129**	[1.094,1.166]
Fertility rate	1.220**	[1.161,1.282]	1.215**	[1.158,1.276]	1.084**	[1.044,1.125]	1.062**	[1.019,1.106]
District random-effects					X		X	

(*p<0.05; **p<0.01).

are also positively correlated with the number of deliveries conducted at the PHC.

Table 3 reports the results from the models that additionally control for facility and staff quality, whether the facility is located in a rural area, and socio-demographic composition of the district. The socio-demographic variables include average adult education level in the district, percentage of population with health insurance, Hindu population, and percentage of population that is poor. For comparison, column 1 reports the results from the last column of Table 2. Column 2 includes indicator variables for location of the facilities (rural/urban), and facility and staff quality. Column 3 shows results from the random-effect model with all the facility variables. Finally, column 4 displays results from a random-effect model that additionally includes socio-demographic controls. In all models, the IRR for rural is less than 1 suggesting that rural PHCs are producing a lower volume of delivery service than urban PHCs, even when adjusting for catchment population size and other demand factors (IRR: 0.88 [95% CI: 0.80–0.97] in column 4). In the full model, including socio-demographic factors and the facility and staff quality variables, RKS is not significantly associated with the outcome, while staff's quality (BEmOC or SBA training) is significantly associated with the volume of delivery services (IRR: 1.05 [95% CI: 1.00–1.11]). Compared to column 1, inclusion of district-level demographic characteristics and random-effects alters the magnitude of several facility-level predictors, such as the drug, equipment, and infrastructure variables, but does not change the directionality or significance substantially. The exception is the number of medical staff, which attains significance in the final model. Most of the other explanatory variables have the expected signs and are statistically significant. As expected, the incidence-rate of delivery in a health facility with a labor room is higher than a facility without a labor room (IRR: 1.81 [95% CI: 1.68–1.95]). It is comforting to note that the main results do not change substantially across models, even after including district-level random-effect, meaning results are not a product of the observed district demographic characteristics, or unobserved factors captured in the random effect.

It is quite possible that availability of labor room might confound the effect of other variables because some of these variables could be largely dependent on the pre-requisite of having a labor room. In theory, presence of a labor room is a pre-requisite to conduct delivery in public facilities, however our analytical data portrays a contrasting picture. In our sample of 8227 facilities, approximately 2591 facilities conducted delivery without a labor room indicating that about 32% of the facilities are providing delivery-care without having access to separate labor room. Nonetheless, as a robustness check, we reestimate eq(1) separately for facilities with and without a labor room to purge out the confounding association between delivery room and other facility characteristics. Results are reported in Table 4. Results are qualitatively similar to Table 3. Availability of paramedical staffs and essential obstetric drugs continues to be significant predictor of delivery-care regardless of availability of a labor room. Availability of beds and obstetric equipment has a larger effect in facilities without a labor room compared to facilities with a labor room. Facility opening hours remain significantly associated with delivery-care in both types of facilities.

Discussion

Despite targeted efforts by government and multinational agencies, close to one-third of the deliveries in India occur at home without any medical supervision. There are many factors that hinder utilization of maternity-care in India. For example, past nationally representative surveys have reported cost to be an important barrier to facility-based delivery and an evaluation of JSY found a significant effect on institutional births in India [22,28]. Similarly, several other studies have identified socioeconomic, demographic, and geographic barriers to an institutional use of maternal-care in India and showed a negative relationship between distance to health facility and in-facility birth in India [8,9,10,29,30]. The majority of the factors examined in these studies are demand-side constraints that mainly operate at the household level. Though it is generally hypothesized that supply-side factors at the facility level have a strong impact on provision and utilization of health services, there exists a surprising scarcity of systematic attempts to understand the association between facility-level bottlenecks and skilled delivery.

Our study explores the association between facility characteristics and the volume of in-facility deliveries performed in India, taking the facility as the unit of analysis. Our main results suggest that availability of labor rooms, opening hours of the facility, and adequacy of general medical equipment and infrastructure are the primary facility-level drivers of institutional delivery at PHCs in India. In contrast, community involvement through RKS, recent relevant staff training, and greater staff numbers had weak or low-magnitude associations. These results are robust to inclusion of district-level socio-demographic factors and a district random effect, indicating that they cannot be explained simply by inter-district variations.

The study has important policy implications because the government has the capabilities and resources to make changes to its health facilities. This is in contrast to efforts of impacting individual-level demand factors, which may require years of complex economic and social change. Our results indicate that equipping more PHCs with labor rooms, and making them meet the requirement of 24/7 service would be important steps to achieving more facility-based deliveries.

The descriptive results of our study also highlight that there is a great deal of room for relevant improvements in these areas. Specifically, only slightly more than half of facilities were open 24 hours a day, and 30% of facilities were not equipped with labor rooms. Beyond the issue of encouraging patients to seek care is the quality and safety of services available at the facility for those who do choose to come. For instance, 625 facilities reported conducting deliveries in the last month despite not having any of the four pieces of equipment available, including a basic delivery kit.

RKS is a strategy to improve the quality of management responses and thereby, facilitate the strengthening of health systems as well as health outcomes. RKS has been an important step under NRHM to increase community participation in the management of the health facilities. However, our results indicate that decentralized decision-making by RKS does not have a strong effect on the provision of delivery care at PHC level. The DLHS-3 report finds that constitution and utilization of untied RKS funds in the CHC and DH have been successfully implemented. However, the implementation of RKS proved problematic at the PHC level. About 70% of the PHC did not spend the RKS untied funds and very few facilities displayed the citizen's charter. Some studies have revealed that inadequate support systems for capacity building and training are constraints which weaken the impact of RKS [31]. This study also reports an absence of regular meeting of stakeholders and autocratic decision-making at many PHCs, thereby diluting the purpose of establishing RKS. Therefore, for RKS to attract users and improve quality of health services, the overall functioning needs to be strengthen at the PHC level by creating a proper grievance redressal system, conducting regular meetings with the stakeholders, and capacity building.

Table 4. Facility-level determinants of institutional deliveries in India.

	Outcome: Number of deliveries performed at the facility			
	Incidence Rate Ratios (IRR) (95% CI)			
	Facilities without labor room (N = 2591)		Facilities with labor room (N = 5636)	
	(1)		(2)	
Health Personnel				
Number of medical staffs	0.96	[0.888,1.038]	1.069**	[1.034,1.105]
Number of paramedic staffs	1.087**	[1.041,1.135]	1.055**	[1.035,1.075]
Drug Availability				
Essential obstetric drugs	1.287**	[1.135,1.458]	1.116**	[1.052,1.185]
Equipment				
Adequate beds	1.328**	[1.170,1.508]	1.155**	[1.074,1.243]
Adequate obstetric equipment	1.297**	[1.225,1.373]	1.050**	[1.025,1.076]
Infrastructure				
Communication infrastructure (phone, computer, internet)	1.148**	[1.072,1.229]	1.068**	[1.039,1.098]
Facility open 24 hours	1.826**	[1.608,2.073]	1.361**	[1.283,1.443]
Access to electricity/generator/invertor	0.986	[0.860,1.130]	1.150**	[1.079,1.226]
Quality variables				
Rogi Kalyan Samiti (RKS)	1.086	[0.826,1.429]	0.845**	[0.765,0.932]
Staff training	1.151*	[1.004,1.320]	1.021	[0.954,1.094]
Rural	0.897	[0.780,1.032]	1.101**	[1.044,1.161]
Average years of school among adults	0.730**	[0.682,0.782]	0.888**	[0.857,0.921]
% population in lowest wealth quintile	0.173**	[0.0970,0.307]	0.699*	[0.512,0.954]
% population insured	1.06	[0.255,4.398]	1.155	[0.693,1.925]
% Hindu population	2.046**	[1.467,2.855]	1.364**	[1.130,1.646]
log catchment population	1.088*	[1.012,1.171]	1.173**	[1.131,1.216]
Fertility rate	1.131**	[1.040,1.229]	1.059*	[1.011,1.110]
District random-effects	X		X	

(*$p<0.05$; **$p<0.01$).

Our study has several strengths. It contributes to the scant literature on the effect of facility characteristics on institutional delivery in India. Given that many births in India are unsafe and home-based, it is important to understand what improvements can be made at the facility level to increase in-facility deliveries. The use of nationally representative data is a strength of this study, and our findings are reliable due to the large sample size. Estimation of a count model, specifically a negative binomial regression model, adds to the strength of this study because a count model is the correct model to apply with this type of outcome variable.

However, our study is not free from limitations. First and foremost, the study is based on cross-sectional data and therefore, causality cannot be inferred. Our analysis may suffer from reverse causality. It is possible that facilities conducting more deliveries are likely to receive more resources or vice-versa. Given the cross-sectional nature of our dataset, pinning down the direction of causality is not possible. A panel data is needed to address the issue of reverse causality or temporality. The dependent variable, the number of deliveries performed at the facility, could suffer from measurement bias as the data quality depends on the specific data management system at each facility. We also do not include activities related to in-home skilled birth attendants, which has been an alternative solution proposed for safe deliveries. Several of the independent variables of interest could also improve in terms of measurement. For example, DLHS-3 only captured a binary indicator for whether each type of personnel was present. Although the PHC standards call for only one individual in each type of position, it would be preferable to capture the total number of personnel working at the facility in case this quota is ever exceeded. It would also be preferable to include a measure of total fertility rather than looking within ever-married women. This was not possible with DLHS-3 data because fertility questions were only asked of ever-married women, and district-level estimates for the time period of interest were not available from other sources.

In India, the private sector plays an important role in delivering healthcare. Due to poor quality of healthcare in public hospitals, many households prefer to visit private clinics to seek maternity-care. Per DLHS 2007-2008, about 17% of the institutional deliveries were performed at private health clinics. However, due to unavailability of data on private facilities, we could not include private clinics/hospitals in our study. But, from a policy perspective, it is more relevant to analyze only public facilities as it is in this sector where government can intervene and improve the quality of healthcare provision because government has limited control over private sector resource allocation.

While we have chosen to focus on the PHC in our analysis, future research could be expanded to examine the role of supply-side factors in other levels of the health system, namely rural and district hospitals. Future studies should also further examine the interaction between supply and demand side factors, to tease out complicated relationships that exist between the two. We attempted to address this by including district-level demographic factors in our final model, but many factors, such as distance to the facility and income are better studied at the individual rather than aggregate level. The supply side factors found to be significant may also interact with demand factors by altering patient perceptions of facility quality, which has been shown to drive demand for health services [32]. Finally, it is important to incorporate the quality of care, mainly the behavior of the providers such as doctors, nurses, and supporting staffs. Unfortunately, our study could not establish the relationship between provider's quality and institutional delivery because the DLHS data did not provide information on quality of the providers. Therefore, future studies should attempt to include measures of quality of care to address concerns that increased volume could affect quality of care.

Acknowledgments

We also acknowledge Kelsey Moore for project management and Nisha Sinha for helpful research assistance.

Author Contributions

Conceived and designed the experiments: SK. Performed the experiments: SK ED. Analyzed the data: SK ED. Contributed reagents/materials/analysis tools: SK ED. Wrote the paper: SK.

References

1. World Bank (2012) World Development Report 2012: Gender Equality and Development. World Bank. Available: https://openknowledge.worldbank.org/handle/10986/4391. Accessed 24 March 2014.
2. WHO UNICEF, UNFPA, World Bank (2012) Trends in maternal mortality: 1990 to 2010. World Health Organization.
3. Department of Health and Family Welfare (2010) Annual Report. Ministry of Health and Family Welfare Government of India.
4. National Health Mission. Ministry of Health and Family Welfare Government of India. Available: http://nrhm.gov.in/. Accessed 24 March 2014.
5. Adamson PC, Krupp K, Niranjankumar B, Freeman AH, Khan M, et al. (2012) Are marginalized women being left behind? A population-based study of institutional deliveries in Karnataka, India. BMC Public Health 12:30.
6. Annual Health Survey (2011) Office of Registrar General of India, New Delhi.
7. WHO UNFPA, UNICEF, World Bank (1999) Reduction of maternal mortality. WHO.
8. Jacobs B, Ir P, Bigdeli M, Annear PL, Van Damme W (2012) Addressing access barriers to health services: an analytical framework for selecting appropriate interventions in low-income Asian countries. Health Policy and Planning 27(4): 288–300.
9. Hanson K, Ranson K, Oliveira-Cruz V, Mills A (2003) Expanding access to priority health interventions: a framework for understanding the constraints to scaling-up. Journal of International Development 15: 1–14.
10. Kesterton AJ, Cleland J, Slogett A, Ronsmans C (2010) Institutional delivery in rural India: the relative importance of accessibility and economic status. BMC Pregnancy & Childbirth 10:30.
11. Borah BJ (2006) A mixed logit model of health care provider choice: analysis of NSS data for rural India. Health Economics 15(9): 915–932.
12. Sarma S (2009) Demand for outpatient healthcare: empirical findings from rural India. Applied Health Economics Health Policy 7(4): 265–277.
13. Ensor T, Cooper S (2004) Overcoming barriers to health service access: influencing the demand side. Health Policy Planning 19(2): 69–79.
14. O'Donnell O (2007) Access to health care in developing countries: breaking down demand side barriers. Cad Saude Publica 23(12): 2820–2834.
15. R . Metcalfe, Adegoke AA (2013) Strategies to increase facility-based skilled birth attendance in South Asia: a literature review. International Health 5(2): 96–105.
16. Peabody JW, Gertler PJ, Leibowitz A (1998) The policy implications of better structure and process on birth outcomes in Jamaica. Health Policy 43(1): 1–13.
17. Olsen OE, Ndeki S, Norheim OF (2005) Human resources for emergency obstetric care in northern Tanzania: distribution of quantity or quality? Hum Resources for Health 29: 3–5.
18. Hong R, Montana L, Mishra V (2006) Family planning services quality as a determinant of use of IUD in Egypt. BMC Health Services Research 6: 79.
19. Mbonye AK, Asimwe JB (2010) Factors associated with skilled attendance at delivery in Uganda: results from a national health facility survey. International Journal of Adolescent Medicine and Health 22(2): 249–255.
20. Stephenson R, Beke A, Tshibangu D (2008) Contextual influences on contraceptive use in the Eastern Cape, South Africa. Health Place 14(4): 841–852.
21. Sharma MP, Soni SC, Bhattacharya M, Datta U, Gupta S, et al. (2009) An assessment of institutional deliveries under JSY at different levels of health care in Jaipur District, Rajasthan. Indian Journal of Public Health 53(3): 177–182.
22. International Institute for Population Sciences (2010) District Level Household and Facility Survey (DLHS-3), 2007–08.
23. Pandian J, Suresh S, Desikachari BR, Padmanaban P (2013) Increased utilization of primary health care centers for birthing care in Tamil Nadu, India: A visible impact of policies, initiatives, and innovations. Journal of Family Medicine and Primary Care 2(4): 329–233.
24. National Health Mission (2012) Indian Public Health Standards Guidelines for PHC. Available:http://www.nrhmassam.in/pdf/guideline2/bulletin/Rural%20Health%20Care%20System%20in%20India.pdf. Accessed 24 March 2014.
25. Winkelmann R (1997) Econometric Analysis of Count Data. Berlin: Springer.
26. Jones AM (2000) Health econometrics. In: Culyer AJ, Newhouse JP, editors. The Handbook of Health Economics. Amsterdam: Elsevier. pp 265–346.
27. Cameron AC, Trivedi PK (2013) Regression Analysis of Count Data. Cambridge: Cambridge University Press.
28. Lim S, Dandona L, Hoisington JA, Spencer JL, Hogan MC, et al. (2010) India's Janani Suraksha Yojana, a conditional cash transfer programme to increase births in health facilities: an impact evaluation. The Lancet 375(9730): 2009–2023.
29. Jat TR, Ng N, Sebastian SM (2011) Factors affecting the use of maternal health services in Madhya Pradesh state of India: a multilevel analysis. International Journal for Equity in Health 10: 59.
30. Stephenson R, Tsui AO (2002) Contextual influences on reproductive health service use in Uttar Pradesh, India. Studies in Family Planning 33(4): 309–320.
31. Adsul N, Kar M (2013) Study of rogi kalian samitis in strengthening health systems under national rural health mission, district pune, maharashtra. Indian Journal of Community Medicine 38(4): 223–228.
32. Rai SK, Dasgupta R, Das MK, Singh S, Devi R, et al. (2011) Determinants of utilization of services under MMJSSA scheme in Jharkhand 'Client Perspective': a qualitative study in a low performing state of India. Indian Journal of Public Health 55(4): 252–259.

16

Microneedle Enhanced Delivery of Cosmeceutically Relevant Peptides in Human Skin

Yousuf H. Mohammed[1,2,3], Miko Yamada[1], Lynlee L. Lin[1], Jeffrey E. Grice[3], Michael S. Roberts[3], Anthony P. Raphael[1], Heather A. E. Benson[2], Tarl W. Prow[1]*

1 Dermatology Research Centre, The University of Queensland, School of Medicine, Translational Research Institute, Brisbane, Queensland, Australia, 2 School of Pharmacy, CHIRI-Biosciences, Curtin University, Perth, Western Australia, Australia, 3 Therapeutics Research Centre, The University of Queensland, School of Medicine, Princess Alexandra Hospital, Brisbane, Queensland, Australia

Abstract

Peptides and proteins play an important role in skin health and well-being. They are also found to contribute to skin aging and melanogenesis. Microneedles have been shown to substantially enhance skin penetration and may offer an effective means of peptide delivery enhancement. The aim of this investigation was to assess the influence of microneedles on the skin penetration of peptides using fluorescence imaging to determine skin distribution. In particular the effect of peptide chain length (3, 4, 5 amino acid chain length) on passive and MN facilitated skin penetration was investigated. Confocal laser scanning microscopy was used to image fluorescence intensity and the area of penetration of fluorescently tagged peptides. Penetration studies were conducted on excised full thickness human skin in Franz type diffusion cells for 1 and 24 hours. A 2 to 22 fold signal improvement in microneedle enhanced delivery of melanostatin, rigin and pal-KTTKS was observed. To our knowledge this is the first description of microneedle enhanced skin permeation studies on these peptides.

Editor: Miguel A. R. B. Castanho, Faculdade de Medicina da Universidade de Lisboa, Portugal

Funding: This project was funded by Australian National Health and Medical Research Council. APR acknowledges The University of Queensland Post-Doctoral Fellowship and Early Career Research Award for funding. YM acknowledges the Australian Postgraduate Award for funding. The funders had no role in study design, data collection and analysis, decision to publish, or preparation of the manuscript.

Competing Interests: The authors have declared that no competing interests exist.

* Email: t.prow@uq.edu.au

Introduction

Peptides have important applications in modulating of skin cell proliferation, cell migration, inflammation, angiogenesis, melanogenesis, and protein synthesis and regulation [1]. With variations in amino acid sequence, number of amino acids and derivatives, the future of peptide based cosmeceuticals is bright [2]. There are three main categories of cosmeceutical peptides: signal peptides, carrier peptides, and neurotransmitter-affecting peptides. The active ingredient must be delivered to the target in stable form and be able to have the desired biological effect in vivo.

The most prevalent and widely used single peptide is lysine-threonine-threonine-lysine-serine (KTTKS) found on type I procollagen. Melanostatin is a novel pseudo-tripeptide with a molecular formula of $C_{19}H_{25}N_5O_5$ and is structurally related to feldamycin. Melanostatin inhibited melanin formation in Streptomyces bikiniensis NRRLB-1049 and B16 melanoma cells. Rigin is a four amino acid peptide that is can reduce inflammation. Specifically, rigin has been shown to down regulate IL-6 [3,4].

The transdermal peptide delivery has attracted interest due to the many biological advantages associated with including avoidance of the first-pass metabolism and sustained therapeutic action. However the stratum corneum barrier has been the greatest challenge for transdermal peptide delivery researchers. Thus, many approaches have been attempted to overcome the skin barrier and enhance the transdermal delivery of peptides for local and systemic effects. The major approaches for enhancing transdermal delivery are physical enhancers, vesicles particulate systems and chemical enhancers. The use of microneedles has been used to overcome the stratum corneum barrier. Microneedles are minimally invasive devices that can drug into or through the skin barrier. Microneedles are generally shorter than 1 mm in length and can breach the stratum corneum barrier. One challenge researchers working in this field face is skin elasticity [5]. Hence microneedle length, manner of insertion and application speed govern the shape and size of the pore formed [6].

The amount of time the pores stay open has been an area of constant debate. Bal *et al.* claim a fast closure of the pores by using a confocal laser scanning microscopy (CLSM) to visualise the amount of a fluorescent dye present in the pores. Visualisation using CLSM is one way to obtain information on morphological parameters of the pores and to monitor the behaviour of a pore and the dye over time. Bal *et al.* reported a quick closure of the pores as there was a strong decrease of the dye present at the skin surface after 10–15 min [6]. Banks *et al.* utilized transepidermal water loss (TEWL) measurements after microneedle treatment and microscopic visualization to determine pore lifetime. They also measured skin permeability of NTXOL (naltrexone analogue 6-β-

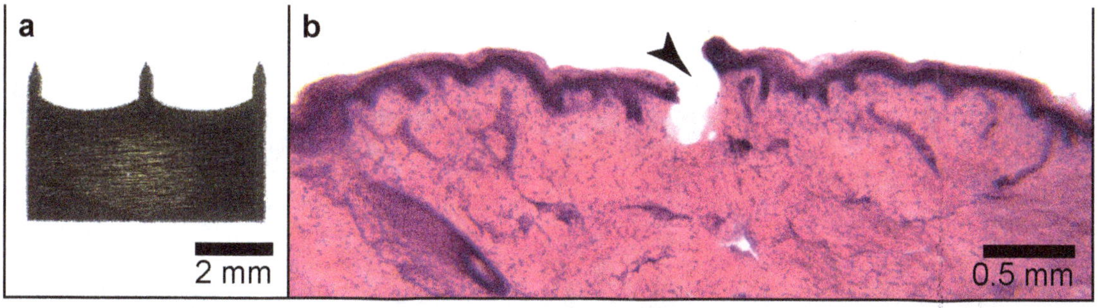

Figure 1. Hematoxylin and eosin image of microneedle hole into excised human skin. The image of microneedle (MN) plate used (with three 700 μm length x 250 μm with MN) is shown (a). Representative image of a 30 μm thick Hematoxylin and eosin (H&E) stained crysection of a microneeedle (MN) penetration site in human skin is shown (b). In this image the microneedle fissure (arrowhead) is 432 μm, reaching the superficial dermis.

naltrexol) over time to determine the pore lifetime. In addition, a staining technique was developed to microscopically visualize microneedle created pores in treated guinea pig skin. Banks *et al.* concluded that microneedle-assisted transdermal delivery appears viable for at least 48 h after microneedle-application [7]. In a subsequent study they showed that the addition of a COX inhibitor, like diclofenac, can keep the microneedle pores open for up to a week [8]. Transport of drug molecules after microneedle application is hypothesized to take place by simple diffusion [9].

The aim of the present study was to evaluate the distribution of fluorescently-tagged peptides, melanostatin, rigin and palmitoyl-pentapeptide (Pal-KTTKS) after microneedle based delivery using CLSM and to determine distribution of the peptides within the skin strata. In particular the effect of peptide chain length (3, 4, 5 amino acid chain length) on passive and microneedle facilitated skin penetration was investigated.

Materials and Methods

2.1 Skin preparation for permeation studies

Human skin was obtained from abdominoplasty patients. All patients signed an informed consent. This study is specifically approved by the Princess Alexandra Hospital Research Committee approval No. 097/090, administered by the University of Queensland Human Ethics Committee (Australia). The subcutaneous fat was removed by dissection and the full thickness skin then stored at −20°C until required. Skin from different donors was used to demonstrate reproducibility of the study. Before commencing the study the skin was thawed to room temperature and carefully dabbed with clean tissue paper to remove excess moisture. The skin was then cut using a circular die to fit Franz cells.

2.2 Microneedles and Microneedle applicator

The microneedles used in this study were cut from a 50 μm thick 304 stainless steel sheet using a LaserPro S290 laser etcher. The microneedle arrays were cut onto a single plate with 700 μm length×250 μm width. Each plate consisted of 3 microneedles separated by a 5 mm distance. These plates were then assembled in banks of 2 with a 3 mm spacing in between. The microneedles were cut in batches with a strict quality control cut-off of 5% standard deviation. A typical batch when observed for quality assurance had an average height of 703.1±16.1 μm and an average width of 257.8±9.4 μm.

The applicator developed for this study was designed to impact the skin surface at 1.5 m/s. After firmly placing the applicator against the skin, the trigger was released to apply the six microneedles.

2.3 Microneedle enhanced peptide delivery in human skin

Microfabrication techniques ensured that the microneedles were long enough to cross the permeability barrier (700 μm) but not so long that they are painful [10]. The peptides used in this

Table 1. Values of integrated density and positive area in epidermis and dermis at 1 hour and 24 hour time points.

	Integrated density				Positive area (μm^2)			
	Epidermis		Dermis		Epidermis		Dermis	
	1 hour	24 hours	1 hour	24 hours	1 hour	24 hours	1 hour	24 hours
Melanostatin	548.7±431.4	1208.0±321.4	137.0±62.2	289.3±171.8	1842±2025	12395±5117	23±97	1094±938
Melanostatin + MN	1463±620.4*	2487.0±1770.0	578.4±316.1**	2970±4026*	15648±5802**	17948±7578	9560±7783**	25032±5390**
Rigin	1325.0±613.8	2172.0±492.4	716.8±504.1	374.0±228.6	9763±3064	16392±2395	1561±906	4269±4172
Rigin + MN	2334.0±781.0*	1264.0±907.1*	768.0±192.7	324.8±237.0	17765±4348*	16594±6218	7683±2887**	2730±2317
Pal-KTTKS	255.8±167.8	3070.0±4101.0	155.3±61.0	196.9±84.1	1902±1525	6578±2441	23±14	205±208
Pal-KTTKS + MN	656.1±272.1	13880±22614	950.7±1403.0	323.1±573.4	977±323	4219±1742	46±54	367±419

* indicates $p<0.05$ and ** indicates $p<0.01$.

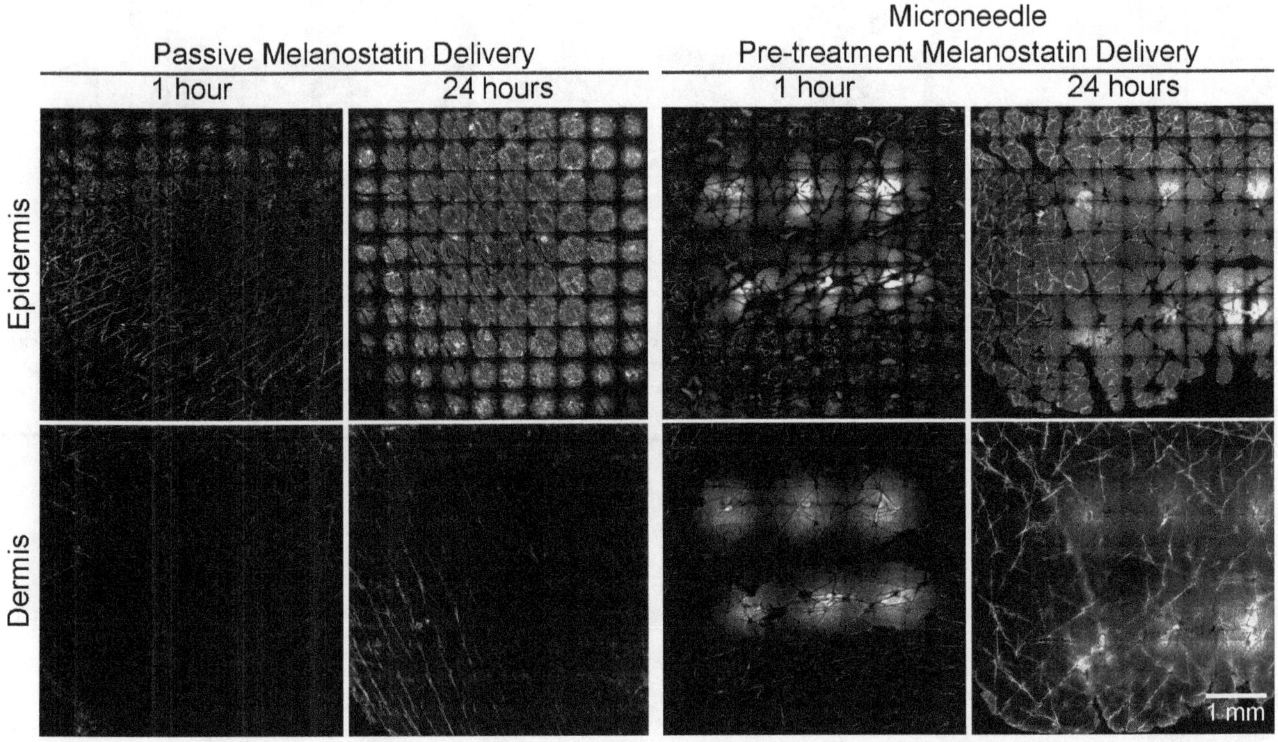

Figure 2. LSCM images of melanostatin delivery into excised human skin. Representative melanostatin (MEL) treated confocal laser scanning microscopy (CLSM) images of viable epidermis and dermis at 1 and 24 hour(s) are shown without and with microneedle (MN) delivery enhancement. Mosaic images of the viable epidermis and dermis (top row and bottom row, respectively) are shown at at 1 and 24 hour(s) after melanstatin delivery with microneedle enhancement. Each mosiac is 5×5 mm^2.

study were selected as cosmetic and therapeutic peptides with increasing chain length and increasing molecular weight. Fluorescein conjugated peptides melanostatin (PLG; MW 803.92 Da; XLOGP calculated log P−1.3), rigin (GQPR; MW 959.04 Da; XLOGP calculated log P−7.7) and Pal-KTTKS (MW 1191.06 Da, log P 3.5) were first dissolved in appropriate solvents. All peptides were purchased from Genscript (Hong Kong). Eight groups were tested in triplicate. Negative controls were vehicle only and vehicles post microneedle application to account for any autofluorescence. Sodium fluorescein, at equal molar levels to that present in the peptide, was used as a positive control in both passive treatment group where microneedles were not applied, and in active treatment group where microneedles were applied (data not shown). The last two treatments included the peptides with and without microneedles applied at a 500 µg/mL concentration. The duration of the study was 1 hour for all treatments. For the peptides a separate 24 hour time point from the same skin donor was also conducted. The replicate experiments on each peptide were conducted using skin from three donors.

2.4 Skin sample confocal microscopy analysis

After completion of the treatment time the skin samples were cut to a smaller size. Before the samples were imaged with CLSM, a dermoscopic image was first taken to identify the exact location of the microneedle fissures. The sample was then mounted with a cover slip. The VivaScope 2500 Multilaser (Caliber I.D., Rochester NY USA) was used for this study as imaging an area large enough to cover the microneedle holes could be done in one tiled image. The excitation wavelength was 445 nm with the laser power (6.8 mW) held constant for all experiments. The images were generated as cubes of tiled images of 8×8 individual images over 20 layers in depth. The cube was generated over 100 µm with images at a step of 5 µm. Similarly cubes were also generated from the same area (depth and location) in reflectance mode. The reflectance image in conjunction with the z-axis profile of the intensity depth was used to determine the top layer of the skin sample. The top 20 µm were designated as the stratum corneum (SC), the following 30 µm were designated as the viable epidermis (VE) and the images from below this (50 µm + deeper) were designated as the dermis (DER) [11]. Mosiacs at 30 and 50 µm were subjected to image analysis and reported as viable epidermis and dermis, respectively.

2.5 Image analysis

Image signal intensity analysis was carried out using Image J software NIH (USA). The raw mosaic images were resized to 10% of the original. The threshold value (54) was derived from pilot experiments with where sodium fluorescein was applied to untreated and microneedle treated skin. The images were opened in ImageJ and a threshold of applied. A circular selection (diameter 750 µm and area 4.42×10^5 µm^2) was centered on the microneedle site. Similarly, the same diameter circular selection was applied to the non-microneedle treated

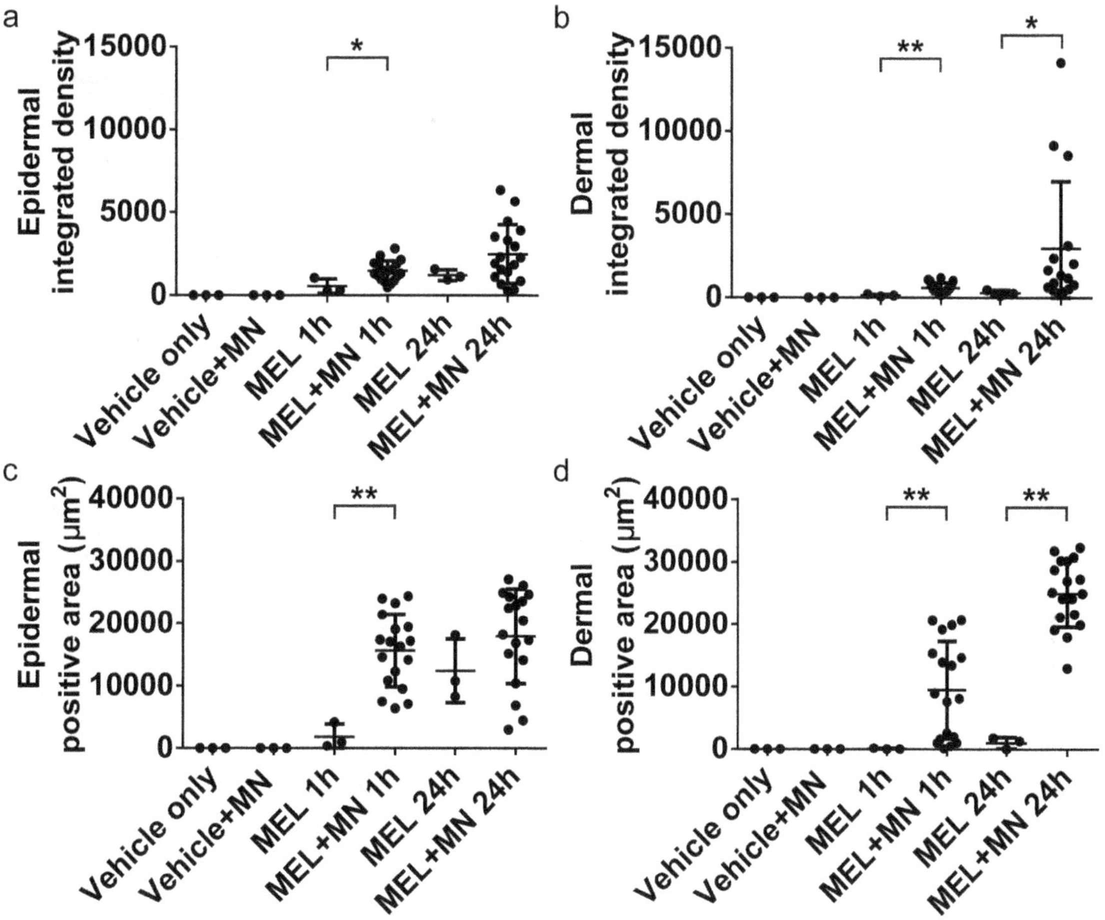

Figure 3. Integrated density and positive area data from melanostatin treated skin. Melanostatin (MEL) delivery characteristics are shown from epidermal (a and c) and dermal (d and d) mosiacs. Both the integrated density (a and b) and positive area (c and d) are shown for each microneedle site (MN). Data are shown for both 1 and 24 hours peptide exposure (1 h and 24 h, respecitvely). * indicates p<0.05. ** indicates p<0.01.

skin groups. The positive area and integrated density values were generated using the measurements function in ImageJ for all images.

2.6 Statistical analysis

The skin permeation data consisted of normalised penetration area and integrated density measurements of active, passive, negative control and positive control taken at 1 and 24 hours within the skin layers, viable epidermis and dermis. Statistical analysis was conducted using GraphPad Prism 5.03 software (GraphPad Software Inc. USA). Mann Whitney test was used to generate p values when comparing two data sets. Significant differences were defined as $p<0.05$. Values for integrated density and positive area are shown as mean ± standard deviation.

Results

3.1. Penetration of microneedle in excised human skin

The design of the microneedles use in this study is shown in **Figure 1.** The microneedles penetrated 304±63 μm deep into human skin. **Figure 1** shows a haematoxylin and eosin stained section of human skin treated with the microneedles. There is a clear puncture site that extends into the superficial dermis. This barrier breach is the best case scenario for enhancing topical peptide delivery.

3.2. Penetration and distribution of microneedle assisted peptides in excised human skin

3.2.1 Melanostatin. Melanostatin penetration into the viable epidermis and dermis with lateral diffusion can be seen in **Figure 2.** The fine lines seen in these images are furrows containing the fluorescently labelled peptide. Each mosaic is composed of 10×10 images at 500×500 μm each. By comparing between 1 hour and 24 hours microneedle assisted delivery, the data shows some increased diffusion of melanostatin to 24 hours. There was minimal penetration of melanostatin in both viable epidermis and dermis without microneedle pre-treatment (**Figure 2**). **Figure 3** shows image analysis outcomes that at 1 hour, microneedles enhanced Melanostatin positive area by 8.5-fold in the viable epidermis (15,648±5,802 μm^2) when compared to without microneedles (1,842±2,025 μm^2). This difference was found to be statistically significant ($p<0.01$). At the same time-point the integrated density in the epidermis was significantly increased by 2.6-fold with microneedles (1,463±620) and without microneedles (549±431) (**Table 1**).

Enhancements of 2.1 and 1.4 fold were seen in the positive area and integrated density at 24 hours with and without microneedles,

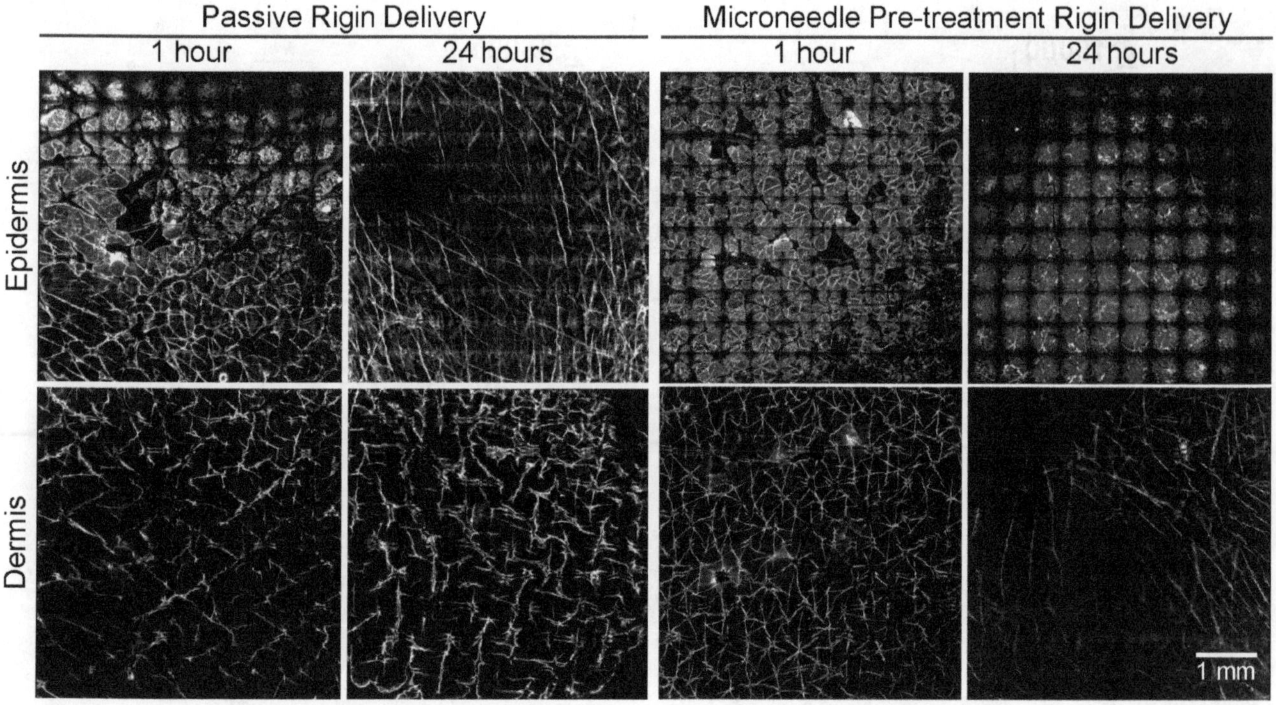

Figure 4. LSCM images of rigin delivery into excised human skin. Representative rigin (RIG) treated confocal laser scanning microscopy (CLSM) images of viable epidermis and dermis at 1 and 24 hour(s) are shown without and with microneedle (MN) delivery enhancement. Mosaic images of the viable epidermis and dermis (top row and bottom row, respectively) are shown at at 1 and 24 hour(s) after rigin delivery with microneedle enhancement. Each mosiac is 5×5 mm^2.

respectively. The trend and deviation intensified with increasing depth. Microneedle enhancement showed a significant increase in the total area of penetration in the dermis (without microneedles: 23±97 μm^2; with microneedles: 9,560±7,783 μm^2) after 1 hour. Although highly variable, the differences were significant ($p<$ 0.0001). At 24 hours the comparison was similar, a 22-fold increase in area was seen in the dermis from 1,094±938 μm^2 without microneedles to 25,032±5,390 μm^2 with microneedles. This was accompanied with a non-significant 1.7-fold increase in dermal integrated density after 24 hours from 196±84 without microneedles to 333±180, with microneedle delivery enhancement. Taken together, these data show that microneedles can indeed enhance topical melanostatin delivery.

3.2.2 Rigin. **Figure 4** shows the 1 and 24 hour(s) images from rigin treated skin with or without microneedle application. There was a slight increase in permeation of rigin in viable epidermis with microneedles at 1 hour compared to that without microneedles. After 24 hours post treatment, there were not substantial differences in rigin permeation at the viable epidermal level with respect to microneedle treatment. The dermal permeation was similar between microneedles and without microneedles at 1 and hours post administration (**Figure 4**). The quantification results (**Figure 5**) show Rigin with microneedles resulted a 1.8-fold increase in the positive area (Rigin 1 hour with microneedles: 17,765±4,348 μm^2; and without microneedles: 9,763±3,064 μm^2) and 1.7-fold increase in the integrated density in the viable epidermis at 1 hour ($p<0.05$). At 24 hours the Rigin positive areas in the viable epidermis were nearly identical with or without microneedles at 16,594±6,218 and 16,392±2,395 μm^2, respectively (**Table 1**). The dermal results were similar in comparison with a ~6-fold drop in Rigin positive area compared to that in the viable epidermis. These data show that microneedle penetration enhancement was effective at 1 hour post treatment, but this effect was not observed at the 24 hour time point.

3.2.3 Pal-KTTKS. Following the microneedle enhanced delivery with Pal-KTTKS, the images (**Figure 6**) showed no obvious change in integrated density or penetration area in the viable epidermis at either 1 or 24 hours with or without microneedles. The outline of the microneedle penetration sites was visible for the most part, but the signal appeared limited to the immediate area.

Image analysis revealed no significant changes in the integrated density or positive area after 1 hour. However, after 24 hours treatment we observed a 4.5 fold increase in integrated density while the Pal-KTTKS positive area remained the same (**Figure 7**). The increase in integrated density was only observed in a subset of microneedle sites (6/18) and was therefore associated with a large standard deviation. At first we suspected the microneedle application was to blame, but this phenomena was only observed with Pal-KTTKS and not melanostatin or rigin. Additionally, the positive area measurements did not show the same trend. Therefore, we hypothesize that this observation may be due to the negligible penetration profile combined with the dynamic nature of skin pore morphology. These increased mean integrated density values were associated with large standard deviations that minimise the relevance of this perceived penetration enhancement (e.g. dermal integrated density increased from 196.9±84.1 to 323.1±573.4 with microneedle pre-treatment at 24 hours) (**Table 1**). Overall, microneedle pre-treatment did not appear to significantly and reproducibly enhance the delivery of Pal-KTTKS.

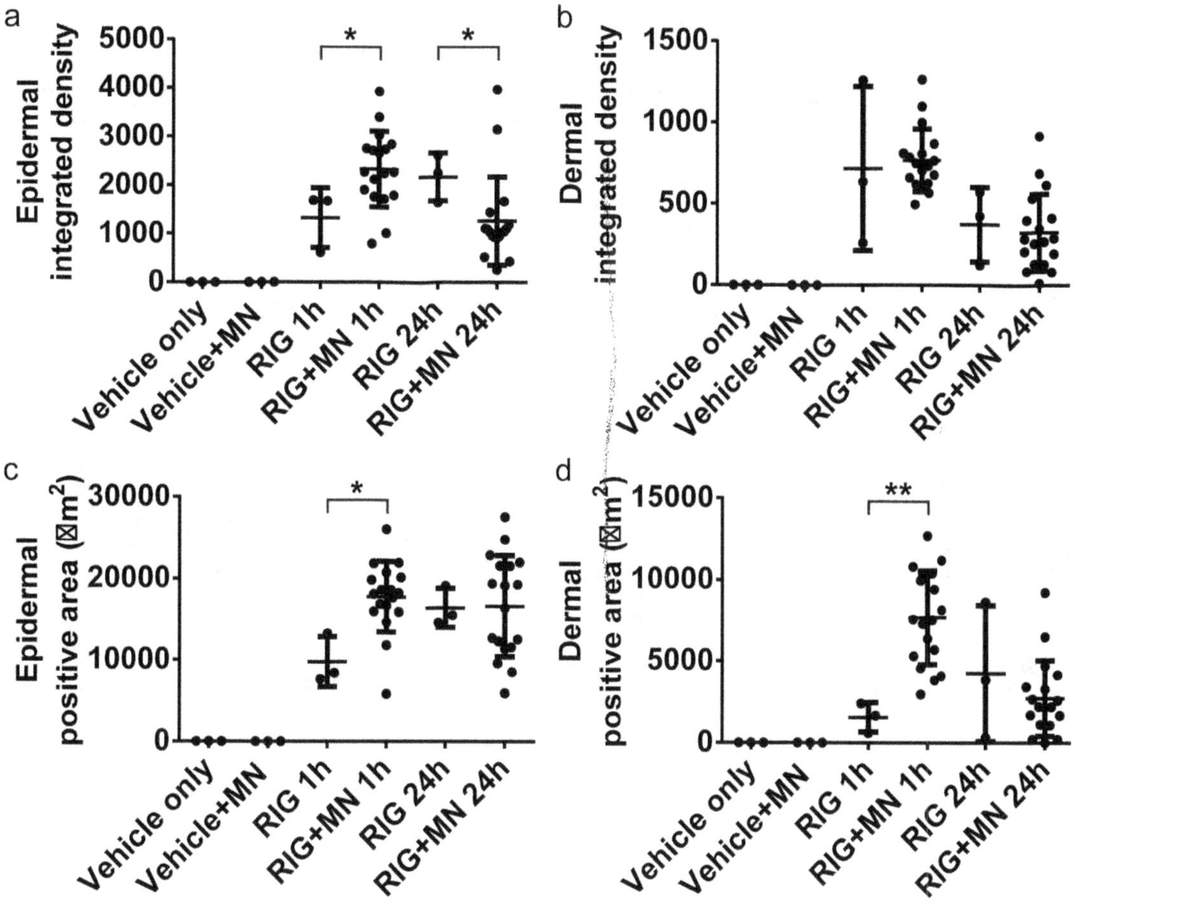

Figure 5. Integrated density and positive area data from rigin treated skin. Rigin (RIG) delivery characteristics are shown from epidermal (a and c) and dermal (d and d) mosiacs. Both the integrated density (a and b) and positive area (c and d) are shown for each microneedle site (MN). Data are shown for both 1 and 24 hours peptide exposure (1 h and 24 h, respecitvely). * indicates $p<0.05$. ** indicates $p<0.01$.

Discussion

There is a balance between microneedles sufficiently long enough to penetrate through the skin barrier for enhanced drug delivery but small enough to cause minimal skin injury and pain. Our study showed the penetration of MN alone into epidermis. Developing clinically feasible microneedle transdermal delivery of peptides is complex. One reason for this is that after the microneedle physically enters the skin, it is almost certain that peptides can get below stratum corneum. However, the diffusion of individual peptides need to be observed so that the potential for clinical/cosmeceutical benefits can be predicted. Positive outcomes from these experiments could result in new devices as skin pre-treatment tools or skin microinjections.

The field of microneedle enhanced protein delivery is largely focused on insulin and vaccine delivery. For a review see Kim *et al.* [12]. Insulin is a protein composed of 51 amino acids that has a molecular weight of 5808 Da. Therefore, comparing microneedle enhanced insulin delivery to even the largest peptide in this study, Pal-KTTKS-fluorescein conjugate at 1191.06 Da, is not relevant. However, there are many reports of enhanced transdermal peptide delivery using approaches other than microneedles (for review see Benson and Namjoshi [13]) and a handful of reports with microneedle enhanced peptide delivery.

A recent report by Sachdeva *et al.* investigated the use of iontophoresis with and without microneedles to enhance the topical delivery of leuprolide [14]. This 9 amino acid containing peptide has a molecular weight of 1209.40 Da, which is similar in mass to our melanostatin (803.92 Da), rigin (959.04 Da) and Pal-KTTKS (1191.06 Da) -fluorescein conjugates. Both peptides require penetration enhancement to cross the skin barrier. Sachdeva *et al.* found that leuprolide penetrated to blood levels of 0.36 ± 0.22 ng/ml after 6 hours without enhancement. The authors subsequently found that microneedle application improved delivery by only 2.7 fold. Similarly, we found that at 1 hour post treatment we observed a 4.2 (melanostatin), 1.1 (rigin) and 6.1 (Pal-KTTKS) fold increase in dermal signal within the microneedle pre-treated groups.

These similarities in fold increase were quite comparable considering differences in the peptide sequences, models, microneeldes and detection approaches. This low level improvement supports the hypothesis that enhancing the transdermal delivery of some peptides requires more than just microneedle holes in the skin.

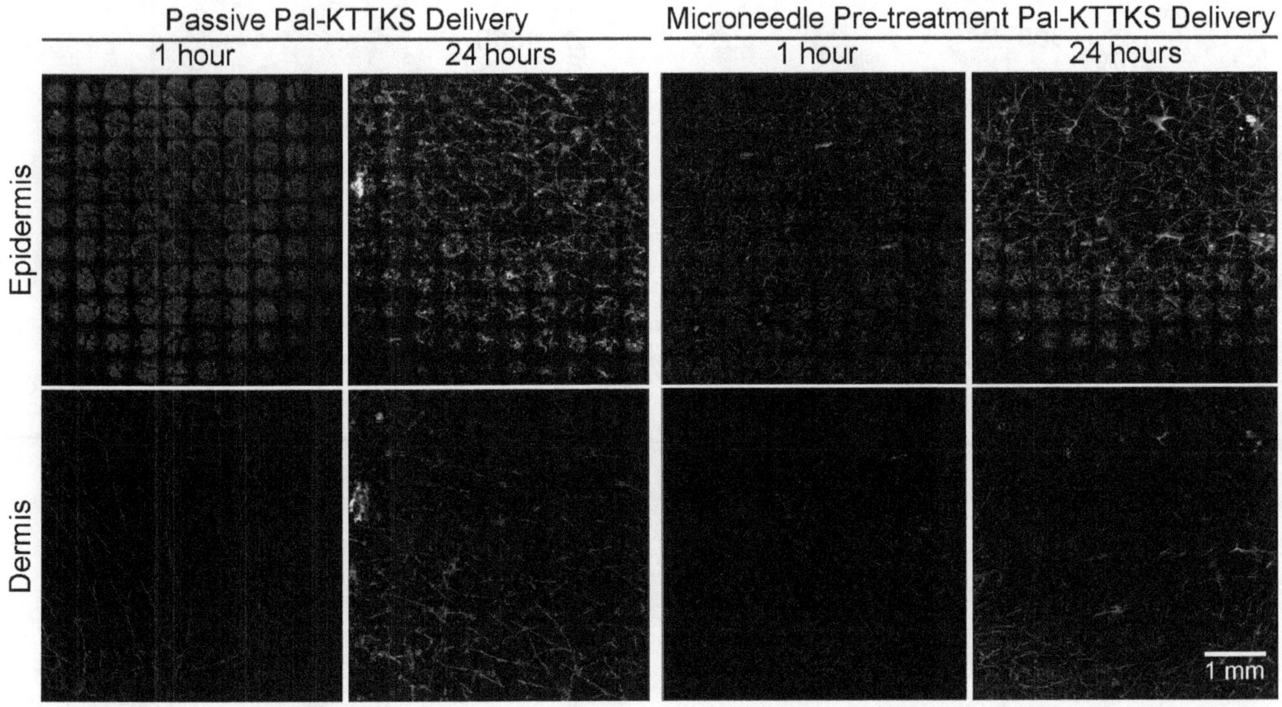

Figure 6. LSCM images of Pal-KTTKS delivery into excised human skin. Representative Pal-KTTKS treated confocal laser scanning microscopy (CLSM) images of viable epidermis and dermis at 1 and 24 hour(s) are shown without and with microneedle (MN) delivery enhancement. Mosaic images of the viable epidermis and dermis (top row and bottom row, respectively) are shown at at 1 and 24 hour(s) after Pal-KTTKS delivery with microneedle enhancement. Each mosiac is 5×5 mm^2.

Sachdeva *et al.* also described iontophoresis as a more effective means to enhance leuprolide delivery across rat skin (9.6 fold enhancement over passive treatment) than microneedles. This suggests that the dissolving microneedles used in the Sachdeva *et al.* study may have been blocking the diffusion of the peptide through the relatively thin rat skin and iontophoresis helped overcome the skin barrier and/or that passive diffusion, even with perforated skin, was still negligible. The combination of the two technologies only improved delivery over iontophoresis alone by 1.02 fold. This modest improvement suggests that iontophoresis was key in moving leuprolide across the rat skin barrier. Iontophoresis may also improve Pal-KTTKS in human skin, but this has yet to be reported. In contrast, we found that microneedles were highly effective in improving transdermal melanostatin delivery, highlighting the necessity to tailor the penetration enhancing technology to the particular peptide of interest.

Desmopressin is a another 9 amino acid long peptide that has been investigated for transdermal delivery with microneedle enhancement and has a molecular weight of 1069.22 Da. Cormier *et al.* used a microneedle array made from titanium that was dry coated with desmopressin formulated in 0.2 wt % polysorbate 20. The study was carried out in hairless guinea pigs. The microneedles were 200 μm long and had a maximal width of 170 μm. Our microneedles were 500 μm longer and 80 μm wider, but we used only 6 microneedles whereas Cormier *et al.* used 642 microneedles. This means that a projected microneedle area impacting the skin for our study was 0.075 mm^2 per group versus 3.8 mm^2 in Cormier *et al.*

Cormier *et al.* did not report desmopressin penetration without microneedles, so we cannot easily compare penetration enhancement. However, they did measure variability in the microneedle experiments. Cormier *et al.* calculated that the microneedle array was capable of delivering 17.5±3.8 μg desmopressin in a single application. The standard deviation equals 21.7% of the mean delivered dose. We found that the integrated density of our 6 microneedle array delivery approach varied from 8.3% (melanostatin), 10.8% (rigin) to 30.9% (Pal-KTTKS) of the mean value after 1 hour in the epidermis. Deviation also increased with depth and time in our study.

There is an evident trend with increasing molecular weight and variability within our data set. There appears to be less variability in the Cormier *et al.* data compared to our Pal-KTTKS and more than we found with rigin and melanostatin. This could be due to peptide diffusion and could also be influenced by the differences in the delivery approaches. Cormier *et al.* used coated microneedles, whereas we employed a "poke and rub" approach. They had over 100 times more microneedles in their device than we had. This could have resulted in a reduced impact of imperfect microneedle penetration. Alternately, the vertical and horizontal diffusion characteristics of the individual peptides within the different skin strata could have also contributed to variability.

Conclusions

In conclusion, we have demonstrated that microneedles can be effective way of enhancing some large and complex pharmaceutically active molecules deep into the skin. The data correlate with previous reports despite considerable technical differences between studies. We observed that the lowest molecular weight peptide was associated with the most improved topical delivery enhancement using microneedle pre-treatment. We also observed that the delivery of a larger molecular weight peptide was not improved by

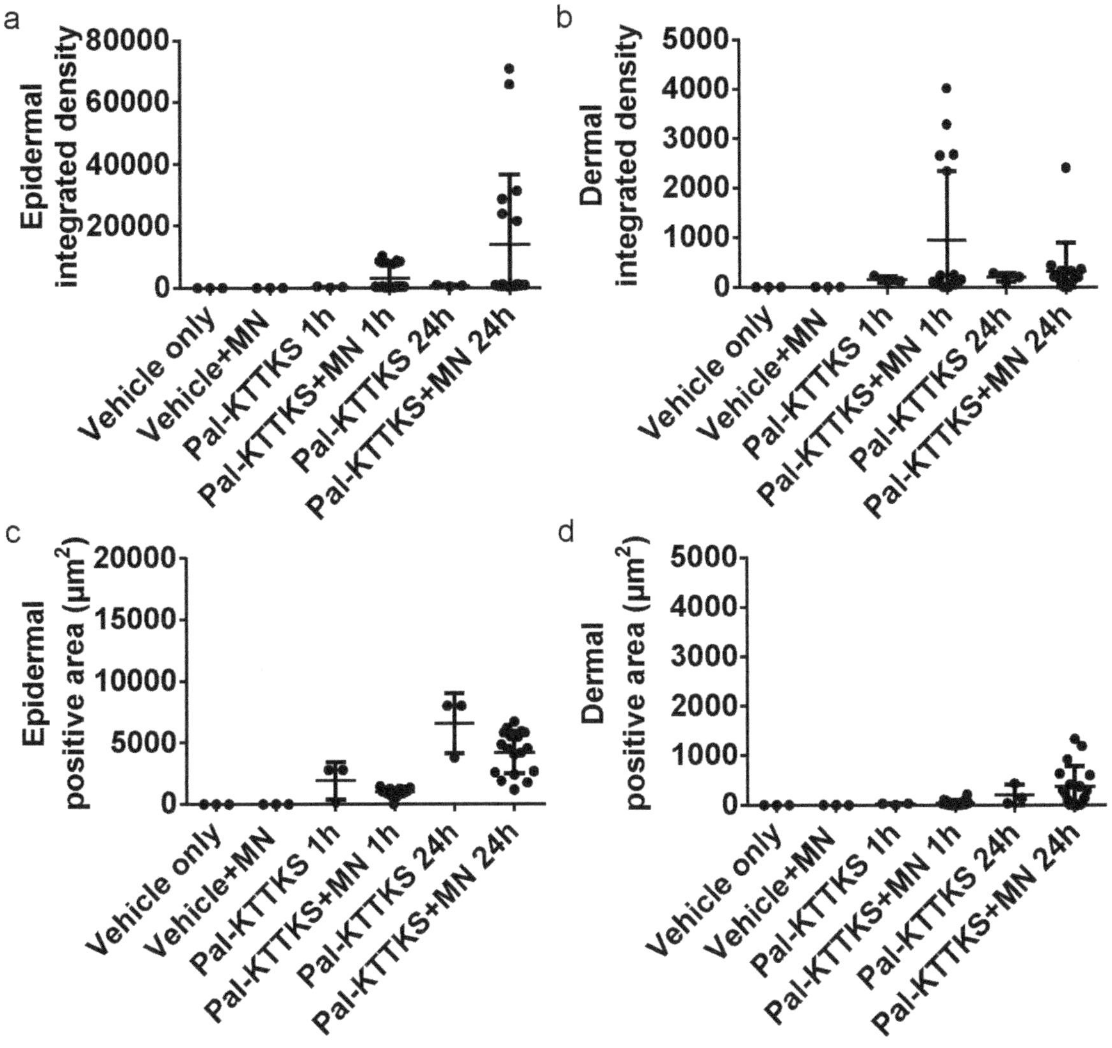

Figure 7. Integrated density and positive area data from Pal-KTTKS treated skin. Pal-KTTKS delivery characteristics are shown from epidermal (a and c) and dermal (d and d) mosiacs. Both the integrated density (a and b) and positive area (c and d) are shown for each microneedle site (MN). Data are shown for both 1 and 24 hours peptide exposure (1 h and 24 h, respecitvely).

microneedle pre-treatment. Therefore, using microneedle penetration enhancement could be effective when delivering some therapeutic peptides, but microneedle pre-treatment is not a one size fits all solution for topical delivery.

Author Contributions

Conceived and designed the experiments: YHM MY LLL JEG MSR APR HAEB TWP. Performed the experiments: YHM LLL APR TWP. Analyzed the data: YHM MY LLL APR TWP. Wrote the paper: YHM MY LLL JEG MSR APR HAEB TWP.

References

1. Zhang X, Hu X, Hou A, Wang H (2009) Inhibitory effect of 2,4,2′,4′-tetrahydroxy-3-(3-methyl-2-butenyl)-chalcone on tyrosinase activity and melanin biosynthesis. Biological & pharmaceutical bulletin 32: 86–90.
2. Donald JE, Shakhnovich EI (2009) SDR: a database of predicted specificity-determining residues in proteins. Nucleic acids research 37: D191–194.
3. Lintner K (2000) Use of peptides as cosmetics or pharmaceuticals for the regulation of immunological dysfunctions and in cutaneous inflammation. In: Application WP, editor. France: SEDERMA S.A.
4. Zhang L, Falla TJ (2009) Cosmeceuticals and peptides. Clinics in dermatology 27: 485–494.
5. Martanto W, Moore JS, Couse T, Prausnitz MR (2006) Mechanism of fluid infusion during microneedle insertion and retraction. Journal of controlled release: official journal of the Controlled Release Society 112: 357–361.
6. Bal SM, Kruithof AC, Zwier R, Dietz E, Bouwstra JA, et al. (2010) Influence of microneedle shape on the transport of a fluorescent dye into human skin in vivo. Journal of controlled release: official journal of the Controlled Release Society 147: 218–224.
7. Banks SL, Pinninti RR, Gill HS, Paudel KS, Crooks PA, et al. (2010) Transdermal delivery of naltrexol and skin permeability lifetime after microneedle treatment in hairless guinea pigs. Journal of pharmaceutical sciences 99: 3072–3080.
8. Banks SL, Paudel KS, Brogden NK, Loftin CD, Stinchcomb AL (2011) Diclofenac enables prolonged delivery of naltrexone through microneedle-treated skin. Pharmaceutical research 28: 1211–1219.
9. Prausnitz MR (2006) A peptide chaperone for transdermal drug delivery. Nature biotechnology 24: 416–417.
10. Gill HS, Prausnitz MR (2008) Pocketed Microneedles for Drug Delivery to the Skin. The Journal of physics and chemistry of solids 69: 1537–1541.
11. Sauermann K, Gambichler T, Wilmert M, Rotterdam S, Stucker M, et al. (2002) Investigation of basal cell carcinoma [correction of carcionoma] by confocal laser scanning microscopy in vivo. Skin research and technology:

official journal of International Society for Bioengineering and the Skin 8: 141–147.

12. Kim YC, Park JH, Prausnitz MR (2012) Microneedles for drug and vaccine delivery. Advanced drug delivery reviews 64: 1547–1568.
13. Benson HA, Namjoshi S (2008) Proteins and peptides: strategies for delivery to and across the skin. Journal of pharmaceutical sciences 97: 3591–3610.
14. Sachdeva V, Zhou Y, Banga AK (2013) In vivo transdermal delivery of leuprolide using microneedles and iontophoresis. Current pharmaceutical biotechnology 14: 180–193.

17

Hydrogel-Forming Microneedles Prepared from "Super Swelling" Polymers Combined with Lyophilised Wafers for Transdermal Drug Delivery

Ryan F. Donnelly[1]*, Maelíosa T. C. McCrudden[1], Ahlam Zaid Alkilani[1,2], Eneko Larrañeta[1], Emma McAlister[1], Aaron J. Courtenay[1], Mary-Carmel Kearney[1], Thakur Raghu Raj Singh[1], Helen O. McCarthy[1], Victoria L. Kett[1], Ester Caffarel-Salvador[1], Sharifa Al-Zahrani[1], A. David Woolfson[1]

1 School of Pharmacy, Queen's University Belfast, Belfast, Co. Antrim, United Kingdom, **2** School of Pharmacy, Zarqa University, Zarqa, Jordan

Abstract

We describe, for the first time, hydrogel-forming microneedle arrays prepared from "super swelling" polymeric compositions. We produced a microneedle formulation with enhanced swelling capabilities from aqueous blends containing 20% w/w Gantrez S-97, 7.5% w/w PEG 10,000 and 3% w/w Na_2CO_3 and utilised a drug reservoir of a lyophilised wafer-like design. These microneedle-lyophilised wafer compositions were robust and effectively penetrated skin, swelling extensively, but being removed intact. In *in vitro* delivery experiments across excised neonatal porcine skin, approximately 44 mg of the model high dose small molecule drug ibuprofen sodium was delivered in 24 h, equating to 37% of the loading in the lyophilised reservoir. The super swelling microneedles delivered approximately 1.24 mg of the model protein ovalbumin over 24 h, equivalent to a delivery efficiency of approximately 49%. The integrated microneedle-lyophilised wafer delivery system produced a progressive increase in plasma concentrations of ibuprofen sodium in rats over 6 h, with a maximal concentration of approximately 179 μg/ml achieved in this time. The plasma concentration had fallen to 71 ± 6.7 μg/ml by 24 h. Ovalbumin levels peaked in rat plasma after only 1 hour at 42.36 ± 17.01 ng/ml. Ovalbumin plasma levels then remained almost constant up to 6 h, dropping somewhat at 24 h, when 23.61 ± 4.84 ng/ml was detected. This work represents a significant advancement on conventional microneedle systems, which are presently only suitable for bolus delivery of very potent drugs and vaccines. Once fully developed, such technology may greatly expand the range of drugs that can be delivered transdermally, to the benefit of patients and industry. Accordingly, we are currently progressing towards clinical evaluations with a range of candidate molecules.

Editor: Masaya Yamamoto, Institute for Frontier Medical Sciences, Kyoto University, Japan

Funding: This study was supported by Biotechnology and Biological Sciences Research Council grant numbers BB/FOF/287 and BB/E020534/1 (http://www.bbsrc.ac.uk/) and Wellcome Trust grant number WT094085MA (http://www.wellcome.ac.uk/). The funders had no role in study design, data collection and analysis, decision to publish, or preparation of the manuscript.

Competing Interests: Ryan Donnelly and David Woolfson are named inventors on a patent application related to hydrogel-forming microneedle arrays (details below). They are working with a number of companies with a view to commercialisation of this technology. They provide advice, through consultancy, to these companies. None of the other authors have any competing interests. Donnelly, R.F., Woolfson A.D., McCarron, P.A., Morrow, D.I.J., Morrissey, A. (2007). Microneedles/Delivery Device and Method. British Patent Application No 0718996.2. Filed September 28th 2007. International publication No WO2009040548. Approved for grant in Japan and China. US, Europe, India and Australia pending.

* Email: r.donnelly@qub.ac.uk

Introduction

Microneedle (MN) arrays, micron scale, minimally-invasive devices that painlessly by-pass the skin's *stratum corneum* barrier, have been shown to be extremely effective in enhancing transdermal delivery of water soluble drugs, biomolecular therapeutics and vaccines [1–3]. The compounds delivered to date have typically been of high potency, meaning only a low dose is required to achieve a therapeutic affect (e.g. insulin) [4,5] or elicit the required immune response [6,7]. Clearly, the majority of marketed drug substances, including many antibodies, are not low dose, high potency molecules. Indeed, many drugs require doses of several hundred milligrams per day in order to achieve therapeutic plasma concentrations in man. Until now, such high doses could not be delivered transdermally from a patch of reasonable size, even for molecules whose physicochemical properties are ideal for passive diffusion across the skin's *stratum corneum* barrier. Therefore, transdermal delivery has traditionally been limited to fairly lipophilic, low molecular weight, high potency drug substances. Since most drugs do not possess these properties, the transdermal delivery market has not expanded beyond around 20 drugs. Marketed MN-based patches are likely to increase this number of drugs in the coming years. However, this increase will only be maximised if high dose molecules can be delivered in therapeutic doses using MN. We have previously shown that suitably-formulated dissolving MN platforms can deliver therapeutic doses of a low potency, high dose drug substance [8]. However, deposition of polymer in skin from a dissolving MN system may be undesirable if the system is to be used on an ongoing basis. The dissolving MN system employed in this previous study would deposit approximately 5–10 mg of polymer per cm^2 in skin [8]. If the patch size were 10 cm^2, then 50–100 mg of polymer would be deposited in the patient's skin every time the product is applied. While vaccines are used infrequently, most therapeutic agents need to be administered regularly. Accordingly, dissolving MN systems may be most appropriate to rapid delivery of low dose vaccines [6,9].

We have recently described novel hydrogel-forming MN arrays, prepared under ambient conditions that contain no drug themselves [10]. Instead, they rapidly imbibe skin interstitial fluid upon insertion to form continuous, unblockable conduits between the dermal microcirculation and an attached patch-type drug reservoir. Such hydrogel-forming MN initially act simply as a tool to pierce the *stratum corneum* barrier. Upon insertion, they function as a rate-controlling membrane, allowing sustained drug delivery at a rate controllable by adjustment of crosslink density, which dictates swelling rate [10,11]. Importantly, such MN are removed intact from skin, leaving no measurable polymer residue behind, but are sufficiently softened, even after 1 minute of skin insertion to preclude reinsertion, thus further reducing the risk of transmission of infection [12]. In the present study, we substantially modified this novel system to facilitate delivery of clinically-relevant doses of a low potency, high dose drug substance and rapid delivery of a model protein by using a modifying agent to increase swelling capabilities [13] and using a hygroscopic lyophilised drug reservoir (**Figure 1**).

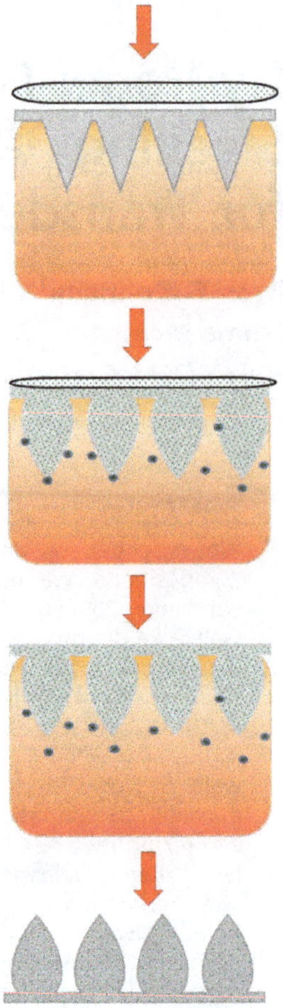
Microneedles inserted into skin
Hygroscopic lyophilised drug reservoir accelerates uptake of skin interstitial fluid into hydrogel-forming microneedles, which swell to allow drug release into skin
Lyophilised drug reservoir dissolves, maximising drug release
Hydrogel-forming microneedles are removed completely intact from skin, leaving no polymer behind

Figure 1. Schematic representation of the concept of combining hydrogel-forming microneedles prepared from super swelling polymers and lyophilised wafer-type drug reservoirs for enhanced transdermal delivery of proteins and high dose low potency drug substances.

Methods and Materials

2.1. Chemicals

Polyethylene glycol (PEG, MW 10,000 Da), ibuprofen-sodium, chicken ovalbumin (OVA, albumin from chicken egg, grade IIV), mouse monoclonal anti-chicken ovalbumin antibody (moAb), Ph. Eur. Gelatin, D-mannitol and tetramethylbenzidine (TMB) substrate were purchased from Sigma-Aldrich, Dorset, UK. Phosphate buffered saline tablets, pH 7.4 (PBS) were obtained from Oxoid Ltd., Hampshire, UK. Rabbit anti-ovalbumin horseradish peroxidase (HRP) conjugated-polyclonal antibody was purchased from Gene Tex Inc Alton Pkwy, Irvine, USA. SuperBlock T20 was purchased from Thermo Scientific, Rockford, Illinois, USA. 50C-Mannitol was supplied by Roquette, Lestrem, France. Gantrez AN-139 and S-97, copolymers of methyl vinyl ether and maleic anhydride and methyl vinyl ether and maleic acid, respectively (PMVE/MAH and PMVE/MA, with molecular masses of 1,080,000 and 1,500,000 respectively) were gifts from Ashland, Kidderminster, UK. Unless otherwise stated, all other chemicals and materials were supplied by Sigma-Aldrich (Dorset, UK) or Fisher Scientific (Loughborough, UK).

2.2. Preparation of hydrogel films

The aim here was to investigate various polymeric compositions in order to find a material capable of rapid swelling, but which would be sufficiently hard in the dry state to penetrate the skin. Importantly, once swollen, the material should maintain structural integrity and be reasonably robust during handling.

Stock solutions of Gantrez S-97 (40% w/w) or AN-139 (30% w/w) [13,14] were prepared using deionised water (**Figure 2A**). Hydrogel films were then prepared using varying concentrations of the co-polymer, PEG 10,000 and the modifying agent, sodium carbonate (Na_2CO_3). The blends were centrifuged at 3,500 rpm for 15 minutes in order to remove any air bubbles. The aqueous blends (30 g) were then slowly poured into moulds consisting of a release liner with the siliconised surface facing upwards (Rayven, Inc., Saint Paul, MN, USA) secured to a Perspex base plate with stainless steel clamps. Once assembled, the internal dimensions available for casting were 100 mm × 100 mm. The aqueous blends were spread evenly across the moulds and these were placed onto a level surface. The cast blend was dried for 48 hours at room temperature. After drying, the films were cured at 80°C for 24 h to induce chemical crosslinking between the PMVE/MA and PEG by ester formation [14,15]. Films were then removed from the mould by simply peeling the release liner, with attached film, off the base.

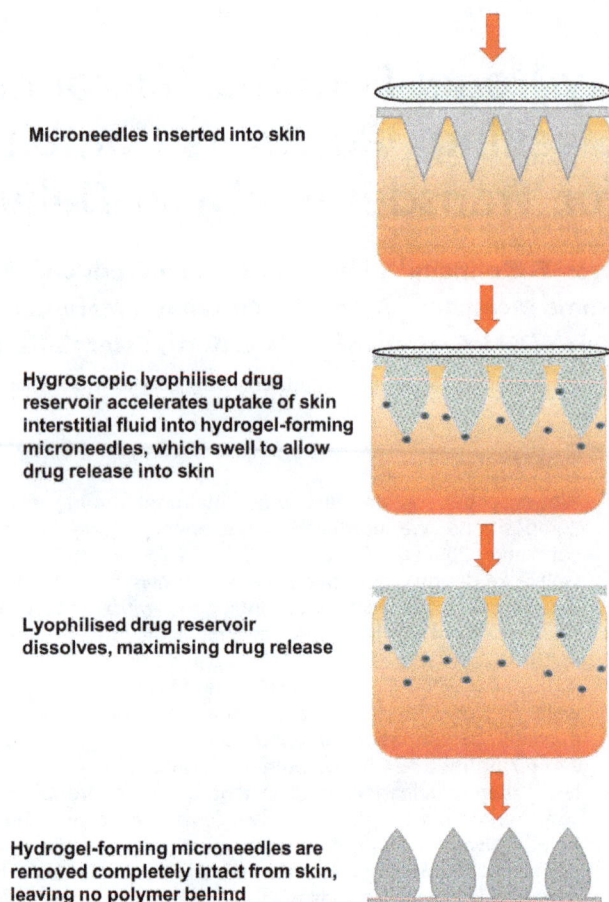

2.3. Swelling of hydrogel films in phosphate-buffered saline (PBS)

For swelling studies, individual film portions (1 cm^2) were weighed at the zero time point in the dry state (m_0) and then placed into a volume of PBS (pH 7.4). The film portions were removed at specific time points, surface fluid was removed between pieces of filter paper and the mass of the swollen film was recorded (m_t). PBS was selected as the swelling medium, as it was deemed to closely resemble/simulate skin interstitial fluid and has been used as the swelling medium in other similar studies [14]. The percentage swelling of the film was determined using

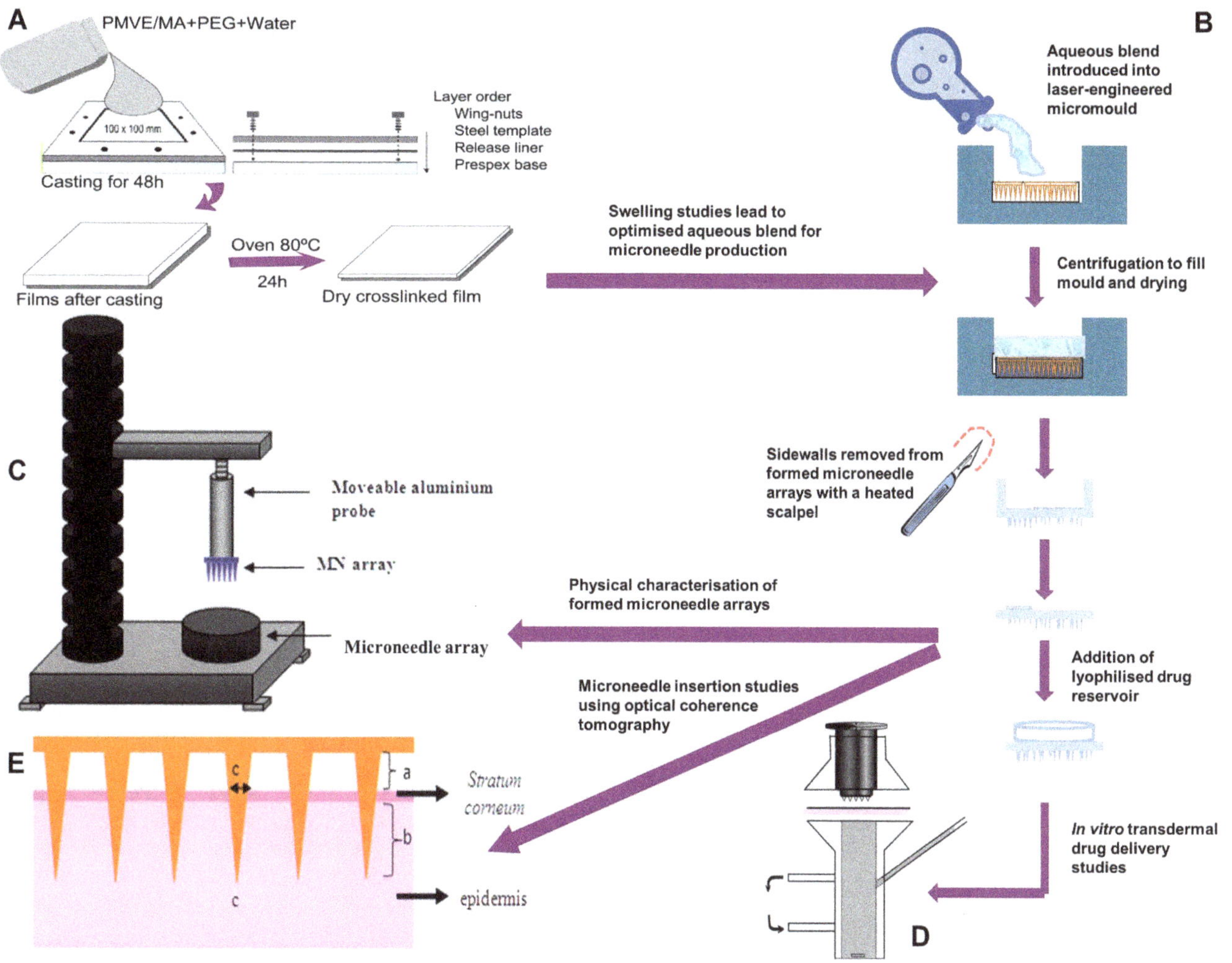

Figure 2. Schematic representation of casting and crosslinking of the super swelling hydrogel films (A), microneedle preparation (B), Texture Analyser set-up for investigation of physical properties of microneedles (C) and Franz cell set-up for *in vitro* transdermal drug release studies (D). Panel (E) shows a diagrammatic representation of the measurements recorded from the optical coherence tomographic images of microneedle penetration into excised neonatal porcine skin *in vitro*, namely; (a) the distance between the lower microneedle base plate and the *stratum corneum*, (b) the depth of microneedle penetration into the skin and (c) the width of the micropore created in the skin.

Equation 1.

$$\% \text{ Swelling} = \left(\frac{m_t - m_o}{m_o}\right) x \ 100\% \qquad (1)$$

To examine the controlled swelling mechanism of the PEG-crosslinked PMVE/MA hydrogels, a second order kinetic model was used to process the experimental data, as outlined in **Equation 2**, where A is the reciprocal of the initial swelling rate of the hydrogel, r_o, or $1/(k_s S_{eq}^2)$, where k_s is the swelling rate constant and B is the inverse of the degree of swelling at equilibrium, S_{eq} [16].

$$\% \text{EWC} = \frac{m_e - m_d}{m_d} \text{ x } 100\% \qquad (2)$$

To analyse the kinetic model, *t/S* versus *t* graphs were plotted and respective swelling rate parameters were determined [14]. The dynamics of the water sorption process are usually investigated either by monitoring the change in physical dimensions of the swelling hydrogel or by knowing the amounts of water imbibed by the hydrogel at various time points. In the current study, the latter procedure was engaged. Analysis of the swelling kinetics of the various films was carried out using **Equation 3** [14]. The portion of the water absorption curve with a fractional water uptake (M_t/M_∞) less than 0.60 was analyzed with **Equation 4**, where M_t is the mass of water absorbed at time t, M_∞ is the water uptake at equilibrium. k is a gel characteristic constant, which depends on the structural characteristics of the polymer and its interaction with the solvent and n is the swelling exponent, describing the mechanism of penetrant transport into the hydrogel. The constants n and k may be calculated from the slopes and intercepts of the plots of $\ln(M_t/M_\infty)$ versus $\ln\ t$ from the experimental data. The value of n provides an indication of the water transport mechanism. When n = 0.5, the swelling process is of Fickian nature and is diffusion controlled while the value of n between 0.5 and 1 suggests non-Fickian diffusion or more specifically anomalous diffusion. When n becomes exactly equal to unity, then the diffusion is termed case II diffusion. In some cases, the value for n has been found to exceed unity and this represents super case II transport [17–19].

$$t/S = A + Bt \quad (3)$$

$$\frac{M_t}{M} = kt^n \quad (4)$$

Hydrogel network structure characterization is a complex procedure because of the many types of possible networks, including, regular, irregular, loosely/highly cross-linked and imperfect networks. As a result of these variations in the network structure, only average values for the cross-linking density and molecular weight (MW) between crosslinks are represented using different experimental or theoretical methods [13,16–19]. In the present study, the number average MW between cross-links, $\bar{M}_C$, was determined using equilibrium swelling theory, $\bar{M}_C$ (Equi), rather than glass transition temperature. The magnitude of $\bar{M}_C$ affected the mechanical and physical properties of crosslinked polymers. The volume fraction of a polymer, ϕ, in the swollen state describes the amount of liquid that can be imbibed into a hydrogel and is described as a ratio of the polymer volume to the swollen gel volume (**Equation 5 and 6**).

$$\bar{M}_C\,(Equi) = \frac{-d_p V_s \phi^{1/3}}{[In(1-\phi)+\phi+\chi\phi^2]} \quad (5)$$

$$\phi = \left[1 + \frac{d_p}{d_s}\left(\frac{m_a}{m_b}\right) - \frac{d_p}{d_s}\right]^{-1} \quad (6)$$

Here, V_s is the molar volume of water (18 cm^3/mol), ϕ is volume fraction of polymer in the hydrogel, χ is the Flory-Huggins polymer-solvent interaction parameter; In the above Equation, m_a and m_b are the mass of polymer before and after swelling and d_p and d_s are the densities of polymer and solvent, respectively. The density of the polymeric films was calculated using the following formula; $d_p = w/SX$, where; X is the average thickness of the film, S is the cross-sectional area and w weight of the film. The polymer water interaction parameter (χ) reflects the thermodynamic interaction in hydrogels, which in turn indicates the change of interaction energy when polymer and solvent mix together. The χ parameters of hydrogels can be obtained experimentally *via* **Equation 7** [13,16–19].

$$\chi = \frac{1}{2} + \frac{\phi}{3} \quad (7)$$

Equation 7 neglects the M_c dependence of the χ parameter, and therefore, this equation indicates that the χ values are always ≥ 0.50. In the present study, crosslink density, V_e, was determined using **Equation 8**. V_e represents the number of elastically effective chains, totally induced in a perfect network, per unit volume. Where, N_A is Avagadro's number (6.023×10^{23} $mole^{-1}$) [13,16–19].

$$V_e = d_p N_A / M_c \quad (8)$$

2.4. Fabrication of hydrogel forming MN arrays

Formulations used to prepare MN were based upon the preceding swelling studies. Aqueous blends containing 15% w/w Gantrez AN-139 and 7.5% w/w PEG, 10,000 (control formulation) [14] were utilized to fabricate MN arrays as previously described [10,11]. The blend (500 mg) was poured into MN moulds (361 (19×19) needles perpendicular to the base and of conical shape, 600 μm high with base width of 300 μm and 50 μm interspacing on a 0.49 cm^2 patch) and these were centrifuged at 3,500 rpm for 15 min and dried at room temperature for 48 h. MN were crosslinked (esterification reaction) by heating at 80°C for 24 hours [10,11,14] and the sidewalls formed by the moulding process were removed using a heated blade (**Figure 2B**). MN arrays were also prepared from a so-called "super swelling" hydrogel formulation containing 20% w/w Gantrez S-97, 7.5% w/w PEG 10,000 and 3% w/w Na_2CO_3.

2.5. Mechanical characterisation of super swelling microneedle arrays

MN were subjected to standard mechanical tests using a TA-XT2 Texture Analyser (Stable Microsystems, Haslemere, UK) in compression mode, as described previously [10,11,20]. Briefly, MN arrays were visualised before testing using a light microscope (GXMGE-5 digital microscope, Laboratory Analysis Ltd, Devon, UK). MN arrays were then carefully placed on the flat stainless steel baseplate of the Texture Analyser with the needles pointing upwards. A flat-faced probe with a diameter of 11.0 mm was lowered at a speed of 0.5 mm s^{-1}. Upon contact with the MN array, the probe continued to travel at a speed of 0.5 mm s^{-1} until the required force had been exerted. Once the target force was reached, the probe was moved upwards at a speed of 0.5 mm s^{-1}. MN arrays were then viewed again under the light microscope.

2.6. Skin insertion studies

Neonatal porcine skin, a good model for human skin [21,22], was obtained from stillborn piglets and immediately (<24 hours after birth) excised, trimmed to a thickness of 700 μm using a dermatome (Integra Life Sciences, Padgett Instruments, NJ, USA) and frozen in liquid nitrogen vapour, as previously described [10,11,20]. Skin was then stored in aluminium foil at −20°C for no more than 7 days prior to use.

Skin was mounted on the baseplate of the Texture Analyser using cyanoacrylate adhesive (Loctite Ltd, Dublin, Ireland) while the MN were this time attached to the probe using double-sided tape (3M, Carrickmines, Ireland). The probe then moved downwards as described above until the required force had been exerted. Once the target force was reached, the probe was moved upwards at a speed of 0.5 mm s^{-1}. The number of MN in an array that had penetrated the skin's *stratum corneum* barrier was counted following visualisation of the pores formed in skin using methylene blue solution (1 mg/ml in PBS pH 7.4).

Optical coherence tomography (OCT), as described previously [23] allowed measurement of the depth of MN insertion for each application force, since the MN are transparent and accordingly can be left in place during OCT studies to mimic their intended use (EX1301 OCT microscope, Michelson Diagnostics, Kent, UK). OCT was also used to visualise the *in situ* swelling of the MN in real time skin at varying time intervals over a 3 h period. OCT data files were exported to Image J (National Institutes of Health, Bethesda, MD, USA) for measurement of insertion depth and false colours were applied using Ability Photopaint (Ability Software International, Horley, UK) for presentation purposes.

2.7. Preparation and characterisation of lyophilised drug reservoirs

A range of lyophilised wafer-type reservoirs loaded with the model compounds ovalbumin (OVA) or ibuprofen sodium were prepared containing varying concentrations of gelatin, mannitol and, in some instances, sodium chloride (NaCl) and sucrose. In the case of the ibuprofen sodium wafers, a variety of different gelatin sources, all at loadings of 10% w/w, were tested in combination with 3% w/w mannitol and 40% w/w ibuprofen sodium in deionised water.

To prepare OVA-containing reservoirs, the protein (0.5% w/w) was dissolved in distilled water, followed by the addition of gelatin, mannitol, NaCl and sucrose. It was then mixed by speed mixer at 3,000 rpm for 60 s and sonicated at 37°C for 60 min. To prepare the ibuprofen sodium-loaded reservoirs, the individual components were mixed by speed mixer at 3,000 rpm for 60 s and sonicated at 37°C for 60 min. The resulting OVA or ibuprofen-sodium formulations were then cast (500 mg in the case of OVA-loaded wafers and 250 mg in the case of ibuprofen sodium-loaded wafers) into cylindrical moulds with one open end moulds (diameter 15 mm, depth 5 mm), frozen at −80°C for a minimum of 60 min and then lyophilised in the freeze-drier (Virtis Advantage Bench top Freeze Drier System, SP Scientific, Warminster PA, USA), according to the following regime: primary drying for forty eight hours at a shelf temperature of −40°C, secondary drying for ten hours at a shelf temperature of 20°C and vacuum pressure of 50 mTorr.

Dried reservoirs were characterised using standard pharmacopoeial tests. Twenty reservoirs were selected randomly, weighed individually and their average weight was calculated to determine the weight uniformity. The percentage deviation of each reservoir from the average weight was determined. The thickness of the reservoirs was determined with a digital micrometer (Digital Calliper, 0–150 mm, Jade Products Rugby Limited, Warwickshire, UK). Five reservoirs were used and average values were calculated. Hardness was determined using a Copley Hardness Tester (Copley Scientific, Nottingham, UK). Twenty reservoirs were weighed (W_0) and then placed in the Friabilitor (Copley Scientific, Nottingham, UK). This was operated at 25 rpm for 4 min. The reservoirs were then weighed again (W). The % friability was then calculated using **Equation 9**. OVA and ibuprofen sodium contents were determined using the ELISA and HPLC methods described below following dissolution of the reservoirs in PBS pH 7.4.

$$\% \text{ Friability} = (W\text{-}W_0/W_0) * 100\% \qquad (9)$$

2.8. *In vitro* release studies

The diffusion of ibuprofen sodium (MW 228.26 g/mol) and OVA (MW 45,000 g/mol) from lyophilised active-loaded tablets through hydrogel MN arrays and across neonatal porcine skin was investigated *in vitro* using modified Franz diffusion cells (FDC-400 flat flange, 15 mm orifice diameter, mounted on an FDCD diffusion drive console providing synchronous stirring at 600 rpm and thermostated at 37±1°C, Crown Glass Co. Inc., Sommerville, NJ, USA), as described previously [4]. Briefly, neonatal porcine skin was obtained from stillborn piglets and immediately (< 24 hours after birth) excised and trimmed to a thickness of 350 μm using an electric dermatome. Skin was then stored in aluminium foil at −20°C until required. Skin barrier function integrity was confirmed in all cases using standard transepidermal water loss measurements (VapoMeter, Delfin Technologies Ltd, Kuopio, Finland), with any damaged skin immediately discarded. Neonatal porcine skin samples were then shaved carefully so as not to damage the skin (again confirmed by TEWL) and were then pre-equilibrated in phosphate buffered saline (PBS), pH 7.4, for 15 minutes prior to the commencement of experimentation. A circular specimen of the skin was secured to the donor compartment of the diffusion cell using cynoacrylate glue (Loctite, Dublin, Ireland) with the *stratum corneum* facing towards the donor compartment. This was then placed on top of dental wax, to give the skin support, and MN arrays inserted into the centre of the skin section, using a spring activated applicator at a force of 11 N/array. The lyophilised active-loaded wafers (which had been trimmed to size using a heated scalpel blade) were placed on the top of the MN, with 20 μl water used to initiate adhesion. A tubular stainless steel weight (diameter 11.0 mm, 3.5 g mass) was then placed on top of this. The donor compartments were mounted onto the receptor compartments and the Franz cell donor compartments covered with laboratory film (Parafilm, Pechiney Plastic Packaging, WI, USA) so as to avoid evaporation of PBS over the course of experimentation. At predetermined time intervals, a 200 μl sample was collected *via* the side arm of the Franz cell and the receiver compartment immediately replenished with an equivalent volume of release medium. OVA was quantified again using ELISA, while ibuprofen sodium was determined using HPLC.

2.9. *In vivo* evaluation of OVA and ibuprofen sodium delivery through super swelling MN

Prior to experimentation, rats were acclimatised to laboratory conditions for a 7 day period. Super swelling hydrogel MN arrays were manually inserted into the skin at a site on the rats' backs. An aliquot of water (20 μl) was applied to the centre of the array and the lyophilised reservoir (again trimmed to size) was placed on top of this. A bespoke adhesive film (Scotchpak 9732, 3M, Carrickmines, Ireland, coated with a 1.0 mm layer of DuroTak 34-416A, National Starch & Chemical Company, Bridgewater, NJ, USA) was applied on top of, and around the edges of, the lyophilised reservoirs to aid retention and provide occlusion. Following application of this integrated system, blood samples were collected at pre-defined time points over 24 h for analysis.

All animal experiments throughout this study were conducted according to the policy of the federation of European Laboratory Animal Science Associations and the European Convention for the protection of vertebrate animals used for experimental and other scientific purposes, with implementation of the principles of the 3R's (replacement, reduction, refinement). Ethical permission specifically for the experiments described here was obtained from the Queen's University Animal Welfare and Ethics Review Board and all researchers carrying out the work had Personal Licences from the UK Home Office. To anaesthetise the animals, isoflurane was used and carbon dioxide was used for euthanisation.

2.10. Extraction of plasma and drug

The following procedure was carried out in the case of ibuprofen sodium-containing samples only. Control rat blood for method development was obtained from healthy Sprague dawley rats. Blood from culled rats was collected via heart puncture with a heparinised syringe into ethylenediaminetetraacetic acid (EDTA)-coated tubes. Plasma separation was performed by centrifuging the blood at 500× g for 10 min in a refrigerated centrifuge (4°C). The plasma was then aliquoted into microtubes and stored at −80°C until required. In the case of standards used in assay development, 10 μl of ibuprofen-sodium working standard solutions were added to 190 μl blank plasma. In the case of plasma samples from MN-treated rats, the drug was extracted from the samples without the addition of any endogenous drug. Samples were then vortex mixed for 10 s in a poly(propylene) microtube and 500 μl each acetonitrile (ACN) was added. The samples were vortex mixed for 10 min and centrifuged at 14,000× g for 10 min at 4°C. The ACN extraction procedure was then repeated to ensure optimum extraction of the drug. The sample mixture was placed in a disposable glass culture tube and the extract dried under a stream of nitrogen at 35°C for 50 min using a Zymark TurboVap LV Evaporator Workstation (McKinley Scientific, Sparta, NJ, USA). The residue was then reconstituted in 200 μl PBS (pH 7.4) and collected into a microtube. This was then vortex mixed for 30 s and centrifuged at 14,000× g for 10 min at room temperature. The supernatant was transferred into an auto sampler vial and 50 μl was injected onto the HPLC column and detection carried out as outlined below. In the case of blood samples collected from OVA- treated rats, plasma was separated from whole blood as outlined and this was then quantified by ELISA experiments.

2.11. Pharmaceutical analysis of ibuprofen sodium

Ibuprofen sodium quantification in PBS (pH 7.4) and rat plasma was performed using reverse-phase high performance liquid chromatography (RP-HPLC) (Agilent 1200 Binary Pump, Agilent 1200, Standard Autosampler, Agilent 1200 Variable Wavelength Detector, Agilent Technologies UK Ltd., Stockport, UK) with UV detection at 220 nm. Gradient separation was achieved using an Agilent Eclipse XDB-C18 (5 μm pore size, 4.6×150 mm) analytical column fitted with a guard cartridge of matching chemistry. The mobile phase was 60%:40% methanol:10 mM potassium phosphate (pH 4.6), with a flow rate of 1 ml min^{-1}, and a run time of 30 min per sample. The injection volume was 50 μl. The chromatograms obtained were analysed using Agilent ChemStation Software B.02.01. Least squares linear regression analysis and correlation analysis were performed on the calibration curves produced, enabling determination of the equation of the line, its coefficient of determination and the residual sum of squares (RSS). To determine the limit of detection (LoD) and limit of quantification (LoQ), an approach based on the standard deviation of the response and the slope of the representative calibration curve was employed, as described in the guidelines from the International Conference on Harmonisation (ICH) [24]. Ibuprofen sodium, either dissolved in PBS (pH 7.4) (standards), or samples collected from the Franz cell apparatus (unknowns), was quantified by injection of the sample, following filter sterilisation through 0.2 μm filters, directly onto the HPLC column. In the case of plasma samples, the drug was first extracted from the plasma as described above and then the resulting sample, which had been reconstituted in PBS (pH 7.4) and filtered through a 0.2 μm filter, was injected onto the column. The method parameters for detection of ibuprofen sodium in PBS (pH 7.4) and plasma were identical.

2.12. Enzyme-linked immunosorbent assay (ELISA) for detection of OVA

An OVA ELISA, developed as described previously [25], was used to detect OVA in samples collected in both *in vitro* and *in vivo* experiments. Briefly, monoclonal anti-chicken egg albumin (ovalbumin) antibody produced in mouse (moAb) was diluted in 0.1 M bicarbonate buffer, pH 9.6 to the optimized concentration of 2.5 μg/ml. An aliquot (50 μl) of anti-ovalbumin was dispensed into the plate and incubated overnight at 4°C. The plate was filled with washing buffer 0.05% v/v Tween-PBS and soaked for 30 seconds before discarded. This process was repeated 5 times. Then, the plate was turned onto absorbance paper to remove any remaining buffer. The plate was blocked with SuperBlock T20 buffer (150 μl/well) and incubated for 2 hours at room temperature. For the calibration curve, OVA solutions were freshly prepared at a concentration of 1 mg/ml in PBS produced concentrations of 1 μg/ml to 10 ng/ml. A 50 μl of sample was dispensed into wells, each sample was analysed in triplicate. The plate was covered and incubated for 1 hour at room temperature. The plate was washed and incubated with rabbit anti chicken OVA polyclonal antibody conjugate with horse-radish peroxidase (HRP) at the optimized concentration of 5 μg/ml in SuperBlock T20 buffer for 1 hour at room temperature. After the plate was washed, 50 μl of TMP was added to each well to detect antibody binding and incubated for 15 min. Colour development was ended using 50 μl/well of 4.0 M HCl and optical density was measured at 450 nm using a microplate reader spectrophotometer (EnSpire Multimode Plate Reader, PerkinElmer, Waltham, MA, USA). In terms of the analysis of blood samples collected during *in vivo* experiments, plasma was separated from whole blood as outlined below and this plasma was then subjected to the ELISA protocol outlined above.

2.13. Statistical analysis

Data was analysed, where appropriate, using the Student's t-test, one-way analysis of variance ANOVA, Mann-Whitney U-test or Wilcoxon test. In each case, a p-value less than 0.05 was considered to denote significance.

Results and Discussion

Microneedles (MN) prepared from hydrogel-forming materials have a range of advantageous characteristics. Firstly, the delivered dose is not limited by what can be loaded into, or onto the surface of the needles themselves, since the drug is contained within an attached patch-type drug reservoir. Secondly, controlled administration is possible for the first time with MN. Finally, since the MN are removed intact, no polymer is deposited in skin, while the inherent antimicrobial properties of the polymer composition used and the fact that the needles are soft upon removal mean transmission of infection from patient to patient is unlikely. To date, we have employed such systems in the effective *in vivo* delivery of potent biomolecules, such as insulin, and for sustained administration of proteins and small molecules over hours or days [10–12]. In order to take this technology to the next stage of development, we must now move beyond simply controlling transdermal permeation to demonstrate its utility in administration of clinically-relevant doses of non-potent drugs and in rapid delivery of large molecules with physicochemical properties similar to vaccine antigens. Accordingly, in the present study, we used our previous experience with hydrogels [13] to alter the MN formulation to enhance its swelling capabilities and changed the drug reservoir from a flexible polymeric patch to a lyophilised wafer-like design. Using a hygroscopic reservoir is likely to have two principal effects. Firstly, its high solid content and porous nature will attract water from skin interstitial fluid by osmosis through the hydrogel-forming MN, whose swelling rate will be enhanced. Secondly, since such lyophilised systems are rapidly soluble in water, the rate of drug dissolution and its subsequent availability for diffusion will also be increased. These theories were examined for the first time here using ibuprofen sodium and ovalbumin as model compounds. Importantly, we also examined MN arrays post removal, since it was possible that excessive swelling would reduce mechanical integrity.

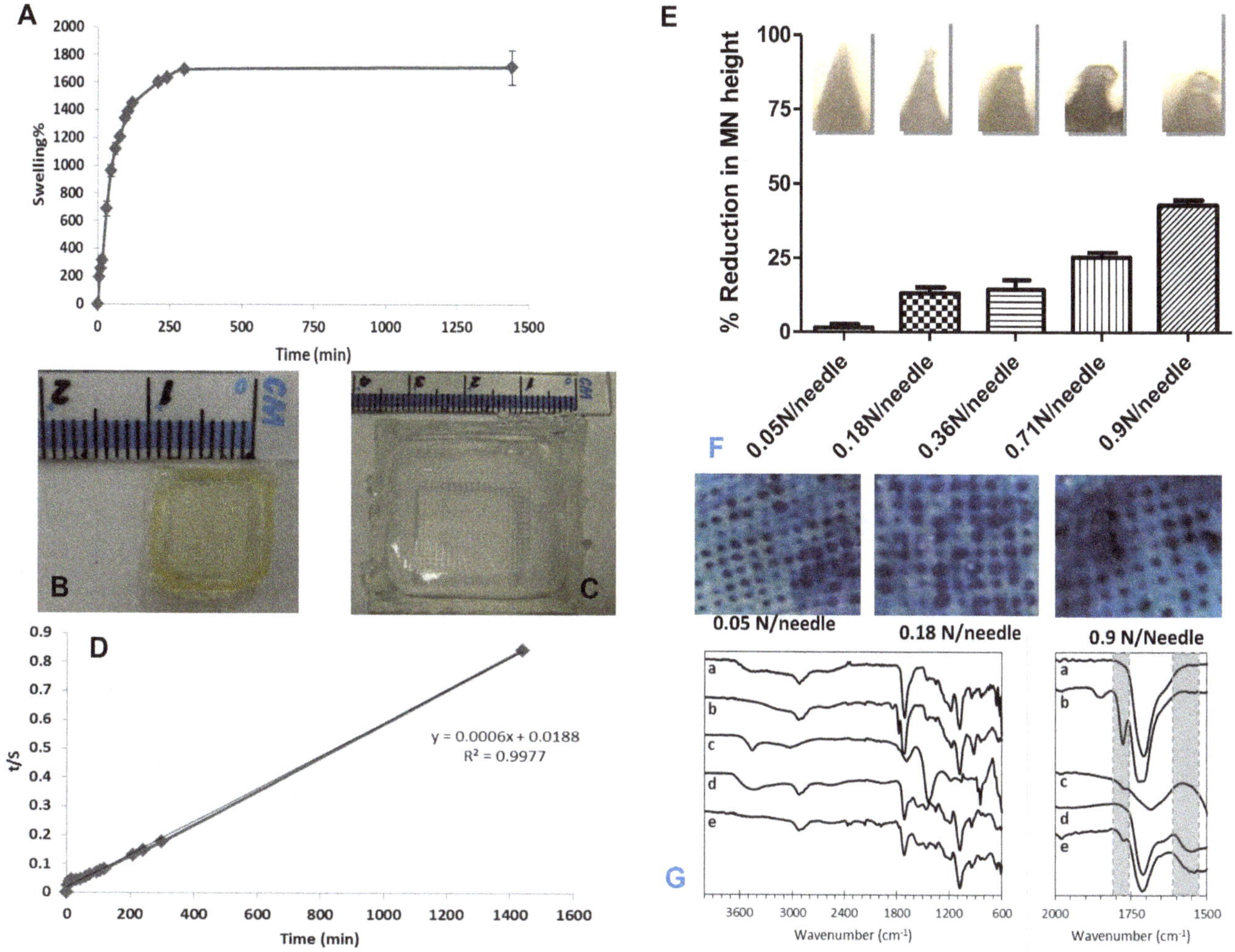

Figure 3. Swelling curve for crosslinked hydrogel films prepared from aqueous blends containing 20% w/w PMVE/MA, 7.5% w/w PEG and 3% Na_2CO_3 based on the increasing mass of the swelling array expressed as a percentage of the mass of a dry array (Means ± SD, n = 3) (A). Super swelling microneedle arrays prepared from aqueous blends containing 20% w/w PMVE/MA, 7.5% w/w PEG and 3% Na_2CO_3 as (**B**) xerogel and (**C**) post-swelling for 3 hours in PBS pH 7.4. t/S versus t swelling curves of super swelling hydrogel prepared from aqueous blends containing 20% w/w PMVE/MA, 7.5% w/w PEG and 3% Na_2CO_3 (Mean ± SD, n = 3) (**D**). Digital microscope images of super swelling hydrogel-forming MN (prepared from aqueous blends containing 20% w/w PMVE/MA, 7.5% PEG 10,000 and 3% Na_2CO_3) following the application of different forces (0.05, 0.18, 0.36, 0.71 and 0.9 N/needle). These images are representative of the percentage reduction in the heights of needles on the MN arrays observed following the application of the different forces (Means+SD, n = 3) (**E**). Digital images showing micropores in excised neonatal porcine skin following application of different forces and subsequent staining with methylene blue solution post microneedle removal (**F**). Attenuated total reflectance (ATR)-Fourier transform infrared (FTIR) spectra of dry hydrogels prepared from aqueous blends containing: 20% w/w Gantrez S-97, 7.5% w/w PEG 10.000 non crosslinked (a) and crosslinked (b) materials; Na_2CO_3 (c) and 20% w/w Gantrez S-97, 7.5% w/w PEG 10.000 and 3% w/w Na_2CO_3 non crosslinked (d) and crosslinked (e) materials. The left panel shows a closer view of the carbonyl region for the same materials. A FTIR Accutrac FT/IR-4100 Series (Jasco, Essex, UK) equipped with MIRacle diamond ATR was used at room temperature. Samples were scanned and recorded in the region of 4000–400 cm^{-1} at a resolution of 4.0 cm^{-1}. The obtained spectra were an average of 64 scans. A standard smoothing process was applied to all the spectra using the equipment software (**G**).

Table 1. Aqueous blends used to prepare hydrogel formulations tested in the current study and the equilibrium swelling of the formed hydrogels (Means ± SD, n = 3).

Formulation no.	Ingredients (pH value of Gantrez gel prior to addition of other ingredients and making up to volume with deionised water)	Percentage swelling at equilibrium
Control formulation	15% w/w Gantrez AN-139 (pH 2) 7.5% w/w PEG 10,000	1071±106
1	15% w/w Gantrez S-97, (pH 2) 7.5% w/w PEG 10,000	918±13
2	20% w/w Gantrez S-97, (pH 2) 7.5% w/w PEG 10,000, 3% w/w Na_2CO_3	1708±125
3	15% w/w Gantrez AN-139, (adjusted to pH 4) 7.5% w/w PEG 10,000, 3% w/w Na_2CO_3	Dissolved
4	16% w/w Gantrez AN-139, (adjusted to pH 4) 6% w/w PEG 10,000, 3% w/w Na_2CO_3	Dissolved

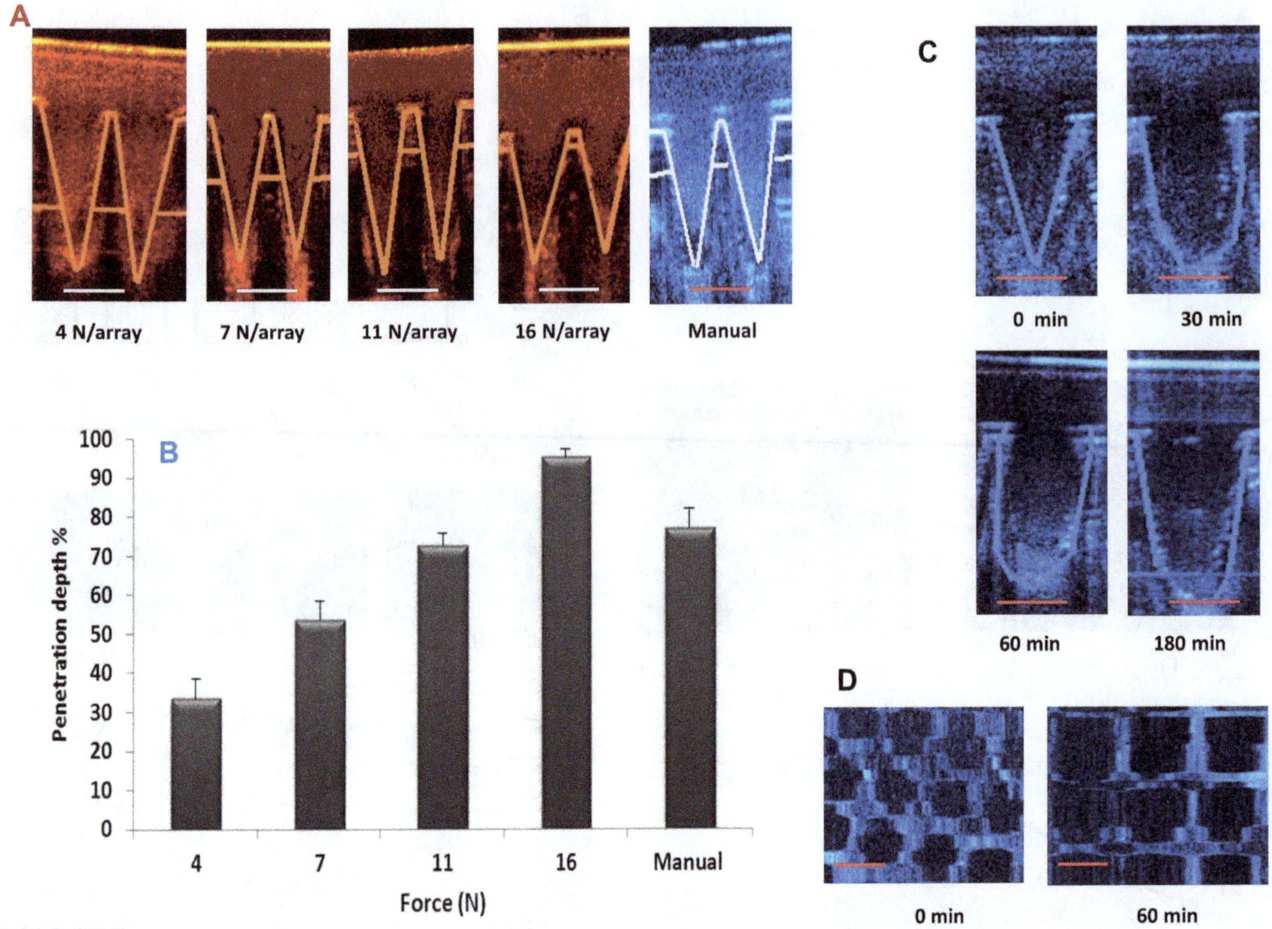

Figure 4. False colour 2D still images of super swelling MN arrays immediately following insertion into excised neonatal porcine skin at application forces of 4, 7, 11 or 16 N/array or using manual application. (Scale bar represents 300 μm in each case) (**A**). The effect of application force (N/array) upon the resultant penetration depth of super swelling MN arrays in neonatal porcine skin *in vitro*, expressed as a p [percentage of MN height (Means+S.D., n = 10)]. The penetration parameters of the MN arrays were quantified using optical coherence tomography (**B**). False colour images of the *in vitro* swelling profile of MN arrays in excised neonatal porcine skin recorded over a 3 h period, as assessed by optical coherence tomography (Scale bar represents 300 μm in each case) (**C**). OCT visualisation of the micropores residing within the skin immediately following MN array insertion (0 min) and following 60 min in skin (Scale bar represents 300 μm. in each case) (**D**).

3.1. Swelling studies

The results outlined in **Figure 3A** display the percentage swelling in PBS pH 7.4 of super swelling hydrogel films cast from aqueous blends of 20% w/w Gantrez S-97, 7.5% w/w PEG 10,000 and 3% w/w Na_2CO_3. The hydrogel formulation incorporating Na_2CO_3 as a modifying agent showed greater initial swelling and reached equilibrium more quickly than the control formula (15% Gantrez AN-139, 7.5% PEG). For example, after 1 hour, the percentage swelling of super swelling hydrogels (20% w/w Gantrez S-97, 7.5% w/w PEG and 3% w/w Na_2CO_3) was 1119%, compared to only 250% for the control formulation. Hydrogels prepared from aqueous blends containing 3% w/w

Table 2. The effect of force of application upon the resultant penetration characteristics of MN arrays cast from 20% w/w Gantrez S-97, 7.5% w/w PEG 10,000 and 3% w/w Na_2CO_3, in the geometry 19×19 with height 600 μm, width 300 μm and interspacing at base 50 μm into neonatal porcine skin, (Means ± SD, n = 10).

Force (N/array)	MN penetration depth (μm)	Pore width (μm)	Base plate/*Stratum corneum* distance (μm)
4	201±31	209±10	398±31
7	322±35	214±17	277±35
11	430±20	219±8	169±20
16	571±8	228±12	29±8
Manual	465±28	211±7	134±28

Table 3. *In vitro* swelling of MN arrays (19×19 MN, 600 μm height, 300 μm width at base, 50 μm interspacing at base) upon insertion into neonatal porcine skin, (Means ± SD, n = 15).

Time (min)	MN depth in skin (μm)
0	465.25±28.25
30	578.08±22.74
60	609.50±35.13
180	697.27±41.63

Na_2CO_3 showed a significant ($p<0.05$) increase in percentage swelling. The percentage swelling at equilibrium was 1071% and 1708% for the control and super swelling formulations, respectively (**Table 1**). **Figure 3** also illustrates the morphology of the MN array as a xerogel (B) and post-swelling in PBS (C). **Figure 3D** is representative of the liner regression plots derived from swelling curves using Equation 3.

Using attenuated total reflectance (ATR)-Fourier transform infrared (FTIR) spectroscopy, the mechanism of action of the modifying agent was confirmed to be due to sodium salt formation on free acid groups on the copolymer, thus reducing ester-based crosslinking (**Figure 3G**). The main difference that can be seen in the spectra of the crosslinked films in contrast with the non crosslinked ones, is the presence of a new band between 1800 and 1750 cm^{-1}. This band can be attributed to the new ester bonds formed between the Gantrez S-97 acid groups and the hydroxyl groups of the PEG molecules. In addition a new band between 1500 and 1600 cm^{-1} can be observed for super-swelling hydrogels that is not present in the other hydrogels. This band is characteristic for the salts of carboxyilic acids [26].

To examine the controlling mechanism of swelling of the super swelling hydrogel materials prepared from aqueous blends of 20% w/w Gantrez S-97, 7.5% w/w PEG and 3% w/w Na_2CO_3, the second order kinetic model (**Equation 4**) was used to process the experimental data. To analyse the kinetic model, *t/S* versus *t* graphs were plotted and respective swelling rate parameters were determined. **Figure 3D** shows representative linear regression plots of the swelling curves derived from **Equation 4**. The diffusional exponent, n, was determined to be 0.76, indicating an anomalous mechanism of water uptake. In addition, the diffusion coefficient (D_i) was 2.47×10^{-6} cm^2 min^{-1}. The volume fraction of polymer, ϕ, determined using **Equation 6** was 0.045, the number average molecular weight between crosslinks, M_c, determined using **Equation 5**, was 6,793,627 g/mol. The crosslink density, V_e, determined using **Equation 8** was 1.08×10^{19}. Due to dissolution of other candidates, the formulation which was selected for continued investigation was that containing 20% w/w Gantrez S-97, 7.5% w/w PEG and 3% w/w Na_2CO_3.

3.2. Mechanical testing

MN arrays formulated using the super swelling formulation (20% w/w Gantrez S-97, 7.5% w/w PEG and 3% w/w Na_2CO_3) and in the geometry, 19×19 (height = 600 μm, width = 300 μm, interspacing = 50 μm) were used to investigate the effects of compression tests on the heights of individual needles on the MN array. The digital microscope images presented in **Figure 3E** are illustrative of the effects, on individual needles of the MN array, of the fracture forces applied by axial load. It is important to note that regardless of the force applied, none of the needles on the MN array broke or shattered upon application into the skin, rather bending. **Figure 3E** also shows the percentage reduction in the height of individual needles on the MN array upon application of increasing fracture forces. The reduction in MN height increased progressively with increases in the force applied. These MN deformed when applied to a stainless steel plate, but were not brittle, which is important from a patient safety point of view. This is especially true considering the relatively high forces applied here (>300 N was the maximal force applied over the 361 MN) and the much softer nature of skin.

Skin penetration of super swelling MN arrays was investigated using dermatomed neonatal porcine skin (approximately 350–450 μm thicknesses) and the percentage of holes (micro-conduits) created by the MN arrays was determined after staining of the skin

Table 4. Physical properties of lyophilised drug reservoirs.

Parameter	Means ± S.D.
Ovalbumin	
Weight (g)	0.32±0.01
Hardness (N)	119.7±5.0
Thickness (mm)	4.12±0.3
Friability	0.47% mass loss
Ibuprofen sodium	
Weight (g)	0.26±0.02
Hardness (N)	178±3
Thickness (mm)	4.96±0.6
Friability	0% mass loss

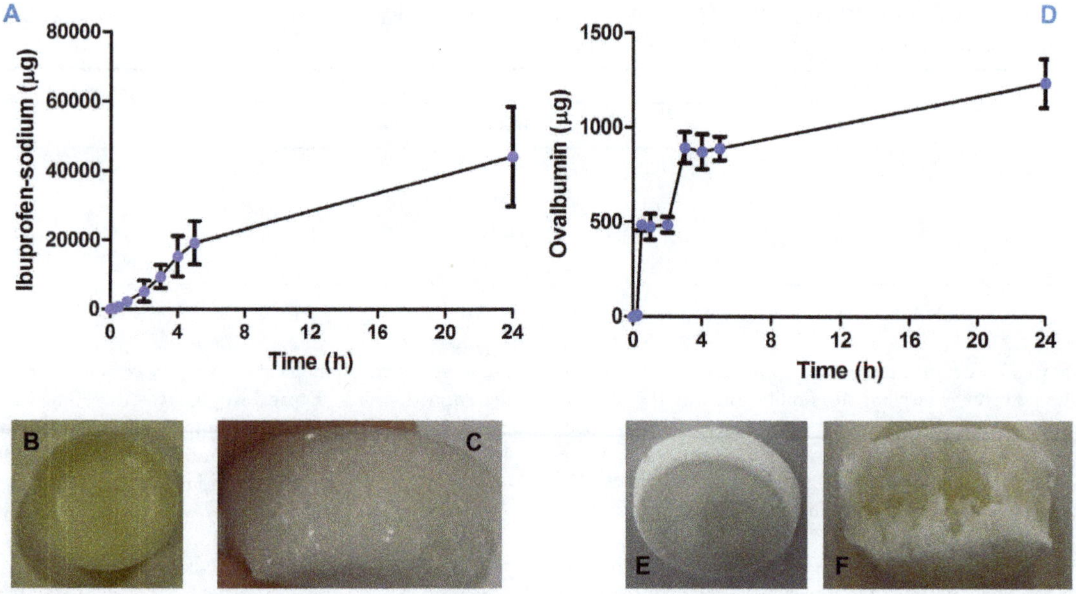

Figure 5. The *in vitro* cumulative permeation profile of ibuprofen sodium across dermatomed 350 μm neonatal porcine skin when delivered using in-dwelling super swelling MN arrays combined with lyophilised drug reservoirs (Means ± S.D., n = 9) (A). Digital images of the ibuprofen sodium-loaded lyophilised wafers used in *in vitro* and *in vivo* experiments and prepared from aqueous blends containing 10% w/w gelatin, 3% w/w mannitol and 40% w/w ibuprofen sodium (**B, C**). The *in vitro* cumulative permeation profile of OVA across dermatomed 350 μm neonatal porcine skin when delivered using in-dwelling super swelling MN arrays combined with lyophilised drug reservoirs (Means ± S.D., n = 5) (**D**). Digital images (**E, F**)of the OVA-loaded lyophilised wafers used in *in vitro* and *in vivo* experiments and prepared from aqueous blends containing 10% w/w gelatin, 40% w/w mannitol, 10% w/w NaCl, 1% w/w sucrose and 0.5% w/w OVA. These active-loaded tablets exhibited high porosities as exemplified in (**G**).

with methylene blue solution. Regardless of force applied,>85% of the MN in each array penetrated the *stratum corneum*, as evidenced by staining of the formed aqueous microconduits by the hydrophilic marker compound. However, with increasing applied forces, the penetration efficiency of the MN also increased (**Figure 3F**). In the case of the 0.9 N/needle applied force, the microconduits created could be traced onto the surface of the laboratory film (Parafilm) placed beneath the skin. This indicated that, at this highest insertion force, which equates to 324.9 N/array as there are 361 needles in each array, the depth of penetration of the needles into the skin was at its greatest. In order to accurately measure miroconduit depth, optical coherence tomography was utilised. The penetration characteristics of MN arrays inserted into neonatal porcine skin using an applicator set to defined forces of 4, 7, 11 or 16 N/array are presented in **Table 2** and **Figure 4B**. Manual force (defined as "gentle finger pressure") was also used to insert the MN arrays and the penetration characteristics are very similar to those quoted when a force of 11 N/array was employed. Increasing force increased penetration depth and decreased distance between the lower MN baseplate and the *stratum corneum*, but microconduit width was largely unaffected.

3.3. In skin swelling

The swelling of the MN arrays upon application into skin was then investigated *in vitro* over 3 hours and in real time. Individual needles on the arrays exhibited an increase in height of approximately 40% by the end of the three-hour testing period (**Figure 4C** and **Table 3**). The microconduits residing within the skin immediately and 60 min post-MN array application were visualised (**Figure 4D**). Importantly, these images confirm that skin under occlusion swells and relaxes with the MN, meaning their increase in volume does not result in the extravasation of the swollen MN from the skin.

3.4. Lyophilised drug reservoirs

Different OVA-loaded and ibuprofen sodium-loaded formulations were prepared and lyophilised. An OVA-loaded formulation containing 10% w/w gelatin (Sigma-Aldrich, Dorset, UK), 40% w/w mannitol (Sigma-Aldrich, Dorset, UK), 10% w/w NaCl, 1% w/w sucrose and 0.5% w/w OVA was determined to be the most suitable, in terms of morphology, strength and dissolution profile of the formed wafers and, hence, was chosen for further characterisation studies. In terms of the ibuprofen sodium, those wafers which were prepared from blends containing 10% w/w gelatin (Cryogel SG3, PB Gelatins, Pontypridd, UK), 3% w/w mannitol (Pearlitol 50C-Mannitol, Roquette, Lestrem, France) and 40% w/w ibuprofen sodium (Sigma-Aldrich, Dorset, UK) were chosen for subsequent investigation, as they were the most homogeneous. There was no loss of active in either case, with recoveries of 100% for ibuprofen sodium and 98±18% for OVA. In addition, the wafers all complied with pharmacopoeial standards [27] for hardness, weight variation, thickness and friability (**Table 4**).

3.5. *In vitro* drug release studies

Ibuprofen sodium exhibited an almost typical first order release profile across excised neonatal porcine skin *in vitro* (**Figure 5A**), with approximately 44 mg delivered in 24 h (range from 9 replicates: 35.2–68.9 mg over 24 h). As the ibuprofen sodium-loaded reservoirs were known to contain a mean loading of 124 mg approximately 37% of this was delivered in 24 h. OVA exhibited a tri-phasic release profile (**Figure 5D**), possibly due to the very different composition and morphology of the lyophilised

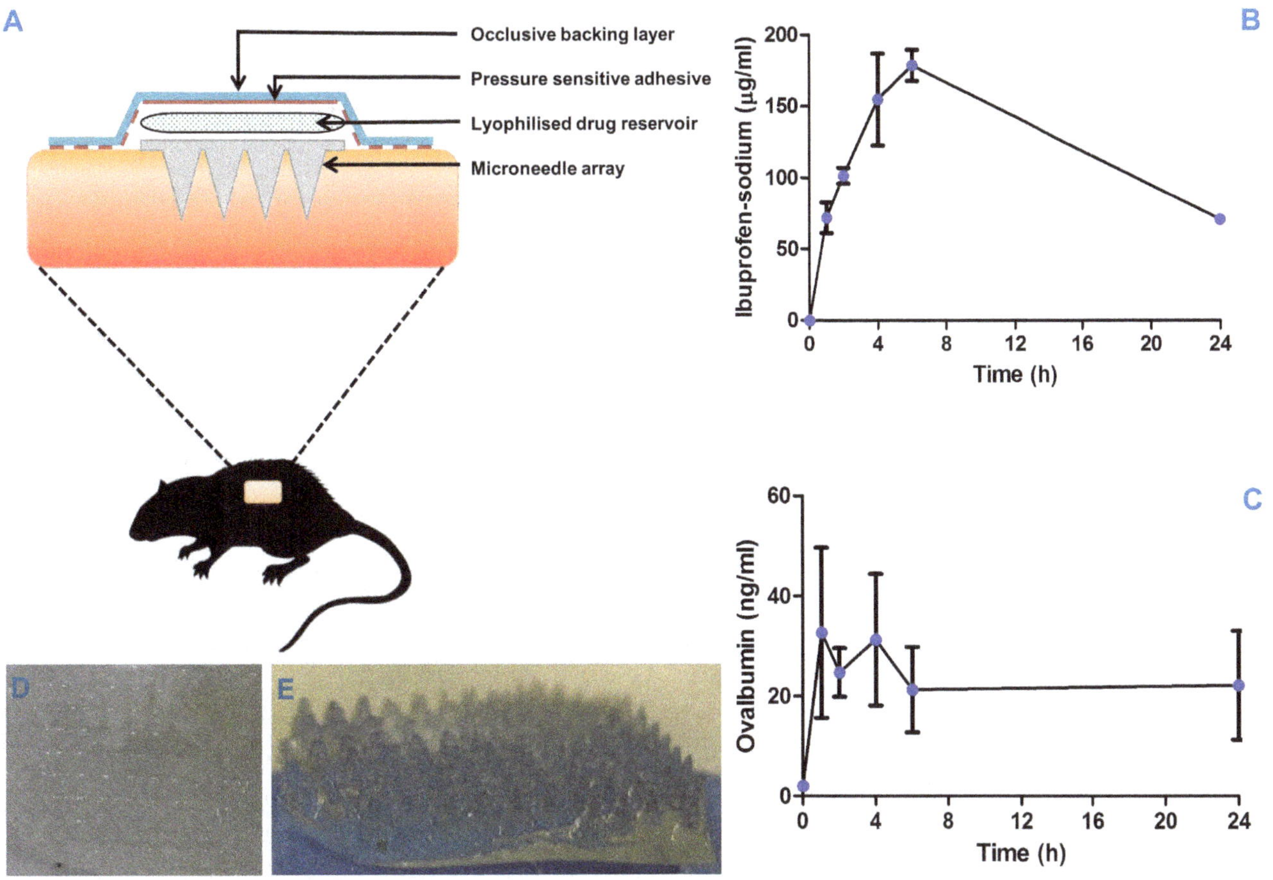

Figure 6. Schematic representation of application and retention strategies for rat experiments designed to evaluate *in vivo* performance of super swelling microneedle arrays (A). The *in vivo* plasma profiles of ibuprofen sodium (**B**) (Means ± S.D., n = 4) and OVA (**C**) (Means ± S.D., n = 3) following transdermal delivery using super swelling microneedle arrays with lyophilised drug reservoirs. Typical morphology of super swelling microneedles upon removal from rat skin *in vivo* after 24 hours insertion indicating that, despite extensive swelling, the microneedles are removed intact (**D**, **E**).

wafers (**Figure 5F**) and the much greater molecular weight and more complex molecular structure, as compared to ibuprofen sodium. The average total OVA content of the lyophilised wafers was 2.5±0.15 mg and it was found that the super swelling MN arrays delivered approximately 1.24 mg OVA over the 24 h experimental period (range from 5 replicates: 1.09–1.36 mg over 24 h). This equates to transdermal delivery of approximately 49% of the OVA loaded into the wafers on average. This is interesting to note, since such effective *in vitro* transdermal delivery has not been seen previously for either high dose low potency molecules or proteins. However, it is unsurprising, given the high molecular weight between crosslinks of the super swelling hydrogel calculated at equilibrium (6,793,627 g/mol) compared to the molecular weights of ibuprofen sodium (229.29 g/mol) and even ovalbumin (44,300 g/mol). Drug permeation is thus likely to be affected more by the dissolution rate of the lyophilised wafers than the hydrogel material, assuming in-skin swelling is complete.

3.6. *In vivo* experiments

In the case of experiments carried out using OVA-loaded reservoirs, two super swelling MN arrays and active-loaded wafers were applied to the backs of the animals (**Figure 6A**). In contrast, four MN arrays and their respective ibuprofen sodium-loaded reservoirs were applied to the backs of the animals in parallel drug delivery experiments. Plasma profiles in the case of both model compounds differed from the patterns of drug permeation profiles seen *in vitro*. This is unsurprising, given that the two experiments are distinct from one another, since the *in vitro* experiments do not have biodistribution, metabolism or excretion components as we have *in vivo*.

For ibuprofen sodium (**Figure 6B**), the integrated MN array delivery system produced a progressive increase in plasma concentrations over 6 h, with a maximal concentration of approximately 179 µg/ml achieved in this time. The plasma concentration had fallen to 71+6.7 µg/ml by 24 h. Therapeutic plasma levels of ibuprofen in humans range between 10 and 15 µg/ml [28] and these levels were achieved within the first hour of MN application. Based on this knowledge and the *in vivo* results, we can approximate the patch size necessary for use in human volunteer studies. An average human male weighs approximately 60 kg [29], which is 286 times greater than the weight of a 210 g rat (the average weight of rat used in these experiments). The peak plasma ibuprofen sodium concentration achieved in the rats at 6 h (179±19 µg/ml) is approximately 18 times greater than the human therapeutic blood levels [28] and this was achieved with MN arrays of total approximate area of 2 cm^2 (4×0.5 cm^2). By this rationale, a MN patch design of no greater than 32 cm^2 could potentially deliver therapeutically-relevant doses of ibuprofen sodium in healthy volunteer studies. Typical commercialised transdermal patches can be as large as 30 or 40 cm^2 (Novartis make Nicotinell nicotine patches of 30 cm^2 [30]; Janssen make Duragesic CII (fentanyl) patches of 32 and 42 cm^2 [31]). Accordingly, it is very reasonable to suggest that a MN product could be successfully developed based on the technology and data presented here. Indeed, we have previously shown that scaling up MN patch size is a relatively straightforward process [8,10].

OVA levels peaked in plasma after only 1 hour (**Figure 6C**) at 42.36±17.01 ng/ml. This represents a significant finding, since macromolecules are normally absorbed quite slowly when administered intradermally [4,5] OVA plasma levels then remained almost constant up to 6 h, dropping somewhat at 24 h, when 23.61±4.84 ng/ml was detected.

Importantly, the super swelling hydrogel MN arrays remained intact over the 24 h application period in all cases, thus allowing their removal as an intact unit at the end of the experiment (**Figure 6D, E**). As can be appreciated, the MN array extensively absorbed interstitial fluid to form a swollen hydrogel matrix, thus enabling delivery of OVA and ibuprofen sodium across the skin and into the systemic circulation. However, the system was sufficiently robust when swollen to ensure that the MN were removed intact.

Conclusions

The work presented here shows, for the first time, that exploitation of so-called "super swelling" hydrogel materials in microneedle-enhanced transdermal drug delivery is a highly promising approach to increasing the range of drugs that can be delivered transdermally. Using such systems in combination with lyophilised wafer-type drug reservoirs facilitated delivery of doses of ibuprofen sodium that could be extrapolated to a useful and usable product for human treatment. Rapid protein delivery using ovalbumin as the model indicated that this technology may also find use in macromolecular drug delivery and vaccine administration. The value to industry is likely to be considerable, since this technology is distinctly different from conventional microneedle systems, which are presently only suitable for bolus delivery of very potent drugs and vaccines. Accordingly, we are currently progressing towards clinical evaluations with a range of candidate molecules.

Author Contributions

Conceived and designed the experiments: RFD MTCM AZA ADW. Performed the experiments: MTCM AZA EM ECS SAZ EL. Analyzed the data: MTCM AZA EM ECS SAZ. Contributed reagents/materials/analysis tools: RFD TRRS HOM VLK ADW. Wrote the paper: RFD MTCM AZA EL EM AJC MCK ECS SAZ ADW.

References

1. Chandrasekhar S, Iyer LK, Panchal JP, Topp EM, Cannon JB, et al. (2013) Microarrays and microneedle arrays for delivery of peptides, proteins, vaccines and other applications. Expert Opin Drug Deliv 10: 1155–1170.
2. Pierre MB, Rossetti FC (2014) Microneedle-based drug delivery systems for transdermal route. Curr Drug Targets 15: 281–291.
3. Gratieri T, Alberti I, Lapteva M, Kalia YN (2013) Next generation intra- and transdermal therapeutic systems: using non- and minimally-invasive technologies to increase drug delivery into and across the skin. Eur J Pharm Sci 50: 609–622.
4. Migalska K, Morrow DIJ., Garland MJ, Thakur RRS, Woolfson AD, et al. (2011) Laser-engineered dissolving microneedle arrays for transdermal macromolecular drug delivery. Pharm Res 28: 1919–1930.
5. Ito Y, Hirono M, Fukushima K, Sugioka N, Takada K (2012) Two-layered dissolving microneedles formulated with intermediate-acting insulin. Int J Pharm 436: 387–393
6. Hong X, Wei L, Wu F, Wu Z, Chen L, et al. (2013) Dissolving and biodegradable microneedle technologies for transdermal sustained delivery of drug and vaccine. Drug Des Devel Ther 7: 945–952.
7. Koutsonanos DG, Compans RW, Skountzou I (2013) Targeting the skin for microneedle delivery of influenza vaccine. Adv Exp Med Biol 785: 121–32.
8. McCrudden MTC, McCrudden C, McAlister E, Zaid Alkilani A, Woolfson AD, et al. (2014) Dissolving microneedle arrays for enhanced transdermal delivery of high dose low potency drug substances. J Cont Rel 180: 71–80.
9. Hirobe S, Azukizawa H, Matsuo K, Zhai Y, Quan YS, et al (2013) Development and clinical study of a self-dissolving microneedle patch for transcutaneous immunization device. Pharm Res 30: 2664–2674
10. Donnelly RF, Thakur RRS, Garland MJ, Migalska K, Majithiya R, et al. (2012) Hydrogel-forming microneedle arrays for enhanced transdermal drug delivery. Adv Funct Mat 22: 4879–4890.
11. Donnelly RF, Morrow DI, McCrudden MT, Alkilani AZ, Vicente-Pérez EM, et al. (2014) Hydrogel-forming and dissolving microneedles for enhanced delivery of photosensitizers and precursors. Photochem Photobiol doi: 10.1111/php.12209.
12. Donnelly RF, Thakur RRS., McCrudden MTC., Zaid-Alkilani A, O'Mahony C, et al. (2013) Hydrogel-forming microneedle arrays exhibit antimicrobial properties: Potential for enhanced patient safety. Int J Pharm 451: 76–91.
13. Thakur RRS, McCarron PA, Woolfson AD, Donnelly RF (2009) Investigation of swelling and network parameters of poly (ethylene glycol)-crosslinked poly (methyl vinyl ether-co-maleic acid) hydrogels. Eur Polym J 45: 1239–1249.
14. Mikolajewska P, Donnelly RF, Garland MJ, Morrow DIJ, Iani V, et al. (2010) Microneedle pre-treatment of human skin improves 5-aminolevulininc acid (ALA) and 5-aminolevulinic acid methyl ester (MAL) induced PpIX production for topical photodynamic therapy without increase in pain or erythema. Pharm Res 27: 2213–2220.
15. McCarron PA, Woolfson AD, Donnelly RF, Andrews GP, Zawislak A, et al. (2004) Influence of plasticiser type and storage conditions on the properties of poly(methyl vinyl ether-co-maleic anhydride) bioadhesive films. J App Polym Sci 91: 1576–1589.
16. Peniche C, Cohen ME, Vázquez B, San Román J (1997) Water sorption of flexible networks based on 2-hydroxyethyl methacrylate-triethylenglycol dimethacrylate copolymers. Polymer 38: 5977–5982.
17. Peppas NA, Korsmeyer RW (1987) Dynamically swelling hydrogels in controlled release applications Hydrogels in Medicine and Pharmacy. Boca Raton, Florida: CRC Press Inc. 109–136 p.
18. Ritger PL, Peppas NA (1987) A simple equation for description of solute release II: Fickian and anomalous release from swellable devices. J Cont Rel 5: 37–42.
19. Bajpai S (2001) Swelling–deswelling behavior of poly(acrylamide-co-maleic acid) hydrogels. J Appl Polym Sci 80: 2782–2789.
20. Donnelly RF, Majithiya R, Thakur RRS, Morrow DIJ, Garland MJ, et al. (2011) Design and physicochemical characterisation of optimised polymeric microneedle arrays prepared by a novel laser-based micromoulding technique. Pharm Res 28: 41–57.
21. Fourtanier A, Berrebi C (1989) Miniature pig as an animal model to study photoaging. Photochem Photobiol 50: 771–784.
22. Woolfson AD, McCafferty DF, McCallion CR, McAdams E, Anderson J (1995) Moisture-activated, electrically conducting bioadhesive hydrogels as interfaces for bioelectrodes: Effect of film hydration on cutaneous adherence in wet environments. J Appl Polym Sci 58: 1291–1296.
23. Donnelly RF, Garland MJ, Morrow DIJ, Migalska K, Thakur RRS, et al. (2010) Optical coherence tomography is a valuable tool in the study of the effects of microneedle geometry on skin penetration characteristics and in-skin dissolution. J Cont Rel 147: 333–341.
24. The International Conference on Harmonisation of Technical Requirements for Registration of Pharmaceuticals for Human Use (ICH) website. Available: http://www.ich.org/. Accessed 2013 Oct 4.
25. McCrudden MTC, Torrisi BM, Al-Zahrani S, McCrudden CM, Donnelly RF et al. (2014) Laser-engineered dissolving microneedle arrays for protein delivery: Potential for enhanced intradermal vaccination. J Pharm Pharmacol doi: 10.1111/jphp.12248.
26. Shevchenko LL (1963) Infrared spectra of salts and complexes of carboxylic acids and some of their derivatives. Russ Chem Rev 32: 201–207.
27. The British Pharmacopoeia 2013 website. Available: http://www.pharmacopoeia.co.uk/2013/. Accessed 2013 Oct 6.
28. Dollery C (1991) Therapeutic Drugs. London: Churchill Livingstone.
29. The National Health Service website. Available: http://www.nhs.uk/Livewell/healthy-living/Pages/height-weight-chart.aspx. Accessed 2013 Oct 5.
30. Nicotinell website. Available: http://www.nicotinell.co.uk/. Accessed 2013 Oct 14.
31. Duragesic website. Available: http://www.duragesic.com/. Accessed 2013 Oct 14.

18

Novel High Efficient Coatings for Anti-Microbial Surgical Sutures Using Chlorhexidine in Fatty Acid Slow-Release Carrier Systems

Andreas Obermeier[1]*, Jochen Schneider[2], Steffen Wehner[1], Florian Dominik Matl[1], Matthias Schieker[3], Rüdiger von Eisenhart-Rothe[1], Axel Stemberger[1], Rainer Burgkart[1]

1 Klinik für Orthopädie und Sportorthopädie, Klinikum rechts der Isar, Technische Universität München, München, Bavaria, Germany, **2** Institut für Mikrobiologie, Immunologie und Hygiene, Klinikum rechts der Isar, Technische Universität München, München, Bavaria, Germany, **3** Experimentelle Chirurgie und Regenerative Medizin, Klinik für Chirurgie, Klinikum der Universität München, München, Bavaria, Germany

Abstract

Sutures can cause challenging surgical site infections, due to capillary effects resulting in bacteria permeating wounds. Anti-microbial sutures may avoid these complications by inhibiting bacterial pathogens. Recently, first triclosan-resistances were reported and therefore alternative substances are becoming clinically relevant. As triclosan alternative chlorhexidine, the "gold standard" in oral antiseptics was used. The aim of the study was to optimize novel slow release chlorhexidine coatings based on fatty acids in surgical sutures, to reach a high anti-microbial efficacy and simultaneously high biocompatibility. Sutures were coated with chlorhexidine laurate and chlorhexidine palmitate solutions leading to 11, 22 or 33 µg/cm drug concentration per length. Drug release profiles were determined in aqueous elutions. Antibacterial efficacy against *Staphylococcus aureus* was assessed in agar diffusion tests. Biocompatibility was evaluated via established cytotoxicity assay (WST-1). A commercially triclosan-containing suture (Vicryl Plus), was used as anti-microbial reference. All coated sutures fulfilled European Pharmacopoeia required tensile strength and proved continuous slow drug release over 96 hours without complete wash out of the coated drug. High anti-microbial efficacy for up to 5 days was observed. Regarding biocompatibility, sutures using 11 µg/cm drug content displayed acceptable cytotoxic levels according to ISO 10993-5. The highest potential for human application were shown by the 11 µg/cm chlorhexidine coated sutures with palmitic acid. These novel coated sutures might be alternatives to already established anti-microbial sutures such as Vicryl Plus in case of triclosan-resistance. Chlorhexidine is already an established oral antiseptic, safety and efficacy should be proven for clinical applications in anti-microbial sutures.

Editor: Ali Al-Ahmad, University Hospital of the Albert-Ludwigs-University Freiburg, Germany

Funding: This work was financially supported by the Heraeus Medical GmbH, Wehrheim, Germany (http://www.heraeus-medical.com/de/home_15.html). Within the Klinikum rechts der Isar, Technische Universität München the external funding number was 8895117_HeraeusCoating. This work was supported by the German Research Foundation (DFG) and the Technische Universität München within the funding programme Open Access Publishing. The funder's financial support does not alter the authors' adherence to PLOS ONE policies on sharing data and materials. The funding organization didn't play any role in the study design, data collection and analysis, decision to publish, or preparation of the manuscript and only provided financial support and research materials.

Competing Interests: The authors have declared that no competing interests exist.

* Email: aobermeier@tum.de

Introduction

Surgical site infections (SSI) are still challenging complications after operations despite of established systemic antibiotic prophylaxis today [1]. Reported rates for SSI are usually in the range of 2–5% [2,3], but can even rise up to 25% e.g. for colorectal surgery [4]. In case of infection, further surgical interventions become necessary followed by a prolongation of hospitalization up to 10 days [2]. In conclusion, this means higher treatment costs of about 50,000 US$ per case on average [5] for the healthcare system as well as an elevated risk profile for the individual patient.

The presence of foreign material increases the risk of infections [6], especially surgical sutures can act as a wick for SSI [7]. So pathogens from the natural skin flora can easily enter wounds via capillary action. After having attached to suture surfaces the pathogens proliferate and are then able to form biofilms difficult to treat [8,9]. One potential solution approach to prevent this process is the use of anti-microbial coated sutures. At present, all commercially available anti-microbial sutures are exclusively coated with triclosan such as Vicryl Plus, Monocryl Plus, and PDS Plus [10].

In vitro studies using triclosan for anti-microbial sutures, e.g. Vicryl Plus, have resulted in a highly efficient defense against various bacterial pathogens [11,12]. *In vivo* studies for sternum surgery [13], abdominal wall closure [14], and cerebrospinal fluid shunting procedures [15] indicate significantly lower infection rates for surgical interventions using triclosan coated anti-microbial sutures [16]. In contrast, for some indications there is an ongoing controversial discussion [10,17], such as appendicitis, breast cancer and colorectal surgery [4,18–20].

The main disadvantage of the so far predominantly used antimicrobial triclosan is its wide non-medical use in cosmetics, hygiene- and household products [21]. First research groups reported resistances of bacteria against triclosan and warnings of

Table 1. Prepared anti-microbial sutures and normalized weights of chlorhexidine.

ratio of chlorhexidine in fatty acid (%)	weight of chlorhexidine (mg)	weight of lauric-/ palmitic acid (mg)	normalized drug weight (µg/cm)	coating type and abbreviation for coated sutures	
20	0.44	1.76	**11**	chlorhexidine-lauric acid	**CL11**
				chlorhexidine-palmitic acid	**CP11**
40	0.88	1.32	**22**	chlorhexidine-lauric acid	**CL22**
				chlorhexidine-palmitic acid	**CP22**
60	1.32	0.88	**33**	chlorhexidine-lauric acid	**CL33**
				chlorhexidine-palmitic acid	**CP33**

Amount of chlorhexidine on anti-microbially coated sutures after preparation. The mean coating weight of 40 cm suture samples were determined at 2.2±0.2 mg. The same amounts of chlorhexidine were calculated for the coating types (CL, CP) inside coating solutions (n = 10). The weights on coated sutures for drug contents, fatty acid carriers and normalized mean drug weight per cm suture are given above.

potential pathogen selections [22,23]. Therefore, we were looking for new alternative substances and chose chlorhexidine to equip surgical sutures anti-microbially. This antiseptic is effective against a broad spectrum of relevant pathogens including clinically problematic bacteria like *Staphylococcus aureus* [24]. Besides the known spectrum chlorhexidine is already approved in a variety of medical applications as coating for medical devices [25–27], skin antiseptic [28,29] or as well as oral antiseptic [30].

In a first feasibility study we could show that chlorhexidine coated sutures demonstrated high efficacy against *S. aureus* with the disadvantage of drug concentration related cytotoxicity [31]. Anti-microbial sutures must fulfill a balancing act between inhibiting bacteria and sustaining biocompatibility to the surrounding eukaryotic tissue cells.

The aim of this study was therefore the optimization of new chlorhexidine fatty acid coating formulations for anti-microbial sutures in regard to their drug concentration. We achieved high anti-microbial efficacy over several days combined with ISO 10993-5 required biocompatibility by variation of drug concentrations at 11, 22 or 33 µg per cm suture. Anti-microbially coated sutures were evaluated by measuring tensile strength, inhibition zones, and drug release profiles. These investigations were compared to commercially available plain sutures and triclosan containing Vicryl Plus, as anti-microbial reference.

Materials and Methods

Surgical sutures

Plain braided sutures (Gunze Ltd., Japan) made of polyglycolic acid (PGA) without the usual fatty acid coating to avoid sewing effects were used for the preparation of the anti-microbial sutures. As reference one triclosan-containing absorbable suture Vicryl Plus (Ethicon GmbH, Germany) and two standard absorbable sutures PGA Resorba (Resorba GmbH, Germany) and Vicryl (Ethicon GmbH, Germany) were used. All sutures used in experiments corresponded to United States Pharmacopeia standard 1 (USP 1).

Anti-microbial coating solutions

Anti-microbial coating solutions were prepared by dissolving a fatty acid (palmitic or lauric acid) and chlorhexidine in 99.8% ethanol (C. Roth GmbH, Germany (CR)). In order to prepare the solutions for suture coatings having a mass content of 5% (w/w), 395.0 mg of the corresponding fatty acid and the antiseptic drug were dissolved in 10.0 ml (7.9 g) ethanol. In particular, two groups of coating types were produced. Group I (**CL**): Chlorhexidine diacetate (Sigma-Aldrich GmbH, Germany) in lauric acid as drug carrier (CR). Group II (**CP**): Chlorhexidine diacetate in the drug carrier palmitic acid (CR). For each type of coating three solutions with 20%, 40% or 60% (w/w) drug concentration were formulated. The percentage of drug was related to the 5% total mass of substances (drug plus drug carrier) dissolved in coating solutions. Components were prepared by weighing, using the precision balance Atilon ATL-224 (Acculab Inc., Massachusetts, USA).

Preparation of anti-microbial sutures

Sutures were cut into 40 cm pieces followed, by coating them in a dip process in flasks under aseptic conditions. The closed flasks were placed on a thermo-shaker (Heidolph Instruments GmbH, Germany) for 2 minutes at 35°C and 150 rpm, in order to achieve reproducible coating weights. After drying for at least 2 hours the coating weight was determined by using the precision balance related to the weight of uncoated sutures. The amount of drug normalized per length of suture (µg/cm) was calculated for each concentration (Table 1).

Tensile strength test

For tensile strength testing the uncoated plain PGA sutures (Gunze), PGA Resorba, Vicryl, Vicryl Plus, and exemplarily novel coated sutures CL22, CP22 were measured. The mechanical strength of individual surgical sutures (n = 5) was determined according to the European Pharmacopoeia (Ph. Eur. 7.0/0667: required minimum for USP 1 sutures is 50.8 N) using the tensile testing instrument Zwicki 8253 (Zwick GmbH, Germany).

Drug release from fatty acid drug delivery coatings

Drug release kinetics of coated sutures were measured over a time period of 96 hours in phosphate-buffered saline (PBS). For this purpose sutures of 2 cm length (n = 3) were eluted in 1 ml PBS inside a thermomixer MHR 23 (HLC-Biotech, Germany) at 37°C and 200 rpm. After 1 h, 3 h, 5 h, 7 h, 24 h, 48 h, 72 h und 96 h, elution media was taken out and replaced by fresh PBS. Amount of released chlorhexidine was measured by absorption at 280 nm in a microplate spectrophotometer Multiskan Go (Thermo Fisher Scientific GmbH, Germany). Measured drug concentrations were normalized to length of suture samples and drug elution profiles were recorded by cumulating the released drug amounts over time. The percentage of released chlorhexidine was calculated referring to loaded drug per cm length.

Table 2. Mean tensile strength values of surgical sutures (USP 1).

Tensile strength	Gunze	PGA Resorba	CL22	CP22	Vicryl	Vicryl Plus
mean F_{max} (N)	73.7	81.6	80.3	75.9	78.3	72.2
± standard deviation (N)	3.0	1.6	1.5	2.2	1.0	2.2

Mean values of the maximum force F_{max} (n = 5) for uncoated, commercial and novel coated sutures CL22 and CP22 in example are given above. The required minimum for USP 1 surgical sutures at 50.8 N according to European Pharmacopoeia, was reached for all tested sutures.

Anti-bacterial efficacy of coated sutures via zones of inhibition

Anti-microbial efficacy was determined in Agar plate diffusion tests by using the strain *Staphylococcus aureus* (ATCC 49230), the main pathogen of implant-associated infections [32,33]. According to CLSI criteria, bacterial suspensions were prepared to 0.5 McFarland standard [34]. On each Agar plate 1 ml of this suspension was uniformly distributed. Coated sutures with 3 cm length (n = 3) were placed onto these inoculated Agar plates and incubated at 37°C for 24 hours. Inhibition zones were measured (in mm), with a calliper perpendicular to the middle of the threads. Novel coated sutures and Vicryl Plus were put on Agar plates every 24 hours with fresh bacterial lawns and incubated overnight. Over the following days we measured the inhibition zones. Analogous to Ming et al. [12] this procedure was repeated by using the same samples for several days to recognize the remaining anti-bacterial activity until no detectable inhibition zone was left.

Cytotoxicity study

According to ISO 10993-5:2009, mouse fibroblasts L-929 (DSMZ, Germany) were used for in vitro cytotoxicity testing of coated sutures. The evaluation was performed by measuring the metabolic activity of cells in the presence of eluates from coated sutures via a WST-1 cell proliferation assay (Roche Diagnostics GmbH, Germany). Cells were cultivated in the corresponding media (D-MEM 4.5 g/l D-glucose, Biochrom AG, Germany) containing 10% fetal bovine serum at 37°C and 5.0% CO2 in a humidified atmosphere. Pre-cultures started at 10.000 cells/well inside 96 well microtiter plates, incubated for 24 hours in 200 µl D-MEM. Simultaneously, eluates were generated by eluting coated sutures of 1 cm length (n = 7) in 1.5 ml D-MEM for 24 hours on a thermomixer at 37°C and 300 rpm. After 24 hours cell media was swapped with eluates. Finally, after 48 hours referred to the WST-1 protocol the metabolic activity was measured by quantitative detection of formazan at 405 nm in a spectral photometer. Metabolic activities obtained were referred to activity of pure L-929 culture. A metabolic activity of 70% represents the limit to claim "biocompatibility" for medical devices.

Statistics

Statistical methods were performed by using the student's t-test (Microsoft Excel 2013) with significant level $p<0.05$. Mean values and standard deviations were calculated from at least 3 measurements. Calculation of mean values from several measurements was accompanied by the Gaussian error propagation law.

Results

Reproducibility of anti-microbial sutures

Coating weight of prepared anti-microbial sutures was an important parameter to estimate weights of drugs per unit length. The weight difference of 40 cm sutures in length between uncoated and coated sutures resulted in a mean coating weight at 2.2 mg±0.2 mg (n = 10) independent from drug concentrations used. The triclosan content on Vicryl Plus sutures was 2.7 µg/cm [35,36].

Tensile strength test

The quasi-static tensile strength values of all sutures tested - uncoated, commercially and novel coated sutures - proved mean maximum tensile strength values higher than the Ph. Eur. required minimum of 50.8 N for USP1 absorbable surgical sutures (Table 2). The strength values showed a moderate but significant increase between Gunze and PGA Resorba ($p<0.05$), similar to novel coated sutures CL22 and CP22 exemplarily. Vice versa for Vicryl Plus sutures, a moderate reduction of tensile strength ($p<0.05$) was observed compared to Vicryl sutures.

Drug release from fatty acid drug delivery coatings

Released drug concentrations in PBS eluates normalized by length were determined. All coated sutures demonstrated continuous drug release within four days of experiment. Chlorhexidine was continuously released from lauric acid (Figure 1A) resulting in a drug concentration at 96 hours of 9.6 µg/ml (CL11), 16.6 µg/ml (CL22) and 23.2 µg/ml (CL33). The coating type chlorhexidine in palmitate achieved a drug concentration of 4.4 µg/ml (CP11), 5.8 µg/ml (CP22) and 15.2 µg/ml (CP33) after 96 h (Figure 1B). Percentage of drug release, the ratios between released drugs after 96 hours and amount of drugs on sutures per cm length were compared to each other for chlorhexidine laurate coatings (Figure 2A) and chlorhexidine palmitate coatings (Figure 2B).

Anti-bacterial efficacy of coated sutures via zones of inhibition

Anti-microbial efficacy of coated sutures was daily assessed by using an Agar diffusion assay over several days (Figure 3A). Sutures coated with chlorhexidine in lauric acid (Figure 3B, a) revealed large *S. aureus* inhibition zones after 24 hours of 7.1 mm (CL11), 8.2 mm (CL22) and 8.7 mm (CL33). Inhibition zones during the first three to four days of experiments averaged up to 1.7 mm for CL11, 3.4 mm for CL22 and 2.5 mm for CL33. After the fifth day no inhibition zones were detectable. Chlorhexidine in palmitic acid coatings showed similar results (Figure 3B, b). Inhibition zones after 24 hours were assessed at 4.9 mm (CP11), 7.1 mm (CP22) and 8.9 mm (CP33). The dimensions and durations of the zones of inhibition were dependent on drug concentrations. CP11 ended up after fourth day of experiment, whereas CP22 and CP33 ended up after the fifth day of experiment. The triclosan containing Vicryl Plus showed large inhibition zones after 24 hours on Agar plates with 19.8 mm (Figure 3B, c) lasting for at least nine days and ending up with 1.7 mm zones. The bioavailability of the antiseptics from the fatty

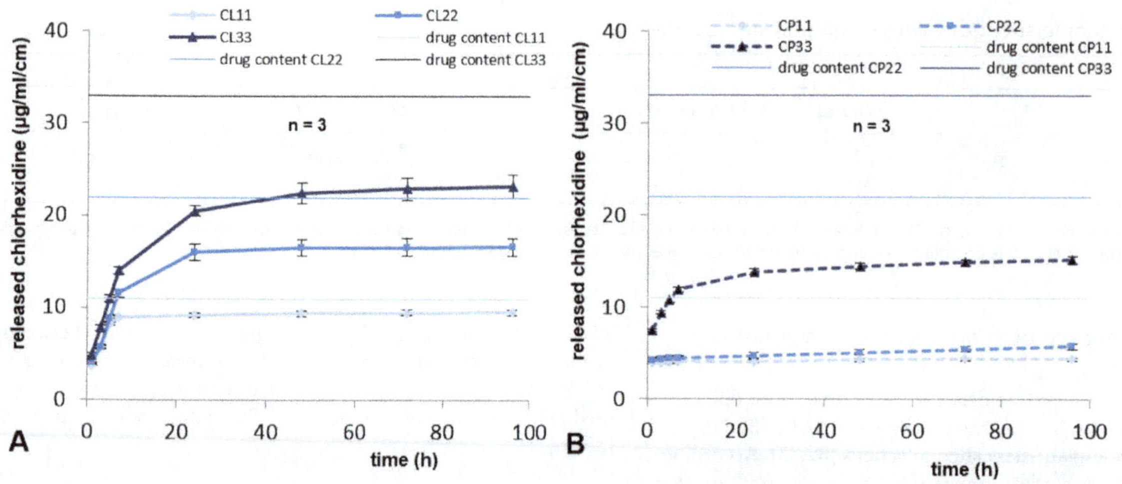

Figure 1. Elution profiles of chlorhexidine coated sutures. Released chlorhexidine in PBS buffer at 37°C for A) chlorhexidine-laurate coatings and B) chlorhexidine-palmitate coated sutures. Elution profiles were determined for each carrier at drug content 11, 22 or 33 µg/cm. The horizontal lines depict the limit of drug release for each concentration, the normalized content of chlorhexidine on coated sutures.

acid delivery systems was corroborated by the microbial experiments.

Cytotoxicity study

Cytotoxicity tests were performed via eluates from individual coated sutures and references. All metabolic activities were referred to L-929 cell samples used as growth reference without sutures. Coatings with chlorhexidine in lauric acid ended with metabolic cell activities at 69.1±7.0% (CL11), 0.9±0.5% (CL22) and 0.3±0.3% (CL33). Chlorhexidine in palmitic acid coatings showed activities at 74.5±29.3% (CP11), 1.1±1.9% (CP22) and no more cell activity for CP33 sutures. The fatty acid coated references identified metabolic activities at 87.8±13.2% and 80.4±13.4% (lauric acid, palmitic acid). Eluates from uncoated sutures reached a metabolic activity at 100.8±9.7% (Gunze). Vicryl Plus eluates demonstrated activities at 98.7±7.1% (Figure 4).

Discussion

Surgical site infection still poses a major complication in surgery. Sutures can cause so called suture-associated infections, induced by proliferation of adhering pathogens. Adhering bacteria enter wounds by capillary action and form infamous biofilms, leading to chronic infections [8]. Anti-microbial coatings for surgical sutures can solve that problem via protecting sutures by inhibiting bacterial growth.

In the present study we developed new anti-microbial suture coatings based on fatty acid carriers using chlorhexidine and adjusting their drug concentrations. The aim was to identify anti-microbial sutures posing effective protection against microbes while being biocompatible in regard to eukaryotic cells. Fatty acids constitute a lubricating film and are state of the art in order to reduce the unwanted sewing effect of sutures. This kind of drug-release system still allows slow-release properties, because of low solubility of fatty acid carriers in aqueous environments [37,38].

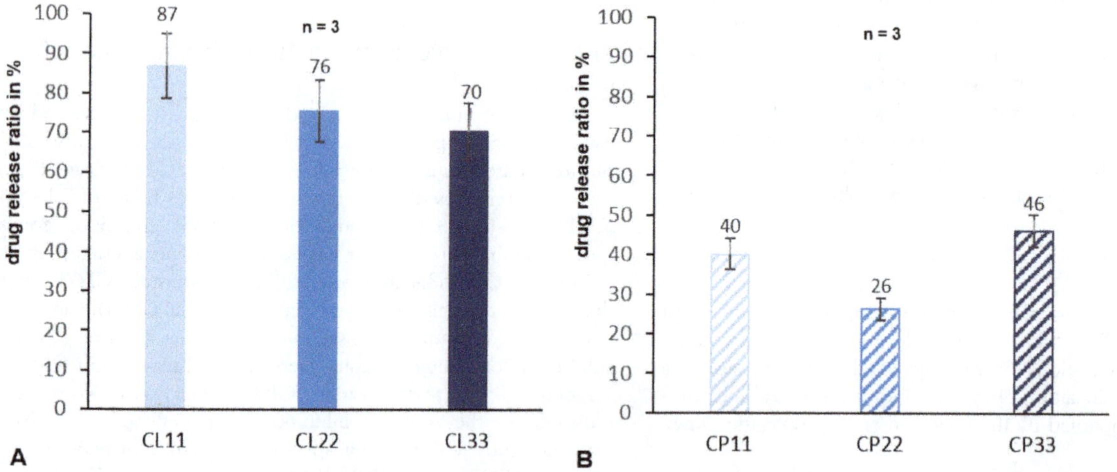

Figure 2. Percentage of chlorhexidine released after 96 hours related to the amount of drug in coated samples. Percentage of chlorhexidine release related to the drug content on coated sutures per cm length at 96 hours of elution in PBS buffer for A) chlorhexidine-laurate and B) chlorhexidine-palmitate coated sutures.

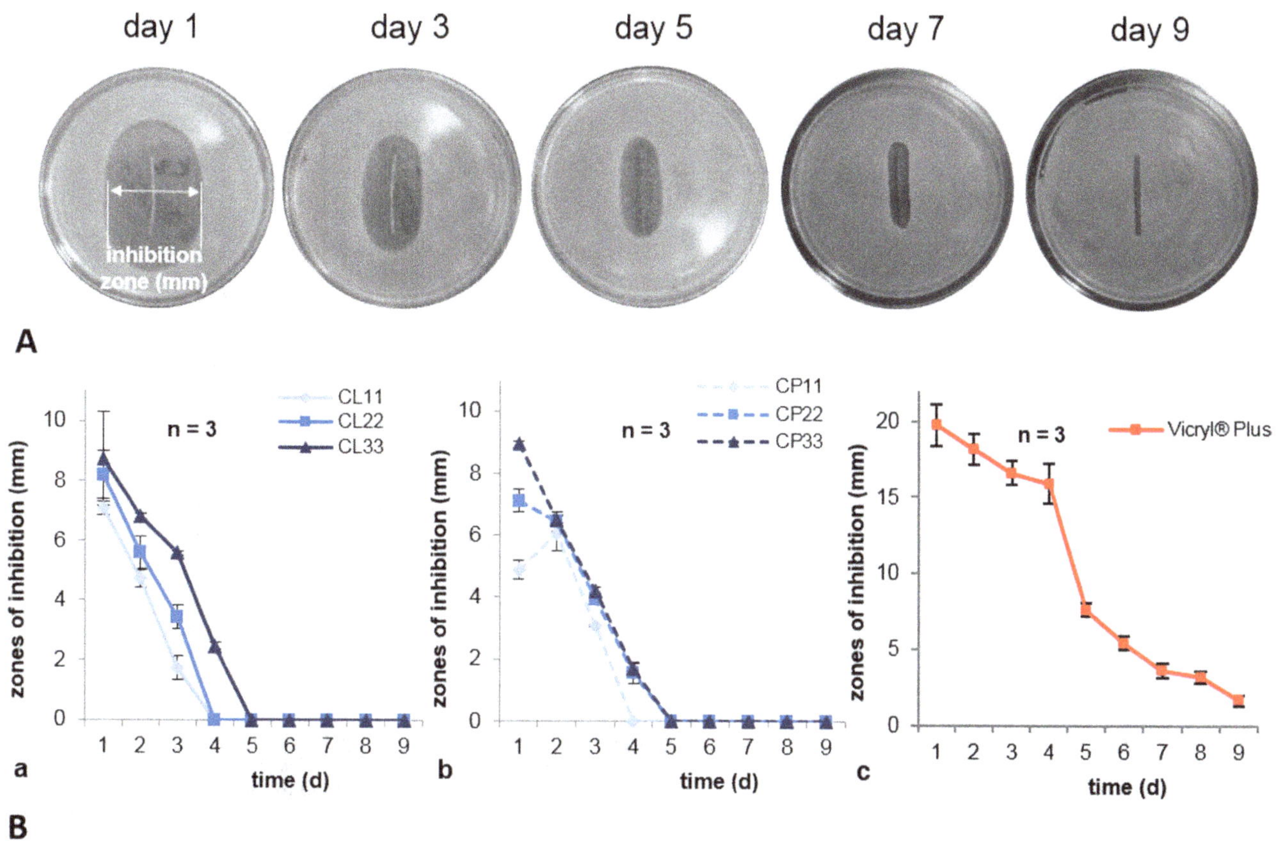

Figure 3. Measuring anti-bacterial efficacy of coated sutures via zones of inhibition. A) Principle of measuring inhibition zones in a longitudinal analysis on the example of a Vicryl Plus suture, in order to achieve anti-microbial effectiveness over several days. B) Anti-microbial efficacies on Agar plates with *S. aureus* lawns (2×10^8 cfu/ml) for a) chlorhexidine lauric acid and b) chlorhexidine palmitic acid coated sutures. Coated suture samples with three different chlorhexidine concentrations 11, 22 and 33 µg/cm. c) Vicryl Plus as reference for commercial anti-microbial sutures.

In a reproducible dip coating process we developed several coating types at various concentrations based on chlorhexidine with lauric or palmitic acid (CL, CP). Coated sutures obtained were tested systematically regarding their tensile strength, drug release, anti-microbial efficacy against *S. aureus*, and cytotoxicity using a WST-1 assay.

Tensile strength of coated PGA sutures was just negligibly influenced by the dip coating process using ethanol. All coated sutures undergoing this process showed much higher maximum strength values than required by the Ph. Eur. standards for USP1 resorbable sutures. The mean strength values of novel coated sutures were comparable to commercially available PGA sutures (PGA Resorba, Vicryl, Vicryl Plus). Therefore, no negative influence of coatings on in vivo degradation time for anti-microbial coated PGA sutures is to be expected. Flexibility of coated sutures remained steady, no delamination was observed after mechanical stress tests. Consequently, no delamination is to be expected while pulling them through the tissue.

Released drug concentration in PBS for chlorhexidine coated sutures showed a continuous drug release for 96 hours with initial rapid release slowing down significantly after 7 hours. In general, drug release should be as slow as possible, however, anti-microbially effective to inhibit pathogens as long as possible, to achieve long-term protection of the coated biomaterial. Drug release is strongly dependent on drug concentration inside coatings. Referring to drug carriers, palmitic acid coatings showed slower drug release values over time than lauric acid coatings with similar anti-microbial efficacies. Moreover, lesser amounts of chlorhexidine were released from palmic acid coatings. Therefore, anti-microbial effects of coated sutures using palmitic acid carrier should have a higher potency for long-term protection in vivo than coatings using lauric acid carriers.

Novel coated sutures showed high anti-microbial efficacy in agar diffusion tests against *S. aureus*. Anti-bacterial tests on agar plates mimic the tissue contact transferring substances by diffusion. All coated sutures generated inhibition zones for more than 24 hours and documented efficacies over several days, similar to Vicryl Plus. Inhibition zones of CP11, on the second day, showed a little increase, presumably a consequence of non-uniform contact of suture samples on Agar surfaces and therefore diffusion problems. The release of chlorhexidine indicated by the inhibition zones is faster during the first days compared to triclosan, because of its much higher solubility in aqueous environments like PBS or Agar. This faster consumption of substances on sutures leads to earlier leaching of inhibition zones. On the one hand, this could be a benefit, because a sufficient release of antiseptics in the wound area in the first days might be an important factor to prevent a potential early wound infection. The long-term efficacy of chlorhexidine coated sutures against *S. aureus* lasted up to 5 days at high levels. Regarding drug concentrations, the dimension of inhibition zones over time did not differ greatly. Thus, even the low drug content of 11 µg/cm can almost be as effective as 22 or

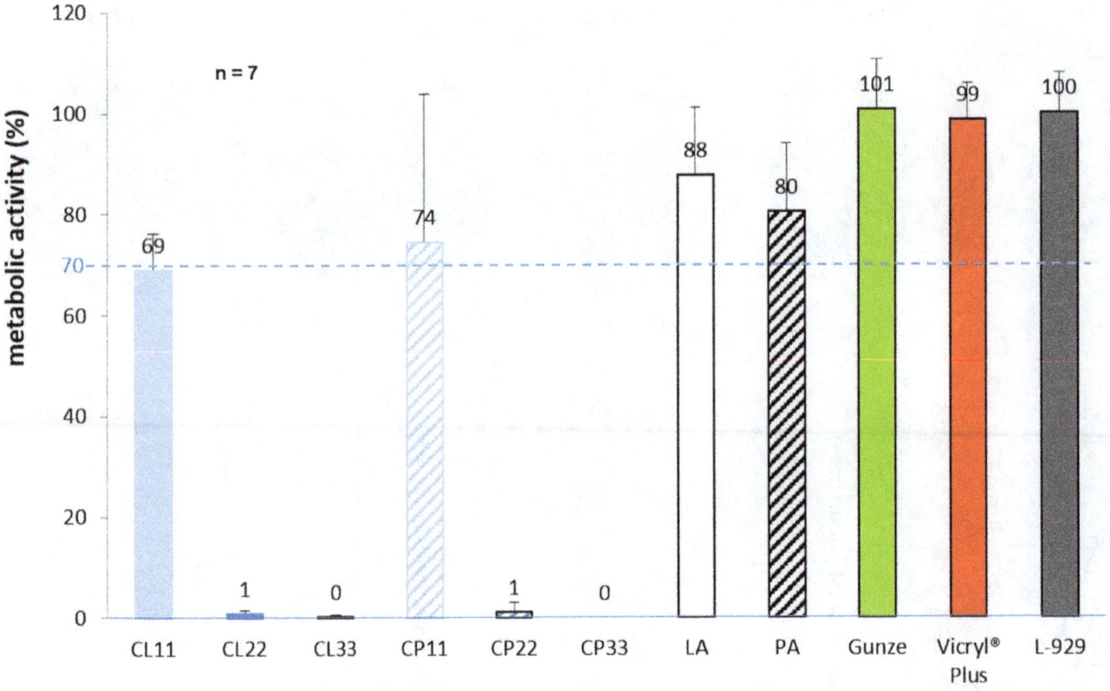

Figure 4. Evaluation of biocompatibility of coated sutures in cytotoxicity tests via WST-1 assay. Metabolic cell activity of fibroblasts in the presence of eluates from coated sutures measured with the WST-1 proliferation assay. Cells were incubated with eluates from coated sutures, suture references: lauric acid (LA), palmitic acid (PA), uncoated suture (Gunze), and Vicryl Plus. All values referred to cellular growth control, pure L-929 mouse fibroblast cultures. Dashed line at 70% pictures the level for acceptable lowering of metabolic activity according to ISO 10993-5:2009 in order to declare biocompatibility of medical devices.

rather 33 μg/cm in protecting surgical sutures, without depletion of the anti-microbial drug on sutures.

Biocompatibility studies on coated sutures demonstrated acceptable cytotoxicities only for the lowest drug concentrations at 11 μg/cm independent from the fatty acid used. Such sutures fulfilled the at least required 70% remaining metabolic activity of L-929 cells to claim non-cytotoxicity according to ISO 10993-5:2009. Nevertheless, those sutures still have a high anti-microbial efficacy. Therefore, 11 μg/cm chlorhexidine coated sutures are potential candidates for further pre-clinical and human in vivo studies. In general, a strong dose-dependent effect for anti-microbial coated sutures was recognized regarding cytotoxicity. To improve biocompatibility a fine tuning with reduction of drug concentration, i.e. from 11 to 9 μg/cm without sacrificing the high anti-microbial efficacies seems promising.

There are limitations of our study, at first, the use of only one bacterial strain, *S. aureus*, for testing efficacy of coated anti-microbial sutures. In vitro tests should be performed to further prove efficacy against other relevant types of pathogens. Second, no effects on biofilms by anti-microbial coated sutures were investigated but bacterial cultures on agar and in suspensions are most common for first evaluation. For that purpose in vitro experiments with microbiological biofilm models are necessary. Third, other antiseptic substances should be identified and investigated regarding biocompatibility and anti-microbial efficacy.

To sum up, we demonstrated a prototypical coating process to provide anti-microbial sutures at high reproducible quality. Mechanical strength tests indicated negligible influences of the coating process comparable to commercial sutures and beyond the Ph. Eur. required strength values for resorbable sutures. Drug release from the novel coated sutures in aqueous media revealed to be dependent on dose, and the entity of the fatty acid carrier. We identified that all used novel chlorhexidine coated sutures proved high anti-bacterial efficacy. Duration of inhibition zones on Agar plates was dependent on the chlorhexidine dose, however there seemed to be no influence from fatty acid carriers. Biocompatibility testing of coated sutures also indicated strong dose dependency.

Conclusions

In this study we developed novel chlorhexidine coatings for anti-microbial surgical sutures with three different antiseptic concentrations based on palmitic and lauric acid carriers. We demonstrated their high anti-microbial efficacy against *S. aureus* in vitro. In particular, chlorhexidine coated sutures with 11 μg/cm concentration proved acceptable cytotoxicity according to ISO 10993-5 and simultaneously high anti-microbial protection over several days. Such coated sutures represent an alternative in the case of triclosan-resistance for prophylactic sutures. The aim is to support surgeons with an effective weapon to reduce suture-associated surgical site infections. However, further pre-clinical and clinical trials are necessary to confirm safety and efficacy in vivo.

Acknowledgments

We would like to express our great appreciation to Dr. K.-D. Kühn (Heraeus Medical GmbH) and Dr. K.-H. Sorg (Resorba GmbH) for their kind supply of materials. Also, many thanks to J. Hintermair (Zentralinstitut für Medizintechnik IMETUM, TU München) for supplying the mouse fibroblastic cell line L-929. Many thanks to J. Tübel (cell culture laboratory, Klinikum rechts der Isar, Klinik für Orthopädie, TU München) for her great assistance in cell biological experiments. Also, many thanks to P. Föhr (biomechanics laboratory, Klinikum rechts der Isar, Klinik für Orthopädie, TU München) for his great guidance in biomechanical testing.

Author Contributions

Conceived and designed the experiments: AO JS SW FDM MS RvER AS RB. Performed the experiments: AO SW JS FDM. Analyzed the data: MS RvER AS RB. Contributed reagents/materials/analysis tools: MS RvER AS RB. Wrote the paper: AO JS SW FDM MS RvER AS RB.

References

1. Young B, Ng TM, Teng C, Ang B, Tai HY, et al. (2011) Nonconcordance with surgical site infection prevention guidelines and rates of surgical site infections for general surgical, neurological, and orthopedic procedures. Antimicrobial agents and chemotherapy 55: 4659–4663.
2. Hranjec T, Swenson BR, Sawyer RG (2010) Surgical site infection prevention: how we do it. Surgical Infections 11: 289–294.
3. Leaper DJ (2010) Surgical-site infection. The British journal of surgery 97: 1601–1602.
4. Baracs J, Huszar O, Sajjadi SG, Horvath OP (2011) Surgical site infections after abdominal closure in colorectal surgery using triclosan-coated absorbable suture (PDS Plus) vs. uncoated sutures (PDS II): a randomized multicenter study. Surgical Infections 12: 483–489.
5. Barnett TE (2007) The Not-So-Hidden Costs of Surgical Site Infections. AORN journal 86: 249–258.
6. Eiff C, Jansen B, Kohnen W, Becker K (2005) Infections Associated with Medical Devices. Drugs 65: 179–214.
7. Geiger D, Debus ES, Ziegler UE, Larena-Avellaneda A, Frosch M, et al. (2005) Capillary activity of surgical sutures and suture-dependent bacterial transport: a qualitative study. Surg Infect (Larchmt) 6: 377–383.
8. Kathju S, Nistico L, Hall-Stoodley L, Post JC, Ehrlich GD, et al. (2009) Chronic surgical site infection due to suture-associated polymicrobial biofilm. Surg Infect (Larchmt) 10: 457–461.
9. Katz S, Izhar M, Mirelman D (1981) Bacterial adherence to surgical sutures. A possible factor in suture induced infection. Ann Surg 194: 35–41.
10. Mingmalairak C (2011) Antimicrobial Sutures: New Strategy in Surgical Site Infections. In: Mendez-Vilas A, editor. Science against Microbial Pathogens: Communicating Current Research and Technological Advances: Formatex Research Center. pp. 313–323.
11. Edmiston CE, Seabrook GR, Goheen MP, Krepel CJ, Johnson CP, et al. (2006) Bacterial adherence to surgical sutures: can antibacterial-coated sutures reduce the risk of microbial contamination? J Am Coll Surg 203: 481–489.
12. Ming X, Rothenburger S, Nichols MM (2008) In vivo and in vitro antibacterial efficacy of PDS plus (polidioxanone with triclosan) suture. Surgical Infections 9: 451–457.
13. Justinger C, Schuld J, Sperling J, Kollmar O, Richter S, et al. (2011) Triclosan-coated sutures reduce wound infections after hepatobiliary surgery—a prospective non-randomized clinical pathway driven study. Langenbeck's Archives of Surgery: 1–6.
14. Justinger C, Slotta JE, Ningel S, Gräber S, Kollmar O, et al. (2013) Surgical-site infection after abdominal wall closure with triclosan-impregnated polydioxanone sutures: Results of a randomized clinical pathway facilitated trial (NCT00998907). Surgery 154: 589–595.
15. Stone J, Gruber TJ, Rozzelle CJ (2010) Healthcare savings associated with reduced infection rates using antimicrobial suture wound closure for cerebrospinal fluid shunt procedures. Pediatr Neurosurg 46: 19–24.
16. Wang ZX, Jiang CP, Cao Y, Ding YT (2013) Systematic review and meta-analysis of triclosan-coated sutures for the prevention of surgical-site infection. British Journal of Surgery 100: 465–473.
17. Fujita T (2010) Antibiotic-coated surgical sutures against surgical site infection. Surgery 147: 464–465; author reply 465–466.
18. Chang WK, Srinivasa S, Morton R, Hill AG (2012) Triclosan-impregnated sutures to decrease surgical site infections: systematic review and meta-analysis of randomized trials. Ann Surg 255: 854–859.
19. Williams N, Sweetland H, Goyal S, Ivins N, Leaper DJ (2011) Randomized trial of antimicrobial-coated sutures to prevent surgical site infection after breast cancer surgery. Surgical Infections 12: 469–474.
20. Mingmalairak C, Ungbhakorn P, Paocharoen V (2009) Efficacy of antimicrobial coating suture coated polyglactin 910 with tricosan (Vicryl plus) compared with polyglactin 910 (Vicryl) in reduced surgical site infection of appendicitis, double blind randomized control trial, preliminary safety report. J Med Assoc Thai 92: 770–775.
21. Cooney CM (2010) Triclosan comes under scrutiny. Environ Health Perspect 118: A242.
22. Yazdankhah SP, Scheie AA, Hoiby EA, Lunestad BT, Heir E, et al. (2006) Triclosan and antimicrobial resistance in bacteria: an overview. Microbial drug resistance 12: 83–90.
23. Aiello AE, Larson EL, Levy SB (2007) Consumer antibacterial soaps: effective or just risky? Clin Infect Dis 45 Suppl 2: S137–147.
24. Segers P, Speekenbrink RG, Ubbink DT, van Ogtrop ML, de Mol BA (2006) Prevention of nosocomial infection in cardiac surgery by decontamination of the nasopharynx and oropharynx with chlorhexidine gluconate: a randomized controlled trial. JAMA 296: 2460–2466.
25. Rupp ME, Lisco SJ, Lipsett PA, Perl TM, Keating K, et al. (2005) Effect of a second-generation venous catheter impregnated with chlorhexidine and silver sulfadiazine on central catheter-related infections: a randomized, controlled trial. Ann Intern Med 143: 570–580.
26. Sanders D, Lambie J, Bond P, Moate R, Steer JA (2013) An in vitro study assessing the effect of mesh morphology and suture fixation on bacterial adherence. Hernia 17: 779–789.
27. Timsit JF, Mimoz O, Mourvillier B, Souweine B, Garrouste-Orgeas M, et al. (2012) Randomized controlled trial of chlorhexidine dressing and highly adhesive dressing for preventing catheter-related infections in critically ill adults. Am J Respir Crit Care Med 186: 1272–1278.
28. Menderes G, Athar Ali N, Aagaard K, Sangi-Haghpeykar H (2012) Chlorhexidine-alcohol compared with povidone-iodine for surgical-site antisepsis in cesarean deliveries. Obstet Gynecol 120: 1037–1044.
29. Suwanpimolkul G, Pongkumpai M, Suankratay C (2008) A randomized trial of 2% chlorhexidine tincture compared with 10% aqueous povidone-iodine for venipuncture site disinfection: Effects on blood culture contamination rates. J Infect 56: 354–359.
30. Hubner NO, Matthes R, Koban I, Randler C, Muller G, et al. (2010) Efficacy of chlorhexidine, polihexanide and tissue-tolerable plasma against Pseudomonas aeruginosa biofilms grown on polystyrene and silicone materials. Skin Pharmacology and Physiology 23 Suppl: 28–34.
31. Matl FD, Zlotnyk J, Obermeier A, Friess W, Vogt S, et al. (2009) New Anti-infective Coatings of Surgical Sutures Based on a Combination of Antiseptics and Fatty Acids. Journal of Biomaterials Science, Polymer Edition 20: 1439–1449.
32. Schierholz JM, Beuth J (2001) Implant infections: a haven for opportunistic bacteria. Journal of Hospital Infection 49: 87–93.
33. Weinstein RA, Darouiche RO (2001) Device-Associated Infections: A Macroproblem that Starts with Microadherence. Clinical Infectious Diseases 33: 1567–1572.
34. CLSI (2012) Methods for Dilution Antimicrobial Susceptibility Tests for Bacteria That Grow Aerobically; Approved Standard—Ninth Edition. CLSI document M07-A9 Clinical and Laboratory Standards Institute.
35. Ethicon (2010) Ihr zusätzlicher Schutz vor postoperativen Wundinfektionen, PLUS Nahtmaterial – ein neues Maβ an Sicherheit Brochures Plus sutures (B-nr 178). Norderstedt, Germany: Ethicon GmbH a Company of Johnson & Johnson.
36. Leaper D, Assadian O, Hubner N-O, McBain A, Barbolt T, et al. (2011) Antimicrobial sutures and prevention of surgical site infection: assessment of the safety of the antiseptic triclosan. International Wound Journal 8: 556–566.
37. Matl FD, Obermeier A, Repmann S, Friess W, Stemberger A, et al. (2008) New anti-infective coatings of medical implants. Antimicrob Agents Chemother 52: 1957–1963.
38. Obermeier A, Matl FD, Schwabe J, Zimmermann A, Kühn KD, et al. (2012) Novel fatty acid gentamicin salts as slow-release drug carrier systems for anti-infective protection of vascular biomaterials. J Mater Sci Mater Med 23: 1675–1683.

A Genetically Modified Protein-Based Hydrogel for 3D Culture of AD293 Cells

Xiao Du[1,2], Jingyu Wang[1,2], Wentao Diao[1,2], Ling Wang[1,3], Jiafu Long[1,2*], Hao Zhou[1,2*]

1 State Key Laboratory of Medicinal Chemical Biology, Nankai University, Tianjin, China, **2** College of Life Sciences, Nankai University, Tianjin, China, **3** College of Pharmacy, Nankai University, Tianjin, China

Abstract

Hydrogels have strong application prospects for drug delivery, tissue engineering and cell therapy because of their excellent biocompatibility and abundant availability as scaffolds for drugs and cells. In this study, we created hybrid hydrogels based on a genetically modified tax interactive protein-1 (TIP1) by introducing two or four cysteine residues in the primary structure of TIP1. The introduced cysteine residues were crosslinked with a four-armed poly (ethylene glycol) having their arm ends capped with maleimide residues (4-armed-PEG-Mal) to form hydrogels. In one form of the genetically modification, we incorporated a peptide sequence 'GRGDSP' to introduce bioactivity to the protein, and the resultant hydrogel could provide an excellent environment for a three dimensional cell culture of AD293 cells. The AD293 cells continued to divide and displayed a polyhedron or spindle-shape during the 3-day culture period. Besides, AD293 cells could be easily separated from the cell-gel constructs for future large-scale culture after being cultured for 3 days and treating hydrogel with trypsinase. This work significantly expands the toolbox of recombinant proteins for hydrogel formation, and we believe that our hydrogel will be of considerable interest to those working in cell therapy and controlled drug delivery.

Editor: Bing Xu, Brandeis University, United States of America

Funding: This work was partially supported by the National Natural Science Foundation of China (31370964 to LW, 31270815 to JL and 31100527 to HZ) and the Open Fund of State Key Laboratory of Medicinal Chemical Biology (20140211 to HZ). The funders had no role in study design, data collection and analysis, decision to publish, or preparation of the manuscript.

Competing Interests: The authors have declared that no competing interests exist.

* Email: haozhou@nankai.edu.cn (HZ); jflong@nankai.edu.cn (JL)

Introduction

By mimicking the biochemical and mechanical properties of native tissue, hydrogels possess hydrated networks of bioactive components [1], such as drugs, proteins, sugars and even cells, leading to contributions to the fields of controllable drug delivery [2,3], tissue engineering [4,5], cell culture [6,7], and others. Within our bodies, cells are known to receive and respond to signals from the crosstalk of extrinsic complexes by proteins, one of the essential building blocks [8]. Thus, protein-based hydrogels can not only provide excellent environments for the cells, but also respond to external stimuli. More and more researchers have focused on the promising applications of protein-based hydrogels, especially in the analytic detection [9,10] and three-dimensional cell culture [11,12]. In comparison with traditional 2D monolayer culture, 3D cell culture clearly approaches the natural physiological conditions of the cell. Besides, cell behaviors including migration, morphology and differentiation can be tailored by the exquisite design of the proteins according to the primary amino acid sequence, which makes protein-based biomaterials stand out among this class of materials [13]. For example, cells exhibit expansion and adhesion in gels by integrating adhesive peptide modules such as RGDS and REDV [14].

Moreover, proteins usually serve as cross-linkers via covalent (Michael addition [15,16], enzyme reaction [17] or site selective conjugation [18,19]) or non-covalent interactions (specific protein-peptide [20], protein-protein [21,22] or protein-polysaccharide interactions [23]) in protein-based hydrogels, which require them to have multiple binding sites to their ligands. Some specific amino acid side chain groups such as the lysine's ε-amine and cysteine's sulphydryl endow favourable targets for cross-linking reactions [24,25].

Recently, Yang's group reported a novel biohybrid hydrogel containing a polymer of 4-armed-PEG-Mal and tetrameric recombinant protein (ULD) for 3D cell culture of NIH 3T3 [11]. In their gel, the cysteines required for hydrogel formation was inherent and exactly coincided at the outer surface of the protein. However, there are no endogenous cysteines available for bioconjugation to the polymers or peptides of many proteins, or the cysteines hide in the inner part of the proteins. Such cases are surely limiting the range of proteins that can be chosen for hydrogel formation and subsequent applications. In order to overcome that problem,we rationally replaced two or four amino acids with cysteine in TIP1 with no inherent cysteines [26] according to its crystal structure and used rheology and SEM to characterise the corresponding hydrogels that were formed by thiol-maleimide reaction. We also incorporated a bioactive peptide, GRGDSP, at the C-terminus of TIP1 2C and uncovered its roles in cell spreading and proliferation in the gel by Live-dead assay and CCK-8 assay.

Materials and Methods

Materials

All molecular cloning reagents were obtained from TIANGEN (Beijing, China). The chemical reagents used for protein purification were obtained from VETEC (Sigma, USA). Maleimide-end-capped four-armed poly (ethylene glycol) was purchased from Laysan Bio (Arab, AL). AD293 (Adeno-X 293) cells were purchased from Clontech (Takara, Japan). Dulbecco's Modified Eagle Medium and fetal bovine serum (FBS) were purchased from GIBCO (Life Technologies, USA) and Hyclone (Thermal Scientific, USA), respectively. Trypsinase (0.25%) + EDTA and penicillin/streptomycin were purchased from Invitrogen (Life Technologies, USA). The Live/Dead Viability Kit was purchased from Invitrogen (Life Technologies, USA). The Cell Counting Kit-8 was obtained from Beyotime (Jiangsu, China). All other commercial chemicals were of reagent grade or better. Ultrapure water was used for all experiments.

Protein expression and purification

The mutated DNA fragment (TIP1 4C, TIP1 2C or TIP1 2C RGD) was first amplified by polymerase chain reaction (PCR) by using the DNA fragment of wild type human TIP1 as the template along with the corresponding mutated primers (Table S1), then the PCR products were ligated into an in-house modification of the pET32a (Novagen) vector. After transformation and screening for the positive clones, the plasmids were extracted for the next protein expression. The Trx-His_6-tag was contained in the resulting proteins' N-termini.

BL21(DE3) *Escherichia coli* cells were cultured in LB medium (10 g/L NaCl, 10 g/L tryptone, 5 g/L yeast extract) at 37°C until the OD_{600} reached 0.6, and then a final concentration of 0.3 mM isopropyl-β-D-thiogalactoside was added to induce protein expression at 16°C for approximately 16 hours. After being centrifuged at 5,000 rpm for 15 minutes, the supernatant was removed and the *Escherichia coli* cells were resuspended in binding buffer (50 mM Tris-HCl, pH 8.0, 200 mM NaCl and 5 mM imidazole). The cells were then lysed by AH-1500 (ATS Engineering Limited) and the lysates were centrifuged at 18,000 rpm for 30 minutes. The supernatant was loaded onto a Ni-NTA-Agarose column that was equilibrated with binding buffer. The Trx-his_6-tagged proteins were eluted with elution buffer (50 mM Tris-HCl, pH 8.0, 200 mM NaCl and 500 mM imidazole). The eluted proteins were then purified by HiLoad 26/60 Superdex 200 column (GE Healthcare) in $T_{50}N_{200}$ buffer (50 mM Tris-HCl, pH 8.0, and 200 mM NaCl). After identifying the protein peak by SDS-PAGE gel, the Trx-his_6-tagged target protein was collected and then the N-terminal Trx-His_6-tag was cleaved overnight with PreScission Protease. The digested protein was passed through a HisTrap HP column (GE Healthcare) to remove the protease and tag. Finally, the target protein was loaded onto a HiLoad 26/60 Superdex 200 size exclusion column and eluted with PBS buffer (NaCl 137 mmol/L, KCl 2.7 mmol/L, Na_2HPO_4 4.3 mmol/L, and KH_2PO_4 1.4 mmol/L, pH 7.4). A Superose 12 10/300 column (GE Healthcare) was used to identify the conformation of the final proteins with different concentrations. By following the above procedure, we acquired the TIP1 4C (T10C, S42C, S101C and S113C), TIP1 2C (S101C and S113C) and TIP1 2C RGD proteins (by incorporating the bioactive peptide GRGDSP into the C-terminus of TIP1 2C).

Hydrogel formation

80 mg/ml of 4-armed-PEG-Mal in PBS buffer and 40 mg/ml of protein TIP1 4C (TIP1 2C or TIP1 2C RGD) in PBS buffer were prepared as stock solutions. For the TIP1 4C gel, 100 μL of PBS buffer and 100 μL of 4-armed-PEG-Mal stock solution were added to 200 μL of TIP1 4C stock solution. A gel of the desired concentration was formed immediately after being kept at room temperature (both final concentrations of the 4-armed-PEG-Mal and the protein in the gel were 2.0 wt%). Other protein-based hydrogels were also formed by this method.

Rheology

A rheology test was performed on an AR 2000ex system (TA instrument). A 40 mm parallel plate was used with a 400 μm gap during the experiment. For the dynamic time sweep, 250 μL of PBS buffer, 250 μL of 4-armed-PEG-Mal stock solution and 500 μL of protein stock solution were directly transferred onto the rheometer and then analysed at the frequency of 1 rad/s and the strain of 1%. The dynamic strain sweep was performed in the 0.1%–10% region at a frequency of 1 rad/s and the strain value in the linear range was chosen for the following dynamic frequency sweep. The gel was also characterised by the dynamic frequency sweep in the 0.1–100 rad/s region at the strain of 1%.

Scanning electron microscopy (SEM)

A thin layer of hydrogel was cast on a silica wafer that was cleaned by sonication in ethanol for 10 minutes and then freeze-dried in a lyophiliser overnight. A layer of gold was spluttered on the sample by vacuum spray to produce a conductive surface. The SEM analysis was conducted on a Hitachi X650 system (Japan) operating at 15 kV.

3D Cell culture

AD293 cells were used in this study. The cells were cultured in complete Dulbecco's Modified Eagle Medium (DMEM) supplemented with 10% fetal bovine serum, 100 units/mL penicillin, and 100 μg/mL streptomycin. Before hydrogel formation, 4-armed-PEG-Mal powder and syringe filters with 0.22 μm apertures were sterilized by UV light on a superclean worktable for 60 minutes, and PBS buffer and protein were then filtered by using the above filters. The cells were separated by trypsinase (0.25%) digestion, followed by centrifugation at 800 rpm for 5 minutes and resuspended in DMEM plus 10% FBS and 1% penicillin/streptomycin. 4-armed-PEG-Mal and cells (the final cell density was 1,000,000 cells/ml hydrogel) in 25 μL of DMEM medium was mixed with an equal volume of protein and then transferred to 96-well plates (50 μL of gel per well). Half an hour later, 100 μL of DMEM medium was added to the top of the hydrogel. The 96-well plate was maintained in a 37°C/5% CO_2 incubator.

Live-dead assay

The viability of encapsulated cells was tested with a live-dead assay at designated times. The cell-gel constructs were washed three times with PBS buffer for the purpose of buffer exchange. After removing the PBS buffer for the last time, 100 μL of live/dead solution containing 4 μM EthD-1 (ethidium homodimer-1) and 2 μM calcein AM was added onto each cell-gel construct. After 30 minutes of incubation at 37°C with 5% CO_2, the staining solution was removed. The constructs were observed by using a Nikon Eclipse TE2000-U inverted fluorescence microscope with excitation filters of 450–490 nm (green, calcein AM) and 510–560 nm (red, EthD-1). The confocal analysis was performed on a Leica TSC SP8 system (Germany).

CCK-8 assay

A CCK-8 assay was performed to quantify cell proliferation in the cell-gel constructs at designated time points. After a 3D culture had been established using the above standard procedure, each cell-gel construct was washed with complete cell culture medium three times and mixed with 100 μL of 10% CCK-8 agent (v/v) in serum-free DMEM. The plates were incubated in a 37°C/5% CO_2 incubator for 4 hours. The absorbance at 450 nm was measured by microplate reader (MultiskaniMark, Bio-Rad, USA). The experiment was performed five times and the SD was then determined.

Cell Recovery

To identify the growth state of AD293 cells that were separated from TIP1 2C RGD gel, we separated the cells from the cell-gel construct by trypsinase digestion. Trypsinase was added onto the gel after 3 days of 3D culture. After incubating for 5 minutes at 37°C, the resulting solution was transferred into an Eppendorf tube and centrifuged for 5 minutes at room temperature at 800 rpm. The supernatant was discarded and 200 μL of the complete cell culture medium was used to resuspend the cells. The individual collected cells were counted and reseeded on a conventional 96-well culture plate at a density of 10,000 cells/well. The cells were observed at 2 days post culture by ordinary inverted microscope.

Results

Protein purification and hydrogel preparation

The protein used for hydrogel formation should be easily purified and have an impressively high yield, such as that of TIP1 [26]. After ensuring that no endogenous cysteine was present and analysing the protein's crystal structure [26], we genetically modified four amino acids to cysteine at the outer surface (T10C, S42C, S101C and S113C) for further hydrogelation (Figure 1). The TIP1 4C protein yield was comparable to that of TIP1; however, if the purified TIP1 4C (Figure S1) was placed at room temperature for approximately 15 minutes, it was unstable and it precipitated, especially when TIP1 4C was present at a high concentration (approximately 10 mg/ml). We also acquired the TIP1 2C (S101C and S113C) gene by employing the above molecular cloning process. When compared with TIP1 4C, TIP1 2C (Figure 2) had better stability at a high concentration (even at approximately 20 mg/ml) because it had fewer thiols in its monomer. To promote cell spreading, we genetically modified a hydrophilic peptide called GRGDSP to the C-terminus of the TIP1 2C protein and the purification of TIP1 2C RGD was shown in Figure S2.

The thiols on the outer surface of genetically mutated TIP1 could react with maleimided PEG by Michael addition [16], as indicated by the high molecular weight polymer in the SDS-PAGE gel (Figure S3), thus leading to hydrogel formation. If we adjusted the final concentration of 4-armed-PEG-Mal to 2.0 wt%, the minimum final concentration of TIP1 4C required for hydrogelation was 0.5 wt%. Upon mixing two solutions of 4-armed-PEG-Mal and TIP1 4C (the final concentration of both components was 2.0 wt%), the TIP1 4C gel was formed rapidly and became turbid after 5 minutes (Figure 3A). Such phase separation indicated it was not suitable for future characterisation and 3D cell culture. The mechanism of TIP1 2C gel formation is similar to that of TIP1 4C gel, and the minimum final concentration of TIP1 2C needed for hydrogel formation was 1.0 wt%. TIP1 2C gel (the final selected concentration of both components was 2.0 wt%) could still stay transparent after 24 hours (Figure 3B), which ensured its promising application in 3D cell culture. TIP1 2C RGD gel exhibited the same characteristics on the minimum final concentration for hydrogelation and appearance (Figure 3C). Besides, If we separately mixed PEG and the above proteins pre-treated with small molecule maleimide (the final concentration of both components was 2.0 wt%), none of them formed hydrogel (Figure S4).

Hydrogel characterization by rheological measurement and scanning electron microscopy

We used rheological measurements to study the kinetics of TIP1 2C gel and TIP1 2C RGD gel containing 2.0 wt% of 4-armed-PEG-Mal and 2.0 wt% of the corresponding proteins, respectively. A dynamic strain sweep at a frequency of 1 rad/s was first performed to set the strain value for the following sweeps (Figure S5). As shown in Figure S6, a dynamic time sweep was then performed at the strain of 1% and the frequency of 1 rad/s. Two types of gels formed rapidly, as indicated by the elasticity (G') values dominating the viscosity (G") values right after mixing the components. The G' values kept slowly increasing and reached a plateau at 1,200 seconds. The final G' values of the gels were approximately 210 Pa and 120 Pa for the TIP1 2C and TIP1 2C RGD gels, respectively. Followed by the dynamic time sweep, the dynamic frequency sweep was conducted at the strain of 1% (Figure 4A). The G' values were almost invariant as the frequency increased, and the G" values were apparently rising from 10–100 rad/s. Moreover, the G' value in the TIP1 2C gel was more than that of the TIP1 2C RGD gel, which implied a weaker hydrogel for the TIP1 2C RGD gel.

Scanning electron microscopy (SEM) provided useful information about the microstructure of freeze-dried hydrogels [27]. Similar to other reports about protein-based hydrogel, both gels in this study possessed a 3D loose and porous structure (Figure 4B and 4C). The pores were approximately 11.5 μm in the TIP1 2C gel, and they were bigger in the TIP1 2C RGD gel at 16.5 μm. These pores interlaced with one another to form three dimensional networks.

3D cell culture and the determination of cell viability and proliferation

We then investigated whether the TIP1 2C gel or the TIP1 2C RGD gel was suitable for 3D cell culture. A DMEM solution containing 1,000,000 cells/ml and 2.0 wt% of 4-armed-PEG-Mal was mixed into PBS solution containing 2.0 wt% of TIP1 2C or TIP1 2C RGD. The mixing-induced hydrogelation process was convenient and rapid, which guaranteed the homogeneous encapsulation of AD293 cells, as demonstrated by the confocal assay (Figure S7). We performed a live-dead assay to determine the cell viability of the gels. Most of the AD293 cells were alive during the 3-day culture period, as indicated by the cells that were stained green, and the dead cells exhibited a red colour (Figure 5). More importantly, cells cultured in the TIP1 2C RGD gel were spreading, polyhedral or spindle-shaped relative to the TIP1 2C gel with cell clusters. The cell densities of both gels kept rising over the 3-day culture period. We quantified the cell proliferation by using a CCK-8 assay. As shown in Figure S8, the number of metabolically active cells persistently increased over the 3-day culture period in TIP1 2C gel. The optical density (OD) in this gel was 1.33, 1.57 and 1.76 at days 1, 2 and 3, respectively. A similar trend was observed in TIP1 2C RGD gel.

TIP1 2C RGD gel could be converted into a clear solution by treating with trypsinase at 37°C for 5 minutes. Therefore, we were able to recovery the AD293 cells after 3 days of culture in gel by

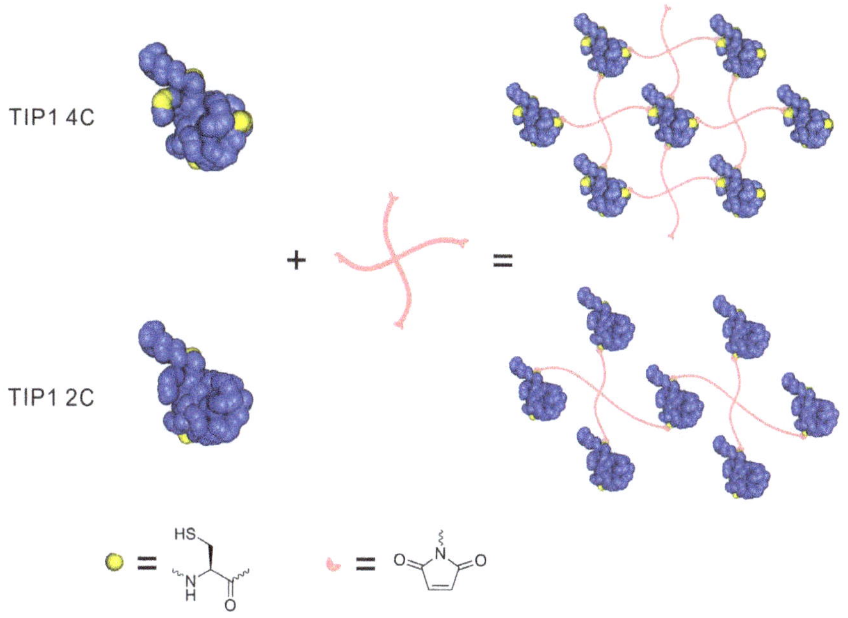

Figure 1. A schematic diagram of hydrogel formation. The Michael addition between maleimides of 4-armed-PEG-Mal and thiols in each mutant protein leads to the formation of 3D networks for hydrogelations. The blue balls represent TIP1 protein. The yellow balls represent amino acids that were replaced by cysteine in TIP1. The pink lines represent 4-armed-PEG-Mal.

trypsinase digestion and centrifugation. The cells that were separated from the cell-gel construct following the above method grew well on normal 96-well culture plates (Figure S9).

Discussion

The Michael addition is attractive for cell encapsulation because of its mildness and close approximation of physiological conditions [28,29]. PEG, which has been conjugated to various proteins to form a hydrogel scaffold, is the most widely used polymer in tissue engineering [30,31]. Among the genetically modified proteins we used, TIP1 4C was unstable, which may have been caused by intermolecular aggregation through nonspecific disulfide bond formation. Although the two mutated serines in TIP1 2C were close to each other in the primary structure, there still existed a certain distance between them in the tertiary structure [26]. Fewer

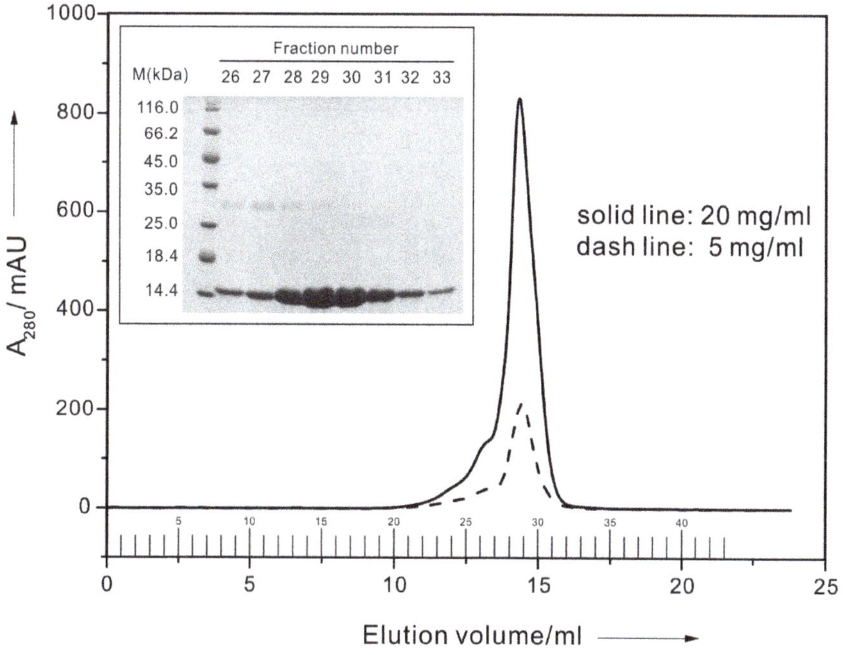

Figure 2. The purification of TIP1 2C. The size-exclusion chromatography of TIP1 2C was performed in a Superose 12 10/300 at two concentrations. Inset: A 20% SDS-PAGE gel result for each fraction.

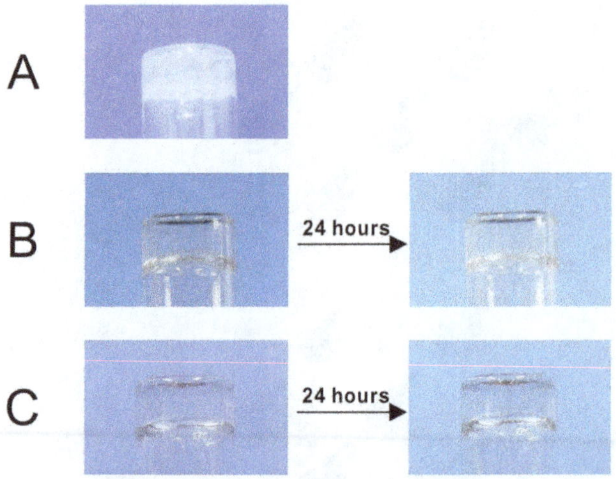

Figure 3. Hydrogel formation and stability. Optical images of three resulting hydrogels formed by 2.0 wt% of 4-armed-PEG-Mal and 2.0 wt% of the corresponding protein. A, TIP1 4C gel; B, TIP1 2C gel; and C, TIP1 2C RGD gel. Both TIP1 2C gel and TIP1 2C RGD gel remained transparent after 24 hours.

cysteines in the protein oligomer rendered more stability to its corresponding hydrogel, which ensured promising applications such as 3D cell culture. Therefore, rationally designing the mutated sites based on the protein structure is crucial.

A suitable mechanical property is essential to the hydrogel for cell culture. Both TIP1 2C and TIP1 2C RGD gels exhibited frequency dependence and weak mechanical properties, which was a universality of protein-based hydrogels [32]. However, these gels exhibited an apparent difference in 3D cell culture. The noticeable difference between the two gels was related to the modified RGD active peptide. Thus far, peptide ligands that promote cell adhesion [33,34] or are sensitive to matrix metalloproteinase cleavage [35,36] have been used extensively to render hydrogels with new features.

Furthermore, when compared with the two gels we used in the CCK-8 assay, the higher OD values in the TIP1 2C RGD gel suggested that incorporating the RGD peptide could partly improve the property of the hydrogel for cell proliferation, adhesion and spreading, which was in accordance with the live-dead assay result. As a result of protein degradation and hydrogel erosion after 3 days of culture, cell recovery should be performed at an appropriate time.

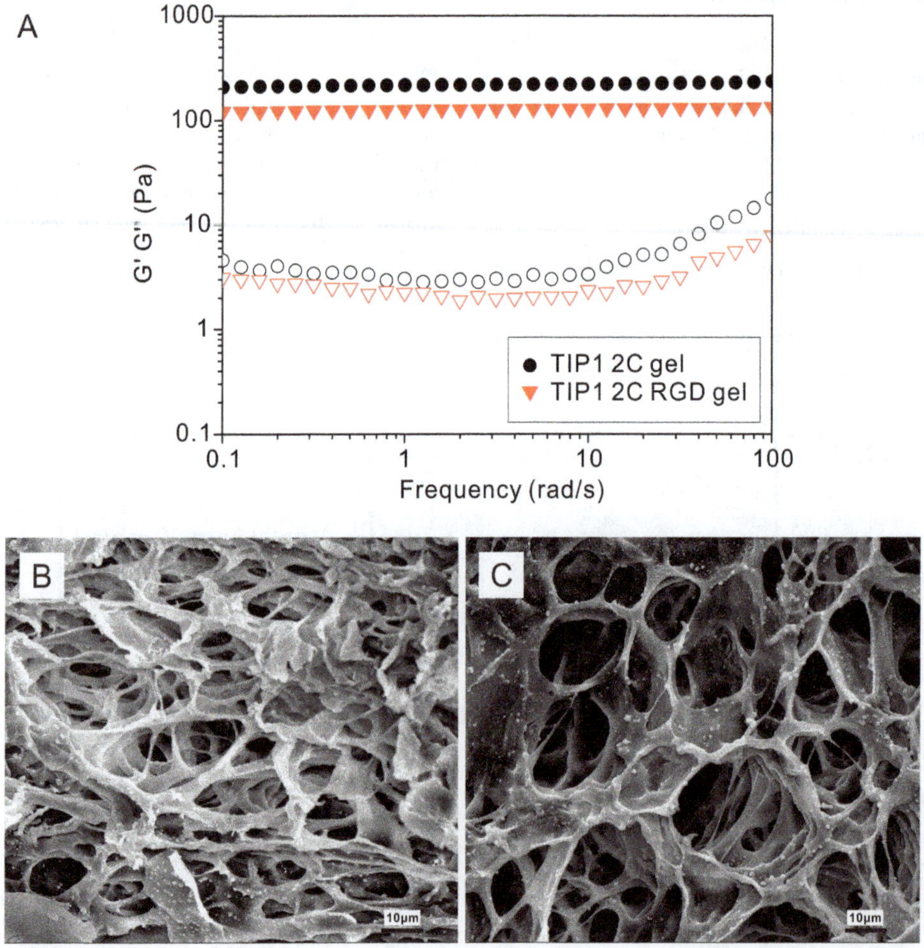

Figure 4. Hydrogel characterization. A, A rheological measurement in dynamic frequency sweep mode at the strain of 1% for each gel containing 2.0 wt% of 4-armed-PEG-Mal and 2.0 wt% of the protein. Closed symbols: elasticity (G') values and open symbols: viscosity (G'') values. Circles: TIP1 2C gel and triangles: TIP1 2C RGD gel. B, An SEM image of the TIP1 2C gel. C, An SEM image of the TIP1 2C RGD gel.

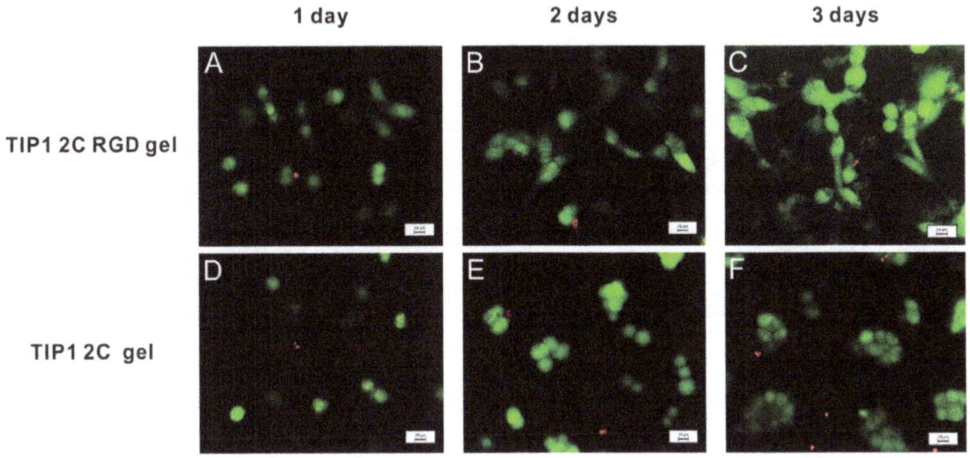

Figure 5. Determining cell viability. A live-dead assay of AD293 cells cultured in TIP1 2C RGD (top) and TIP1 2C (down) hydrogels at different time points. A and D, day 1; B and E, day 2; and C and F, day 3. Live cells were stained green and dead cells were stained red. Magnification: 20×.

Conclusions

In summary, we have successfully produced in situ gelating hybrid hydrogels composed of genetically modified recombinant proteins and 4-armed-PEG-Mal. Although the AD293 cells continuously divided over the 3-day culture period in the both TIP1 2C and TIP1 2C RGD gels, they displayed a spreading morphology in the latter one, which demonstrated that the TIP1 2C RGD gel could provide an excellent and biocompatible microenvironment for the 3D cell culture of AD293 cells. The cells that were recovered from the TIP1 2C RGD gel grew well in the conventional 2D cell culture, suggesting its great potential for large-scale culture. We anticipated that this hydrogel would have broad applications in many areas, such as the delivery of cells for cell therapy, controlled drug delivery, and tissue engineering, which was studied in the next step.

Supporting Information

Figure S1 The purification of TIP1 4C. The size-exclusion chromatography of TIP1 4C was performed in a Superose 12 10/300 at two concentrations. Inset: A 20% SDS-PAGE gel result for each fraction.

Figure S2 The purification of TIP1 2C RGD. The size-exclusion chromatography of TIP1 2C RGD was performed in a Superose 12 10/300 at two concentrations. Inset: A 20% SDS-PAGE gel result for each fraction.

Figure S3 Identifying the Michael addition reaction. A 20% SDS-PAGE gel result for purified proteins and their corresponding hydrogels.

Figure S4 Hydrogel formation test. Optical images of three mixtures containing PEG and corresponding proteins pre-treated with small molecule maleimide. A, TIP1 4C; B, TIP1 2C; and C, TIP1 2C RGD.

Figure S5 A dynamic strain sweep of the gels. A rheological measurement in dynamic strain sweep mode at the frequency of 1 rad/s for each gel containing 2.0 wt% of 4-armed-PEG-Mal and 2.0 wt% of the protein. Closed symbols: elasticity (G') values and open symbols: viscosity (G'') values. Circles: TIP1 2C gel and triangles: TIP1 2C RGD gel.

Figure S6 A dynamic time sweep of the gels. A rheological measurement in dynamic time sweep mode at the frequency of 1 rad/s and the strain of 1% for each gel containing 2.0 wt% of 4-armed-PEG-Mal and 2.0 wt% of the protein. Closed symbols: elasticity (G') values and open symbols: viscosity (G'') values. Circles: TIP1 2C gel and triangles: TIP1 2C RGD gel.

Figure S7 The cell distribution in both gels. Confocal images of 3D cell cultures in the hydrogels at day 1. Cells were distributed evenly in both gels. A, TIP1 2C gel and B, TIP1 2C RGD gel.

Figure S8 Determining cell proliferation. The cell proliferation rate of AD293 was evaluated by CCK-8 assay. Two asterisks (**) indicate a p value smaller than 0.01 ($p<0.01$). Three asterisks (***) indicate a p value smaller than 0.001 ($p<0.001$), $n=5$.

Figure S9 Cell Recovery. A, 200 μL of the TIP1 2C RGD gel was treated with 100 μL of trypsinase (2.5 μg/mL) for 5 minutes, and then 200 μL of PBS was added. B, The solution was then centrifuged at 1000 rpm for 5 minutes and no precipitation was observed. C, The AD293 cells were separated from the cell-gel construct by adding trypsinase and then centrifuging. The cells could grow well on a conventional 96-well culture plate.

Table S1 The primers used for mutations in this study. The restriction sites are underlined.

Author Contributions

Conceived and designed the experiments: XD LW HZ. Performed the experiments: XD JW WD. Analyzed the data: XD WD. Contributed reagents/materials/analysis tools: XD JW. Contributed to the writing of the manuscript: XD JL HZ.

References

1. Kopecek J (2007) Hydrogel biomaterials: a smart future? Biomaterials 28: 5185–5192.
2. Branco MC, Pochan DJ, Wagner NJ, Schneider JP (2010) The effect of protein structure on their controlled release from an injectable peptide hydrogel. Biomaterials 31: 9527–9534.
3. Yang C, Li D, Fengzhao Q, Wang L, Yang Z (2013) Disulfide bond reduction-triggered molecular hydrogels of folic acid-Taxol conjugates. Org Biomol Chem 11: 6946–6951.
4. Drury JL, Mooney DJ (2003) Hydrogels for tissue engineering: scaffold design variables and applications. Biomaterials 24: 4337–4351.
5. Nicodemus GD, Bryant SJ (2008) Cell encapsulation in biodegradable hydrogels for tissue engineering applications. Tissue Eng Part B Rev 14: 149–165.
6. Lv L, Liu H, Chen X, Yang Z (2013) Glutathione-triggered formation of molecular hydrogels for 3D cell culture. Colloids Surf B Biointerfaces 108: 352–357.
7. Yang C, Li D, Liu Z, Hong G, Zhang J, et al. (2012) Responsive small molecular hydrogels based on adamantane-peptides for cell culture. J Phys Chem B 116: 633–638.
8. Yu D, Kim M, Xiao G, Hwang TH (2013) Review of Biological Network Data and Its Applications. Genomics Inform 11: 200–210.
9. Wang H, Liu J, Han A, Xiao N, Xue Z, et al. (2014) Self-Assembly-Induced Far-Red/Near-Infrared Fluorescence Light-Up for Detecting and Visualizing Specific Protein-Peptide Interactions. ACS Nano 8: 1475–1484.
10. Gu Z, Zhao M, Sheng Y, Bentolila LA, Tang Y (2011) Detection of mercury ion by infrared fluorescent protein and its hydrogel-based paper assay. Anal Chem 83: 2324–2329.
11. Wang H, Han A, Cai Y, Xie Y, Zhou H, et al. (2013) Multifunctional biohybrid hydrogels for cell culture and controlled drug release. Chem Commun (Camb) 49: 7448–7450.
12. Wang J, Zhang J, Zhang X, Zhou H (2013) A protein-based hydrogel for in vitro expansion of mesenchymal stem cells. PLoS One 8: e75727.
13. Sengupta D, Heilshorn SC (2010) Protein-engineered biomaterials: highly tunable tissue engineering scaffolds. Tissue Eng Part B Rev 16: 285–293.
14. Liu JC, Heilshorn SC, Tirrell DA (2004) Comparative cell response to artificial extracellular matrix proteins containing the RGD and CS5 cell-binding domains. Biomacromolecules 5: 497–504.
15. Yuan W, Yang J, Kopeckova P, Kopecek J (2008) Smart hydrogels containing adenylate kinase: translating substrate recognition into macroscopic motion. J Am Chem Soc 130: 15760–15761.
16. Sui ZJ, King WJ, Murphy WL (2007) Dynamic materials based on a protein conformational change. Advanced Materials 19: 3377–3380.
17. Mosiewicz KA, Johnsson K, Lutolf MP (2010) Phosphopantetheinyl transferase-catalyzed formation of bioactive hydrogels for tissue engineering. J Am Chem Soc 132: 5972–5974.
18. Esser-Kahn AP, Iavarone AT, Francis MB (2008) Metallothionein-cross-linked hydrogels for the selective removal of heavy metals from water. J Am Chem Soc 130: 15820–15822.
19. Esser-Kahn AP, Francis MB (2008) Protein-cross-linked polymeric materials through site-selective bioconjugation. Angew Chem Int Ed Engl 47: 3751–3754.
20. Zhang X, Chu X, Wang L, Wang H, Liang G, et al. (2012) Rational design of a tetrameric protein to enhance interactions between self-assembled fibers gives molecular hydrogels. Angew Chem Int Ed Engl 51: 4388–4392.
21. Wong Po Foo CT, Lee JS, Mulyasasmita W, Parisi-Amon A, Heilshorn SC (2009) Two-component protein-engineered physical hydrogels for cell encapsulation. Proc Natl Acad Sci U S A 106: 22067–22072.
22. DiMarco RL, Heilshorn SC (2012) Multifunctional materials through modular protein engineering. Advanced Materials 24: 3923–3940.
23. Yamaguchi N, Zhang L, Chae BS, Palla CS, Furst EM, et al. (2007) Growth factor mediated assembly of cell receptor-responsive hydrogels. J Am Chem Soc 129: 3040–3041.
24. Straley KS, Heilshorn SC (2009) Independent tuning of multiple biomaterial properties using protein engineering. Soft Matter 5: 114–124.
25. Lim DW, Nettles DL, Setton LA, Chilkoti A (2007) Rapid cross-linking of elastin-like polypeptides with (hydroxymethyl)phosphines in aqueous solution. Biomacromolecules 8: 1463–1470.
26. Yan X, Zhou H, Zhang J, Shi C, Xie X, et al. (2009) Molecular mechanism of inward rectifier potassium channel 2.3 regulation by tax-interacting protein-1. J Mol Biol 392: 967–976.
27. Wang H, Yang Z (2012) Short-peptide-based molecular hydrogels: novel gelation strategies and applications for tissue engineering and drug delivery. Nanoscale 4: 5259–5267.
28. Hoyle CE, Bowman CN (2010) Thiol-Ene Click Chemistry. Angewandte Chemie-International Edition 49: 1540–1573.
29. Mather BD, Viswanathan K, Miller KM, Long TE (2006) Michael addition reactions in macromolecular design for emerging technologies. Progress in Polymer Science 31: 487–531.
30. Almany L, Seliktar D (2005) Biosynthetic hydrogel scaffolds made from fibrinogen and polyethylene glycol for 3D cell cultures. Biomaterials 26: 2467–2477.
31. Gonen-Wadmany M, Oss-Ronen L, Seliktar D (2007) Protein-polymer conjugates for forming photopolymerizable biomimetic hydrogels for tissue engineering. Biomaterials 28: 3876–3886.
32. Grove TZ, Osuji CO, Forster JD, Dufresne ER, Regan L (2010) Stimuli-responsive smart gels realized via modular protein design. J Am Chem Soc 132: 14024–14026.
33. Chien HW, Tsai WB, Jiang SY (2012) Direct cell encapsulation in biodegradable and functionalizable carboxybetaine hydrogels. Biomaterials 33: 5706–5712.
34. Zhu JM, He P, Lin L, Jones DR, Marchant RE (2012) Biomimetic Poly(ethylene glycol)-Based Hydrogels as Scaffolds for Inducing Endothelial Adhesion and Capillary-Like Network Formation. Biomacromolecules 13: 706–713.
35. Lutolf MP, Lauer-Fields JL, Schmoekel HG, Metters AT, Weber FE, et al. (2003) Synthetic matrix metalloproteinase-sensitive hydrogels for the conduction of tissue regeneration: Engineering cell-invasion characteristics. Proc Natl Acad Sci U S A 100: 5413–5418.
36. Bahney CS, Hsu CW, Yoo JU, West JL, Johnstone B (2011) A bioresponsive hydrogel tuned to chondrogenesis of human mesenchymal stem cells. Faseb Journal 25: 1486–1496.

20

In Vitro and *In Vivo* Evaluation of a Hydrogel Reservoir as a Continuous Drug Delivery System for Inner Ear Treatment

Mareike Hütten[1,2], Anandhan Dhanasingh[3,4], Roland Hessler[3], Timo Stöver[5], Karl-Heinz Esser[2], Martin Möller[4], Thomas Lenarz[1], Claude Jolly[3], Jürgen Groll[4,6]*, Verena Scheper[1,7]*

1 Department of Otolaryngology, Hannover School of Medicine, Hannover, Germany, **2** University of Veterinary Medicine Hannover, Foundation, Institute of Zoology, Hannover, Germany, **3** MED-EL Innsbruck, Research & Development, Innsbruck, Österreich, **4** Interactive Materials Research–DWI e.V. and Institute of Technical and Macromolecular Chemistry, RWTH Aachen University, Aachen, Germany, **5** J.W. Goethe University Hospital and Faculty of Medicine, Department of Otolaryngology, Frankfurt am Main, Germany, **6** University of Würzburg, Department of Functional Materials in Medicine and Dentistry, Würzburg, Germany, **7** Institute of Audioneurotechnology, Hannover School of Medicine, Hannover, Germany

Abstract

Fibrous tissue growth and loss of residual hearing after cochlear implantation can be reduced by application of the glucocorticoid dexamethasone-21-phosphate-disodium-salt (DEX). To date, sustained delivery of this agent to the cochlea using a number of pharmaceutical technologies has not been entirely successful. In this study we examine a novel way of continuous local drug application into the inner ear using a refillable hydrogel functionalized silicone reservoir. A PEG-based hydrogel made of reactive NCO-sP(EO-*stat*-PO) prepolymers was evaluated as a drug conveying and delivery system *in vitro* and *in vivo*. Encapsulating the free form hydrogel into a silicone tube with a small opening for the drug diffusion resulted in delayed drug release but unaffected diffusion of DEX through the gel compared to the free form hydrogel. Additionally, controlled DEX release over several weeks could be demonstrated using the hydrogel filled reservoir. Using a guinea-pig cochlear trauma model the reservoir delivery of DEX significantly protected residual hearing and reduced fibrosis. As well as being used as a device in its own right or in combination with cochlear implants, the hydrogel-filled reservoir represents a new drug delivery system that feasibly could be replenished with therapeutic agents to provide sustained treatment of the inner ear.

Editor: Bernd Sokolowski, University of South Florida, United States of America

Funding: This study was supported by the DFG within the SPP 1259 "Intelligent hydrogels" (RWTH Aachen) and the European Community 6th Framework Programme on Research, Technological Development and Demonstration (Nanotechnology based Drug Delivery. Contract Number: NMP4-CT-2006-026556, Project acronym: NANOEAR; Hannover Medical School, MED-EL, RWTH Aachen). The funders had no role in study design, data collection and analysis, decision to publish, or preparation of the manuscript.

Competing Interests: The data and results presented within this manuscript are in total obtained with MEDEL as a research partner having no financial interest on the outcome of the study. No products exactly comparable to the one used in this study will be released to the market. AD, RH and CJ are employed by MED-EL Corporation.

* Email: juergen.groll@fmz.uni-wuerzburg.de (JG); scheper.verena@mh-hannover.de (VS)

These authors contributed equally to this work.

Introduction

Hearing loss affects approximately 278 million people worldwide. Next to infectious causes like meningitis, measles, mumps and chronic ear infections, hearing impairment is commonly triggered by exposure to excessive noise, head and ear injury, ageing and the use of ototoxic drugs [1]. Since sensory cells of the inner ear develop exclusively during embryogenesis and are not programmed to regenerate postnatally in mammals [2], in many cases hearing ability can only be regained by the insertion of a cochlear implant (CI) [3].

After CI surgery the acuity of residual hearing and that of CI-mediated hearing are often affected by postoperative intra-cochlear fibroblast growth and a delayed degeneration of neuronal tissue. A histological evaluation of human temporal bones from cochlear implant patients showed fibrous growth formation in 57% of examined cases. The fibrous growth formation were believed to be as a result of intra-cochlear mechanical trauma to the fine structures caused by electrode insertion as well as a foreign body reaction of the host tissue to the implant [4]. As a consequence, increased impedance, reduced speech perception and functional derogation of the device itself may take place [5].

Locally applied glucocorticoid receptor agonists like dexamethasone suppress inflammation in the inner ear and consequently prohibit growth of fibrosis related connective tissue expanse, cell degeneration and loss of residual hearing [6,7]. Due to the relative difficulty in accessing the inner ear, the maintenance of sufficient therapeutic levels of this agent over a prolonged period has been problematic. Available application aids like pump systems and intra-cochlear electrode array loaded with dexamethasone have limited delivery duration, are not rechargeable and/or have to be detached after entirely emitting the drug (reviewed by [8]). Polyethylene glycol (PEG) based hydrogels are one of the widely studied biomaterial as tissue culture scaffold and as drug loading and delivery system [9–11]. Briefly, hydrogels are three dimensionally cross-linked hydrophilic polymer chains that exhibit strong swelling in water and available as degradable or non-degradable depending on the polymer chain chemistry [12]. Non-degradable hydrogel in the free form state loaded with any water soluble low molecular weight drug molecules will be diffused out completely within 24–48 hours depending on how big is the volume of release medium. For the delayed release of drug for at least 4 week time for inner ear treatment, the drug loaded hydrogel has to be physically restricted from release medium which can be achieved by incorporating the drug loaded hydrogel within the thin electrode array. The electrical impedance of the CI which is a hint of fibrous tissue growth is largely taking place in the first 4 weeks of implantation [13].

We have previously shown that six-arm star shaped poly-(ethylene oxide-*stat*-propylene oxide) prepolymers with 80% ethylene oxide (EO) content in the backbone and reactive isocyanate groups at the distal ends of the arms (NCO-sP(EO-stat-PO) can be used to prepare ultra-thin biocompatible coatings that very efficiently minimize unspecific protein adsorption [14]. We have also shown that NCO-sP(EO-stat-PO) may be used to prepare physiologically stable three-dimensional hydrogels [15] and as cross-linker to polysaccharides [16].

In this study, we evaluated the physiologically stable NCO-sP(EO-stat-PO) hydrogel as drug carrier of dexamethasone 21-phosphate disodium salt (referred to as DEX in the manuscript), a hydrophilic modification of dexamethasone with high water solubility, in silicone tubes that connect the inner ear with an external potentially refillable drug reservoir. In order to evaluate the potential use of this hydrogel system together with an implant, we have assessed the processes regarding its filling into silicone tubes, drying for shelf-storage, heat-treatment for sterilization and re-swelling after time to examine tight fit at the inner lumen of the silicone tube. Drug release from the hydrogels was first examined as free gels without outer steric restriction in order to show pure diffusion controlled release. Subsequently, drug release kinetics were examined with the hydrogel filled into a silicone tube with one end open and PBS (pH 7.4) as the release medium. Additionally, the hydrogel was studied as drug diffusion gateway for a drug reservoir made of silicone tubing. In order to understand the drug diffusion behaviour, the hydrogel was primed and replenished with DEX. For *in vivo* evaluation, hydrogel reservoirs were used to deliver DEX into the inner ear in a guinea pig model. Reservoirs primed with PBS only as well as reservoirs being implanted and immediately explanted served as control. The response of the cochlea in terms of foreign body reaction and hearing loss were examined four weeks following the implantation procedure.

Materials and Methods

1. *In vitro* experiments

Star-shaped poly-ethers with a backbone of statistically copolymerized 80% ethylene oxide and 20% propylene oxide, molecular weight of 18000 g/mol (PD = 1.15) with isocyanate (NCO) end groups (NCO-sP(EO-stat-PO) was synthesized as described previously [17]. An overview on the chemical structure of the gel precursor and the cross-linking reaction is shown in Fig. S2. Dexamethasone 21-phosphate disodium salt (DEX; molecular weight 516.4 g/mol) was purchased from Sigma-Aldrich Germany. Silicone tubes of 6 cm length with an internal diameter of 0.31 mm and an outer diameter of 0.64 mm were kindly provided by MED-EL GmbH, Austria.

1.1. Hydrogel preparation and determination of the swelling ratio. Hydrogels were prepared by dissolution of the reactive NCO-sP(EO-*stat*-PO) precursors in water as described before [15]. The cross-linked hydrogels were dried to xerogel condition in triplets in a vacuum chamber overnight and the dry weights were measured. Xerogels were then placed in an excess of phosphate buffered saline (PBS; pH 7.4) at 37°C for studying its swelling kinetics. The weight of the swollen gel was measured at specific time intervals until it reached its equilibrium swelling state. The swelling ratio is determined by the ratio of dry weight of the gel (W_d) to the swollen weight of the gel (W_s): swelling ratio = $(W_d/W_s) \times 100$.

1.2. Drug release studies from free 3D hydrogels. NCO-sP(EO-stat-PO) was dissolved in a 50 mg/mL (w/v) DEX solution in PBS (pH 7.4) to a final concentration of 20% (w/v). Subsequently, 0.5 mL of this solution (containing 25 mg DEX) was placed into a Teflon mould of 15 mm diameter and 3 mm depth and covered airtight for 24 hours. After completed cross-linking, the DEX-loaded hydrogel was dried to zerogel in a vacuum chamber and then placed in PBS at 37°C for swelling and release of the drug molecules. The amount of drug released in to the PBS was measured by CARY 100 Bio UV-visible spectrophotometer at selected time intervals until the minimum detection limits were reached. The wavelength used to detect DEX was 238–242 nm.

1.3. Drug release from hydrogels in silicone tubes. PBS solution containing DEX (50 mg/mL) was used to dissolve homogenously the hydrogel precursor to obtain a 20% w/v concentration. By use of an insulin syringe avoiding air bubbles, the gellifying solution was sucked inside the silicon tubes of length 60 mm and an inner diameter of 0.31 mm with one end open and the other end closed. The silicone tubes were sealed for 24 hours to allow complete gelation and to prevent drying. Subsequently the silicone tubes containing the hydrogel were placed in PBS at 37°C to examine the release of DEX as mentioned in section 1.1.2.

1.4. Hydrogel as diffusion gate in drug reservoir. NCO-sP(EO-*stat*-PO) was dissolved in PBS and sucked inside a silicone tube from the open end for a length of 10, 5 and 2 mm and maintained undisturbed for 24 hours. After cross-linking of the hydrogel, the remaining length of the silicone tube between the closed end and the hydrogel was filled with DEX solution (100 mg/mL) using an insulin syringe. This set-up was again placed in PBS at 37°C to investigate the release profile of DEX as mentioned in section 1.1.2.

2. *In vivo* experiments

Normal hearing Dunkin Hartley guinea pigs (n = 28; Harlan-Winkelmann GmbH, Borchen, Germany) of both sexes, weighing about 400 g were used. All experiments were carried out in accordance with the institutional guidelines for animal welfare of Hannover Medical School following the standards described by both German laws on protecting animals (Tierschutzgesetz) and the European Communities Council Directive 86/609/EEC for the protection of animals used for experimental purposes. The experiments of this study were approved by the regional government (Niedersächsisches Landesamtes für Verbraucherschutz und Lebensmittelsicherheit, LAVES, registration no. 10/0137).

2.1. Hydrogel reservoir. Using a syringe, the NCO-sP(EO-stat-PO) solution was filled into the hollow silicone reservoirs

(4.32 µL total volume). One end of the reservoir was equipped with a silicone septum which could be perforated with a tuberculin syringe with a needle diameter of 0.5 mm for sterile injection of DEX solution. To allow for a less traumatic implantation, each reservoir tip was smoothed down but remained unsealed in order to release DEX from the hydrogel. After being filled the reservoir was sterilized using ethylene oxide. DEX priming was performed during surgery immediately before reservoir insertion into the inner ear.

DEX sodium phosphate (Spectrum chemical MFG. Corp., Gardena, California, USA) was dissolved in PBS (PBS tablets, Invitrogen Corporation, Paisley, Scotland, UK). The DEX concentration in PBS was 50 µg/ µL for both HPLC and *in vivo* studies which necessitated a loading of 216 µg DEX per reservoir.

2.2. Acoustically evoked auditory brainstem response measurement. Before surgery (day 0) and subsequently on day 3, 7, 14, 21 and 28, animals were anesthetized (diazepam 2.5 mg/kg p.o., atropine sulfate 0.05 mg/kg s.c., ketamine 30 mg/kg i.m., xylazine 7.5 mg/kg i.m.) in order to perform frequency-specific acoustically evoked auditory brainstem response measurements (AABR). All animals were treated with subcutaneous (s.c.) injections of carprofen (0.5 mg/kg), and atropine (0.05 mg/kg) for analgesia and reduction of secretion respectively.

Four needle electrodes were inserted s.c.: a positive pole at the vertex, a ground electrode in the neck, and negative poles postauricularily on the mastoids. The guinea pigs were placed in a soundproof box positioned on a heating pad with a temperature of 37°C. Speakers were connected to the acoustic meatus by calibrated pipette tips.

For frequency-specific acoustic stimulation and measurement, hardware and software from Tucker-Davis Technologies (Alachua, FL, USA) were used. Stimuli were 10 ms pure tones with a cosine-squared rise-fall time of 1 ms (24-bit Sigma-Delta D/A conversion at 200 kHz sampling rate). Six different frequencies (1, 4, 8, 16, 32, and 40 kHz) generated in 10 dB steps from 20 to 90 dB SPL (decibel sound pressure level) were presented using the TDT software (BioSigRP). The recorded neural signals were digitized at 24 kHz sampling rate (16-bit) and bandpass filtered between 0.3 to 3 kHz. The measurements of every frequency and sound intensity were recorded 270 times and averaged.

For evaluation purposes, data were exported into Microsoft Excel (Microsoft Corporation, Redmond, Washington, Seattle, USA) where the recordings were graphed and the triple standard deviation (SD) of background noise of each measurement, recorded in a phase of non-stimulation was calculated and plotted graphically. Hearing threshold was defined as the lowest stimulus level that generated a visually detected peak 3 exceeding three times SD. In the case where no hearing threshold could be detected at the systems limit of 90 dB SPL, the hearing threshold was set to 100 dB SPL. For every individual, frequency specific hearing thresholds of every measurement were compared to the related hearing threshold determined before surgery on day 0. The difference between the pre-surgical hearing threshold and those following was defined as hearing loss.

2.3. Surgical procedures. Before surgery DEX solution and PBS were prepared freshly and filled into the reservoirs (for details see section 2.1.1).

Anaesthesia was performed similarly to that used for AABR but the dosage of ketamine and xylazine was higher (40 mg/kg i.m., respectively 10 mg/kg i.m.) and animals were supplied with enrofloxacine (10 mg/kg s.c.) for prevention of infection. Following initial AABR measurement on day 0 the postauricular area was bilaterally sheared placed under analgesia (1 ml prilocaine) and disinfected. Under sterile conditions a postauricular approach was performed to visualize the *Bulla tympanica*. The periosteum was abscised and the middle ear was opened with scalpel and forceps. Using an OP-MI microscope (Carl Zeiss AG, Oberkochen, Germany) the cochlea was identified and ventral to the round window a cochleostomy was drilled in the basal turn of the cochlea (drilling head 600 µm diameter). The reservoir was inserted 3 mm deep into the perilympathic space of the *Scala tympani* and left in situ. In an additional set of animals, reservoirs were inserted and withdrawn immediately to serve as a control trauma group. In all other groups the implant was fixed and the cochleostomy and fenestration of the middle ear were sealed with carboxylate cement (Durelon Carboxylate Cement, 3 M ESPE AG, 82229 Seefeld, Germany). Thereafter, the protruding part of the reservoir was rolled-up and secured s.c. and the wound was sutured in two layers.

Animals were treated bilaterally but some ears had to be excluded from the study due to e.g. reservoir displacement after tissue harvesting. To summarize the treatments, 11 animals (14 ears used) were treated with DEX administered by the hydrogel reservoir, 10 animals (12 ears used) received PBS released from the hydrogel reservoir and 7 animals (12 ears used) served as trauma group.

2.4. Exploitation of specimens. On day 28 guinea pigs were anesthetised (ketamine 40 mg/kg i.m., xylazine 10 mg/kg i.m., atropine 0.05 mg/kg s.c.), the final AABR measurement was performed after which the sternal area of the animal was placed under analgesia with 4 ml prilocaine (2%). The chest was opened and the animal was perfused intracardially with 200 ml PBS and then fixed with 200 ml of modified Wittmaack fixing solution. The inner ears were extracted while the end section of the reservoirs remained inside the *Scala tympani*.

The *fenestra ovalis* and the apex were pierced with a lancet and the specimens were fixed in advanced Wittmaack fixing solution for up to 24 hours, rinsed for 10 hours with a 4% solution of lithium sulphate (Merck KGaA, Darmstadt, Germany) and dehydrated (2 hours per concentration) in ascending ethanol concentrations (50% v/v, 70% v/v 90% v/v and 100%) or optionally overnight in 70% v/v ethanol. Afterwards they were dried at room temperature and embedded in 5 parts epoxy resin and 2 parts hardening agent (SpeciFix-40 Kit, Struers GmbH, Ballerup, Denmark). Resin was adjusted by the addition of titanium oxide for whitening and reduction of transparency. Specimens and resin were filled into self-made silicone moulds with an inner diameter of 3 cm and a height of 4 cm (silicone source: SORTA Clear 40, Kaupo, Spaichingen, Germany) and placed into vacuum until all spaces in the specimens were filled with epoxy resin. The vaccum was slowly released and the samples were left to harden overnight at room temperature.

2.5. Grinding, Histology. All specimens were grinded with a grinding machine (PowerPro 4000, Bühler, Lake Bluff, Illinois, USA) and abrasive paper. After reaching the cochlea with coarse sand paper (grain size 800) the process was then continued with fine sandpaper (grain size 1200). For every layer of the cochlea, 20 µm were abraded and the section was stained for two minutes with each eosine and toluidine (Merck KGaA, Darmstadt, Germany). The freshly stained surface of the specimen was photographically documented at 30-, 150- and 200-times magnification using a Keyence system (VHX-600 DSO, Osaka, Japan).

For assessment of tissue response inside the *Scala tympani*, Keyence software was used to measure the area occupied with connective tissue in the first and the last mid-modiolar plane section as well as that arithmetically lying in between those two sections. The 7 cross sections of the *Scala tympani* per section were titled as lower basal turn, upper basal turn, first middle turn,

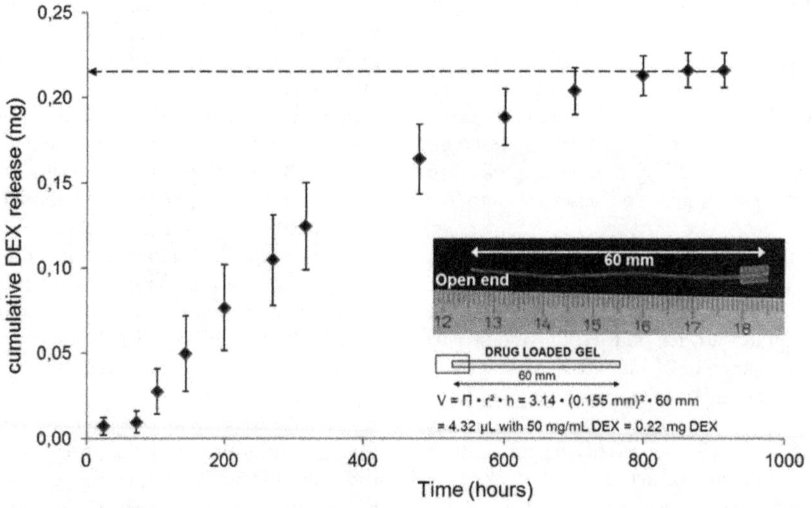

Figure 1. Image of a hydrogel reservoir with one end closed by a silicone septum for fluid injections (right end), while the other end is open in order to release the drug into the area to be addressed (left end) and calculation of the amount of drug inside the hydrogel filled tube. Drug release from this arrangement is shown in the diagram. The data points result from nine experiments from three different NCO-sP(EO-*stat*-PO) batches, each of them used for the preparation of three release setups.

second middle turn, third middle turn, forth middle turn and apical turn [18]. Connective tissue span was set into a ratio to the area of the *Scala tympani* which were measured by tracking the inner outline of the Scala tympani using the Keyence software. Additionally, for every single layer and every part of the *Scala tympani* (lower basal to apical turn) a subjective evaluation using a ranking system was performed in order to monitor the distribution of connective tissue in relation to the point of cochleostomy and the turns of the cochlea. The rationale for subjective ranking was: score 0: no connective tissue; score 1: less than one quarter of the scala tympani is filled with connective tissue; score 2: less than half but more than one quarter of the scala has to be filled with tissue and/or the whole surface of the implants crosscut has to be covered; and score 3: more than half of the scala tympani is filled with connective tissue; see Fig. S1)

In order to correlate results from fibrosis evaluation and AABR measurements, averages of the single values of every group were composed and compared to the averaged results of hearing loss on day 28.

2.6. Statistical Analysis. Statistical analysis was performed using GraphPad Prism 5 (GraphPad Software Inc., La Jolla, California, USA). Since animals were treated bilaterally, the correlation of left and right ears of same individuals were excluded, before using One-way ANOVA in combination with the Tukey post-test to compare mean hearing loss and measurement or ranking of tissue response within the turns for each group or for grouped comparison of tissue formation in the turns. Unpaired students t-test was used to calculate differences between results of mean tissue growth ranking and measurement between groups. Correlation assessment between tissue growth determined by ranking and hearing threshold shift was performed using a nonparametric correlation test (Spearman). Significance was defined as p-values with * = $p<0.05$, ** = $p<0.01$, *** = $p<0.001$.

Results

3.1. *In vitro* results - Drug release studies from DEX loaded free form hydrogels

As reported previously [19], the free-form hydrogel reached the EWC state from dry state within 360 minutes and cryo-SEM pictures shows the macro-porous morphology of the hydrogel in the EWC state. (Fig. S2 and S2C). However, the pores are not inter-connected and the molecular mesh size of the hydrogel network remains decisive for diffusion of drug molecules through the hydrogel. The drug release from free standing 3D hydrogels is fully diffusion controlled and almost quantitative within 24 hours (Fig. S3).

3.2. *In vitro* results - Drug release studies from hydrogels in silicone tubes

In this configuration, the release of drug may logically occur only through the open end of the silicone tube. The walls of the silicone tube will restrict the hydrogel to swell to its full equilibrium state, hence at every point of time the hydrogel will exert a swelling force against the inner wall of the silicone tube by which the hydrogel adjusts tightly to the inside wall of the silicone tube. The exact dimension of the silicone tube reservoir with the amount of drug molecule inside the hydrogel and the cumulative release profile is shown in Fig. 1. Reproducibility of the hydrogel packing inside the silicone tube reservoir and the kinetics of the drug release were performed with three batches of separately prepared DEX loaded hydrogels with each of the batches inserted in three different tubes. Although the release of the drug happens by diffusion process, the geometrical constraint result in a time of about 900 hours or 38 days until DEX is quantitatively released. Interestingly, there was only negligible release in the first 50 hours. This may be explained by the initial diffusion of water inside the gel such that maximal water content in the tube is reached allowing the diffusion controlled release to start.

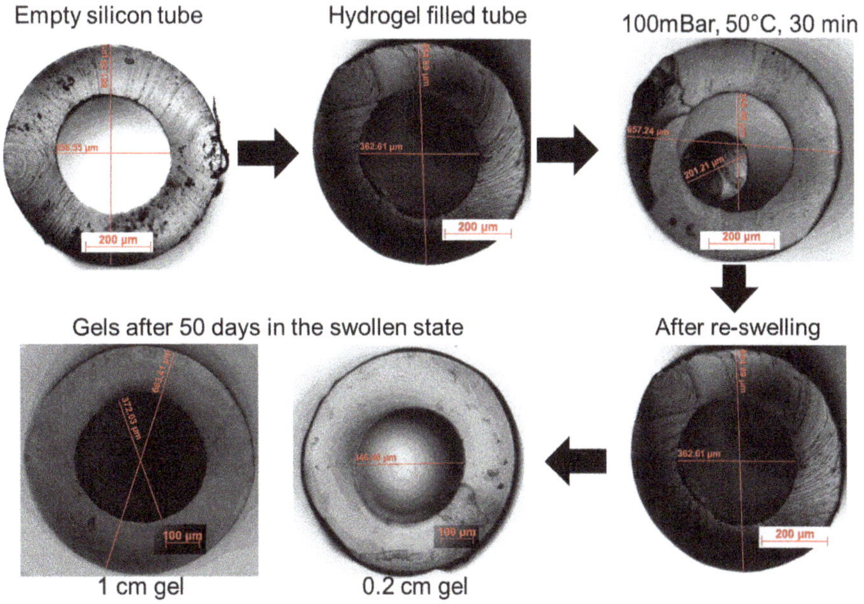

Figure 2. Cross-section images of silicone tubes before and after filling between 2 and 10 mm with with 20% (w/v) NCO-sP(EO-stat-PO) gels (top left and middle), after drying of the gel (top right), re-swelling (bottom right) and after maintaining the gels in a swollen condition for 50 days (bottom left).

3.3. *In vitro* results - Drug release studies from hydrogel as diffusion gate for drug reservoir

In this configuration, the open end of the silicone tube is filled hydrogel for a certain length, so as to create a diffusion gate that could possibly separate the inner ear from an externally accessible drug reservoir. We also evaluated the possibility to dry and re-swell the set-up and whether this would lead to a tight fit of the re-swollen gel inside the tubes. Fig. 2 presents a series of images showing cross-sections of silicone tubes before and after filling with gel. In order to evaluate whether the gels remain in the tubes after drying and re-swelling, the gels in the tubes were warmed to 50°C under reduced pressure (100 mbar) for 30 minutes which resulted in a strong shrinkage of the hydrogel. However, the gels remained at the place in the tubes where they had been placed and after re-swelling the gels tightly closed the inner lumen of the tubes without any visible gaps, this being independent of the hydrogel gate length.

We also checked whether longer incubation times affected the hydrogels within the tubes with regard to signs of degradation or morphological changes. Our results show that at least for 50 days, no changes of the hydrogel within the tubes could be observed.

We then prepared the aforementioned hydrogel gate arrangement in triplets and loaded the free space in the tubes with DEX solutions (100 mg/mL) to study the drug release kinetics. During this procedure (see Fig. S4 for details) it was necessary to create a pinhole at one place in the side wall of the silicone tube. In order to assess whether this pinhole did not result in uncontrolled release during the studies, we checked its tightness by using a dye solution (Fig. S5). This control experiment showed that the pinhole closes tightly after removal of the needle and no uncontrolled release occurs. Fig. S6 shows images of three samples with hydrogel gates of 10, 5 and 2 mm length as well as the calculation of drug loading and the drug release profiles. Again an initial lag-time was observed, however with about 100 hours being twice as long. This results from the need for DEX to diffuse through the hydrogel gates before release can occur. Quantitative release of DEX was reached in all three gate-length cases after approximately 1200 hours (= 50 days).

Since DEX release started earlier in the completely gel filled tubes and the diffusion time of DEX out of those fully filled tubes remained for 38 days, which covers the critical time period in cochlear implant patients, these results encouraged us to examine whether this system would demonstrate beneficial effects *in vivo*.

3.4. *In vivo* results - AABR measurements

On experimental day 0, prior to surgery, all animals were possessing normal hearing. No significant differences in mean AABR thresholds, given as lowest sound intensity where the brainstem response exceeded the triple standard deviation of the background noise, were observed between experimental groups across all frequencies (data not shown). Postoperatively, all groups suffered from an initial loss of hearing detected in the average of all frequencies measured three days after surgery: the mean ± SEM difference compared to the day 0 threshold was: 8.33±4.52 dB SPL in the reservoir + DEX group, 16.94±7.04 dB SPL in the reservoir + PBS group and 39.03±7.28 dB SPL in the trauma group (Fig. 3).

This hearing loss stayed statistically stable within every group over the whole experimental time but it significantly differed among the four groups over this time period. Significantly better results in comparison to all other groups from day 3 until day 28 were detected in animals implanted with the reservoir applying DEX (hearing loss on experimental day 28: 14.42±1.54 (mean ± SEM) dB SPL; $p_{\text{reservoir + DEX vs. trauma}} < 0.001$, $p_{\text{reservoir + DEX vs. reservoir + PBS}} < 0.01$), whereas the highest hearing loss (43.17±1.08 (mean ± SEM) dB SPL) was measured in the trauma group ($p_{\text{trauma vs. reservoir + DEX}} < 0.001$, $p_{\text{trauma vs. reservoir + PBS}} < 0.001$) (Fig. 3)

Concerning the frequency specific hearing loss within each experimental group, differences are only seen between the 1 kHz and 8 kHz spectrum of the trauma group (hearing loss at 1 kHz: 28±4.55; at 8 kHz: 56.5±6.36 dB SPL (mean ± SD); $p < 0.05$;

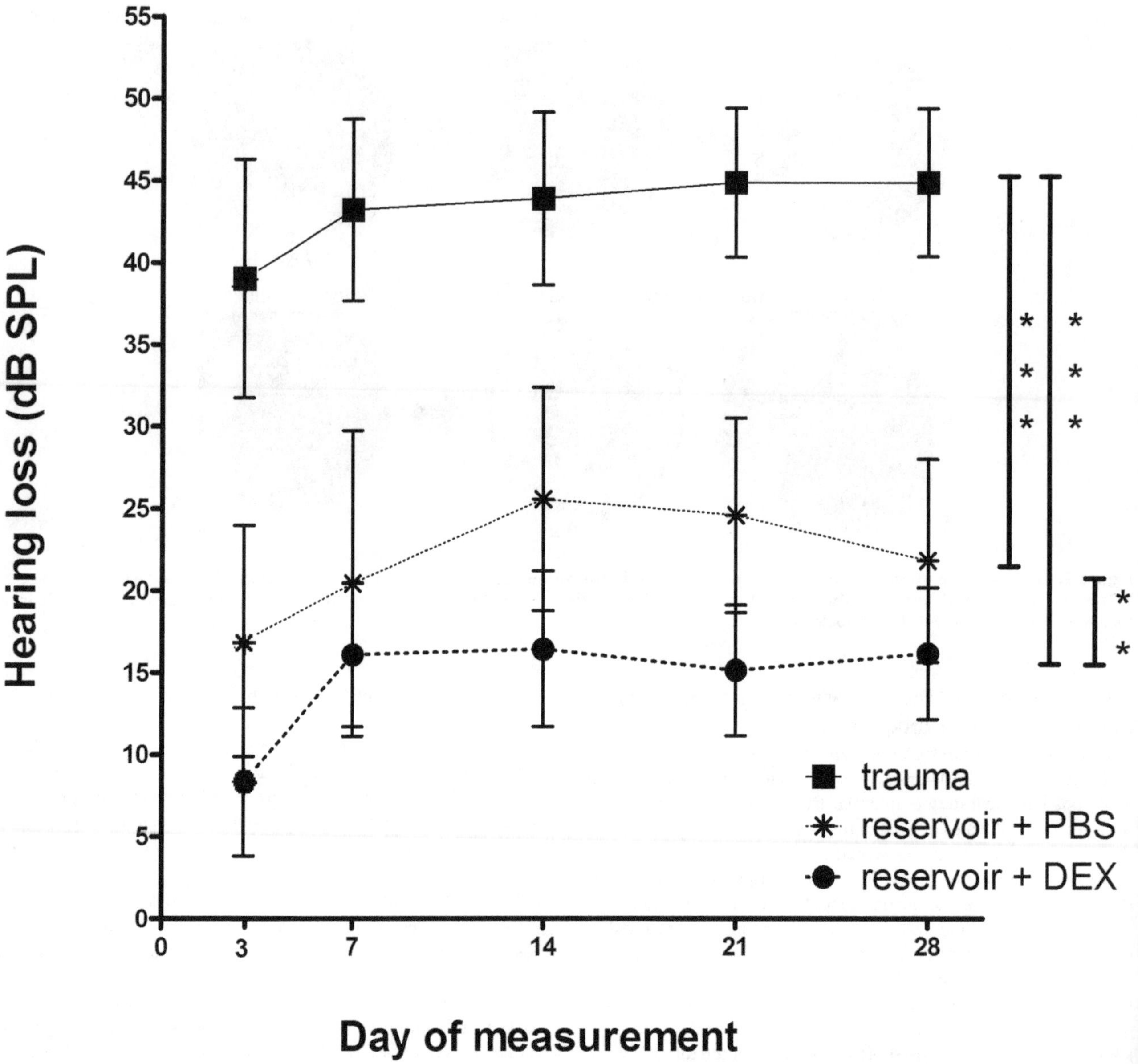

Figure 3. Mean and SEM of hearing loss (difference between the experimental days hearing threshold and hearing threshold before implantation) development from day 3 to day 28 for all experimental groups. Cochleae of the trauma group (n = 12) suffered from highest hearing loss compared to all other experimental groups. Additionally, individuals implanted with a PBS releasing reservoir (n = 12) lost hearing more significantly compared to the group having been implanted with the DEX filled reservoir (n = 14). The statistical differences using ANOVA test examined on experimental day 28 are plotted at the right side of the graph, demonstrating, that the reservoir + DEX treatment resulted in the significantly best hearing thresholds. (** = p<0.01; *** = p<0.001).

Figure S7), or in the averaged results of all animals of all groups, where the mean hearing loss at 1 kHz was 15.94±3.35 SD dB SPL and thus statistically lower than hearing loss at 8 kHz (36.95±4.02 SD dB SPL, $p<0.01$), 16 kHz (31.47±4.22 SD, $p<0.05$) and 32 kHz (31.45±3.81 SD, $p<0.05$) (data not shown).

3.5. *In vivo* results - Tissue response

3.5.1. Ranking of tissue growth – whole cochlea length. Using student's t-test the evaluation of fibrotic tissue response in the whole cochlea by use of a subjective scoring system revealed significant differences between the three experimental groups (Fig. 4A). The trauma group suffered from a more intense tissue response (score: 0.83±0.12 SEM) which can be statistically underscored with a p-value of 0.0133 when compared to the reservoir + PBS group, and $p<0.001$, when matched with reservoir + DEX. The group treated with the reservoir and PBS (0.47±0.08) also achieved a higher ranking score than the reservoir + DEX treated ones (0.25±0.05 SEM; $p<0.05$).

3.5.2. Ranking of tissue growth - Distribution across scalae. In all experimental groups tissue growth was significantly worse in the basal half turns of the cochleae (Fig. 5 and S8) compared to the apical region or the middle turns ($p<0.001$) (Fig. S8). Concerning this characteristic, all groups achieved similar tendencies. In the trauma group basal turns (lower and upper basal turn) achieved a ranking score of 2.04±0.25. Middle turns a score

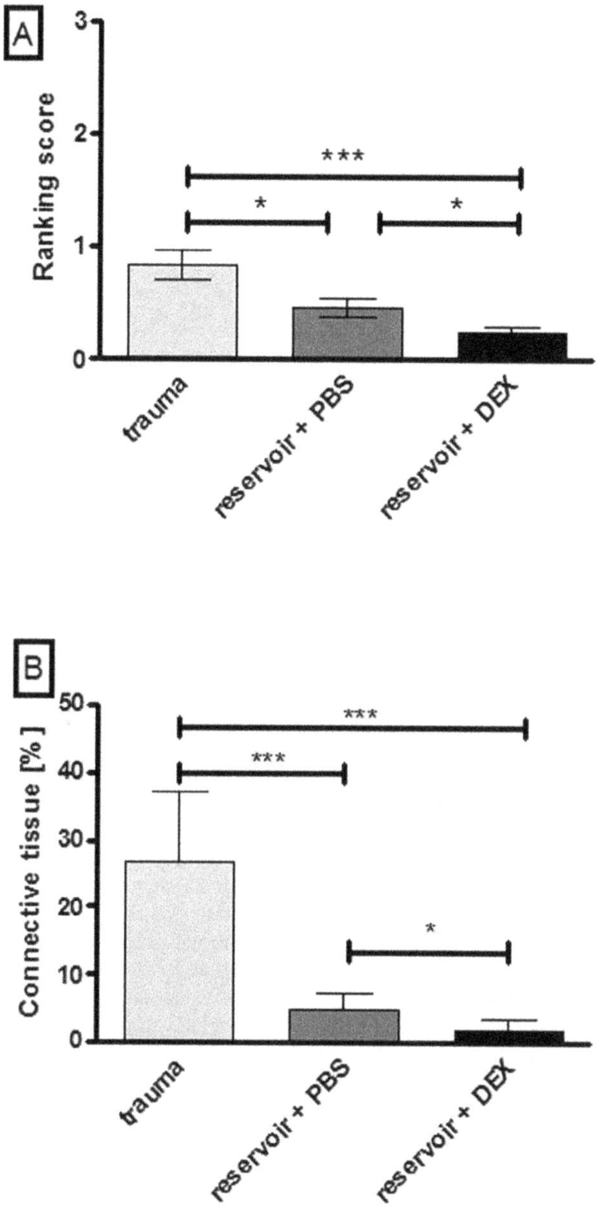

Figure 4. Graphed t-test results of tissue growth ranking (A) and measurement (B) for the whole cochlea length. Using both evaluation methods the tissue growth in the trauma group was significantly increased compared to the reservoir and DEX group with a p value <0.001. When applying the ranking score the difference between reservoir + PBS and trauma or reservoir + DEX was significant with p<0.05 (A). Comparing the tissue growth of the reservoir + PBS group with those of the trauma group or the DEX group using the measuring method, the p value is <0.001 (PBS vs. trauma) and <0.05 (PBS vs. DEX). Error bars: SEM. * = p<0.05, *** = p<0.001.

of 0.42±0.19 and apical turns a value of 0.08±0.08 (p<0.001; Fig S8A). Basal turns of the reservoir + PBS group showed tissue growth with a ranking score of 1.45±0.16 (Fig. S8B). Middle turns of 0.09±0.05 and basal turns of the reservoir + DEX group had a score of 0.88±0.11, while middle turns received a score of 0.0004±0.0004 (Fig. S8C). Both of the reservoir groups exhibited no fibrotic tissue response in the apical turns Comparison of fibrotic tissue reaction in middle and apical turns did not show any significant differences (Fig. S8A–C).

Differences between the experimental groups were also demonstrated most clearly in their disparity of tissue growth in the basal regions and the 1st middle turn. Fig. 5, illustrating tissue growth ranking in all turns of all experimental groups, reveals the trauma group to undergo significantly more tissue growth in the basal turn (2.41±0.23 SEM) than both reservoir groups ($p_{trauma\ vs.\ reservoir+PBS}<0.001$, $p_{trauma\ vs.\ reservoir+DEX}<0.001$). The amount of newly formed tissue in the upper basal turns of all groups did not differ but the tissue in the first middle turn of the trauma group was significantly increased compared to the reservoir + DEX treated ones (p<0.05). In all scales more apical to this, no statistical relevant difference could be demonstrated among the groups and no significant differences were observed between PBS and DEX supported cochleae at all.

3.5.3. Quantitative measurement of tissue growth-whole cochlea length. When measuring the area of fibrotic tissue growth and relating it to the matching area of the *Scala tympani*

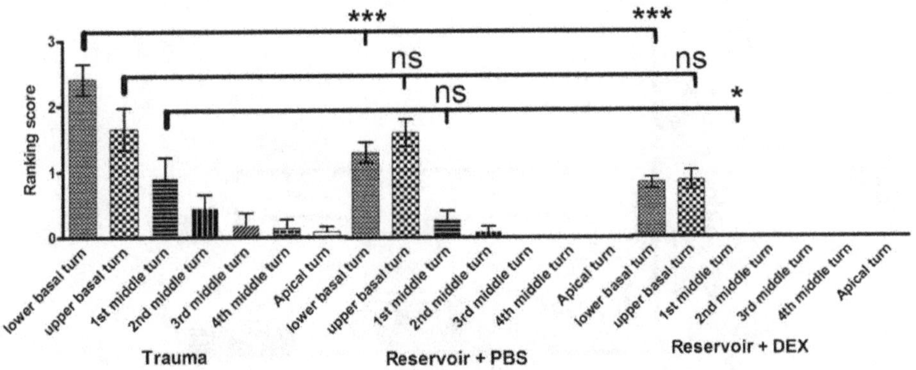

Figure 5. Distribution of fibrosis regarding subjective ranking for all inner ear turns and all experimental groups. In all groups the highest extend of connective tissue growth was detected in the basal turns. Fibroblast growth in more apical turns was only detected in the trauma group and did not take place in reservoir groups at all. Significant differences between the groups were detected (plotted above the SEM bars: * = $p < 0.05$, *** = $p < 0.001$; reference of the significance is marked by the thick bar) and were most prominent in the lower basal turns ($p < 0.001$). Even though there seems to be a tendency of increased tissue formation in the PBS group compared to the DEX group there is no statistical relevance detectable using One-way ANOVA in combination with the Tukey post-test to compare the means between groups.

we detected the highest tissue formation in the trauma group where 26.78±4.17% (mean ± SEM) of the *Scala tympani* area was covered with fibrotic tissue or bony structures (Fig. 4B). In comparison to cochleae provided with the reservoir + PBS (4.74±1.11%) and reservoir + DEX (2.14±0.55%) the trauma control group suffered from significantly higher tissue proliferation ($p<0.001$). A relevant difference in tissue formation was detected in reservoir + PBS treated animals compared to DEX treated ones as well ($p<0.05$).

3.5.4. Quantitative measurement of tissue growth – Distribution across scalae. The significantly most affected location of the cochlea are the basal turns when compared to more apical regions (p between <0.05 and <0.001; Fig. S9A–C). Fig. 6 and Fig. S9 illustrate the decrease of tissue growth from the basal to the apical parts of the cochleae. Comparisons of tissue growth within the turns of each experimental group are plotted in Fig. S9 A–C.

Additionally, the groups showed different amounts of tissue in the individual parts of the cochlea. In the lower basal turn trauma group reached a tissue fraction of mean ± SEM of 65.41±9.32% with a p-value of <0.001 compared to the tissue response found in the lower basal turns of reservoir + PBS group (16.17±4.01%), and reservoir + DEX group (8.25±2.46%) (Fig. 6). Similar findings are seen in the upper basal turn where the trauma group suffered from a tissue growth of 52.36±10.64%, and thus a statistically higher tissue reaction than the reservoir + PBS group (11.86±3.88, $p<0.001$) and reservoir + DEX group (6.67±1.95%, $p<0.001$). In the 1st middle turn the differences are found in p-values <0.01 between trauma group with a score of 39.95±12.92%, and reservoir + PBS group with a score of 3.7±2.91% and <0.001 for the reservoir + DEX group with 0.05±0.05%. Evaluation of the 2nd middle turn reveals a p-value of <0.05 for the difference between the trauma group (27.87±12.27%) and reservoir + PBS group (1.43±1.43%) and the reservoir + DEX (0%). In the 3rd middle turn of the trauma group 1.83±1.59% of the scala tympani area was filled with tissue, which was compared to the 3rd middle turns of the PBS or DEX treated groups, where no tissue growth was observed at all, although this tissue reaction was not statistically relevant. In all turns more apical to this point, no statistical distinction was found since no tissue growth was detected apical to the 3rd turn in any of the experimental groups (Fig. 6). Comparing the tissue growth measured in PBS treated animals to those in DEX treated ones no statistically relevant difference was observed even though the tendency of higher fibrosis rate in PBS treated animals (lower basal: 16.17±4.01%; upper basal 6.67±1.95%; 1st middle 3.70±2.91%; 2nd middle: 1.43±1.43%) compared to DEX treated guinea pigs (lower basal: 8.25±2.46%; upper basal 11.86±3.88%; 1st middle 0.05±0.05%; 2nd middle: 0%) (Fig. 6) was clearly seen.

3.5.5. Differences in ranking and quantitative measurement. Results from subjective ranking of tissue reaction in all images taken from the scala tympani of all experimental animals and the findings from the tissue growth measurement performed in three pictures of each cochlea are very similar but significances differed between both methods when comparing the mean values of the experimental groups. More precisely, ranking showed a p-value of <0.05 for the difference between the trauma and the reservoir + PBS group (Fig. 4A), which is $p<0.001$ according to the measurement technique (Fig. 4B). Next to this, the statistical results were equal.

3.5.6. Correlation of tissue growth and hearing impairment. Tissue growth concurred with the results of AABR measurements. A profound correlation between mean values of the amount of tissue, determined by subjective ranking, and the averaged hearing loss of all frequencies of the individual animal was ascertained. It was demonstrated that with increasing tissue growth hearing loss increased (Fig. 7A). Using the Spearman-Rho-tests a correlation with $r=0.6338$ ($p<0.001$) was detected.

Correlation between the location of new tissue formation in the scala tympani and hearing loss at specific frequencies was detected as well, that is to say, accumulation of tissue growth in basal parts of the cochlea were associated with loss of hearing in high frequencies, equally, tissue formation in the more apical cochlear turns did accompany loss of hearing in. lower frequencies. For example, the fibrous tissue expanse in the upper basal turn of all evaluated cochleae corresponded significantly ($p=0.0225$) to the hearing loss detected at 32 kHz ($r=0.3742$). And the other way around, the amount of tissue detected in the 3rd middle turn correlated significantly to the hearing loss at 1 kHz ($p=0.00231$; $r=0.3727$ (Fig. 7B and C).

The trauma group, which showed almost no residual hearing on day 28 (hearing threshold: 93.75±2.24 dB SPL) and thus the most severe hearing loss (44.86±4.52 dB), was marked by the most

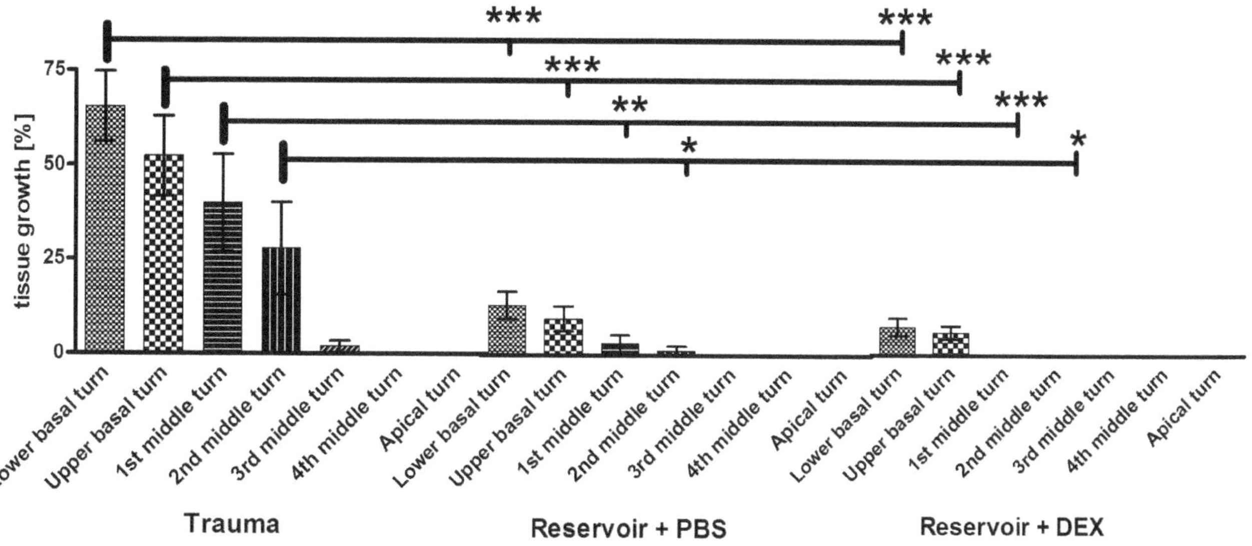

Figure 6. In this graph the mean and SEM percentage of measurement of connective tissue growth in the scala tympani of all experimental groups for each cochlear turn from basal to apical are plotted. The comparison of tissue growth between the groups is illustrated by horizontal lines. Reference of the significance is marked by the thick bar. Highly significant differences were observed between tissue growth in the trauma group and groups receiving PBS or DEX by reservoir. No differences were measured between PBS or DEX treated groups even though a slightly increased connective tissue growth seems to be apparent in the PBS group compared to DEX treated animals. In cochleae implanted with a PBS releasing reservoir tissue growth could be measured from basal up to the 2nd middle turn whereas in the reservoir and DEX treated cochleae connective tissue formation was only visible in the lower and upper basal region. One-way ANOVA in combination with the Tukey post-test was used to compare means between groups: * = $p<0.05$; ** = $p<0.01$; *** = $p<0.001$.

intense new tissue formation especially in the lower basal turn of the cochlea (ranking score for whole cochlea: 0.83±0.12; measurement: 26.78±10.21%). Animals provided with the reservoir plus PBS showed less tissue growth (ranking: 0.47±0.08; measurement: 4.74±2.49%) and reduced hearing loss (21.81±6.18 dB) and cochleae that were treated with the DEX reservoir developed minimal fibrotic outgrowth (ranking score: 0.25±0.05; measurement: 2.14±1.38%) associated with a minimal loss of hearing ability 28 days after implantation (16.15±4 dB).

3.5.7. Angiogenesis and osteogenesis. Additionally to fibrotic tissue growth, an organisation of the tissue in terms of angiogenesis was detected in 5 cochleae of the trauma group and one ear of the reservoir + PBS group. Furthermore, in two cochleae of the trauma group initial signs of osteogenesis were visible (see Fig. S1D).

Discussion

The aim of this study was the evaluation of a novel hydrogel reservoir for inner ear drug delivery *in vitro* and *in vivo*. The hydrogel precursor NCO-sP(EO-*stat*-PO) possesses highly reactive

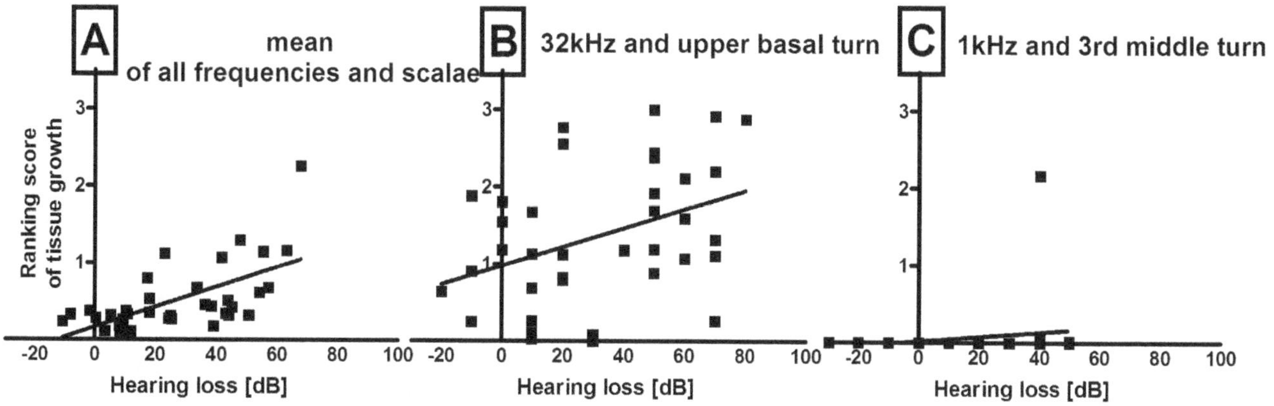

Figure 7. Correlation of hearing loss measured on day 28 and tissue reaction determined by ranking. Graph A illustrates that with the amount of tissue reaction evaluated over the whole cochlea length the loss of residual hearing in all frequencies increases ($p<0.001$; $r = 0.6338$). This effect is detectable in lower and higher frequency regions of the cochleae as well. In figure 7B the detected tissue reaction and hearing loss at the upper basal turn and at 32 kHz are plotted as an example for the correlation in higher frequency areas ($p<0.05$; $r = 0.3742$). Fig. C is an example for correlation of tissue reaction and hearing loss in lower frequency areas of the cochlea. Here we correlated hearing loss at 1 kHz and tissue growth in the 3rd middle turn ($p<0.05$; $r = 0.3727$).

isocyanate (NCO) groups which can potentially react with the alcohol groups of DEX. However, the presence of the phosphate groups and the two sodium counter ions render the molecule extremely hydrophilic while the isocyante groups are placed at relatively hydrophobic iosphorne-rings. Moreover, the hydroxyl groups of the drug molecule are directly attached to the aromatic ring. These various properties prevent permanent covalent binding of DEX to the hydrogel network to any detectable level [19].The free form hydrogels exhibited the fastest release kinetics within 24 hours as the release medium could have access to all the 3D surface of the hydrogels by which the diffusion of entrapped drug molecules in all the direction. The drug release was by swelling controlled diffusion process. The system where the hydrogel was completely filled inside the silicone tube, only the open end of the silicone tube have access to the release medium to the hydrogel. In this configuration, the wall of the silicone tube restricted the swelling kinetics of the hydrogel. In this system, the drug release was purely by diffusion controlled process which took almost 900 hours to release the loaded drug completely. In the other system where, the hydrogel without any drug in it was only acting as the diffusion gate, the drug from the reservoir had to diffuse through the hydrogel gate to reach the release medium; it took almost 1200 hours to release the drug completely. In the 1200 hours, the initial 100 hours was the lag time during which the drug had to diffuse through the gel gate. All these three configurations explain how the release of the drug can be controlled precisely by checking the access of the release medium to the hydrogels. Finally, examination of the hydrogel as a drug delivery matrix in a medical device used for inner ear treatment *in vivo* was carried out.

DEX was chosen for this drug delivery study as model drug because of its well-known anti-inflammatory and hair cell protective effects [6,7,20–22]. DEX suppresses apoptotic activities in response to TNF-α. Studies performed by Messmer and colleagues demonstrate that this effect can be achieved even up to 12 hours after TNF-α application. DEX retards the down-regulation of inhibitors of apoptosis proteins [23], blocks transcription of pro-inflammatory molecules and increases transcription of anti-inflammatory factors and reduces leukocyte migration through decreasing the adherence of these cells to the vascular endothelium [24]. Synthetic glucocorticoids are also able to decrease vascular permeability and vasodilatation, prominent features of the inflammatory reaction and necessary for the emigration of immune cells. Consequently, glucocorticoids reduce oedema and fibrin formation, inhibit capillary and fibroblast proliferation and enhance collagen breakdown [24].

These effects play an essential role in the neutralisation of foreign bodies or bacteria raising the consideration regarding the use of DEX in cases where infection may be likely or is actually present. Conversely, all of these properties are necessary in the suppression of inflammation concerning cochlear implantation. Hence, although a precautious use of DEX is essential, it is a noteworthy ally for offering protection of hearing ability following cochlear implantation [25–27].

The extent of tissue response was determined both by ranking and direct measurement. The results from both the methods were not equal but did tend to deliver the same information. While the measurement of 3 slices per scale per cochlea brought the quality of objective evaluation, the subjective ranking of tissue growth in every single slice covered a quantitative assessment. Since the measurement was performed on 1 mid-modiolar image and the one directly before and one directly after the modiolus, the measured area was identical in all cochleae. This leads to a high comparability between the cochleae but also implies that alteration could only be detected in this specific region. Although the ranking underlay a subjective assessment, it was exclusively performed by one person who obliterates variation due to diverging assessment criteria of various individuals. In addition, scoring between 0 and 3 only allowed for an unrefined classification although as a positive factor, it involves the whole cochlea. As such, it is considered that the subjective ranking of all slices leads to a more comprehensive and accurate estimate of the level of tissue reaction.

Probably all distinctions between ranking results and measurement results concerning p-values are based on the alteration of modiolus-near or modiolus-distant evaluation and the fact that three images per scale used for objective measurement may not give a synopsis on the status of the whole cochlea. Nevertheless, ranking and measurement methods led to similar results in most cases, indicating that measurement can be used to support the coarser ranking score with more detailed values.

The reservoirs remained inside the *Scala tympani* and interacted with the inner ear in terms of foreign bodies over a time period of four weeks. Nevertheless, AABR results and the distribution of tissue growth along the cochlea length have shown that producing a trauma as performed on animals in the trauma group, has a more devastating influence on the structures of the inner ear. An initial hearing loss after surgery was observed on day 3 which remained stable over time. We consider that this initial hearing loss is brought about by the implantation procedure as well as the physical presence of the implant itself in the *Scala tympani* which may modify the fluid and basilar membrane movement and induce inflammatory reactions. An additional reason may be due to mechanical damage of hair cells although this would occur only in the basal region of the cochlea where the implant is located and would consequently affect only the higher frequency regions. Due to the fact that no differences in hearing loss between lower and higher frequencies were observed, this seems unlikely.

In contrast to Braun and colleagues who reported DEX-dependent hearing preservation without tissue reduction [28], we observed a correlation of hearing ability and fibrosis which has recently been reported by O'Leary [29]. These parameters depend on the same factor, inflammation, which lends to the concept that the tissue growth modifies the influence of the travelling wave towards the basilar membrane which in turn reduces exhibition of hair cells. Reduction of the nutrition requirement of sensory cells in this area may also occur as a consequence. Additionally, tissue proliferation inside the *Scala tympani* may disturb the travelling wave on its way towards the apical turns and consequently prohibit the stimulation of more apical sensory cells. As a result of this, hearing of higher frequencies is reduced as well as the sensation of low frequencies albeit the inflammation bring localised mostly in the basal turns.

All animals of the trauma group suffered from significantly increased hearing loss and tissue reaction compared to the other experimental groups. We believe that the double movement of the reservoir inside the cochlea of trauma group specimens, insertion as the first manipulation and explantation as the second, is a valid reason for this finding. In contrast, cochleae of the other groups had to sustain only one traumatic manipulation.

These results indicate that common application aids that have to be removed after usage may lead to traumatic changes of the inner ear. Consequently we suggest that an application aid, at least if its properties are comparable to the hydrogel reservoirs tested in this study, should be bound to the CI and remain inside the cochlea. Further studies concerning this topic would be necessary to evaluate if the findings from this study are generally representative for removable drug delivery systems. In addition to the different mechanical stimuli, it is important to consider whether more immunologically active cells arrived from the blood into the *Scala tympani* after the necessary rupture of the *Stria vascularis* during cochleostomy in cochleae of the trauma group. Although the opening of the cochleostomy was filled with carboxylate cement, it was not blocked with a close-fitting implant like the silicone reservoir and as a result the blood vessels inside the *Stria* may not have been compressed. Additional irritation by the cement may be assumed with respect to reports concerning pulpa irritation in dental medicine [30,31] and to a newly published study stating that dental cement, applied on guinea pig inner ears, leads to a strong new bone formation [32], even though this method is a widely used [33,34] and other reports have also assessed carboxylate cement to be non-irritating [35,36].

Luttikhuizen and colleagues stated in 2006 that inflammatory processes are related to components of the blood stream; not only immune cells like macrophages but, for example, proteins like fibrinogen, the complement system, antibodies and various inflammatory factors [37]. They are attracted by chemotactic factors that are secreted from injured tissue or by cells stressed by the presence of foreign bodies [4,38]. Although materials of current implants are biologically inert, they still trigger inflammatory responses of the surrounding tissue. This is based upon endogenous proteins that attach to the surface of the implant and attract components of the nonspecific immune system. In the later stages of the inflammatory process, following earlier leucocytic invasion, fibroblasts migrate towards the implant and build a tissue coating around the foreign material in order to protect the healthy tissue. This step is clearly seen in many specimens with implanted reservoirs (see Section 3.2.2).

Angiogenesis, another cardinal sign of inflammation, is seen in cochleae of the trauma and reservoir + PBS group. In cochleae of the trauma group angiogenesis had already progressed into a stage of osteogenesis. Subsequent to fibrotic tissue growth, angiogenesis follows as a consequence of the coagulation cascade and hypoxia and is incited by locally released histamine and fibrin fragment E [37]. Since most of these cells and substances are bound to the blood stream, the correlation between the effluence of blood into the cochlea and higher levels of inflammation must be considered.

Furthermore, the diameter and related rigidity as well as the material composition of the inserted piece of the reservoir, played an accessory role for the severity of the inflammatory reaction. Previous reports by Jolly and colleagues [26] demonstrated that electrode trauma depends on the size and flexibility of the array and that reduction of trauma can be achieved by flexible implants that easily adapt to the angulations of the cochlear turns. This information can be transferred to the implantation of silicone reservoirs that appear to be flexible which according to Jolly [26] should provoke less irritation in the tissue of the cochlea. This depends strongly on the composition of the material. The process of implantation and fixation of the reservoirs explains similarities between the impact administrated by reservoirs with either PBS or DEX. Nevertheless, significant higher fibrosis in PBS treated ears discovered over the whole length of the cochleae and the distinct angiogenesis in these cochleae prove the influence of DEX applied via the reservoir.

Conclusions

In this study, the technical feasibility of incorporating hydrogels prepared from NCO-sP(EO-*stat*-PO) pre-polymers within the silicone tube for sustained release of DEX for several weeks through diffusion process into the inner ear was demonstrated which encouraged the *in vivo* studies.

Animal experiments using normal hearing Dunkin Hartley guinea pigs followed by treatment and regular measurement of hearing loss showed significantly lower fibrosis in case of DEX loaded hydrogel reservoir as compared to a PBS releasing control-reservoir and pure trauma. Most importantly, the hearing loss was significantly lower in case of the DEX loaded hydrogel reservoirs as compared to the other groups. In contrast, considerable functional and morphological changes were detected in the trauma group. We hypothesize that the insertion and immediate explantation of a delivery device is even more destructive to the inner ear than the impact of a foreign body in terms of a reservoir.

Our results strongly suggest that the NCO-sP(EO-*stat*-PO) hydrogel reservoir is a promising drug delivery device to apply water-soluble drugs in therapeutically relevant doses into the inner ear for a sustained treatment period. We conclude that the hydrogel used in combination with a rechargeable design of reservoir is a promising alternative of drug delivery device. This method might be optimized by adapting the reservoir to the cochlear implant in order to combine its insertion with the inevitable implantation of the CI, and thus avoiding additional trauma. This would allow surgeons to decide on the execution of drug application during surgery.

Supporting Information

Figure S1 Representative images of tissue response scores A) representatively depicts the score 0 mainly detected in animals of the reservoir + DEX group. Images B) and C) illustrate score 1 and 2 representative for the reservoir + PBS or trauma groups. Score 3 is shown in D) which is taken from an animal of the trauma group. In this figure the reorganization of fibrotic tissue response (black arrow) in terms of ossification (white arrow) is clearly seen. Asterixes: hydrogel; black arrow head: silicone reservoir, missing in image D), taken from the trauma group, where the tubing was implanted and subsequently explanted.

Figure S2 Relevant chemical structure (A) Hydrogel precursor and the chemical reaction of isocyanates with H_2O, (B) shows the swelling kinetics of the hydrogel from its dry state to its fully swollen state, (C) microporous structure of the swollen hydrogel.

Figure S3 Structure of dexamethasone 21-phosphate disodium salt (DEX) and its complete release profile from the free form hydrogel.

Figure S4 Experimental procedure for sample preparation of the release studies from the silicone tubes with hydrogel gates.

Figure S5 Control experiment using a dye-solution showing that the pin-hole created in the silicone tube during loading of the DEX solution does not result in uncontrolled release.

Figure S6 Picture of hydrogel-gates with three different lengths in silicone tubes (top left), calculation of the amount of DEX in each of the tubes (top right) and result of the release studies (bottom).

Figure S7 Frequency specific hearing loss. The mean and SD of hearing loss of all experimental groups after 28 days of implantation is plotted for each frequency tested. In all groups the hearing loss seems to be less affected in the lower frequencies but statistical evaluation did not show any significant differences between the frequency specific hearing loss in any of the experimental groups.

Figure S8 Tissue growth evaluated by ranking. The mean ± SEM results of subjective ranking of tissue formation in the cochlea turns of each experimental group are plotted. In all groups the tissue reaction is significantly increased in the basal regions compared to the middle and apical regions. Fibrotic tissue response in more apical turns was only detected in the trauma group (A) and did not take place in reservoir groups treated with PBS (B) or DEX (C). One-way ANOVA in combination with the Tukey post-test was used to compare the tissue growth within the different cochlea turns of each experimental group: ** = $p<0.01$; *** = $p<0.001$. Reference of the significance is marked by the thick bar.

Figure S9 Tissue growth evaluated by measurement. The mean ± SEM percentage of scala tympani area of each cochlea turn covered with tissue is plotted for each experimental group. In all groups the tissue reaction is significantly increased in the basal regions compared to the middle and apical regions. Fibroblast growth in more apical turns was only detected in the trauma group (A) and did not take place in reservoir groups treated with PBS (B) or DEX (C). One-way ANOVA in combination with the Tukey post-test was used to compare the fibrous tissue growth within the different cochlea turns of each experimental group: ** = $p<0.01$; *** = $p<0.001$. Reference of the significance is marked by the thick bar.

Acknowledgments

We thank Dr. Henning Voigt, Hannover School of Medicine, for his support in quality management, and Peter Erfurt, Hannover School of Medicine, for his technical advice in grinding techniques.

Author Contributions

Conceived and designed the experiments: MH AD RH TS KE MM TL CJ JG VS. Performed the experiments: MH AD RH JG VS. Analyzed the data: MH AD CJ JG VS. Contributed reagents/materials/analysis tools: TS KE MM TL CJ JG VS. Contributed to the writing of the manuscript: MH AD RH CJ JG VS.

References

1. WHO (2014). http://www.who.int/mediacentre/factsheets/fs300/en/.
2. Ruben RJ (1967) Development of the inner ear of the mouse: a radioautographic study of terminal mitoses. Acta Otolaryngol: Suppl 220: 221–244.
3. Lenarz T (1998) Cochlear implants: selection criteria and shifting borders. Acta Otorhinolaryngol Belg 52: 183–199.
4. Nadol JB Jr., Eddington DK (2004) Histologic evaluation of the tissue seal and biologic response around cochlear implant electrodes in the human. Otol Neurotol 25: 257–262.
5. Birman CS, Sanli H, Gibson WP, Elliott EJ (2014) Impedance, Neural Response Telemetry, and Speech Perception Outcomes After Reimplantation of Cochlear Implants in Children. Otol Neurotol.
6. Abi-Hachem RN, Zine A, Van De Water TR (2010) The injured cochlea as a target for inflammatory processes, initiation of cell death pathways and application of related otoprotectives strategies. Recent Pat CNS Drug Discov 5: 147–163.
7. Eshraghi AA, Adil E, He J, Graves R, Balkany TJ, et al. (2007) Local dexamethasone therapy conserves hearing in an animal model of electrode insertion trauma-induced hearing loss. Otol Neurotol 28: 842–849.
8. Borenstein JT (2011) Intracochlear drug delivery systems. Expert Opin Drug Deliv 8: 1161–1174.
9. Merrill EW (1993) Poly(ethylene oxide) star molecules: synthesis, characterization, and applications in medicine and biology. J Biomater Sci Polym Ed 5: 1–11.
10. Peppas NA, Keys KB, Torres-Lugo M, Lowman AM (1999) Poly(ethylene glycol)-containing hydrogels in drug delivery. J Control Release 62: 81–87.
11. Kim P, Kim DH, Kim B, Choi SK, Lee SH, et al. (2005) Fabrication of nanostructures of polyethylene glycol for applications to protein adsorption and cell adhesion. Nanotechnology 16: 2420–2426.
12. Hoffman AS (2002) Hydrogels for biomedical applications. Adv Drug Deliv Rev 54: 3–12.
13. Paasche G, Bockel F, Tasche C, Lesinski-Schiedat A, Lenarz T (2006) Changes of postoperative impedances in cochlear implant patients: the short-term effects of modified electrode surfaces and intracochlear corticosteroids. Otol Neurotol 27: 639–647.
14. Groll J, Amirgoulova EV, Ameringer T, Heyes CD, Rocker C, et al. (2004) Biofunctionalized, ultrathin coatings of cross-linked star-shaped poly(ethylene oxide) allow reversible folding of immobilized proteins. J Am Chem Soc 126: 4234–4239.
15. Dalton PD, Hostert C, Albrecht K, Moeller M, Groll J (2008) Structure and properties of urea-crosslinked star poly[(ethylene oxide)-ran-(propylene oxide)] hydrogels. Macromol Biosci 8: 923–931.
16. Dhanasingh A, Salber J, Möller M, Groll J (2010) Tailored hyaluronic acid hydrogel through hydrophilic prepolymer cross-linkers. Soft Matter 6: 618–629.
17. Goetz H, Beginn U, Bartelink C F, Gruenbauer H J M, Möller M (2002) Preparation of isphorone diisocyanate terminated star polyethers. Macromol Mater Eng 287: 223–230.
18. Scheper V, Paasche G, Miller JM, Warnecke A, Berkingali N, et al. (2009) Effects of delayed treatment with combined GDNF and continuous electrical stimulation on spiral ganglion cell survival in deafened guinea pigs. J Neurosci Res 87: 1389–1399.
19. Dhanasingh A, Groll J (2012) Polysaccharide based covalently linked multimembrane hydrogels. Soft Matters Advance article.
20. James DP, Eastwood H, Richardson RT, O'Leary SJ (2008) Effects of round window dexamethasone on residual hearing in a Guinea pig model of cochlear implantation. Audiol Neurootol 13: 86–96.
21. Kim HH, Addison J, Suh E, Trune DR, Richter CP (2007) Otoprotective effects of dexamethasone in the management of pneumococcal meningitis: an animal study. Laryngoscope 117: 1209–1215.
22. Takemura K, Komeda M, Yagi M, Himeno C, Izumikawa M, et al. (2004) Direct inner ear infusion of dexamethasone attenuates noise-induced trauma in guinea pig. Hear Res 196: 58–68.
23. Messmer UK, Pereda-Fernandez C, Manderscheid M, Pfeilschifter J (2001) Dexamethasone inhibits TNF-alpha-induced apoptosis and IAP protein downregulation in MCF-7 cells. Br J Pharmacol 133: 467–476.
24. Tizard IR (2004) Veterinary Immunology: An Introduction. Saunders.
25. Chandrasekhar SS, Rubinstein RY, Kwartler JA, Gatz M, Connelly PE, et al. (2000) Dexamethasone pharmacokinetics in the inner ear: comparison of route of administration and use of facilitating agents. Otolaryngol Head Neck Surg 122: 521–528.
26. Jolly C, Garnham C, Mirzadeh H, Truy E, Martini A, et al. (2010) Electrode features for hearing preservation and drug delivery strategies. Adv Otorhinolaryngol 67: 28–42.
27. Meltser I, Canlon B (2011) Protecting the auditory system with glucocorticoids. Hear Res 281: 47–55.
28. Braun S, Ye Q, Radeloff A, Kiefer J, Gstoettner W, et al. (2011) Protection of inner ear function after cochlear implantation: compound action potential measurements after local application of glucocorticoids in the guinea pig cochlea. ORL J Otorhinolaryngol Relat Spec 73: 219–228.
29. O'Leary SJ, Monksfield P, Kel G, Connolly T, Souter MA, et al. (2013) Relations between cochlear histopathology and hearing loss in experimental cochlear implantation. Hear Res 298: 27–35.
30. Ito M, Yagasaki H (2001) Bone substitute product and method of producing the same. United States Patent US 6,214,048 B1.
31. Seltzer S, Maggio J, Wollard RR, Brough SO, Barnett A (1976) Tissue reactions to polycarboxylate cements. J Endod 2: 208–214.
32. Burghard A, Lenarz T, Kral A, Paasche G (2014) Insertion site and sealing technique affect residual hearing and tissue formation after cochlear implantation. Hear Res 312C: 21–27.
33. Scheper V, Wolf M, Scholl M, Kadlecova Z, Perrier T, et al. (2009) Potential novel drug carriers for inner ear treatment: hyperbranched polylysine and lipid nanocapsules. Nanomedicine (Lond) 4: 623–635.
34. Vivero RJ, Joseph DE, Angeli S, He J, Chen S, et al. (2008) Dexamethasone base conserves hearing from electrode trauma-induced hearing loss. Laryngoscope 118: 2028–2035.
35. el-Kafrawy AH, Dickey DM, Mitchell DF, Phillips RW (1974) Pulp reaction to a polycarboxylate cement in monkeys. J Dent Res 53: 15–19.

36. Lervik T (1978) The effect of zinc phosphate and carboxylate cements on the healing of experimentally induced pulpitis. Oral Surg Oral Med Oral Pathol 45: 123–130.
37. Luttikhuizen DT, Harmsen MC, Van Luyn MJ (2006) Cellular and molecular dynamics in the foreign body reaction. Tissue Eng 12: 1955–1970.
38. Nadol JB, Jr., Hsu WC (1991) Histopathologic correlation of spiral ganglion cell count and new bone formation in the cochlea following meningogenic labyrinthitis and deafness. Ann Otol Rhinol Laryngol 100: 712–716.

21

Elucidation of the Interaction Mechanism with Liposomes of gH625-Peptide Functionalized Dendrimers

Annarita Falanga[1], Rossella Tarallo[2], Thomas Carberry[2], Massimiliano Galdiero[3], Marcus Weck[2], Stefania Galdiero[1]*

1 Department of Pharmacy & CIRPEB & DFM Scarl, University of Naples "Federico II", Naples, Italy, 2 Molecular Design Institute and Department of Chemistry, New York University, New York, New York, United States of America, 3 Department of Experimental Medicine, Second University of Naples, Naples, Italy

Abstract

We have demonstrated that amide-based dendrimers functionalized with the membrane-interacting peptide gH625 derived from the herpes simplex virus type 1 (HSV-1) envelope glycoprotein H enter cells mainly through a non-active translocation mechanism. Herein, we investigate the interaction between the peptide-functionalized dendrimer and liposomes composed of PC/Chol using fluorescence spectroscopy, isothermal titration calorimetry, and surface plasmon resonance to get insights into the mechanism of internalization. The affinity for the membrane bilayer is very high and the interaction between the peptide-dendrimer and liposomes took place without evidence of pore formation. These results suggest that the presented peptidodendrimeric scaffold may be a promising material for efficient drug delivery.

Editor: Valentin Ceña, Universidad de Castilla-La Mancha, Spain

Funding: Financial support was provided by MIUR - PON01_02388 "Verso la medicina personalizzata: nuovi sistemi molecolari per la diagnosi e la terapia di patologie oncologiche ad alto impatto sociale" SALUTE DELL'UOMO E BIOTECNOLOGIE. The funders had no role in study design, data collection and analysis, decision to publish, or preparation of the manuscript.

Competing Interests: The authors have declared that no competing interests exist.

* Email: stefania.galdiero@unina.it

Introduction

The cellular membrane plays an essential role in controlling the transport of external molecules into the cell interior. It acts as a selective barrier that only allows the passage of selected molecules. Non-specific and non-disruptive penetration across the membrane without protein mediation is typically achievable only by small molecules, while larger ones generally induce significant disruption of the lipid bilayer structure [1]. Thus, there is considerable interest to pave the way to strategies able to translocate synthetic molecules into and through the membrane for drug delivery, biosensing, and other biomedical applications, without permanently disrupting the membrane and the risk of inducing cell death [2]. The success of novel strategies for health care therapies relies on the development of delivery vehicles capable of improving the therapeutic index of biologically active molecules as well as diagnosing at the disease site of interest. At the present, most active compounds are not deemed therapeutically effective due to their inability to reach the target tissue. A variety of drug delivery carriers including polymer microcapsules, liposomes, polymer conjugates, and nanoparticles are in pre-clinical and clinical development to improve many drug bioavailability, especially for cancer treatment [3,4]. Most drug carriers lack the potential for orthogonal multi-functionalization, a prerequisite for theranostics and are often not well-defined compounds but polydisperse mixtures, rendering the analysis of structure-property relationships challenging. These drawbacks limit their potential use in theranostics. One class of biomaterials that can serve as drug carrier or, more generally as a platform for theranostics, and that has the potential to overcome these limitations is dendrimers.

Dendrimers are well-defined synthetic hyperbranched macromolecules which possess a high number of active termini that defines their properties and functions [5]. As a result of perfect branching, dendrimers have the highest number of terminal functionalities of any polymeric material at a given molecular weight and are monodisperse. Comparing the features of dendrimers with those of linear polymers, it was shown that the dendrimer architecture presents several advantages for drug delivery [6,7]: (i) low polydispersity allowing for reproducible pharmacokinetic behavior; ii) globular shape of higher generation dendrimers affecting their biological and rheological properties; and iii) controlled multivalency which can be used to attach several molecules, e.g. drugs, imaging agents, cell-penetrating peptides, targeting groups, and/or solubilizing moieties. The possibility to introduce several functionalities into the dendrimer structures has opened the door for their applications in theranostics [8]. Over the past decade, the relationships between dendrimer architecture, biocompatibility, circulation time, and release kinetics have been partially elucidated allowing the development of general principles for the design of dendrimers as "ideal" drug delivery carriers. These include PEGylation to increase water solubility, permeability, stability and dendrimer size (leading to tunable retention and biodistribution characteristics), the internalization of therapeutic agents into the void space between the branches or the covalent attachment of them to surface groups, and the addition of targeting moieties bound to the dendrimer surface can be used to preferentially treat disease cells with specific over-expressed receptor targets.

Dendrimers usually cross cell barriers by endocytosis [9,10], thus they are entrapped in endososomes and only a small amount of the active drug is able to reach the intracellular target. We recently reported that virally derived peptides could significantly help in solving this problem as many viruses have evolved rather efficient systems for endosomal release. Viruses can enter cells either through an endosomal pathway or via direct fusion of the plasma membrane through the activity of membranotropic peptides [11,12]. Great attention has been devoted to the study of hydrophobic peptides that efficiently traverse biological membranes, promoting lipid-membrane reorganizing processes, such as fusion or pore formation, and involving temporary membrane destabilization and subsequent reorganization [13,14,15,16,17,18,19,20]. These peptides are significantly different from the well-known cell penetrating cationic peptides such as TAT, which do not translocate spontaneously across bilayers but rather are taken up by cells via endocytosis [21]. According to our previously reported data [22,23], coupling of a poly(amide)-based dendrimer [24,25] to viral peptide gH625 enabled the non-specifically crossing of the membrane bilayer through an energy-independent process, without showing evidence of endocytosis, poration, or cytotoxicity. Translocation mediated by gH625 may be very useful in the delivery of drugs; the mechanism of spontaneous translocation is not yet well understood.

The translocation of gH625 dendrimers through lipid bilayers could provoke changes in the bilayer which need to be taken into account in the design of a drug controlled release delivery system. To understand the mechanism of our HSV-1 derived peptide-dendrimer to mediate the cell membrane crossing, it is necessary to understand its interactions with lipid bilayers [26]. Liposomes are excellent model systems for biological experiments because of their simple and membrane-like composition, easy preparation, biodegradability, biocompatibility and acceptable stability over time. By examining the interactions between liposomes and dendrimers, conclusions can be drawn about biological processes such as membrane fusion and translocation and ultimately transport pathways for drug delivery. In the literature, several modes of interactions between dendrimers and liposomes are described [27,28,29,30,31,32,33,34,35,36,37,38]. Dendrimers can either pass through the lipid bilayer or dendrimer-lipid micelles are created [39]. Some dendrimers can interact with lipids by hydrophobic interactions between lipid acyl chains and the hydrophobic dendrimer interior [40,41]. It was shown that the strength of the interaction mainly depends on the size and charge of the molecule [42,43,44] and the phase of lipids [45].

This contribution describes the effect of the gH625 dendrimer on lipid bilayers composed of cholesterol (Chol) and neutral phospholipids such as phosphatidylcholine (PC). Surface plasmon resonance (SPR), fluorescence spectroscopy, and isothermal titration calorimetry (ITC) were used to elucidate the dendrimer/membrane interactions in order to push further the design of new drug delivery systems that consist of dendrimers incorporating bioactive molecules. These studies are of interest in understanding the interaction of gH625-dendrimer with native cell membranes, and complement previous studies showing that the gH625-dendrimer is able to pass through and does not disrupt the biological membrane.

Materials and Methods

Materials

Fmoc-protected amino acids, coupling reagents, and Rink- amide *p*-methylbenzhydrylamine (MBHA) resin were purchased from Calbiochem-Novabiochem (San Diego, CA, USA). Fmoc-l-propargylglycine (Fmoc-PrA-OH) was purchased from NeoSystem (Tysons Corner, VA, USA). The phospholipid phosphatidylcholine (PC), 1-hexadecanoyl-2-(6,7-dibromooctadecanoyl)-sn-glycero-3-phosphocholine (6,7 Br-PC), 1-hexadecanoyl-2-(9,10-dibromooctadecanoyl)-sn-glycero-3-phosphocholine (9,10 Br-PC), 1-hexadecanoyl-2-(11,12-dibromooctadecanoyl)-sn-glycero-3-phosphocholine (11,12 Br-PC) were purchased from Avanti Polar Lipids (Birmingham, AL, USA). Cholesterol, Triton-X100 and 3-propyl-2-(5-(3-propyl)-2(3H)-benzothiazolidene-1,3-pentadienyl), iodide (diS-C_3-5) were obtained from Sigma (St. Louis, MO, USA). All other chemicals were purchased from Sigma-Aldrich (St Louis, MO, USA), Alfa Aesar (Ward Hill, MA, USA), or TCI International (Portland, Oregon, USA). Ultrafiltration membranes were purchased from Millipore. Analytical and semi-prep reverse-phase high-performance liquid chromatography (HPLC) was performed on a Shimadzu LC8 pump setup using Phenomenex C4 (4.6×150 mm-5 μm, 10×250 mm-10 μm) columns.

gH625-dendrimer preparation

The dendrimer and the peptide have been synthesized as previously reported [22,23]. To obtain the peptidodendrimer, a 1:1 methanol/water solution of peptide gH625–PrA (660 μl, 36 equiv), an aqueous solution of $CuSO_4 \cdot 5H_2O$ (10 μl, 1.46 mM, 1 equiv), and an aqueous solution of sodium ascorbate (50 μl, 1.17 mM, 4 equiv) were added to the dendrimer (50 μg, 0.0146 μmol) in a 1:1 water/methanol solution (280 μl). The mixture was left stirring for one hour at 40°C and for two days at RT. The compound was purified twice by ultrafiltration in water:methanol:DMSO 50:48:2 versus 30,000 molecular weight cut-off membranes and then by reverse phase HPLC on a C4 column with water (0.1% TFA) and acetonitrile (0.1% TFA) from 30 to 95% over 20 min at 5 mL/min. IR (cast on poly(ethylene)): $\tilde{\nu} = 3295, 1658, 1545, 1471, 1203\ cm^{-1}$. No peak at 2098 cm^{-1} was observed. The functionalization of the gH625-dendrimer was confirmed by determining the amount of peptide attached via UV analysis ($\varepsilon_{gH625} = 7000\ M^{-1}cm^{-1}$ at $\lambda = 280$ nm) and comparing the result to the amount of dendrimer and peptide initially used for the reaction (18 mol peptide per mol dendrimer). The functionalization of the peptidodendrimer, and thus the reaction between the azide and the alkyne, was also confirmed by following the ^1H NMR (MeOD, 600 MHz) chemical shift of the triplet representing the CH_2N_3 protons of the dendrimer from 3.37 to 5.34 ppm after reaction.

Liposome preparation

Phospholipids and fluorescent probes were dissolved in organic solvents. Then the solvent was evaporated to obtain a lipid film which was hydrated with an appropriate volume of 10 mM HEPES buffer at pH 7.4. Small unilamellar vesicles (SUVs) was prepared from dry lipid films were suspended in buffer by vortexing for 1 h, then the lipid suspension was sonicated for 30 minutes. Lipid concentrations of liposome suspensions were determined by phosphate analysis as previously reported [16]. The final lipid concentration was 1 mM.

Tryptophan fluorescence measurements

Tryptophan fluorescence increases with an increase of the environment hydrophobicity and a blue shift of the emission maxima was observed. Emission spectra of the gH625 peptide and of the gH625-dendrimer (4 μM in peptide), containing the tryptophan residue, in the absence or presence of target vesicles (PC/Chol = 55/45) were recorded between 300 and 400 nm with an excitation wavelength of 295 nm.

The degree of association with the lipid vesicles was determined by adding lipid vesicles to 4 μM of the desired compounds. Fluorescence intensity was measured as a function of the lipid/peptide molar ratio, in three to four separate experiments. The fluorescence values were corrected by taking into account the dilution factor corresponding to the addition of microliter amounts of liposomes and by subtracting the corresponding blank. The lipid/peptide molar ratio was 200:1.

The binding of gH625 and gH625-dendrimer to membranes can be described as a partition equilibrium: $X_b = K_p C_f$ where K_p is the apparent partition coefficient in units of M^{-1}, X_b is the molar ratio of bound molecules per total lipid and C_f is the equilibrium concentration of the free molecules in solution. In order to calculate X_b, we estimated F_∞, the fluorescence signal obtained when all the molecules are lipid-bound, either from the plateau region of the titration curve or from a double reciprocal plot of F (total molecule fluorescence) versus C_L (total concentration of lipids), as previously suggested by Schwarz et al. [46]. (F_∞ was obtained by extrapolation of a double reciprocal plot of the total molecule fluorescence vs. the total lipid concentration in the outer leaflet, i.e. $1/F$ vs. $1/0.6C_L$). Knowing the fluorescence intensities of the free and bound forms of the molecules of interest, the fraction of membrane-bound molecules, f_b, can be determined from $f_b = (F\text{-}F_0)/(F_\infty\text{-}F_0)$, where F represents the fluorescence of molecules after the addition of the vesicles and F_0 represents the fluorescence of the unbound molecules. Determining f_b allows us to calculate the equilibrium concentration of free molecules in solution, C_f, as well as the extent of molecules binding X_b. It was assumed that the molecules were initially partitioned only over the outer leaflet of the SUV (60% of the total lipid). Therefore, values of X_b were corrected as follows: $X_b^* = X_b/0.6$.

The curve resulting from plotting X_b^* versus the concentration of the free molecules, C_f, is referred to as the conventional binding isotherm. Plots of X_b^* versus C_f yield straight lines with the slope corresponding to K_p if a simple partition equilibrium is observed. A deviation is expected for the binding of molecules that self-associate at the membrane surface corresponding to binding isotherms that are not straight lines but deviate to increased binding at higher molecule concentrations. If enough data points of C_f can be collected at very low free molecule concentrations, the surface partition coefficients, K_p, can be estimated from the initial slopes of the curves (Figure 1).

Tryptophan quenching by acrylamide

Aliquots of a 4 M solution of the water-soluble quencher acrilamide were added to the solution containing gH625 or gH625-dendrimer (4 μM in peptide) in the absence or presence of liposomes (PC:Chol 55:45, $8 \cdot 10^{-4}$ M) at a lipid/peptide molar ratio of 200: 1. The maximal concentration of acrylamide is 0.2 mM. Fluorescence was measured at an excitation wavelength of 295 nm to reduce acrylamide absorbance (and the resulting inner filter effect), and emission at a wavelength of 340 nm to eliminate interference from the Raman band of water. The data were analyzed according to the Stern-Volmer equation [47], $F_0/F = 1 + K_{sv} [Q]$, where F_0 and F represent the fluorescence intensities in the absence and the presence of the quencher (Q), respectively, and K_{sv} is the Stern-Volmer quenching constant, which is a measure of the accessibility of tryptophan to acrylamide. Considering that acrylamide does not significantly partition into the membrane bilayer, the value for K_{sv} can be considered to be a reliable reflection of the bimolecular rate constant for collisional quenching of the tryptophan residue present in the aqueous phase. Accordingly, K_{sv} is determined by the amount of non-vesicle-associated free molecule as well as the fraction of the molecule residing on the surface of the bilayer.

Tryptophan quenching experiments with Br-PC

Tryptophan is sensitive to its environment and has been previously utilized to evaluate peptide localization in the membrane [48]. Emission spectra of the gH625-dendrimer in the absence or presence of target vesicles (PC/Chol = 55/45) were recorded between 300 and 400 nm with an excitation wavelength of 295 nm. Br-PC employed as quencher of tryptophan fluorescence is suitable for probing membrane insertion of peptides, since it acts over a short distance and does not drastically perturb the membrane [20]. The peptidodendrimer was added (final concentration of 222 nM) to 2 mL of SUVs, thus establishing a lipid:peptide molar ratio of 100:1. After two minutes of incubation at room temperature, an emission spectrum of the tryptophan was recorded with the excitation set at 295 nm. SUVs composed of PC/Chol that contained 25% of either 6,7 Br-PC, or 9,10 Br-PC or 11,12 Br-PC were used. Three separate experiments were conducted. In control experiments, the peptidodendrimer in PC/Chol (55/45) SUVs without Br-PC were used.

Membrane permeability studies

Membrane destabilization, in the form of diffusion potential collapse, was detected fluorimetrically as described previously [49]. Briefly, a liposome suspension (SUV = PC:Chol 55:45, 0.1 mM), prepared in "K^++buffer", (50 mM K_2SO_4, 25 mM HEPES-SO_4 pH 6.8) was added to an isotonic buffer, K^+-free buffer (50 mM Na_2SO_4, 10 mM HEPES-SO_4 pH 6.8), to which the dye diS-C_3-5 (final concentration 1×10^{-6} M) was added. Subsequent addition of valinomycin (final concentration 1×10^{-7} M) creates a negative diffusion potential inside the vesicles by a selective efflux of K^+ ions, resulting in a quenching of the dye's fluorescence. The addition of a permeable compound induces membrane permeability toward all the ions in solution causing dissipation of the diffusion potential, monitored by an increase of fluorescence. Compound concentrations varied from 5 10^{-6} M to 7 10^{-5} M. Fluorescence was monitored using excitation at 620 nm and emission at 670 nm. The percentage of fluorescence recovery (F_t) was defined as shown in Equation 1.

$$F_t = [(I_t\text{-}I_0)/(I_f\text{-}I_0)]100\% \qquad \text{(Eq.(1))}$$

I_t is the fluorescence observed after addition of the dendrimer-peptide at time t, I_0 is the fluorescence after addition of valinomycin, and I_f is the total fluorescence prior to addition of valinomycin. The peptide melittin was used as a positive control in this experiment.

Binding analysis by surface plasmon resonance (SPR)

SPR experiments were carried out with a BIAcore 3000 analytical system (Biacore, Uppsala, Sweden) using the HPA sensor chip. The HPA sensor chip contains hydrophobic alkanethiol chains, which are covalently bound to its gold surface, and a lipid heteromonolayer created by introducing liposomes to the chip. The complete coverage of the surface with a polar lipid monolayer generates a membrane-like environment where analytes in aqueous buffer interact with a lipid monolayer. The experimental protocol used, was previously described by Mozsolits *et al.* [50]. The running buffer used for all experiments was 5 mM HEPES 100 mM NaCl (pH 7.4); the washing solution was 40 mM

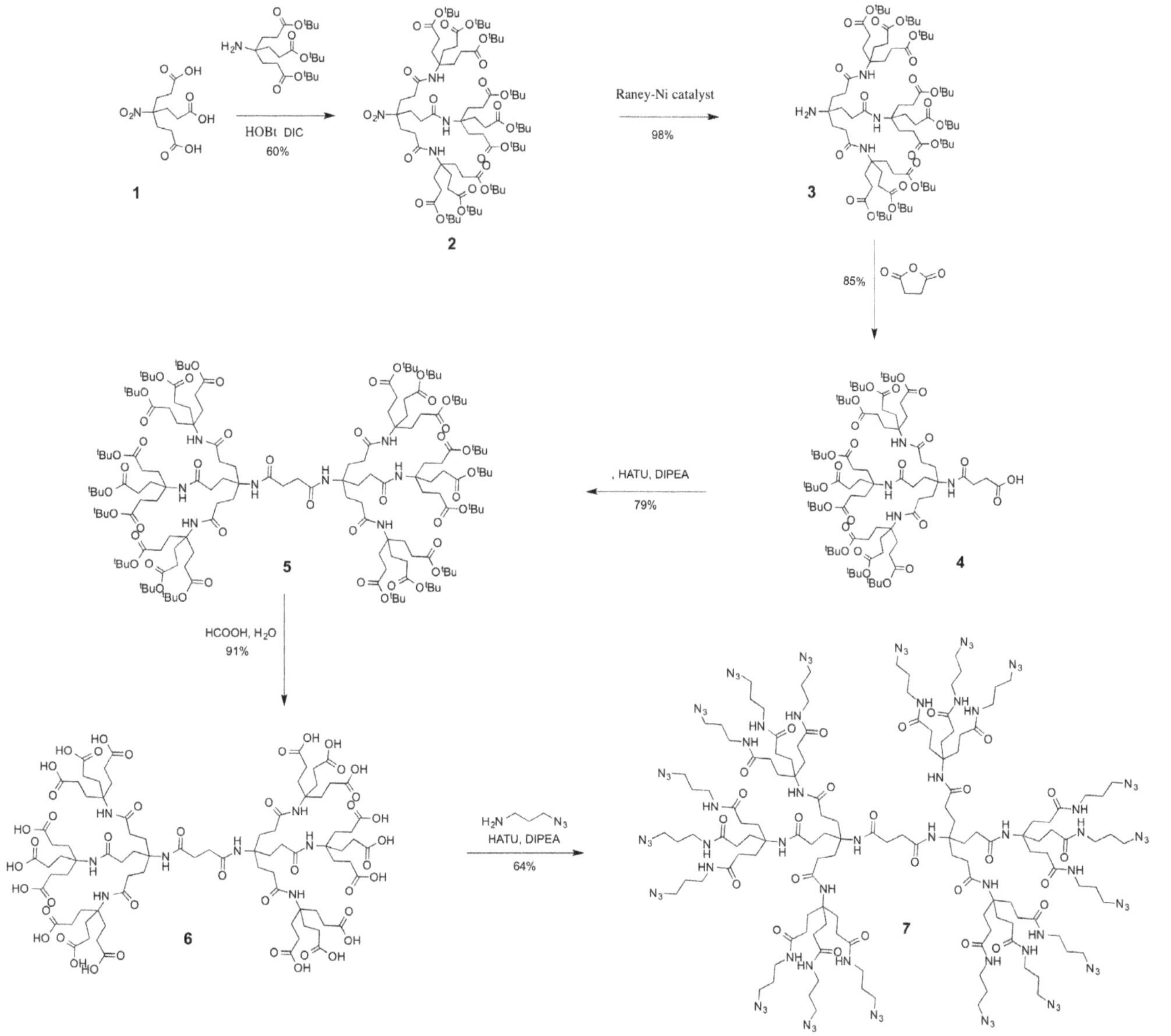

Figure 1. Scheme of the octadecaazide dendrimer synthesis.

N-octyl *β*-D-glucopyranoside. All solutions were freshly prepared, degassed, and filtered through 0.22 μm pores. The operating temperature was 25°C. After cleaning as indicated by the manufacturers, the BIAcore 3000 instrument was left running overnight using Milli-Q water as eluent to thoroughly wash all liquid-handling parts of the instrument. The HPA chip was then installed, and the alkanethiol surface was cleaned by an injection of the nonionic detergent N-octyl *β*-D-glucopyranoside (25 μl, 40 mM) at a flow rate of 5 μl/min. PC/Chol (55/45 w/w) SUVs (80 μl, 0.5 mM) were then applied to the chip surface at a flow rate of 2 μl/min. To remove any multilamellar structures from the lipid surface, we used NaOH 10 mM and increased the flow rate to 50 μl/min, which resulted in a stable baseline corresponding to the lipid monolayer linked to the chip surface. The negative control albumin bovine serum (BSA) was injected (25 μl, 0.1 mg/μl in PBS) to confirm complete coverage of the nonspecific binding sites. gH625-dendrimer solutions at the concentration of 0.07, 0.11, 0.22, 0.28, 0.33, 0.44, 0.55 nM (75 μl at a flow rate of 30 μl/min) were injected onto the lipid surface. HEPES alone then replaced the peptide solution for 15 min to allow gH625-dendrimer dissociation. SPR detects changes in the reflective index of the surface layer of peptidodendrimer and lipids in contact with the sensor chip. A sensorgram is obtained by plotting the SPR angle against time. This change in the angle is then translated to response units. Analysis of the peptidodendrimer lipid binding event was performed from a series of sensorgrams collected at different peptide concentrations.

The sensorgrams for each gH625-dendrimer lipid interaction were analyzed by curve fitting using numerical integration analysis. The BIA evaluation was used to perform complete kinetic analyses of the gH625-dendrimer sensorgrams and results were compared with those obtained for the peptide alone which were previously reported [18].

Isothermal calorimetry

Isothermal titration calorimetry was carried out on a MicroCal-ITC 200 calorimeter. Solutions were degassed under vacuum for ten minutes with gentle stirring prior to use. The heat of dilution values were obtained in control experiments by injecting either the peptidodendrimer or the lipid solutions into buffer and the heats of dilution were substracted from the heats determined in the corresponding peptidodendrimer-lipid experiments. Two kinds of experiments were performed; in the first the calorimeter cell contains lipid vesicles and the peptidodendrimer is injected into the cell (lipid 0.033 mM and gH625-dendrimer 17 μM); while in the second, the two solutions are exchanged (gH625-dendrimer 2.8 μM was placed in the 280 μL reaction cell, while SUVs 2 mM (PC:Chol 55:45) in 5 mM Hepes 100 mM NaCl (pH 7.4) were placed in a 40 μL syringe). In the second experiment the LUVs were added into the gH625-dendrimer solution via 20 injections of 2 μl per injection. The injections were pre-programmed at 150 sec intervals and were performed automatically at 25°C under stirring at 1000 rpm. The exotermic heat flow (dQ/dt) data were collected every second for the first 100 sec after each injection and every 5 sec for the remaining time interval and were analysed using the inbuilt Origin software.

Results

Synthesis of the gH625-dendrimer

The octadecaazide dendrimer was synthetized as previously reported [22] and as shown in Figure 1. Briefly, the second generation Newkome-style dendron 2 was first functionalized at the amine terminus with succinic anhydride to afford the hemisuccinate dendron 3. Coupling dendrons 2 and 3 by using 2-[7-aza-1H-benzotriazol-1-yl]-1,1,3,3-tetramethyluronium hexafluorophosphate (HATU) as coupling agent afforded the symmetrical dendrimer 4. Acidic deprotection of the terminal tert-butyl esters resulted in the formation of the octadecaacid dendrimer 5. Reaction between the terminal carboxylic acid groups and an azido-terminated amine and an azido-terminated amine linker afforded the octadecaazide dendrimer 6 (Figure 1).

The gH625 peptide sequence was synthesized with a propargylglycine residue (PrA) at the C terminus to provide a handle for the copper-catalyzed azide–alkyne cycloaddition (CuAAC). Functionalization of the dendrimer was performed in a water/methanol solution (1:1 v/v) by using $CuSO_4{\cdot}5H_2O$ as catalyst and sodium ascorbate as reducing agent. The obtained peptide-dendrimer was purified by HPLC as reported in the experimental section. The obtained profiles are reported in Figure 2. The amount of peptide functionalization was determined to be 71% by UV analysis ($\varepsilon = 7000\ M^{-1}\ cm^{-1}$ at $\lambda = 280$ nm). IR analysis showed the disappearance of the azide stretch at 2098 cm^{-1} suggesting that all azides were consumed within the instrumental error range, thus suggesting high functionalization of the dendrimer with peptides. Analysis of the NMR spectrum suggested at least 57% functionalization, corresponding to 10–11 peptides per dendrimer, however the actual value is higher due to the peak at 3.37 ppm overlapping with residual solvent and peptide backbone peaks, and possible suppression of the triazole ring due to aggregation of the dendrimers in solution. These three methods suggest that the degree of functionalization is above 70% and potentially quantitative.

Tryptophan fluorescence measurements

In order to evaluate the degree of penetration of the gH625-dendrimer into the membrane bilayer we compared the intrinsic fluorescence of gH625 alone and of gH625-dendrimer due to the presence of a tryptophan residue in the middle of the peptide sequence. For both of them, we compared the fluorescence emission spectra in the presence of PC/Chol vesicles with that in buffer (Figure 3).

It is widely accepted that the fluorescence emission of tryptophan residues increases when the amino acid penetrates a more hydrophobic environment and the maximal spectral position may be shifted toward shorter wavelengths (blue shift) [48]. For both molecules, we observed changes in the spectral properties, suggesting that the tryptophan residue of each of them is located in a less polar environment upon interaction with lipids. Emission intensity was enhanced and the maxima shifted to lower wavelengths; blue shifts of this magnitude have been observed when amphiphilic tryptophan-containing peptides interact with phospholipid bilayers and are consistent with the indole moiety becoming partially immersed in the membrane, further suggesting that the two molecules are capable of penetrating a lipid bilayer [48]. A lipid-exposed tryptophan residue located at the center of the hydrocarbon core of a bilayer exhibits a characteristic highly blue shifted emission, with a λ_{max} in the range of 315–318 nm http://pubs.acs.org/cgi-bin/article.cgi/bichaw/2003/42/i11/html/bi026697d.html - bi026697db00003#bi026697db00003. As a tryptophan residue moves toward the more polar membrane surface, λ_{max} gradually shifts to 335–340 nm. A smaller blue shift of the fluorescence for a tryptophan at the bilayer center can also be detected upon helix oligomerization inside the membrane. This shift presumably reflects the change in local environment upon replacement of contacts between tryptophan and lipid with contacts between tryptophan and polypeptide. Our data support the hypothesis that the tryptophan is located inside the membrane and moreover that oligomerization processes may have taken place.

The increase in fluorescence for tryptophan binding to membrane phospholipids was used for the binding isotherms for gH625 and the gH625-dendrimer, from which partition coefficients could be calculated. The concentrations of peptides used were low enough to cause minimal aggregation in the aqueous phase and were assumed to not disrupt the bilayer structure. SUV vesicles were used in the assay in order to minimize light scattering effects.

To determine the surface partition coefficient, the fluorescence intensities were converted to moles of bound peptide per moles of lipid and plotted as a function of the free peptide concentration as described in material and methods (Figure 3).

As partition coefficients depend on the concentration of lipid accessible to peptide, the curves obtained by plotting X_b^* (the molar ratio of bound peptide per 60% of the total lipid) vs C_f (the equilibrium concentration of free peptide in the solution) are referred to as the conventional binding isotherms. We observed a non-linear relationship indicating accumulation of the two compounds on the surface which cannot be explained as a simple phenomenon without cooperative association. This behavior is the hallmark for peptides that self-associate at membrane surfaces upon partitioning. If aggregation occurred only in water but not in the bilayer phase, the opposite course of the isotherms should be expected: a steep rise at the origin, followed by pronounced flattening; thus, the shape of the isotherms obtained could be interpreted as reflecting a process whereby peptides first incorporate into the membrane and then aggregate there within. Moreover, there was no evidence of aggregation in water at the concentration used in this experiment. In the isotherms obtained, the total extent of incorporation (X_b^*) slowly increases until a critical concentration is reached, where massive internal aggregation apparently starts to develop.

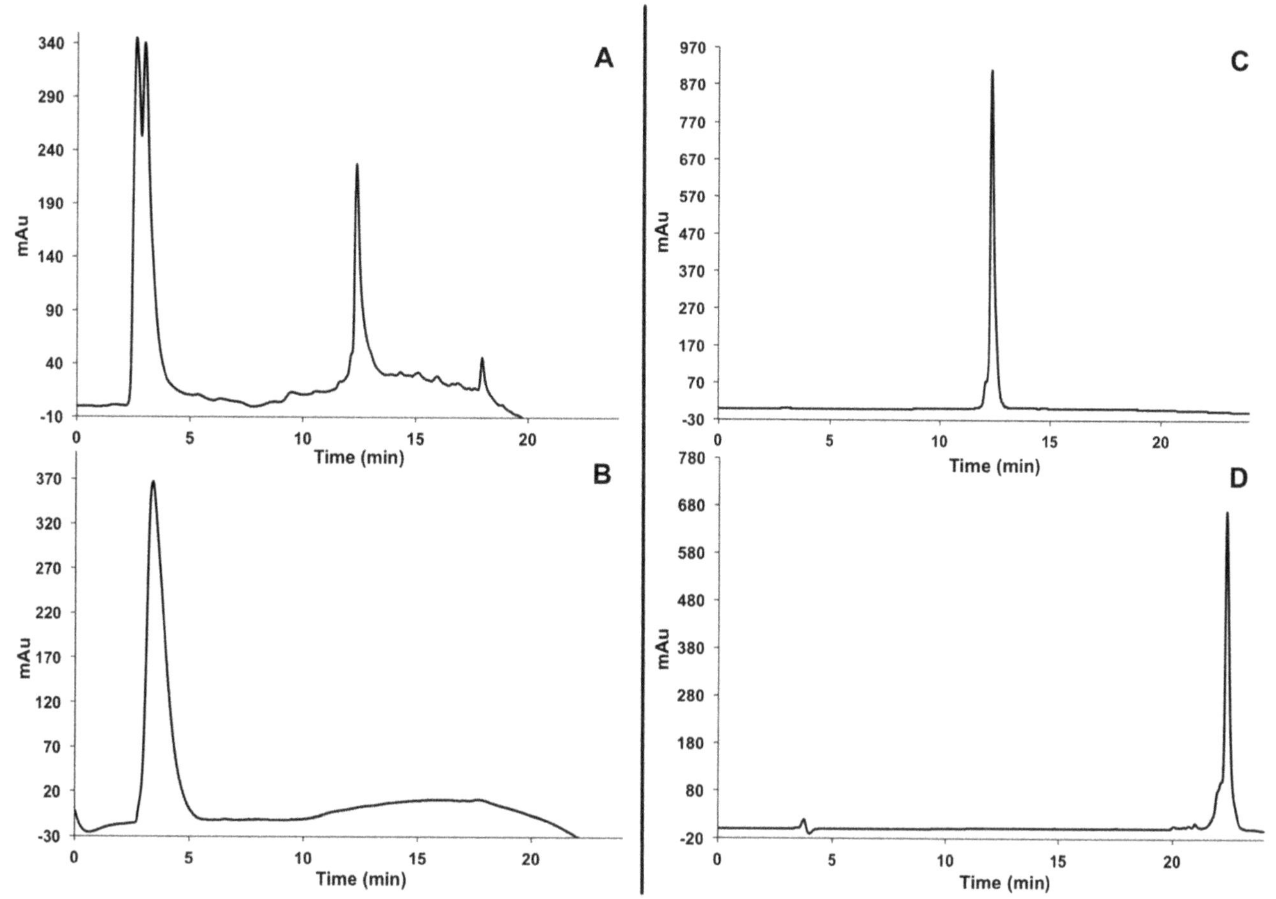

Figure 2. HPLC traces of gH625-Dendrimer crude (panel A), gH625-Dendrimer pure (panel B), gH625 pure (panel C) and dendrimer pure (panel D).

The surface partition coefficients K_p were estimated by extrapolating the initial slopes of the curves to C_f values of zero; curves are shown in Figure 3.

The K_p values for gH625 and gH625-Dendrimer are shown in Table 1. The K_p value obtained for gH625 is 2.8 10^4, indicating that the tryptophan in gH625 is embedded in the bilayer and thus that most of the peptide gH625 is located inside the bilayer. The K_p value for gH625-dendrimer is 3.4 10^4, indicating that also in the functionalized dendrimer the tryptophan residue of the peptide is stably inserted inside the bilayer.

Quenching of tryptophan by acrylamide

The changes in the tryptophan fluorescence spectra upon binding of gH625 and gH625-dendrimer to lipid vesicles indicate their insertion into the hydrophobic bilayer. We further determined the accessibility of the tryptophan residue to acrylamide, a neutral, water-soluble, highly efficient quenching molecule that is unable to penetrate into the hydrophobic core of the lipid bilayer. The more deeply a tryptophan residue is buried, the less strongly it is quenched by acrylamide. Stern-Volmer plots for the quenching of tryptophan by acrylamide in buffer and in PC/Chol LUVs are shown in Figure 4.

Fluorescence of tryptophan decreased in a concentration dependent manner by the addition of acrylamide to the peptide solution both in the absence and presence of liposomes, without other effects on the spectra. However, in the presence of liposomes, less decrement in fluorescence intensity was evident, thus revealing that tryptophan is less accessible to the quencher in the presence of LUVs. K_{sv} values are reported in Table 2.

Analysis of the obtained values confirm that the gH625-dendrimer tryptophans are more exposed than those of gH625 in buffer; in fact the K_{sv} of gH625-dendrimer is higher. On the contrary, the K_{sv} value in LUVs of gH625-dendrimer is lower, suggesting that tryptophans are more buried in the bilayers, becoming more inaccessible for quenching by acrylamide. Comparison of the plots (Figure 4) and of the values of K_{sv} (Table 2) confirms that the tryptophans in gH625-dendrimer are more deeply inserted than in the isolated peptide.

Membrane permeability studies

Increasing concentrations of gH625 and gH625-dendrimer were mixed with the same amount of PC/Chol SUVs pretreated with the fluorescent dye and valinomycin. We did not observe any enhanced recovery of fluorescence (quenched by the addition of valinomycin) with increasing amounts of the two molecules. Our results indicate that there is no electroporation effect due to the peptide or the peptide-dendrimer interactions with the SUVs.

Tryptophan quenching experiments with Br-PC

The position and the depth of the two molecules inside the bilayer can be investigated by measuring the relative quenching of the fluorescence of the Trp residue by the probes 11,12-Br-PC,

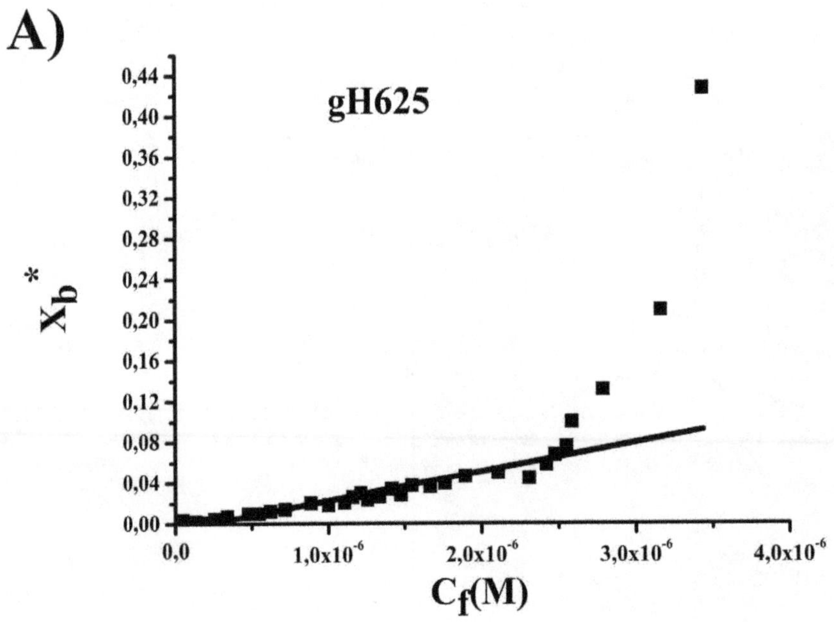

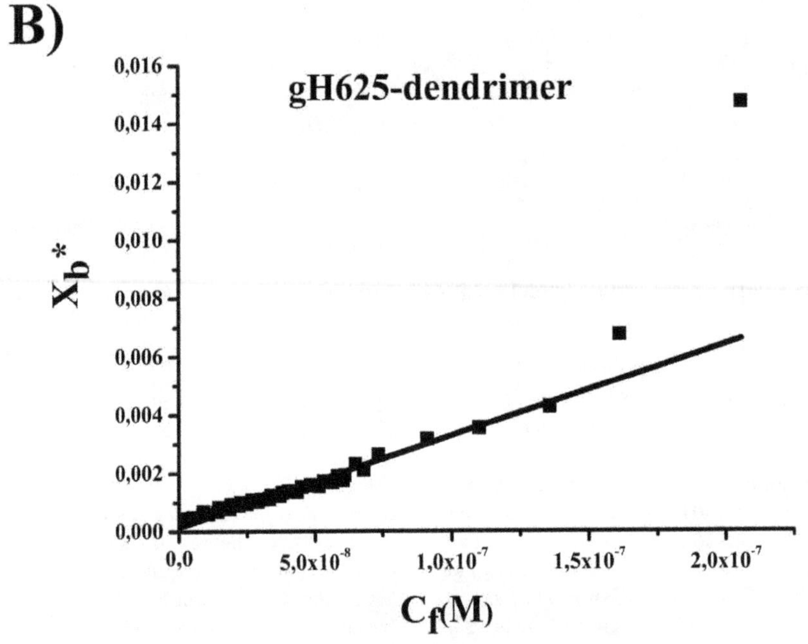

Figure 3. Binding isotherms obtained plotting X_b^* versus C_f for gH625 and gH625-Dendrimer.

9,10-Br-PC, and 6,7-Br-PC, which differ in the position of the quencher moiety along the hydrocarbon chain. 6,7-Br-PC is a better quencher for molecules near or at the interface, while the other two are better probes for molecules buried deeply inside a membrane. We previously reported that the largest quenching of tryptophan fluorescence for gH625 was observed with 11,12- Br-PC vesicles and 9,10-Br-PC, while slightly less quenching was observed with 6,7-Br-PC [20]. These results indicate that, upon binding to vesicles, gH625 inserted into the membrane bilayer with the tryptophan side chain pointing toward the bilayer

Table 1. Partition coefficient for the binding of gH625 and gH625-dendrimer with PC/Chol obtained by fluorescence studies.

	gH625	gH625-dendrimer
K_p	2.8 $10^4 \pm 0.2$	3.4 $10^4 \pm 0.1$

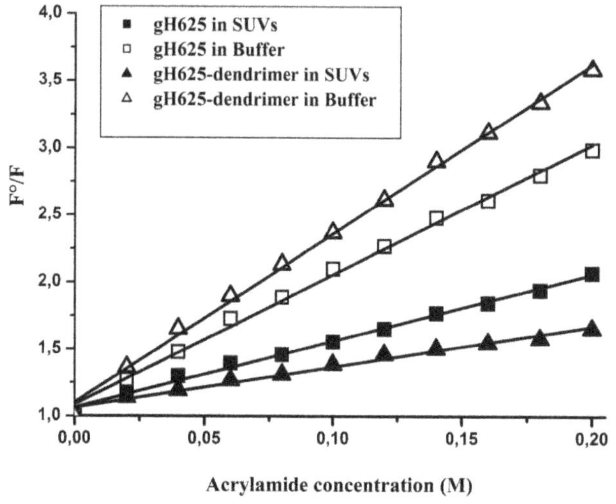

Figure 4. Stern-Volmer plots of acrylamide quenching of gH625 and gH625-Dendrimer in buffer (open symbols) and in LUVs (closed symbols).

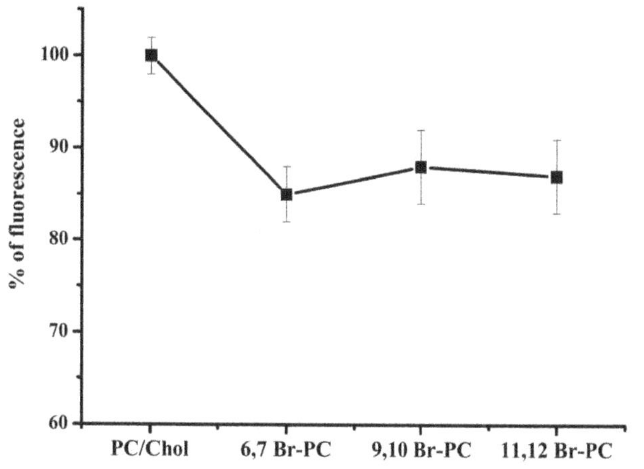

Figure 5. Percentage of tryptophan fluorescence for gH625–dendrimer in PC/Chol and in the presence of the probes 11,12-Br-PC, 9,10-Br-PC, and 6,7-Br-PC.

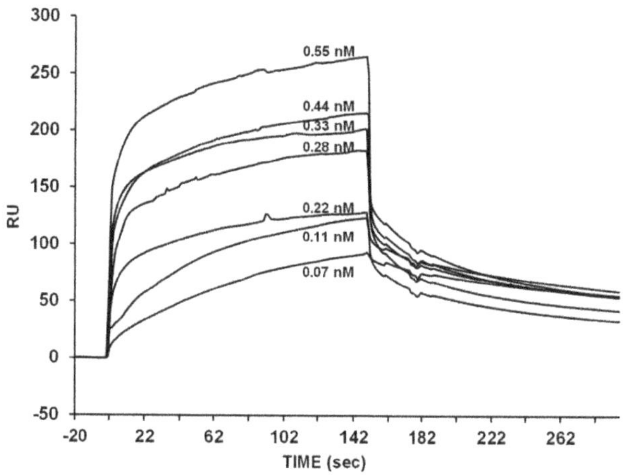

Figure 6. Sensorgrams of the binding between various concentrations of gH625-dendrimer with the HPA chip.

interior. We observed a different result for the gH625-dendrimer. There is a significant change compared to the control but the three spectra are superimposable, indicating that there is probably a distribution of the molecule inside the bilayer with the tryptophan localized at various depths (Figure 5).

Binding Analysis by Surface Plasmon Resonance (SPR)

We utilized a BIAcore biosensor to investigate the mode of action of gH625-dendrimer and compared it with gH625 [18,19]. PC/Chol monolayers were absorbed onto the HPA. Sensorgrams of the binding with monolayers are shown in Figure 6.

The sensorgrams revealed that the RU signal intensity increased as a function of the molecule concentration. This indicates that the amount of molecule bound to the lipids is proportional to its concentration. We employed numerical integration analysis that uses nonlinear analysis to fit an integrated rate equation directly to the sensorgrams [51]. When fitting the sensorgrams globally with the simplest 1:1 Langmuir binding model, a poor fit was obtained (χ^2>50), confirming that this model does not represent the lipid binding mechanism of the gH625-dendrimer. However, a significantly improved fit was obtained using numerical integration of the two-state reaction model of the binding sensorgrams, suggesting that, in analogy with the data previously obtained for the peptide alone [19], there are likely to be at least two steps involved in the interaction between the gH625-dendrimer and the hybrid bilayer membrane surface. In analogy with previous studies of peptide-membrane interactions using SPR [19,50,52], the first step may correspond to the actual binding to the surface, while the second step might be the insertion into the hydrophobic core of the membrane. A set of sensorgrams with different gH625-dendrimer concentrations was used to estimate the kinetic parameters. The average values for the rate constants obtained from the two-state model analysis are listed in Table 3 along with the affinity constant

Table 2. Stern-Volmer (K_{sv}) quenching constant calculated from the equation $F^o/F = 1+K_{sv}[Q]$ (Q, quencher) for gH625 and gH625-dendrimer.

	$K_{sv}(M^{-1})$
gH625 in Buffer	9.70±0.21
gH625 in LUVs	4.98±0.14
gH625-dendrimer in Buffer	12.60±0.22
gH625-dendrimer in SUVs	3.04±0.14

Table 3. Association (k_{a1}, k_{a2}) and dissociation (k_{d1}, k_{d2}) rate constants obtained for the HPA chip using the two state model.

	gH625	gH625-dendrimer
k_{a1}	$(5.11\pm0.03)10^{1}$	$(6.57\pm0.02)10^{3}$
k_{d1}	$(2.51\pm0.05)10^{-2}$	$(6.95\pm0.03)10^{-2}$
K_1	$2.0\ 10^{3}$	$9.4\ 10^{4}$
k_{a2}	$(5.22\pm0.05)10^{-3}$	$(1.61\pm0.05)10^{-2}$
k_{d2}	$(110\pm0.06)\ 10^{-4}$	$(4.93\pm0.09)10^{-3}$
K_2	47	3.2
K_A	$1.00\ 10^{5}$	$4.03\ 10^{5}$

The affinity constants K_1 and K_2 are for the first ($K_1 = k_{a1}/k_{d1}$) and for the second ($K_2 = k_{a2}/k_{d2}$) steps respectively, and the affinity constant (K_A) determined as $(k_{a1}/k_{d1}) \times (k_{a2}/k_{d2})$ is for the complete binding process. Standard deviations are reported in brackets.

values (K_A) and compared with the data previously obtained for the peptide gH625 [18].

The data indicate the main influence on the overall binding constant of the fast association rate and slow dissociation rate of the first step. If this step corresponds to the electrostatic interaction, these results suggest that electrostatic forces play an important role in the binding of membrane-active peptides.

It is interesting to note that gH625 and gH625-dendrimer have high K_1, indicative of the first step corresponding to the electrostatic interaction is important for the binding and the higher value for gH625-dendrimer is probably influenced by the presence of several peptide molecules on the same dendrimer. The overall binding to the membrane bilayer is thus stronger for the gH625-dendrimer.

Isothermal calorimetry

Isothermal calorimetry can be applied to study membrane interactions in two different modes. In the first, the calorimeter cell contains lipid vesicles and the ligand is injected into the calorimeter cell, while in the second, the two solutions are exchanged. The two experiments provide different thermodynamic parameters. The first type of experiment allows to measure the reaction enthalpy ΔH (Figure 7).

In the second experiment, after each addition of lipid, the ligand is bound to the lipid vesicles and removed from bulk solution; as a consequence, with increasing lipid concentration in the reaction vessel, less and less ligand is available for binding and the heat of reaction is no longer constant but decreases with each lipid injection. The ΔH values determined in the two experiments should be identical, but the additional advantage of the second type of experiment is the ability to measure the binding isotherm and to evaluate the binding constant K.

The enthalpy change upon binding of the gH625-dendrimer to lipid vesicles was measured from the first type of experiment by injecting small aliquots of a gH625-dendrimer solution into concentrated SUVs. Under these conditions, the lipid is in large excess over the ligand during the whole experiment and the injected ligand is completely bound to the membrane surface if the binding constant is sufficiently large. Each injection experiment thus produces the same heat of reaction, Δh. Figure 7 shows the result of the injection of 2 μl aliquots of the 0.017 mM gH625-dendrimer solution (buffer: Hepes 5 mM, NaCl 100 mM, pH 7.4) into 0.033 mM PC:Chol (55:45) SUVs at 25°C. The average heat of reaction observed after subtraction of the heat of dilution (measured in control experiments of peptidodendrimer into buffer injection) was −1.5 μcal. The analysis of the heat of reactions shows that the reaction is exothermic. Dividing the heat of reaction by the amount of injected molecule yields the molar enthalpy of binding, ΔH (−47.5 Kcal/mol) (Figure 7).

In the second experiment, the gH625-dendrimer was contained in the calorimeter cell and lipid vesicles were injected. This allowed the determination of the binding isotherm. The molecule was employed at a concentration of 2.8 μM and each titration peak corresponds to a 2 μl injection of a 2 mM SUVs (20 injections) except the first one that corresponds to a 0.4 μl

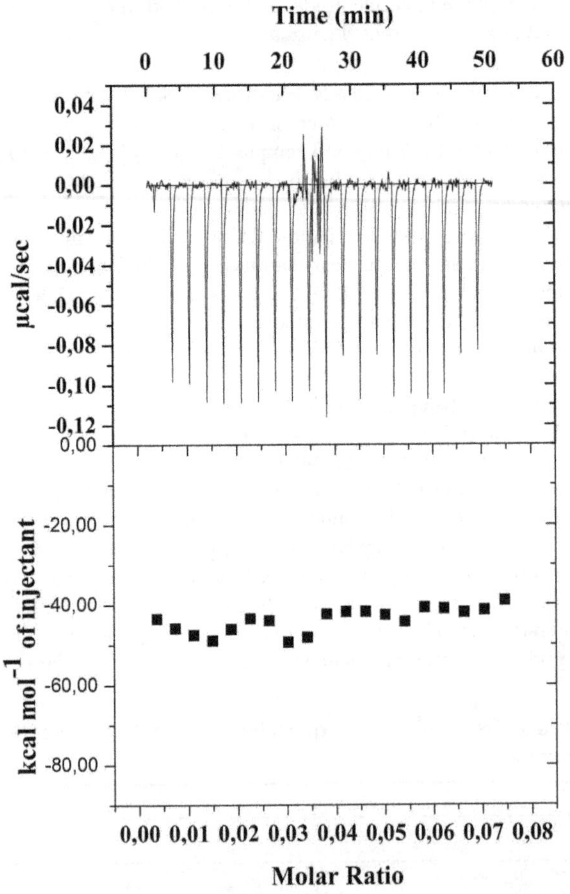

Figure 7. Isothermal titration calorimetry of SUVs with gH625-dendrimer at 25°C. The upper panel shows the calorimeter trace; the lower panel shows the molar enthalpy as evaluated by integration of the calorimeter traces.

injection. The amount of heat released decreases with increasing injection number as less and less gH625-dendrimer remains free in solution. The heat of reaction values are shown in Figure 8 after subtraction of the heats of dilution obtained in control experiments of vesicle-into-buffer titrations.

If we denote with Δh the experimentally measured heat of reaction at the kth injection, then $\Sigma^{k}{}_{1}\Delta h_k$ is the *cumulative* heat of the first k injections and $\Sigma^{n}{}_{1}\Delta h_k$ is the *total* heat of injection provided Δh_k, the last injection step, is zero. It is possible to calculate the molar heat of reaction, ΔH, according to:

$$\Delta H = \Sigma_1^n \Delta h_k / n\ p.$$

where n is the molar amount of the molecule in the calorimeter cell after n injections.

The ΔH values determined in the two experiments should be identical. However, the additional advantage of the second type of titration experiment is the possibility to measure the binding isotherm and to evaluate the binding constant K. The binding isotherm reports the dependence of the molar ratio of bound molecule per total lipid, X_b, on the free molecule concentration in solution, C_f, and can be derived using established procedures [53]. As for the fluorescence data, X_b^* was calculated on the basis of the lipid present in the outer leaflet of the bilayer only since the molecule cannot cross the bilayer under the present experimental conditions.

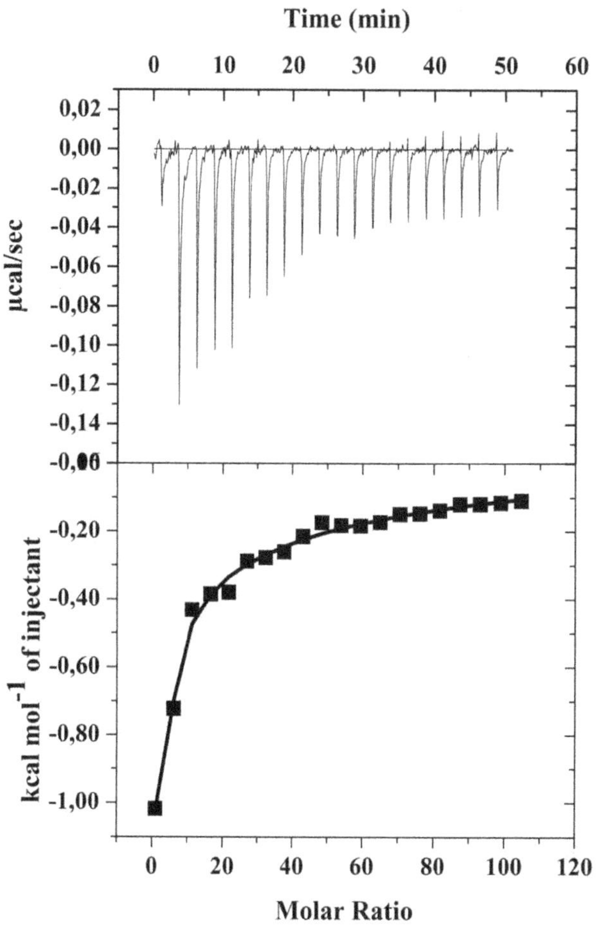

Figure 8. Isothermal titration calorimetry of gH625-dendrimer with SUVs at 25°C. The upper panel shows the calorimeter trace; the lower panel shows the molar enthalpy as evaluated by integration of the calorimeter traces.

The two essential parameters which constitute the binding isotherm, namely the degree of binding X_b^* and the corresponding free molecule concentration C_f can thus be determined in a single titration experiment.

Hence the peptidodendrimer lipid-binding equilibrium is $X_b^* = f(C_f)$, where $f(C_f)$ describes the functional dependence of X_b^* on C_f. The exact form of the functional dependence depends on the nature of the problem and provides information on the organization of the molecule within the membrane as was previously discussed for fluorescence data. A linear relationship is the exception rather than the rule; a straight line indicates a simple adhesion process. The shape of the binding isotherm was not linear indicating that the gH625-dendrimer accumulation at the surface is a complex phenomenon. In particular, also from isothermal calorimetry we obtained a binding isotherm characterized by a flattening at the origin, followed by steep rise, which could be interpreted as reflecting a process whereby peptides first incorporate into the membrane and then aggregate within. In our isotherms, the total extent of incorporation (X_b^*) slowly increases until a critical concentration is reached, where massive internal aggregation apparently starts to develop (Figure 9).

The surface partition coefficient K_p was estimated by extrapolating the initial slopes of the curves to C_f values of zero. The values of K_p (4.3 10^4) obtained are within the range of those obtained for membrane-permeating bioactive peptides and its high value indicates that the tryptophans of gH625-dendrimer are embedded in the bilayer. Knowledge of the partition constant allows the calculation of the free energy of binding according to ΔG = -RTln(55.5 K), yielding ΔG = -8.6Kcal/mol (Table 4). The factor 55.5 corrects the cratic contribution since the concentration of the macromolecule in solution is measured in moles per liter and that in the membrane phase in moles of macromolecule per mole of lipid [54]. The relation $\Delta G = \Delta H - T\Delta S$, allows the calculation of $\Delta S = -130$ cal/mol K. Considering the complex interaction of the gH625-dendrimer with the bilayer, we may consider that this constant is model independent and describes the overall behavior. We obtained a considerably favorable enthalpic contribution and a unfavorable entropic contribution. This

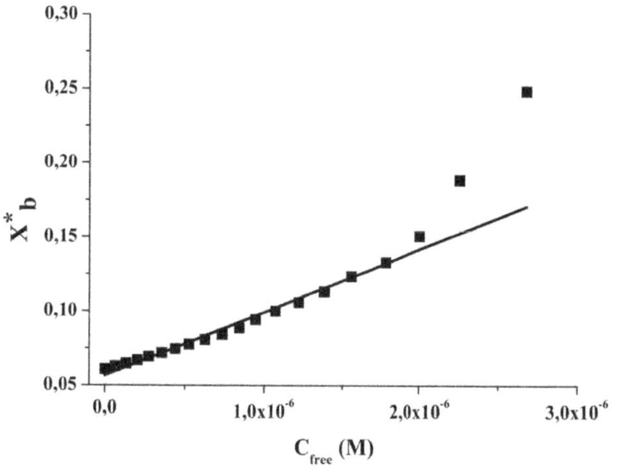

Figure 9. Binding isotherms for binding of gH625-dendrimer to SUVs at 25°C. Binding isotherms were derived from lipid into peptidodendrimer titrations as described in the text. The degree of binding is plotted against the free peptidodendrimer concentration. The solid line corresponds to the theoretical binding isotherm.

unfavorable entropy change may be attributed to the conformational change of gH625 from an unordered structure in aqueous solution to an ordered α-helix upon interaction with the membrane as previously shown by circular dichroism data in membrane mimetic environment [22] and as reported in literature for other peptides [55,56]. Nevertheless, the overall free energy change is still large.

In analogy with the SPR analysis, we decided to interpolate the experimental data reported in Figure 7 with two different models: the one site binding and the sequential binding site. From the one binding site we obtained a high χ^2 and thus thermodynamic parameters similar to those obtained from the isothermal binding curve but with a high standard deviation. When we used the sequential binding (for 2 sites) we obtained lower χ^2. The thermodynamic parameters are indicative of an initial interaction with the bilayer with a negative enthalpic change (−6.3 Kcal/mol) which is in the typical range of membrane interactions (from −2 to −10) [53] and a small favorable entropic component (1 Kcal/mol) which may be attributed to the partition from water into a nonpolar environment due to the release of the hydration shell. The second step may correspond to the insertion and the conformational change inside the bilayer. The enthalpic contribution is very favorable while the entropic contribution is negative. These results are similar to those obtained for membrane interacting peptides and has been previously attributed to the formation of an α -helix in the membrane bilayer [57]. The high binding constant for this step may allow us to conclude that membrane-facilitated helix formation is a strong driving force for the gH625-dendrimer binding to the lipid membrane.

Conclusions

Dendrimers are well-defined highly branched structures that have attracted much interest in the biomedical field [58,59,60,61]. Among their potential biomedical applications are drug delivery across the cell membrane, a complex structure composed of lipids and embedded proteins. In order to understand dendrimer's mechanism of action and to increase their targeting efficiency, the interaction with lipid bilayers needs to be unravelled. Model membranes, like liposomes, represent outstanding models due to their simple composition, ease of preparation and good stability.

Many reports are dedicated to the study of interactions between dendrimers and biological membranes. The type and strength of the interaction is dependent on charge and size of the molecule. Evidences suggest that dendrimers either create holes in a bilayer [29,30,31,32,33,39,62,63,64] or can be incorporated into lipid structure [35,37,45,65]. Higher generation dendrimers cause greater disturbances in a lipid bilayer and positively charged dendrimers interact more effectively with liposomes [28,35,42,43,44,45]. It has been proposed that at low concentrations, dendrimers can traverse the bilayer, whereas at higher concentrations, dendrimer: lipid micelles are created [63,66].

The toxicity of PAMAM dendrimers generally increases with increasing generation number, which has been attributed to the increased number of positive charges per molar concentration and thus increased contact area of the dendrimer with the cell membrane [29]. The electrostatic interactions of cationic dendrimers with cell membranes probably induces nano-scale hole formation and membrane destabilization mechanisms [29,30,67]. It is thus necessary to remove positive charges, through the functionalization of external groups, from the surface of the dendrimer [68] to achieve better cytotoxicity profiles. In this contribution, we present a dendrimer with the external termini modified by a peptide, which has been proved to enhance cell membrane crossing [14,69,70].

The peptide gH625 has been previously characterized [16,17,18], indicating its strong interaction with LUVs without the formation of pores inside the bilayer, therefore able to reduce toxicity problems. We have previously shown that the peptidodendrimer is more effective than the native peptide at interacting and fusing with lipid membranes, showing its efficacy as a membrane-perturbing agent [22]. We proposed that the peptidodendrimer translocates across the bilayer without involving essentially the endocytic mechanism.

The mechanism of internalization has direct implications for the design of drug delivery, cell transfection and gene therapy agents. In order to gain a better understanding of this mechanism for the peptide functionalized dendrimer, it was essential to investigate possible disruption of cell membranes. Delivery agents that have the ability to pass through membranes without causing leakage are desirable as drug delivery vehicles.

All the results from the complementary techniques such as fluorescence spectroscopy, surface plasmon resonance and isothermal calorimetry, obtained in this contribution, indicate that the gH625-dendrimer has a high affinity for the membrane bilayer; moreover, we were able to determine via tryptophan quenching experiments with Br-PC that the molecule is deeply inserted inside the bilayer. We proved that the molecule is able to cause membrane fusion but not holes in the bilayer. The peptide coupled to the dendrimer is also able to assume a helical conformation when in membrane mimetic environment. The data obtained further support the hypothesis that the binding to the membrane bilayer can be divided at least into two steps. The first step is an adsorption process that leads to an increased macromolecule concentration on the membrane. The second step is a hydrophobic insertion which is characterized by penetration into the lipid bilayer and probably a conformational change of the peptide coupled to the dendrimer. The first step has a higher binding constant compared to the second step as obtained both from surface plasmon resonance and isothermal calorimetry. These data further support the view that the mechanism of lipid

Table 4. Partition coefficient for the binding of gH625-dendrimer with PC/Chol obtained by isothermal calorimetry.

Method used for calculations	ΔH (Kcal/mol)	K	ΔG (Kcal/mol)	TΔS (Kcal/mol)	ΔS (cal/mol K)
Isothermal binding curve	−47.5±0.9[a]	4.3 10^4	−8.6	−38.7	−130
One site Binding	−48±3	1.0 10^4	−5.4	−42.6	−143
Sequential site binding	−6.3±0.5	7.6 10^4	−6.6	+0.3	1
	−47.3±0.3	2.9 10^3	−4.7	−42.6	−143

[a]This value is the one obtained from the titration of the lipid with the macromolecule.

association plays a key role in the translocation activity and the hypothesis that gH625-dendrimer cellular uptake is associated with its ability to interact with membrane lipids and to temporarily affect membrane organization, thereby facilitating insertion into the membrane and translocation.

The translocating ability of our peptidodendrimer is different from the most commonly used cell penetrating peptides (such as the HIV derived TAT peptide) and from the mechanism hypothesized for PAMAM dendrimers, which do not translocate spontaneously across bilayers but rather are taken up by cells via endocytosis [21,71].

Our peptido-dendrimer presents a very efficient membrane penetration ability and our findings could prove helpful for a better understanding of the advantages of combining dendrimers and peptides to design and develop new and effective drug delivery tools.

Acknowledgments

The authors thank Maurizio Amendola and Luca De Luca for excellent technical assistance.

Author Contributions

Conceived and designed the experiments: SG MW MG. Performed the experiments: AF RT TC. Analyzed the data: SG. Wrote the paper: SG MW MG. Contributed reagents/materials/analysis tools: SG.

References

1. Lipinski CA, Lombardo F, Dominy BW, Feeney PJ (1997) Experimental and computational approaches to estimate solubility and permeability in drug discovery and development settings. Advanced Drug Delivery Reviews 23: 3–25.
2. Torchilin VP (2006) Recent approaches to intracellular delivery of drugs and DNA and organelle targeting. Annual Review of Biomedical Engineering. Palo Alto: Annual Reviews. pp. 343–375.
3. Accardo A, Tesauro D, Morelli G (2013) Peptide-based targeting strategies for simultaneous imaging and therapy with nanovectors. Polym J 45: 481–493.
4. Sanna V, Pala N, Sechi M (2014) Targeted therapy using nanotechnology: focus on cancer. Int J Nanomedicine 9: 467–483.
5. Newkome GR, Moorefield CN, Vögtle F (2001) Dendrimers and Dendrons: Concepts, Synthesis, Applications. Weinheim: Wiley-VCH.
6. Lee CC, MacKay JA, Fréchet JMJ, Szoka FC (2005) Designing dendrimers for biological applications. Nature Biotech 23: 1517–1526.
7. Gillies ER, Frechet JMJ (2005) Dendrimers and dendritic polymers in drug delivery. Drug Discovery Today 10: 35–43.
8. Pearson RM, Sunoqrot S, Hsu HJ, Bae JW, Hong S (2012) Dendritic nanoparticles: the next generation of nanocarriers? Therapeutic delivery 3: 941–959.
9. Seib FP, Jones AT, Duncan R (2007) Comparison of the endocytic properties of linear and branched PEIs, and cationic PAMAM dendrimers in B16f10 melanoma cells. J Control Release 117: 291–300.
10. Saovapakhiran A, D'Emanuele A, Attwood D, Penny J (2009) Surface modification of PAMAM dendrimers modulates the mechanism of cellular internalization. Bioconjug Chem 20: 693–701.
11. Galdiero S, Vitiello M, Falanga A, Cantisani M, Incoronato N, et al. (2012) Intracellular delivery: exploiting viral membranotropic peptides. Curr Drug Metab 13: 93–104.
12. Falanga A, Cantisani M, Pedone C, Galdiero S (2009) Membrane fusion and fission: enveloped viruses. Protein Pept Lett 16: 751–759.
13. Falanga A, Tarallo R, Vitiello G, Vitiello M, Perillo E, et al. (2012) Biophysical characterization and membrane interaction of the two fusion loops of glycoprotein B from herpes simplex type I virus. PLoS One 7: e32186.
14. Tarallo R, Accardo A, Falanga A, Guarnieri D, Vitiello G, et al. (2011) Clickable Functionalization of Liposomes with gH625 Peptide from Herpes Simplex Virus type I for Intracellular Delivery. Chem Eur J 17: 12659–12668.
15. Falanga A, Vitiello M, Cantisani M, Tarallo R, Guarnieri D, et al. (2011) A peptide derived from HSV1gH: membrane translocation and applications to delivery of QDs. Nanomedicine 7: 925–934.
16. Galdiero S, Falanga A, Vitiello M, Browne H, Pedone C, et al. (2005) Fusogenic Domains in Herpes Simplex Virus Type I Glycoprotein H. J Biol Chem 280: 28632–28643.
17. Galdiero S, Falanga A, Vitiello M, Raiola L, Fattorusso R, et al. (2008) Analysis of a Membrane Interacting Region of Herpes Simplex Virus Type I Glycoprotein H. J Biol Chem 283: 29993–30009.
18. Galdiero S, Falanga A, Vitiello M, Raiola L, Russo L, et al. (2010) The Presence of a Single N-terminal Histidine Residue Enhances the Fusogenic Properties of a Membranotropic Peptide Derived from Herpes Simplex Virus type I Glycoprotein H. J Biol Chem 285: 17123–17136.
19. Galdiero S, Falanga A, Vitiello G, Vitiello M, Pedone C, et al. (2010) Role of membranotropic sequences from herpes simplex virus type I glycoproteins B and H in the fusion process. Biochim Biophys Acta 1798: 579–591.
20. Galdiero S, Russo L, Falanga A, Cantisani M, Vitiello M, et al. (2012) Structure and orientation of the gH625-644 membrane interacting region of herpes simplex virus type 1 in a membrane mimetic system. Biochemistry 51: 3121–3128.
21. Mae M, Langel U (2006) Cell-penetrating peptides as vectors for peptide, protein and oligonucleotide delivery. Curr Opin Pharmacol 6: 509–514.
22. Carberry TP, Tarallo R, Falanga A, Finamore E, Galdiero M, et al. (2012) Dendrimer functionalization with a membrane-interacting domain of herpes simplex virus type 1: towards intracellular delivery. Chemistry 18: 13678–13685.
23. Tarallo R, Carberry TP, Falanga A, Vitiello M, Galdiero S, et al. (2013) Dendrimers functionalized with membrane-interacting peptides for viral inhibition. Int J Nanomedicine 8: 521–534.
24. Roberts JC, Bhalgat MK, Zera RT (1996) Preliminary biological evaluation of polyamidoamine (PAMAM) Starburst dendrimers. Biomed Mater Res 30: 53–65.
25. Ornelas C, Pennell R, Liebes LF, Weck M (2011) Construction of a Well-Defined Multifunctional Dendrimer for Theranostics. Org Lett 13: 967–979.
26. Ruzza P, Biondi B, Marchiani A, Antolini N, Calderan A (2010) Cell-Penetrating Peptides: A Comparative Study on Lipid Affinity and Cargo Delivery Properties. Pharmaceuticals 3: 1045–1062.
27. Castile JD, Taylor KMG, Buckton G (1999) A high sensitivity differential scanning calorimetry study of the interaction between poloxamers and dimyristoylphosphatidylcholine and dipalmitoylphosphatidylcholine liposomes. International Journal of Pharmaceutics 182: 101–110.
28. Purohit G, Sakthivel T, Florence AT (2001) Interaction of cationic partial dendrimers with charged and neutral liposomes. International Journal of Pharmaceutics 214: 71–76.
29. Hong S, Bielinska AU, Mecke A, Keszler B, Beals JL, et al. (2004) Interaction of poly(amidoamine) dendrimers with supported lipid bilayers and cells: Hole formation and the relation to transport. Bioconjugate Chemistry 15: 774–782.
30. Hong S, Leroueil PR, Janus EK, Peters JL, Kober MM, et al. (2006) Interaction of polycationic polymers with supported lipid bilayers and cells: Nanoscale hole formation and enhanced membrane permeability. Bioconjugate Chemistry 17: 728–734.
31. Mecke A, Uppuluri S, Sassanella TM, Lee DK, Ramamoorthy A, et al. (2004) Direct observation of lipid bilayer disruption by poly(amidoamine) dendrimers. Chemistry and Physics of Lipids 132: 3–14.
32. Mecke A, Lee DK, Ramamoorthy A, Orr BG, Holl MMB (2005) Synthetic and natural polycationic polymer nanoparticles interact selectively with fluid-phase domains of DMPC lipid bilayers. Langmuir 21: 8588–8590.
33. Mecke A, Majoros IJ, Patri AK, Baker Jr JR, Banaszak Holl MM, et al. (2005) Lipid bilayer disruption by polycationic polymers: The roles of size and chemical functional group. Langmuir 21: 10348–10354.
34. Klajnert B, Epand RM (2005) PAMAM dendrimers and model membranes: Differential scanning calorimetry studies. International Journal of Pharmaceutics 305: 154–166.
35. Klajnert B, Janiszewska J, Urbanczyk-Lipkowska Z, Bryszewska M, Epand RM (2006) DSC studies on interactions between low molecular mass peptide dendrimers and model lipid membranes. International Journal of Pharmaceutics 327: 145–152.
36. Gardikis K, Hatziantoniou S, Viras K, Wagner M, Demetzos C (2006) A DSC and Raman spectroscopy study on the effect of PAMAM dendrimer on DPPC model lipid membranes. International Journal of Pharmaceutics 318: 118–123.
37. Ionov M, Garaiova Z, Wróbel D, Waczulikova I, Gomez-Ramirez R, et al. (2011) The carbosilane dendrimers affect the size and zeta potential of large unilamellar vesicles. Acta Phys Univ Comenianae 52: 33–39.
38. Wrobel D, Kłys A, Ionov M, Vitovic P, Waczulikowa I, et al. (2012) Cationic carbosilane dendrimers–lipid membrane interactions. Chemistry and Physics of Lipids 165: 401–407.
39. Lee H, Larson RG (2008) Coarse-grained molecular dynamics studies of the concentration and size dependence of fifth- and seventh-generation PAMAM dendrimers on pore formation in DMPC bilayer. Journal of Physical Chemistry B 112: 7778–7784.
40. Smith PES, Brender JR, Dürr UHN, Xu J, Mullen DG, et al. (2010) Solid-state NMR reveals the hydrophobic-core location of poly(amidoamine) dendrimers in biomembranes. Journal of the American Chemical Society 132: 8087–8097.
41. Kelly CV, Liroff MG, Triplett LD, Leroueil PR, Mullen DG, et al. (2009) Stoichiometry and structure of poly(amidoamine) dendrimer- Lipid complexes. ACS Nano 3: 1886–1896.
42. Tiriveedhi V, Kitchens KM, Nevels KJ, Ghandehari H, Butko P (2011) Kinetic analysis of the interaction between poly(amidoamine) dendrimers and model

lipid membranes. Biochimica et Biophysica Acta - Biomembranes 1808: 209–218.
43. Ottaviani MF, Matteini P, Brustolon M, Turro NJ, Jockusch S, et al. (1998) Characterization of starburst dendrimers and vesicle solutions and their interactions by CW- and pulsed-EPR, TEM, and dynamic light scattering. Journal of Physical Chemistry B 102: 6029–6039.
44. Ottaviani MF, Daddi R, Brustolon M, Turro NJ, Tomalia DA (1999) Structural modifications of DMPC vesicles upon interaction with poly(amidoamine) dendrimers studied by CW-electron paramagnetic resonance and electron spin-echo techniques. Langmuir 15: 1973–1980.
45. Wrobel D, Ionov M, Gardikis K, Demetzos C, Majoral JP, et al. (2011) Interactions of phosphorus-containing dendrimers with liposomes. Biochimica et Biophysica Acta - Molecular and Cell Biology of Lipids 1811: 221–226.
46. Schwarz G, Stankowski S, Rizzo V (1986) Thermodynamic analysis of incorporation and aggregation in a membrane: application to the pore-forming peptide alamethicin. Biochim Biophys Acta 861: 141–151.
47. Eftink MR, Ghiron CA (1976) Exposure of tryptophanyl residues in proteins. Quantitative determination by fluorescence quenching studies. Biochemistry 15: 672–680.
48. Yau WM, Wimley WC, Gawrisch K, White SH (1998) The preference of tryptophan for membrane interfaces. Biochemistry 37: 14713–14718.
49. Shai Y, Bach D, Yanovsky A (1990) Channel formation properties of synthetic pardaxin and analogues. J Biol Chem 265: 20202–20209.
50. Mozsolits H, Wirth HJ, Werkmeister J, Aguilar MI (2001) Analysis of antimicrobial peptide interactions with hybrid bilayer membrane systems using surface plasmon resonance. Biochim Biophys Acta 1512: 64–76.
51. Papo N, Shai Y (2003) Exploring peptide membrane interaction using surface plasmon resonance: differentiation between pore formation versus membrane disruption by lytic peptides. Biochemistry 42: 458–466.
52. Shai Y (1999) Mechanism of the binding, insertion and destabilization of phospholipid bilayer membranes by alpha-helical antimicrobial and cell non-selective membrane-lytic peptides. Biochim Biophys Acta 1462: 55–70.
53. Seelig J (1997) Titration calorimetry of lipid-peptide interactions. Biochim Biophys Acta 1331: 103–116.
54. Cantor CR, Schimmel PR (1980) Biophysical chemistry: W. H. Freeman.
55. Andrushchenko VV, Aarabi MH, Nguyen LT, Prenner EJ, Vogel HJ (2008) Thermodynamics of the interactions of tryptophan-rich cathelicidin antimicrobial peptides with model and natural membranes. Biochim Biophys Acta 1778: 1004–1014.
56. Wenk MR, Seelig J (1998) Magainin 2 amide interaction with lipid membranes: calorimetric detection of peptide binding and pore formation. Biochemistry 37: 3909–3916.
57. Wieprecht T, Beyermann M, Seelig J (1999) Binding of antibacterial magainin peptides to electrically neutral membranes: thermodynamics and structure. Biochemistry 38: 10377–10387.
58. Klajnert B, Sadowska M, Bryszewska M (2004) The effect of polyamidoamine dendrimers on human erythrocyte membrane acetylcholinesterase activity. Bioelectrochemistry 65: 23–26.
59. Klajnert B, Cortijo-Arellano M, Cladera J, Bryszewska M (2006) Influence of dendrimer's structure on its activity against amyloid fibril formation. Biochemical and Biophysical Research Communications 345: 21–28.
60. Smith DK (2008) Dendrimers and the double helix - From DNA binding towards gene therapy. Current Topics in Medicinal Chemistry 8: 1187–1203.
61. Svenson S, Tomalia DA (2005) Dendrimers in biomedical applications - Reflections on the field. Advanced Drug Delivery Reviews 57: 2106–2129.
62. Shcharbin D, Drapeza A, Loban V, Lisichenok A, Bryszewska M (2006) The breakdown of bilayer lipid membranes by dendrimers. Cell Mol Biol Lett 11: 242–248.
63. Lee H, Larson RG (2006) Molecular dynamics simulations of PAMAM dendrimer-induced pore formation in DPPC bilayers with a coarse-grained model. Journal of Physical Chemistry B 110: 18204–18211.
64. Yan LT, Yu X (2009) Enhanced permeability of charged dendrimers across tense lipid bilayer membranes. ACS Nano 3: 2171–2176.
65. Kelly CV, Leroueil PR, Orr BG, Holl MMB, Andricioaei L (2008) Poly(amidoamine) dendrimers on lipid bilayers II: Effects of bilayer phase and dendrimer termination. Journal of Physical Chemistry B 112: 9346–9353.
66. Leroueil PR, Hong S, Mecke A, Baker JR, Jr., Orr BG, et al. (2007) Nanoparticle interaction with biological membranes: does nanotechnology present a Janus face? Acc Chem Res 40: 335–342.
67. Hong S, Rattan R, Majoros IJ, Mullen DG, Peters JL, et al. (2009) The role of ganglioside GM1 in cellular internalization mechanisms of poly(amidoamine) dendrimers. Bioconjug Chem 20: 1503–1513.
68. Jain K, Kesharwani P, Gupta U, Jain NK (2010) Dendrimer toxicity: Let's meet the challenge. Int J Pharm 394: 122–142.
69. Guarnieri D, Falanga A, Muscetti O, Tarallo R, Fusco S, et al. (2013) Shuttle-mediated nanoparticle delivery to the blood-brain barrier. Small 9: 853–862.
70. Smaldone G, Falanga A, Capasso D, Guarnieri D, Correale S, et al. (2013) gH625 is a viral derived peptide for effective delivery of intrinsically disordered proteins. Int J Nanomedicine 8: 2555–2565.
71. Wimley WC, Hristova K (2011) Antimicrobial peptides: successes, challenges and unanswered questions. J Membr Biol 239: 27–34.

The Effect of Nanoemulsion as a Carrier of Hydrophilic Compound for Transdermal Delivery

Ming-Jun Tsai[1,2]⁹, Yaw-Syan Fu[3]⁹, Yu-Hsuan Lin[4], Yaw-Bin Huang[4], Pao-Chu Wu[4]*

1 Department of Neurology, China Medical University Hospital, School of Medicine, Medical College, China Medical University, Taichung, Taiwan, ROC, **2** Department of Neurology, Tainan Municipal An-Nan Hospital, Tainan, Taiwan, ROC, **3** Department of Biomedical Science and Environmental Biology, Kaohsiung Medical University, Kaohsiung, Taiwan, ROC, **4** School of Pharmacy, Kaohsiung Medical University, Kaohsiung, Taiwan, ROC

Abstract

The purpose of the present study was to investigate the effect of nanoemulsions as a carrier vehicle of hydrophilic drug for transdermal delivery. The response surface methodology with a mixture design was used to evaluate the effect of ingredient levels of nanoemulsion formulations including cosurfactant (isopropyl alcohol, 20~30%), surfactant (mixed of Brij 30 and Brij 35, 20~30%), and distilled-water (34.5~50.0%) on properties of the drug-loaded nanoemulsions including physicochemical characters and drug permeability through rat skin. The result showed that the hydrophilic drug in aqueous solution with or without penetration enhancer could not transport across rat skin after 12 h of application. Used nanoemulsions as carrier vehicle, the permeation rate of drug was significantly increased from 0 to 63.23 μg/cm²/h and the lag time was shortened from more than 12 h to about 2.7~4.0 h. Moreover, the drug-loaded nanoemulsion formulation also showed physicochemical stability after 3 month storage at 25°C and 40°C.

Editor: Vipul Bansal, RMIT University, Australia

Funding: This work was supported by a Grant from the National Science Council of Taiwan (NSC 102-2320-B-037-006-MY2 and NSC101-2320-B-037-33). The funders had no role in study design, data collection and analysis to publish, or preparation of the manuscript.

Competing Interests: The authors have declared that no competing interests exist.

* Email: pachwu@kmu.edu.tw

⁹ These authors contributed equally to this work.

Introduction

Transdermal drug delivery offers many benefits over other traditional routes of administration including non-invasiveness, accessibility, avoidance of first-pass metabolism, compliance, ease of drug input termination in problematic cases, and controllable drug delivery rates [1,2]. Ropinirole hydrochloride (RHCl) is a selective non-ergoline dopamine D2 receptor agonist, which can stimulate striatal dopamine receptors to produce dopamine, hence it has been prescribed for Parkinson's disease treatment [3,4]. It is a potent drug with a dose of 2 mg to be administered 3–4 times daily. In view of the characteristics of RHCl including small oral dosage (3–9 mg daily), low molecular weight (MW = 260), short elimination half-life (about 6 h), and low bioavailability (approximately 50%) because of extensive first-pass metabolism, oral administration is problematic [3–6]. In additional, dysphagia is a frequent and potentially serious complication of Parkinson's disease [7]. RHCl seems to be a good candidate for transdermal administration; hence, it was used as a model drug in this study.

The greatest obstacle for drug transdermal delivery is the barrier property of stratum corneum, a 10 μm to 20 μm thick tissue layer composed of a structured lipid/protein matrix [8,9]. Numerous strategies including used carrier vehicle, chemical penetration enhancers, and physical technologies such as electroporation, iontophoresis, ultrasound, and microneedle technologies either singly or in combination, have been used to facilitate the permeability of therapeutical compounds through the skin [10–13]. A previous study [14] pointed out that small droplet size provides a better chance for adherence to biological membranes transporting therapeutic compounds in a controlled manner. Hence, nano- or micro- carriers such as ethosomes, nanoemulsions, liposomes, and polymeric nanoparticles have been widely used to improve permeability of therapeutic agents through skin in recent years [1,15–17]. Nanoemulsion is an isotropic and thermodynamically stable colloidal system with a mean droplet size in range of 10–100 nm [18]. In general, a nanoemulsion formulation contains the four major ingredients of water, oil, surfactant, and cosurfactant. The surfactant is used to decrease the interfacial tension between oil and aqueous phase, and then form a nanoemulsion. Cosurfactant could provide further decrease in interfacial tension and to fluidize the interfacial surfactant film. Moreover, it can decrease the used amount of surfactant in nanoemulsion preparation and influence the drug-loaded nanoemulsion transportation through the skin [19,20]. The four ingredients may decrease the diffusion barrier of the skin by acting as penetration enhancer [20]. Many studies have reported that using nanoemulsion as vehicle can enhance the transportation of drug through the skin over conventional topical products such as ointments, gels, and creams [21–24]. Furthermore, nanoemulsions can be manufactured by a spontaneous emulsifying method which provides some advantages over other carriers such as polymeric nanoparticles and liposome, including low cost preparation procedure, high hydrophilic and lipophilic drug loading, and long shelf life for therapeutic agents [25–27]. Hence, the nanoemulsions were used as the vehicle to facilitate the transportation rate of the hydrophilic model drug RHCl through rat skin in this study.

Materials and Methods

Materials

Ropinirole hydrochloride (RHCl) was purchased from Glenmark Generics Limited (Mumbai, India). Polyoxyl 23 lauryl ether (Brij 35) and Polyoxyl 4 lauryl ether (Brij 30) were from Acros Organic (Pennsylvania, USA). Sorbitan monolaurate (Span 20, HLB = 8.6) was from Tokyo Chemical Industry (Tokyo, Japan). Polyoxyethylene sorbitan monooleate (Tween 80, HLB = 15) was acquired from Showa Corporation (Saitama, Japan). Isopropyl myristate (IPM) and isopropyl alcohol (IPA) were purchased from Merck Chemicals (Darmstadt, Germany). Caffeine was from Wako Pure Chemical Industries Ltd, (Tokyo, Japan). All other chemicals and solvents were of analytical reagent grade.

Preparation of drug-loaded Nanoemulsions

The RHCl-loaded nanoemulsions were prepared by spontaneous emulsion method. The mixture surfactants were mixed well in advance. Oil phase (IPM) was mixed thoroughly with mixture surfactants and cosurfactant by a vortex at room temperature. Subsequently, distilled water was slowly added to the mixture and mixed evenly with a vortex. After the clarity and transparency of blank nanoemulsions were formed, RHCl was dissolved in the blank nanoemulsions by a shaker for 10 min. There was no precipitate observed in the final RHCl-loaded nanoemulsion.

In order to estimate the degree of effects of the formulation factors and obtain an optimal formulation, the response surface methodology [28–30] was applied in this study. RHCl of 0.5% nanoemulsions were prepared. According to preliminary study, the amount of IPM was fixed at 5% because RHCl is a hydrophilic compound (133 mg/m L), and the amount of oil phase can't influence the solubility. The other level of ingredients in nanoemulsions such as cosurfactant of IPA (20~30%), mixture surfactant of Brij 30 and Brij 35 (20~30%), and double-distilled water (34.5~50.0%) were selected as formulation variables. The ranges of formulation variables were set according to our preliminary study. The total amount of the three ingredients was fixed at 95% of total amount of nanoemulsion formulation. Ten model RHCl-loaded nanoemulsions were arranged randomly, based on the constrained mixture model (Design-Expert software). The compositions of RHCl-loaded nanoemulsions are listed in Table 1.

Nanoemulsion characterization. Viscosities of drug-loaded nanoemulsions were determined in triplicate using a cone-plate of viscometer (Brookfield, Model LVDV-II, USA). A sample of 0.5 mL was placed in the plate, the temperature of which was maintained at 37°C by thermostatic pump for 3 mins. The rotation rate of viscometer was set at 120 rpm. The viscosity value was recorded 20 s after measurement had begun.

Mean droplet size and droplet size distribution of RHCl-loaded nanoemulsions were measured by a photo correlation spectroscopy equipped with laser light scattering (Zetasizer 3000HSA, Malvern, UK). The intensity of the light scattering was observed at a fixed angle of 90°. The helium-neon laser of λ was set at 633 nm. A sample of 3 mL was loaded in a cuvette and placed in the scattering chamber to measure the mean droplet size and droplet size distribution.

Table 1. The composition, physicochemical properties, and permeability parameters of RHCl-loaded nanoemulsions.

	MS %	CoS %	IPM %	Drug %	Size (nm)	Viscosity (cps × 10^3)	Flux (μg/cm^2/h)	LT (h)
F1	20B	30E	5	0.5	14.73 ± 1.16	8.99 ± 0.12	44.21 ± 5.73	4.3 ± 1.2
F2	25B	30E	5	0.5	12.73 ± 1.50	9.71 ± 0.11	48.53 ± 5.16	3.0 ± 0.0
F3	30B	30E	5	0.5	21.03 ± 7.60	9.79 ± 0.07	25.94 ± 3.51	4.3 ± 0.6
F4	30B	20E	5	0.5	14.10 ± 0.66	19.10 ± 0.56	20.25 ± 4.23	5.3 ± 0.6
F5	20B	30I	5	0.5	14.40 ± 2.79	6.67. ± 0.04	65.45 ± 13.2	3.7 ± 0.6
F6	30B	20I	5	0.5	12.67 ± 0.81	13.33. ± 0.06	30.61 ± 2.71	3.7 ± 0.6
F7	15T	30E	5	0.5	107.93 ± 7.14	11.37 ± 0.21	13.08 ± 0.57	4.0 ± 0.0

RHCl: ropinirole hydrochloride, MS: Mixture surfactant, CoS: Cosurfactant, IPM: Isopropyl myristate,
B: Brij30/Brij35 (4/1); T: Tween80/Span20 (2/3), E: Ethanol, I: Isopropyl alcohol.
LT: lag time

Skin permeation study

The skin permeation experimental protocol was approved by the Institutional Animal Care and Use Committee of Kaohsiung Medical University (Kaohsiung, Taiwan). The committee confirmed that the permeation experiment followed the guidelines as set forth by the Guide for Laboratory Fact lines and Care. The *in vitro* skin permeation of RHCl from nanoemulsion formulations and control groups determined using a modified transdermal Franz diffusion cell [31] (Fig. 1) with an effective diffusion area of the cell was 3.46 cm^2 and receptor compartment volume of 20 mL. The abdominal skin of excised Wistar albino rat (275–300 g) was mounted on the receptor compartment with the stratum corneum side facing upward to the donor cell. The donor cell was loaded with 1 mL of samples and occluded by para film. The temperature of receiver vehicle of pH 7.4 phosphate buffer containing 40% PEG400 (drug solubility of 67.2 ±0.5 mg/mL) was maintained at 37±0.5 °C by thermostatic pump and was constantly stirred at 600 rpm by a magnetic stirrer during the experiment. At specific intervals, *i.e.*,1, 2, 3, 4, 5, 6, 8,10, and 12 h, one milliliter of receptor medium was withdrawn via the sampling port and was analyzed for drug content by modified HPLC method [32]. All experiments were repeated three times and averaged.

Chromatographic condition HPLC analysis of RHCL

A Hitachi L-7100 series HPLC system and a LiChroCART RP-18e column (125×4 mm I.D., particle size 5 μm) were used for RHCl analysis. A mixture of 60% 0.05 M ammonium acetate buffer containing 0.05% triethylamine (adjusted to pH 7.0 by hydrochloride) and 40% methanol was used as mobile phase. The flow rate and detection wavelength were 1 mL/min and 250 nm respectively. Internal standard was caffeine of 100 μg/mL. The concentration of RHCl ranged from 3 to 200 μg/mL with a linearity of ($r^2 = 0.9998$). The limit of quantitation was 1 μg/mL. The precision, as coefficient of variation (CV, %), was calculated for all the calibration standards. Accuracy was calculated as relative error (RE, %). The CV and RE values were less than 1.7% and 6.7% respectively.

Data analysis

The cumulative amount of RHCl transported through rat skin was plotted as a function of time, and the linear regression analysis was used to determine the permeation rate (flux) of RHCl. The

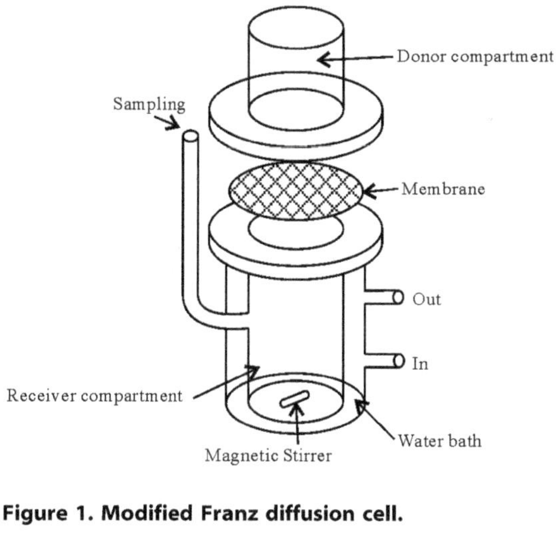

Figure 1. Modified Franz diffusion cell.

Table 2. The composition, physicochemical properties, and permeability parameters of model RHCl-loaded nanoemulsions provided mixture design.

	X_1%	X_2%	X_3%	Size (nm)	PI	Viscosity (cps×10^3)	Flux (μg/cm^2/h)	LT (h)
F01	20.0	30.0	44.5	12.1 ± 1.1	0.36 ± 0.07	12.73 ± 0.21	33.04 ± 2.72	4.0 ± 0.6
F02	25.9	30.0	38.6	12.5 ± 1.6	0.45 ± 0.06	9.79 ± 0.07	33.98 ± 3.71	3.7 ± 0.6
F03	20.0	30.0	44.5	12.6 ± 0.2	0.41 ± 0.06	12.67 ± 0.06	33.76 ± 4.54	4.0 ± 1.0
F04	25.9	25.9	42.7	24.5 ± 1.5	0.32 ± 0.04	8.82 ± 0.07	45.67 ± 4.93	3.7 ± 0.6
F05	30.0	30.0	34.5	53.2 ± 7.3	0.57 ± 0.12	8.52 ± 0.02	35.53 ± 2.31	3.7 ± 0.6
F06	30.0	25.7	38.8	24.4 ± 3.6	0.30 ± 0.03	7.80 ± 0.05	56.93 ± 13.16	3.0 ± 1.0
F07	30.0	30.0	34.5	55.5 ± 3.8	0.61 ± 0.03	8.60 ± 0.11	41.23 ± 5.91	3.7 ± 0.6
F08	30.0	20.0	44.5	15.4 ± 0.8	0.32 ± 0.06	6.55 ± 0.00	63.23 ± 6.32	3.0 ± 0.0
F09	24.5	20.0	50.0	16.1 ± 0.8	0.26 ± 0.05	7.75 ± 0.03	59.91 ± 5.30	2.7 ± 0.6
F10	20.0	24.5	50.0	14.3 ± 1.2	0.34 ± 0.06	10.99 ± 0.06	49.80 ± 2.13	3.0 ± 0.0

The amounts of RHCl and IPM in formulations were fixed at 0.5% and 5% respectively.
The total amount of three variables of X_1 (isopropyl alcohol, 20~30%), X_2(mixture surfactant of Brij30/Brij35 at ratio of 4/1, 20~30%), and X_3 (distilled water, 34.5~50.0%) was 95%. $X_1+X_2+X_3=0.95$.
LT: lag time; PI: polydispersity index.

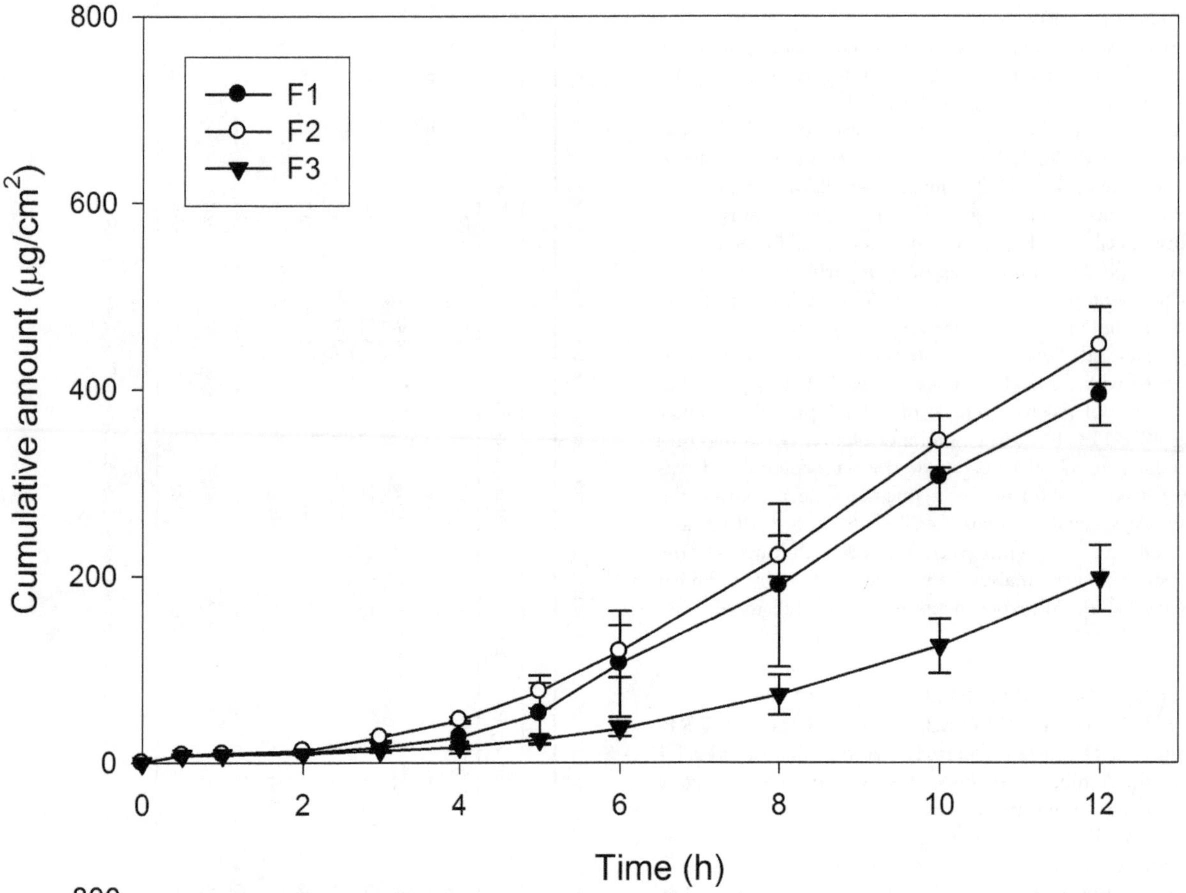
800
600
400
200
0
Cumulative amount (μg/cm²)
F1
F2
F3
0
2
4
6
8
10
12
Time (h)

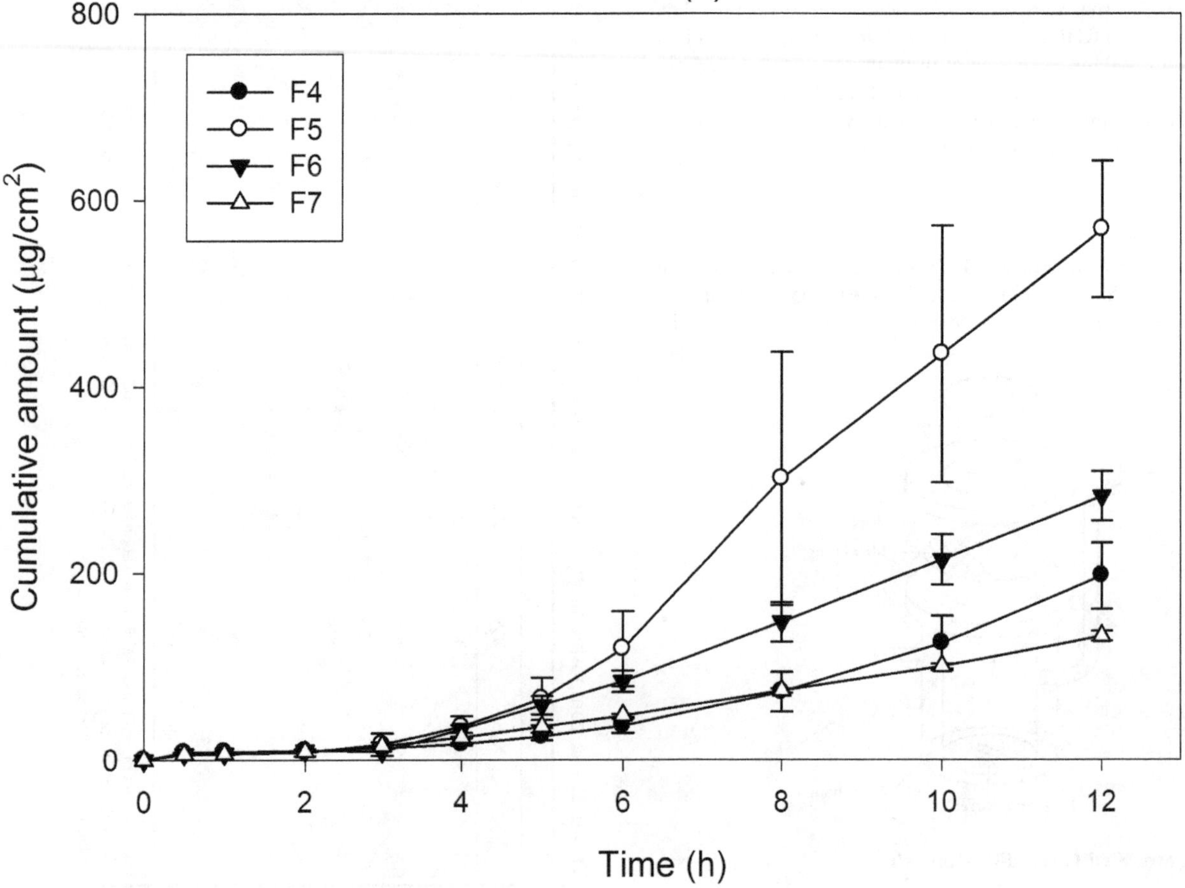
800
600
400
200
0
Cumulative amount (μg/cm²)
F4
F5
F6
F7
0
2
4
6
8
10
12
Time (h)

Figure 2. In vitro penetration-time profile of RCHl-loaded nanoemulsions with different combinations through rat skin. (n = 3).

time of first-detected RHCl was set as lag time (LT). The formulation variables (X_1, X_2 and X_3) and responses (flux and LT) of model RHCl-loaded nanoemulsions were analyzed by using Design-Expert® software. Polynomial equations of linear, quadratic, and cubic forms were utilized to depict the relationship between independent variables and responses. The statistical parameters: the multiple correlation coefficient, the adjusted multiple correlation coefficient, the coefficient of variation, and the *p* value of model as well as lack of fit were used to confirm the suitable model equation for representing the relationship of formulation variables and responses.

Stability

The RHCl-loaded nanoemulsion was stored in dark-brown bottles for protection from light. The stability of drug-loaded nanoemulsion formulation was evaluated via clarity and phase separation observation, and drug content at 25°C and 40°C.

Results and Discussion

Physicochemical characteristics of drug-loaded nanoemulsion

The mean droplet size and droplet size distribution (polydispersity index) and viscosity of experimental RHCl formulations are listed in Tables 1 and 2. The mean droplet size ranged from 14.5 to 107.9 nm, demonstrating all experimental nanoemulsion formulations were submicron emulsions. The polydispersity index ranged from 0.33 to 0.47, indicated a narrow deviation of average size. The viscosity of drug-loaded formulations ranged from 7.53 to 13.07×10^3 cps at 37°C. It was found that the viscosity slightly increased when higher levels of surfactant were incorporated. A previous study pointed that the progress of emulsification is yielded by viscous liquid crystalline gel building at the interface between surfactant and water at high surfactant levels [33]. Nanoemulsions with higher levels of ethanol showed lower viscosity. The result might be attributed to the cosurfactant being able to decrease surface tension, and this then led to increased liquidity of the interfacial layer [19,20]. In addition, it can be seen that the viscosity of nanoemulsion with IPA was lower than that of nanoemulsion with ethanol, demonstrating that cosurfactant type will influence the characteristics of the nanoemulsion [19,20].

Skin permeation study

The permeation profiles of RHCl-loaded nanoemulsions through the skin are plotted in Fig. 2. The permeation parameters including flux and lag time (LT) of RHCl-loaded nanoemulsions with different composition and proportion are listed in Table 1. The 2.5% RHCl of aqueous solution and aqueous solution containing 40% ethanol were used as control groups. In permeation study, no drug was detected at end time point of the experiment (12 h) indicating that the hydrophilic compound RHCl has difficulty in being transported through the skin barrier, even using 40% ethanol as a penetration enhancer. As shown in Table 1, when used nanoemulsion as the carrier vehicle, the permeability of the hydrophilic compound RHCl through skin was significantly improved. The result was in accordance with previous studies reporting that nanoemulsions could modify the surface electrical charge of an ionic drug and then enhance the permeability of a hydrophilic drug [34–37].

In comparing the effect of composition and proportion of formulation on the permeation capacity of the drug, it was found that flux increased by decrease in the amount of surfactant incorporated (F1~F3). The result might be due to the thermodynamic activity of drug decreased and viscosity increased in formulation containing higher levels of surfactant [14]. When the level of ethanol in nanoemulsions increased from 20% to 30% (F3 vs F4, p>0.05), the flux slightly increased from 20.25 to 25.94 µg/cm²/h, and lag time decreased from 5.3 h to 4.3 h. Used IPA instead of ethanol as cosurfactant (F4 vs F6, F1 vs F5), the viscosity decreased and flux increased. Therefore, IPA was used in the follow-up experiment. In using mixed surfactants of Tween80/Span20 instead of mixture surfactant of Brij30/Brij35 (F1 vs F7,

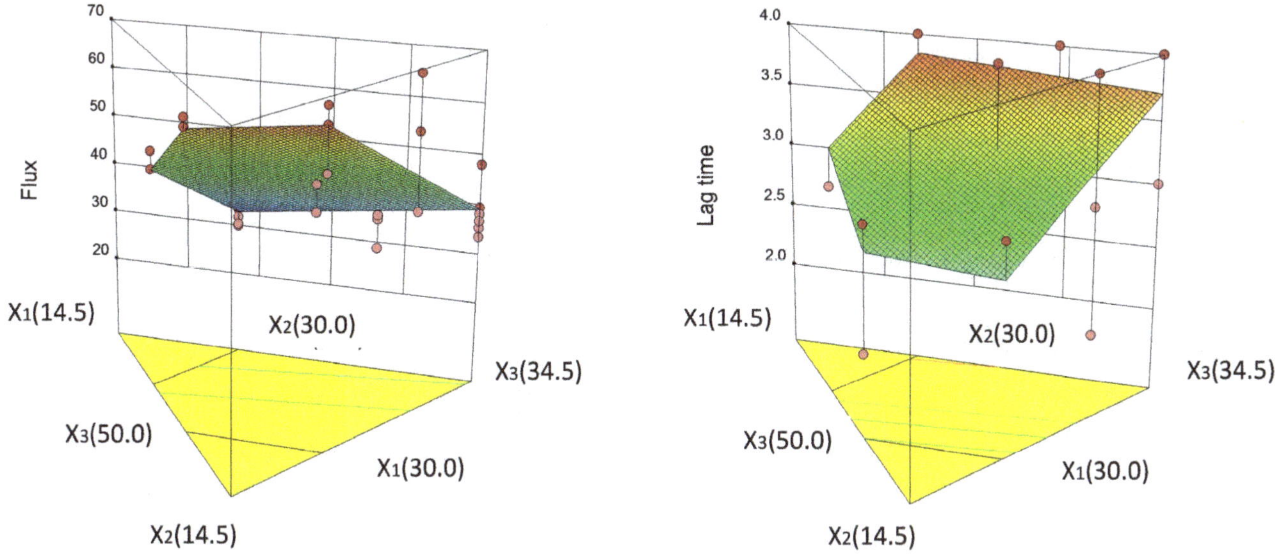

Figure 3. Three dimensional response surface plots illustrating the effect of IPA (X_1), mixture surfactant (X_2) and distilled water (X_3) on the flux and lag time (LT) of RCHl-loaded nanoemulsions.

$p<0.05$), the flux of drug decreased, hence the mixture surfactant of Brij30/Brij35 was chosen as surfactant for subsequent experiments.

In order to evaluate the degree of effect of each component and the interaction components of nanoemulsion formulation on the permeation capacity of the drug and to acquire an optimal formulation, response surface methodology [28–30] was used in the present study. According to the above result, the oil amount was fixed at 5%, while the other ingredients of cosurfactant of IPA, mixture surfactant of B30/B35 and distilled water were set as variable factors and range of 20~30%, and 20~30% and 34.5~50% respectively in this study. Ten model 0.5% RHCl-loaded nanoemulsions were prepared based on the mixture design provided by Design-Expert® software. The permeation parameters of the drug were estimated by in vitro permeation study. The permeation parameters of all RHCl-loaded nanoemulsions are summarized in Table 2. The flux and LT of RHCl-loaded nanoemulsions ranged from 33.04 to 63.23 $\mu g/cm^2/h$ and 2.7 to 4.0 h respectively, indicating that the permeability of RHCl from nanoemulsions was significantly influenced by the composition proportion of formulations.

The flux and LT of RHCl-loaded nanoemulsions were set as responses, and the level of component of formulations set as variable factors were statistically analyzed using the RSM provided Design-Expert software.

The polynomial equation to depict the flux may be indicated thus: $Flux = 1.64X_1 - 1.55X_2 + 1.05X_3$.

The *p*-value of the model polynomial equation was less than 0.001, demonstrating that the model was adequate to describe the relationship between independent and dependent variables. The *p*-value of the lack of fit was 0.2909, revealing no indication of significance, and further verified the satisfactory fitness of the model. The coefficients value of X term presented the effect degree of the independent factors on the dependent factors (responses). A positive sign displays a synergistic effect while a negative term shows an antagonistic effect on the dependent factors. The response surface plots illustrating the simultaneous effect of the independent factors on dependent variables (Flux and LT) are represented in Fig 3. The result showed that the IPA (X_1) and mixture surfactant (X_2) had similar effect on the drug permeation rate, followed by aqueous phase (X_3). The flux increased with an increasing level of IPA and water and a decreasing level of mixture surfactant (Fig. 3).

To describe the LT, the mathematical polynomial equation might be written thus: $LT = -0.016X_1 + 0.108X_2 + 0.011X_3$.

The *p*-values of the model and lack of fit were <0.0001 and 0.4969 respectively, which demonstrated that the mathematical polynomial equation can describe the relationship between the formulation variables and LT. The three dimensional surface plot was graphed according to the mathematical polynomial equation and is shown in Fig. 3. It was found that the surfactant (X_2) showed the greatest effect, followed by cosurfactant (X_1) and distilled water (X_3). The cosurfactant showed that the negative effect indicated lag time could be shortened by the increase in the level of IPA. The reason might be attributed to the cosurfactant decreasing the viscosity, and this then led to the increased diffusivity of the drug (reduction in the lag time) [19]. To validate the predictive ability of the hypothesized mathematical model, an optimal nanoemulsion with flux and LT values of 57.90 $\mu g/cm^2/h$ and 2.98 h respectively, when level of X_1, X_2 and X_3 were 30%, 22.7% and 41.8% respectively was predicted by the response surface methodology. A new RHCl-loaded nanoemulsion was prepared and obtained flux as well as LT values of 58.55 ± 5.75 $\mu g/cm^2/h$ and 3.0 ± 0.0 h respectively. The predicted and observed values showed no significant difference, indicating that the response surface methodology can be used to design RHCl-loaded nanoemulsions.

Stability

After 3 months storage at 25°C and 40°C, the apparent RHCl-loaded nanoemulsion had no obvious change, and no drug crystal was observed. After storage, mean droplet size showed non-significant change, from 19.0±5.0 nm to 22.3±3.1 nm for 25°C storage and 23.5±4.2 nm for 40°C storage. The residual drug contents tested drug-loaded nanoemulsions at 25°C and 40°C storage were 98.89±3.90% and 98.46±2.56% respectively, indicated that RHCl-loaded nanoemulsion was stable.

Conclusions

The permeation rate of hydrophilic compound increased from 0 to 63.23 $\mu g/cm^2/h$ and the lag times were also shortened from more than 12 h to 2.7 h by using nanoemulsions as carrier vehicle, suggesting a promising role of nanoemulsions in enhancing the permeability of RHCl. An appropriate combination and proportion of nanoemulsion formulation including the type and level of oil, surfactant, cosurfactant, and water is a major consideration for the transdermal drug delivery.

Author Contributions

Conceived and designed the experiments: MJT PCW YBH. Performed the experiments: YHL YSF. Analyzed the data: MJT PCW. Contributed reagents/materials/analysis tools: MJT. Contributed to the writing of the manuscript: PCW YSF YBH.

References

1. Azeem A, Khan ZI, Aqil M, Ahmad FJ, Khar RK, et al. (2009) Microemulsions as a surrogate carrier for dermal drug delivery. Drug Dev Ind Pharm 35: 525–547.
2. Brown MB, Martin GP, Jones SA, Akomeah FK (2006) Dermal and transdermal drug delivery systems: current and future prospects. Drug Deliv 13: 175–187.
3. Kaye CM, Nicholls B (2000) Clinical pharmacokinetics of ropinirole. Clin Pharmacokinet 39: 243–254.
4. Matheson AJ, Spencer CM (2000) Ropinirole: a review of its use in the management of Parkinson's disease. Drugs 60: 115–137.
5. Alonso Canovas A, Luquin Piudo R, Garcia Ruiz-Espiga P, Burguera JA, Campos Arillo V, et al. (2011) Dopaminergic agonists in Parkinson's disease. Neurologia.
6. Tompson DJ, Vearer D (2007) Steady-state pharmacokinetic properties of a 24-hour prolonged-release formulation of ropinirole: results of two randomized studies in patients with Parkinson's disease. Clin Ther 29: 2654–2666.
7. Fuh JL, Lee RC, Wang SJ, Lin CH, Wang PN, et al. (1997) Swallowing difficulty in Parkinson's disease. Clin Neurol Neurosurg 99: 106–112.
8. Cevc G (2004) Lipid vesicles and other colloids as drug carriers on the skin. Adv Drug Deliv Rev 56: 675–711.
9. Schreier H, Bouwstra J (1994) Liposomes and niosomes as topical drug carriers: dermal and transdermal drug delivery. J Control Release 30: 1–15.
10. Kim HM, Lim YY, An JH, Kim MN, Kim BJ (2012) Transdermal drug delivery using disk microneedle rollers in a hairless rat model. Int J Dermatol 51: 859–863.
11. Nair A, Vyas H, Shah J, Kumar A (2011) Effect of permeation enhancers on the iontophoretic transport of metoprolol tartrate and the drug retention in skin. Drug Deliv 18: 19–25.
12. Ryan E, Garland MJ, Singh TR, Bambury E, O'Dea J, et al. (2012) Microneedle-mediated transdermal bacteriophage delivery. Eur J Pharm Sci 47: 297–304.
13. Tsai YH, Chang JT, Huang CT, Chang JS, Huang YB, et al. (2012) Electrically-Assisted Skin Delivery of Buspirone Submicron Emulsions. J Food Drug Anal 20: 22–26.
14. Kogan A, Garti N (2006) Microemulsions as transdermal drug delivery vehicles. Adv Colloid Interface Sci 123–126: 369–385.
15. Chen Y, Wu Q, Zhang Z, Yuan L, Liu X, et al. (2012) Preparation of curcumin-loaded liposomes and evaluation of their skin permeation and pharmacodynamics. Molecules 17: 5972–5987.

16. Fang YP, Huang YB, Wu PC, Tsai YH (2009) Topical delivery of 5-aminolevulinic acid-encapsulated ethosomes in a hyperproliferative skin animal model using the CLSM technique to evaluate the penetration behavior. Eur J Pharm Biopharm 73: 391–398.
17. Shi J, Ma F, Wang X, Wang F, Liao H (2012) Formulation of liposomes gels of paeonol for transdermal drug delivery by Box-Behnken statistical design. J Liposome Res 22: 270–278.
18. Wang L, Dong J, Chen J, Eastoe J, Li X (2009) Design and optimization of a new self-nanoemulsifying drug delivery system. J Colloid Interface Sci 330: 443–448.
19. El Maghraby GM (2008) Transdermal delivery of hydrocortisone from eucalyptus oil microemulsion: effects of cosurfactants. Int J Pharm 355: 285–292.
20. Peltola S, Saarinen-Savolainen P, Kiesvaara J, Suhonen TM, Urtti A (2003) Microemulsions for topical delivery of estradiol. Int J Pharm 254: 99–107.
21. Mostafa DM, Ammar NM, Abd El-Alim SH, El-anssary AA (2014) Transdermal microemulsions of Glycyrrhiza glabra L.: characterization, stability and evaluation of antioxidant potential. Drug Deliv 21: 130–139.
22. Fouad SA, Basalious EB, El-Nabarawi MA, Tayel SA (2013) Microemulsion and poloxamer microemulsion-based gel for sustained transdermal delivery of diclofenac epolamine using in-skin drug depot: in vitro/in vivo evaluation. Int J Pharm 453: 569–578.
23. El Maghraby GM, Arafa MF, Osman MA (2013) Microemulsion for simultaneous transdermal delivery of benzocaine and indomethacin: in vitro and in vivo evaluation. Drug Dev Ind Pharm.
24. Teichmann A, Heuschkel S, Jacobi U, Presse G, Neubert RH, et al. (2007) Comparison of stratum corneum penetration and localization of a lipophilic model drug applied in an o/w microemulsion and an amphiphilic cream. Eur J Pharm Biopharm 67: 699–706.
25. Azeem A, Rizwan M, Ahmad FJ, Iqbal Z, Khar RK, et al. (2009) Nanoemulsion components screening and selection: a technical note. AAPS PharmSciTech 10: 69–76.
26. Heuschkel S, Goebel A, Neubert RH (2008) Microemulsions–modern colloidal carrier for dermal and transdermal drug delivery. J Pharm Sci 97: 603–631.
27. Azeem A, Ahmad FJ, Khar RK, Talegaonkar S (2009) Nanocarrier for the transdermal delivery of an antiparkinsonian drug. AAPS PharmSciTech 10: 1093–1103.
28. Tsai PJ, Huang CT, Lee CC, Li CL, Huang YB, et al. (2013) Isotretinoin oil-based capsule formulation optimization. ScientificWorldJournal 2013: 856967.
29. Makraduli L, Crcarevska MS, Geskovski N, Dodov MG, Goracinova K (2013) Factorial design analysis and optimisation of alginate-Ca-chitosan microspheres. J Microencapsul 30: 81–92.
30. Pabari RM, Ramtoola Z (2012) Application of face centred central composite design to optimise compression force and tablet diameter for the formulation of mechanically strong and fast disintegrating orodispersible tablets. Int J Pharm 430: 18–25.
31. Kimura C, Nakanishi T, Tojo K (2007) Skin permeation of ketotifen applied from stick-type formulation. Eur J Pharm Biopharm 67: 420–424.
32. Aydogmus Z (2008) Highly sensitive and selective spectrophotometric and spectrofluorimetric methods for the determination of ropinirole hydrochloride in tablets. Spectrochim Acta A Mol Biomol Spectrosc 70: 69–78.
33. Zidan AS, Sammour OA, Hammad MA, Megrab NA, Habib MJ, et al. (2007) Quality by design: understanding the product variability of a self-nanoemulsified drug delivery system of cyclosporine A. J Pharm Sci 96: 2409–2423.
34. Osborne DW, Ward AJ, O'Neill KJ (1991) Microemulsions as topical drug delivery vehicles: in-vitro transdermal studies of a model hydrophilic drug. J Pharm Pharmacol 43: 450–454.
35. Piemi MP, Korner D, Benita S, MartyJp (1999) Positively and negatively charged submicron emulsions for enhanced topical delivery of antifungal drugs. J Control Release 58: 177–187.
36. Wu H, Ramachandran C, Weiner ND, Roessler BJ (2001) Topical transport of hydrophilic compounds using water-in-oil nanoemulsions. Int J Pharm 220: 63–75.
37. Raza K, Negi P, Takyar S, Shukla A, Amarji B, et al. (2011) Novel dithranol phospholipid microemulsion for topical application: development, characterization and percutaneous absorption studies. J Microencapsul 28: 190–199.

Permissions

All chapters in this book were first published in PLOS ONE, by The Public Library of Science; hereby published with permission under the Creative Commons Attribution License or equivalent. Every chapter published in this book has been scrutinized by our experts. Their significance has been extensively debated. The topics covered herein carry significant findings which will fuel the growth of the discipline. They may even be implemented as practical applications or may be referred to as a beginning point for another development.

The contributors of this book come from diverse backgrounds, making this book a truly international effort. This book will bring forth new frontiers with its revolutionizing research information and detailed analysis of the nascent developments around the world.

We would like to thank all the contributing authors for lending their expertise to make the book truly unique. They have played a crucial role in the development of this book. Without their invaluable contributions this book wouldn't have been possible. They have made vital efforts to compile up to date information on the varied aspects of this subject to make this book a valuable addition to the collection of many professionals and students.

This book was conceptualized with the vision of imparting up-to-date information and advanced data in this field. To ensure the same, a matchless editorial board was set up. Every individual on the board went through rigorous rounds of assessment to prove their worth. After which they invested a large part of their time researching and compiling the most relevant data for our readers.

The editorial board has been involved in producing this book since its inception. They have spent rigorous hours researching and exploring the diverse topics which have resulted in the successful publishing of this book. They have passed on their knowledge of decades through this book. To expedite this challenging task, the publisher supported the team at every step. A small team of assistant editors was also appointed to further simplify the editing procedure and attain best results for the readers.

Apart from the editorial board, the designing team has also invested a significant amount of their time in understanding the subject and creating the most relevant covers. They scrutinized every image to scout for the most suitable representation of the subject and create an appropriate cover for the book.

The publishing team has been an ardent support to the editorial, designing and production team. Their endless efforts to recruit the best for this project, has resulted in the accomplishment of this book. They are a veteran in the field of academics and their pool of knowledge is as vast as their experience in printing. Their expertise and guidance has proved useful at every step. Their uncompromising quality standards have made this book an exceptional effort. Their encouragement from time to time has been an inspiration for everyone.

The publisher and the editorial board hope that this book will prove to be a valuable piece of knowledge for researchers, students, practitioners and scholars across the globe.

List of Contributors

Feng-Yi Yang
Department of Biomedical Imaging and Radiological Sciences, National Yang-Ming University, Taipei, Taiwan
Biophotonics and Molecular Imaging Research Center, National Yang-Ming University, Taipei, Taiwan

Yi-Li Lin, Lun-Wei Chang and Ling Hsieh
Department of Biomedical Imaging and Radiological Sciences, National Yang-Ming University, Taipei, Taiwan

Fong-In Chou
Nuclear Science and Technology Development Center, National Tsing Hua University, Hsinchu City, Taiwan
Institute of Nuclear Engineering and Science, National Tsing Hua University, Hsinchu City, Taiwan

Yen-Wan Hsueh Liu
Institute of Nuclear Engineering and Science, National Tsing Hua University, Hsinchu City, Taiwan

Hong Chen, Cherry C. Chen, Camilo Acosta, Shih-Ying Wu and Tao Sun
Department of Biomedical Engineering, Columbia University, New York, New York, United States of America

Elisa E. Konofagou
Department of Biomedical Engineering, Columbia University, New York, New York, United States of America
Department of Radiology, Columbia University, New York, New York, United States of America

Sheng-Feng Hung, Chen, Yu-Chun Wang, Hsiu-O Ho and Ying-Chen Chen
School of Pharmacy, College of Pharmacy, Taipei Medical University, Taipei, Taiwan

Chien-Ming Hsieh
School of Pharmacy, College of Pharmacy, Taipei Medical University, Taipei, Taiwan
Department of Cosmetic Science, Providence University, Taiwan Boulevard, Shalu, Taichung, Taiwan, ROC

Ming-Thau Sheu
School of Pharmacy, College of Pharmacy, Taipei Medical University, Taipei, Taiwan
Clinical Research Center and Traditional Herbal Medicine Research Center, Taipei
Medical University Hospital, Taipei, Taiwan

Domenica Capasso
Department of Pharmacy, University of Naples "Federico II", Naples, Italy

Ivan de Paola, Annarita Del Gatto, Sonia Di Gaetano and Laura Zaccaro
Institute of Biostructures and Bioimaging -CNR, Naples, Italy, 3 Diagnostic and Molecular Pharmaceutics -Scarl, Naples, Italy

Annamaria Liguoro
Diagnostic and Molecular Pharmaceutics -Scarl, Naples, Italy

Daniela Guarnieri
Center for Advanced Biomaterials for Health Care @ CRIB- Italian Institute of Technology, Naples, Italy

Michele Saviano
Institute of Crystallography -CNR, Bari, Italy

Sun Min Park, Jae Min Cha, Jungyong Nam, Min Sang Kim, Sang-Jun Park, Eun Sung Park and Hyun Ryoung Kim
Drug Delivery System Group, Bio Research Center, Samsung Advanced Institute of Technology (SAIT), Yongin, Gyeonggi-do, South Korea

Hwankyu Lee
Department of Chemical Engineering, Dankook University, Yongin, Gyeonggi-do, South Korea

Yarong Liu, Jinxu Fang and Kye-Il Joo
Mork Family Department of Chemical Engineering and Materials Science, University of Southern California, Los Angeles, California, United States of America

Michael K. Wong
Division of Medical Oncology, Norris Comprehensive Cancer Center, Keck School of Medicine, University of Southern California, Los Angeles, California, United States of America

Pin Wang
Mork Family Department of Chemical Engineering and Materials Science, University of Southern California, Los Angeles, California, United States of America
Department of Biomedical Engineering, University of Southern California, Los Angeles, California, United States of America
Department of Pharmacology and Pharmaceutical Sciences, University of Southern California, Los Angeles, California, United States of America

Xiangru Wen
Jiangsu Key Laboratory of Brain Disease Bioinformation, Xuzhou Medical College, Xuzhou, Jiangsu Province, China
School of Basic Education Sciences, Xuzhou Medical College, Xuzhou, Jiangsu Province, China

Kai Wang, Yifang Zhang and Tingting Sun
College of Animal Science and Technology, Yunnan Agricultural University, Yunnan, Kunming Province, China

Fang Zhang, Jian Wu, Yanyan Fu, Yang Du and Hongzhi Liu
Research Center for Neurobiology and Department of Neurobiology, Xuzhou Medical College, Xuzhou, Jiangsu Province, China

Lei Zhang, Ying Sun and YongHai Liu
Department of Neurology, Affiliated Hospital of Xuzhou Medical College, Xuzhou, Jiangsu Province, China, 7 Department of Medical
Information, Xuzhou Medical College, Xuzhou, Jiangsu Province, China

Kai Ma
School of Basic Education Sciences, Xuzhou Medical College, Xuzhou, Jiangsu Province, China
Department of Medical Information, Xuzhou Medical College, Xuzhou, Jiangsu Province, China

Yuanjian Song
Jiangsu Key Laboratory of Brain Disease Bioinformation, Xuzhou Medical College, Xuzhou, Jiangsu Province, China
Research Center for Neurobiology and Department of Neurobiology, Xuzhou Medical College, Xuzhou, Jiangsu Province, China

Marwan Moussa, Gaurav Kumar and Muneeb Ahmed
Laboratory for Minimally Invasive Tumor Therapies, Department of Radiology, Beth Israel Deaconess Medical Center/Harvard Medical School, Boston, MA, United States of America

S. Nahum Goldberg
Laboratory for Minimally Invasive Tumor Therapies, Department of Radiology, Beth Israel Deaconess Medical Center/Harvard Medical School, Boston, MA, United States of America
Division of Image-guided Therapy and Interventional Oncology, Department of Radiology, Hadassah Hebrew University Medical Center, Jerusalem, Israel

Rupa R. Sawant, Tatyana Levchenko and Vladimir P. Torchilin
Department of Pharmaceutical Sciences and Center for Pharmaceutical Biotechnology and Nanomedicine, Northeastern University, Boston, MA, United States of America

Yuling Zhao, Matthew J. Haney, Richa Gupta, Zhijian He and Elena V. Batrakova
Center for Nanotechnology in Drug Delivery, University of North Carolina at Chapel Hill, Chapel Hill, North Carolina, United States of America
Eshelman School of Pharmacy, University of North Carolina at Chapel Hill, Chapel Hill, North Carolina, United States of America

John P. Bohnsack
Eshelman School of Pharmacy, University of North Carolina at Chapel Hill, Chapel Hill, North Carolina, United States of America

Alexander V. Kabanov
Center for Nanotechnology in Drug Delivery, University of North Carolina at Chapel Hill, Chapel Hill, North Carolina, United States of America
Eshelman School of Pharmacy, University of North Carolina at Chapel Hill, Chapel Hill, North Carolina, United States of America
Department of Chemical Enzymology, Faculty of Chemistry, M.V. Lomonosov Moscow State University, Moscow, Russia

Shi-Ting Feng, Yanji Luo, Huasong Cai, Zhi Dong and Zi-Ping Li
Department of Radiology, The First Affiliated Hospital, Sun Yat-Sen University, Guangzhou, China

Jingguo Li, Xintao Shuai and Yong Wang
PCFM Lab of Ministry of Education, School of Chemistry and Chemical Engineering, Sun Yat-Sen University, Guangzhou, China, 3 Department of Medical Ultrasonic, The Third Affiliated Hospital of Sun Yat-Sen University, Guangzhou, China

Jian Jin, Bowen Sui, Jingshuo Liu and Xiangqun Jin
Department of Pharmaceutics, College of Pharmacy Sciences, Jilin University, Changchun, People's Republic of China

Jingxin Gou, Xing Tang, Hui Xu and Yu Zhang
Department of Pharmaceutics, Shenyang Pharmaceutical University, Shenyang, People's Republic of China

Kirtee D. Wani, Prakash Mansara and Ruchika Kaul-Ghanekar
Cell and Translational Research Laboratory, Interactive Research School for Health Affairs (IRSHA), Bharati Vidyapeeth University Medical College Campus, Dhankawadi, Pune, Maharashtra, India

Brijesh S. Kadu and Rajeev C. Chikate
Nanoscience Group, Department of Chemistry, Post-graduate and Research Center, MES Abasaheb Garware College, Pune, Maharashtra, India

Preeti Gupta and Pankaj Poddar
Physical and Material Chemistry Division, CSIR-National Chemical Laboratory, Pune, Maharashtra, India

Avinash V. Deore and Sanjay D. Dhole
Department of Physics, University of Pune, Pune, Maharashtra, India

Yang Xia and Mingpo Yang
Institute of Neuroscience, State Key Laboratory of Neuroscience, Shanghai Institutes for Biological Sciences, Chinese Academy of Sciences, Shanghai, P. R. China

Yuan Zhao and Shaoqun Zeng
Britton Chance Center for Biomedical Photonics, Wuhan National Laboratory for Optoelectronics-Huazhong University of Science and Technology, Wuhan, P. R. China

Yousheng Shu
State Key Laboratory of Cognitive Neuroscience and Learning & IDG/McGovern Institute for Brain Research, Center for Collaboration and Innovation in Brain and Learning Sciences, Beijing Normal University, Beijing, P. R. China

Etienne van Bracht, Luuk R. M. Versteegden, René Raavé, Theo Hafmans, Roland Brock, Toin H. van Kuppevelt and Willeke F. Daamen
Department of Biochemistry, Radboud Institute for Molecular Life Sciences, Radboud university medical centre, Geert Grooteplein 28, 6525 GA, Nijmegen, The Netherlands

Sarah Stolle
Current address: Department of Pediatrics, Center for Liver, Digestive and Metabolic Disease, University Medical Center Groningen, Hanzeplein 1, 9713 GZ Groningen, The Netherlands

Wouter P. R. Verdurmen
Current address: Department of Biochemistry, University of Zurich, Winterthurerstrasse 190, 8057 Zurich, Switzerland

Rob Woestenenk
Department of Laboratory Medicine, Laboratory of Hematology, Radboud university medical centre, Geert Grooteplein 8, 6525 GA, Nijmegen, The Netherlands

Egbert Oosterwijk
Department of Urology, Radboud Institute for Molecular Life Sciences, Radboud university medical centre, Geert Grooteplein 28, 6525 GA, Nijmegen, The Netherlands

Santosh Kumar
Department of Economics & International Business, Sam Houston State University, Huntsville, Texas, United States of America
Institute for Health Metrics and Evaluation, University of Washington, Seattle, Washington, United States of America

Emily Dansereau
Institute for Health Metrics and Evaluation, University of Washington, Seattle, Washington, United States of America

Yousuf H. Mohammed
Dermatology Research Centre, The University of Queensland, School of Medicine, Translational Research Institute, Brisbane, Queensland, Australia
School of Pharmacy, CHIRI-Biosciences, Curtin University, Perth, Western Australia, Australia
Therapeutics Research Centre, The University of Queensland, School of Medicine, Princess Alexandra Hospital, Brisbane, Queensland, Australia

Miko Yamada1, Lynlee L. Lin, Anthony P. Raphael and Tarl W. Prow
Dermatology Research Centre, The University of Queensland, School of Medicine, Translational Research Institute, Brisbane, Queensland, Australia

Jeffrey E. Grice and Michael S. Roberts
Therapeutics Research Centre, The University of Queensland, School of Medicine, Princess Alexandra Hospital, Brisbane, Queensland, Australia

Ahlam Zaid Alkilani
School of Pharmacy, Queen's University Belfast, Belfast, Co. Antrim, United Kingdom
School of Pharmacy, Zarqa University, Zarqa, Jordan

Ryan F. Donnelly, Maelíosa T. C. McCrudden, Eneko Larrañeta, Emma McAlister, Aaron J. Courtenay, Mary-Carmel Kearney, Thakur Raghu Raj Singh, Helen O. McCarthy, Victoria L. Kett, Ester Caffarel-Salvador, Sharifa Al-Zahrani and A. David Woolfson
School of Pharmacy, Queen's University Belfast, Belfast, Co. Antrim, United Kingdom

Andreas Obermeier, Steffen Wehner, Florian Dominik Matl, Rüdiger von Eisenhart-Rothe, Axel Stemberger and Rainer Burgkart
Klinik für Orthopädie und Sportorthopädie, Klinikum rechts der Isar, Technische Universität München, München, Bavaria, Germany

Jochen Schneider
Institut für Mikrobiologie, Immunologie und Hygiene, Klinikum rechts der Isar, Technische Universität München, München, Bavaria, Germany

Matthias Schieker
Experimentelle Chirurgie und Regenerative Medizin, Klinik für Chirurgie, Klinikum der Universität München, München, Bavaria, Germany

Xiao Du, Jingyu Wang, Wentao Diao, Jiafu Long and Hao Zhou
State Key Laboratory of Medicinal Chemical Biology, Nankai University, Tianjin, China
College of Life Sciences, Nankai University, Tianjin, China

Ling Wang
State Key Laboratory of Medicinal Chemical Biology, Nankai University, Tianjin, China
College of Pharmacy, Nankai University, Tianjin, China

Mareike Hütten
Department of Otolaryngology, Hannover School of Medicine, Hannover, Germany
University of Veterinary Medicine Hannover, Foundation, Institute of Zoology, Hannover, Germany

Anandhan Dhanasingh
MED-EL Innsbruck, Research & Development, Innsbruck, Österreich
Interactive Materials Research–DWI e.V. and Institute of Technical and Macromolecular Chemistry, RWTH Aachen University, Aachen, Germany

Roland Hessler and Claude Jolly
MED-EL Innsbruck, Research & Development, Innsbruck, Österreich

Timo Stöver
J.W. Goethe University Hospital and Faculty of Medicine, Department of Otolaryngology, Frankfurt am Main, Germany

Karl-Heinz Esser
University of Veterinary Medicine Hannover, Foundation, Institute of Zoology, Hannover, Germany

Martin Möller
Interactive Materials Research–DWI e.V. and Institute of Technical and Macromolecular Chemistry, RWTH Aachen University, Aachen, Germany

Thomas Lenarz
Department of Otolaryngology, Hannover School of Medicine, Hannover, Germany

Jürgen Groll
Interactive Materials Research–DWI e.V. and Institute of Technical and Macromolecular Chemistry, RWTH Aachen University, Aachen, Germany
University of Würzburg, Department of Functional Materials in Medicine and Dentistry, Würzburg, Germany

Verena Scheper
Department of Otolaryngology, Hannover School of Medicine, Hannover, Germany
Institute of Audioneurotechnology, Hannover School of Medicine, Hannover, Germany

Annarita Falanga and Stefania Galdiero
Department of Pharmacy & CIRPEB & DFM Scarl, University of Naples "Federico II", Naples, Italy

Rossella Tarallo, Thomas Carberry and Marcus Weck
Molecular Design Institute and Department of Chemistry, New York University, New York, New York, United States of America

Massimiliano Galdiero
Department of Experimental Medicine, Second University of Naples, Naples, Italy

Ming-Jun Tsai
Department of Neurology, China Medical University Hospital, School of Medicine, Medical College, China Medical University, Taichung, Taiwan, ROC
Department of Neurology, Tainan Municipal An-Nan Hospital, Tainan, Taiwan, ROC

Yaw-Syan Fu
Department of Biomedical Science and Environmental Biology, Kaohsiung Medical University, Kaohsiung, Taiwan, ROC

Yu-Hsuan Lin, Yaw-Bin Huang and Pao-Chu Wu
School of Pharmacy, Kaohsiung Medical University, Kaohsiung, Taiwan, ROC

Index

N

P

R

S

T

www.ingramcontent.com/pod-product-compliance
Lightning Source LLC
Chambersburg PA
CBHW061252190326
41458CB00011B/3654
* 9 7 8 1 6 3 2 4 2 4 7 8 5 *